# Current Research in Epilepsy

# Current Research in Epilepsy

Editor: Noel Day

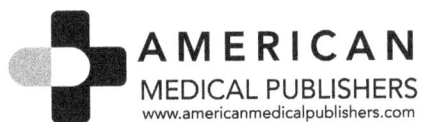

AMERICAN
MEDICAL PUBLISHERS
www.americanmedicalpublishers.com

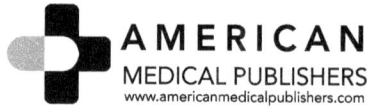

**AMERICAN**
MEDICAL PUBLISHERS
www.americanmedicalpublishers.com

### Cataloging-in-Publication Data

Current research in epilepsy / edited by Noel Day.
   p. cm.
Includes bibliographical references and index.
ISBN 978-1-63927-286-0
1. Epilepsy. 2. Epilepsy--Research. 3. Spasms. 4. Convulsions. I. Day, Noel.
RA645.E64 C87 2022
616.853--dc23

American Medical Publishers,
41 Flatbush Avenue,
1st Floor, New York,
NY 11217, USA

ISBN 978-1-63927-286-0 (Hardback)

# Contents

# Preface

Epilepsy is a disorder of the central nervous system that is characterized by recurring epileptic seizures. The brain activity becomes abnormal, causes seizures and periods of sensations and unusual behavior. It affects people of all ages. These epileptic seizures are the result of excessive and abnormal neuronal activity in the cortex of the brain. These seizures range from undetectable shorter to longer periods of time. They do not have an immediate underlying cause. Some of the causes can be stroke, brain tumors, brain injury and birth defects. Epilepsy can be diagnosed through the use of electroencephalogram. Its treatment involves the use of medications in most of the cases. Surgery, neurostimulation and dietary changes are further measures of treatment. This book provides comprehensive insights into this disorder. Different approaches, evaluations and advanced research on epilepsy have been included herein. Those in search of information to further their knowledge will be greatly assisted by this book.

The information contained in this book is the result of intensive hard work done by researchers in this field. All due efforts have been made to make this book serve as a complete guiding source for students and researchers. The topics in this book have been comprehensively explained to help readers understand the growing trends in the field.

I would like to thank the entire group of writers who made sincere efforts in this book and my family who supported me in my efforts of working on this book. I take this opportunity to thank all those who have been a guiding force throughout my life.

Editor

# Sesamin ameliorates oxidative stress and mortality in kainic acid-induced status epilepticus by inhibition of MAPK and COX-2 activation

Peiyuan F Hsieh[1,2*], Chien-Wei Hou[3*], Pei-Wun Yao[3], Szu-Pei Wu[3], Yu-Fen Peng[3], Mei-Lin Shen[1], Ching-Huei Lin[1], Ya-Yun Chao[1], Ming-Hong Chang[1] and Kee-Ching Jeng[4,5†]

## Abstract

**Background:** Kainic acid (KA)-induced status epilepticus (SE) was involved with release of free radicals. Sesamin is a well-known antioxidant from sesame seeds and it scavenges free radicals in several brain injury models. However the neuroprotective mechanism of sesamin to KA-induced seizure has not been studied.

**Methods:** Rodents (male FVB mice and Sprague-Dawley rats) were fed with sesamin extract (90% of sesamin and 10% sesamolin), 15 mg/kg or 30 mg/kg, for 3 days before KA subcutaneous injection. The effect of sesamin on KA-induced cell injury was also investigated on several cellular pathways including neuronal plasticity (RhoA), neurodegeneration (Caspase-3), and inflammation (COX-2) in PC12 cells and microglial BV-2 cells.

**Results:** Treatment with sesamin extract (30 mg/kg) significantly increased plasma $\alpha$-tocopherol level 50% and 55.8% from rats without and with KA treatment, respectively. It also decreased malondialdehyde (MDA) from 145% to 117% ($p = 0.017$) and preserved superoxide dismutase from 55% of the vehicle control mice to 81% of sesamin-treated mice, respectively to the normal levels ($p = 0.013$). The treatment significantly decreased the mortality from 22% to 0% in rats. Sesamin was effective to protect PC12 cells and BV-2 cells from KA-injury in a dose-dependent manner. It decreased the release of $Ca^{2+}$, reactive oxygen species, and MDA from PC12 cells. Western blot analysis revealed that sesamin significantly reduced ERK1/2, p38 mitogen-activated protein kinases, Caspase-3, and COX-2 expression in both cells and RhoA expression in BV-2 cells. Furthermore, Sesamin was able to reduce $PGE_2$ production from both cells under KA-stimulation.

**Conclusions:** Taken together, it suggests that sesamin could protect KA-induced brain injury through anti-inflammatory and partially antioxidative mechanisms.

**Keywords:** Status epilepticus, PC12 cells, BV-2 cells, sesamin, kainic acid, reactive oxygen species, thiobarbituric acid reactive substances, nitric acid, superoxide dismutase, mitogen-activated protein kinases, COX-2

## Background

Status epilepticus (SE) is defined as a period of continuous seizure activity [1,2]. Prolonged febrile seizures and SE have been implicated as a major predisposing factor for the development of mesial temporal sclerosis and temporal lobe epilepsy [1,3]. This emergency condition requires a prompt and appropriate treatment to prevent brain damage and eventual death. In animal models, similar pathologic changes can be observed with electrically and chemically induced seizures [4-7]. Animal studies show that SE causes recurrent spontaneous seizures (epilepsy) [6,8,9] and releases free radicals from experimental models of kainic acid (KA), pilocarpine, pentylenetetrazole, and ferric chloride [10-14].

KA, a glutamate related chemical, induces neuronal excitability, reactive oxygen species (ROS) production and lipid peroxidation in neurons [15-17]. It triggers neuronal membrane depolarization by the release of calcium ions which are involved in nerve impulse

* Correspondence: pfhsieh@vghtc.gov.tw; rolis.hou@mail.ypu.edu.tw
† Contributed equally
[1]Division of Neurology, Taichung Veterans General Hospital, Taichung, Taiwan
[3]Department of Biotechnology, Yuanpei University, Hsinchu, Taiwan
Full list of author information is available at the end of the article

transmission as the calcium action potential reaches the synapse [15]. The apoptosis of nerve cells can be triggered by a large number of intracellular calcium influx [18]. Mitogen-activated protein kinases (MAPKs) and Rho kinases are also associated with seizures, inflammation and apoptosis [19-21].

Sesamin and sesamolin are the major lignans from sesame seeds. Previously, we and others report that sesamin can protect against hypoxia-, $H_2 O_2$ -or 1-methyl-4-phenyl-pyridine (MPP$^+$)-induced brain and PC12 cells injuries [22,23]. Various plant antioxidants have been shown to protect brain form KA-induced calcium ions and ROS [24-26]. Sesamin also inhibits nitric oxide (NO) and cytokine production in lipopolysaccharide (LPS)-and oxidative-stressed BV-2 microglia [27,28].

It is perceivable that sesamin could protect animal from KA-induced SE as in other brain injury models. Therefore, this study investigated the effect of sesamin on the KA-induced SE animals as well as the protective mechanism in neuronal PC12 cells and microglial BV-2 cells.

## Methods

### Reagents

Pure sesamin and sesamin extract (90% sesamin and 10% sesamolin, as determined by HPLC) were purchased from Joben Bio-medical co. (Kaohsiung, Taiwan). Kainic acid (KA) was obtained from Sigma-Aldrich (Steinheim, Germany) and Cayman Chemical (Ann Arbor, MI, USA), 2', 7'-dichlorodihydrofluorescein diacetate ($H_2$ DCF-DA) was obtained from Molecular Probes (Eugene, OR, USA).

### Oxidative Stress in mice

Adult male FVB mice, 23-25 g of weight, were used for the study. SE was induced with KA (30 mg/ml in phosphate-buffered saline (PBS), 30 mg/kg, s.c.). Sesamin extract was diluted with corn oil (30 mg/ml). The animals were fed with 2 different dosages of sesamin extract (15 mg/kg or 30 mg/kg) by gavage for 3 days before the KA experiment. The vehicle control group was fed with equal volume of corn oil. The procedures were approved by the Institutional Animal Care and Use Committee, Taichung Veterans General Hospital (IACUC Approval No. LA-97490) and all possible steps were taken to avoid animals' suffering at each stage of experiments.

Diazepam at lethal dosage, 60 mg/kg i.p., was given to stop seizures 2 h after KA injection and the animal was sacrificed by decapitation under $CO_2$ asphyxia. The naïve animal serves as a control. The whole brain was removed and immediately frozen in liquid nitrogen and stored at-70°C until use.

Malondialdehyde (MDA) as a part of thiobarbituric acid reacting substances (TBARS) was used as an indicator of lipid peroxidation. To estimate oxidative stress, the amount of TBARS in the brain from each group was measured. Manual homogenization of brains was carried out at 4°C with a cold buffer. Protein concentration of the homogenate was determined by BCA protein assay using bovine serum albumin as a standard. The detection of TBARS was from the modified method of Ohkawa [29]. Briefly, the sample (0.2 ml) was mixed with the same volume of 20% (w/v) trichloroacetic acid and 1% (w/v) thiobarbituric acid in 0.3% (w/v) NaOH. The mixture was heated in the water bath at 95°C for 40 min, cooled to room temperature and centrifugation at 5000 rpm for 5 min at 4°C. The fluorescence of the supernatant was determined by a spectrophotometer with excitation at 544 nm and emission at 590 nm.

Superoxide dismutase (SOD) activity was determined by a RANSOD kit (Randox, USA). This method was based on the formation of red formazan from the reaction of 2-(4-iodophenyl)-3-(4-nitrophenol)-5-phenyltetrazolium chloride and superoxide radical and assayed in a spectrophotometer at 505 nm. The inhibition of the produced chromogen was proportional to the activity of the SOD present in the sample. A 50% inhibition was defined as one unit of SOD, and specific activity was expressed as units per milligram protein.

### Measurement of tocopherols

Plasma α-tocopherol was determined by HPLC method. Briefly, plasma was treated with anti-oxidant reagent (0.25% BHT and 0.2% vitamin C in methanol, 1:7), mixed and centrifuged for 10 min × 12000 $g$. Sample (20 μl) or internal control was then injected to HPLC system (BAS PM-80) with C18 column (4.6 × 150 mm, 5 μm; mobile phase, 95% methanol, flow rate: 1.0 ml/min) and fluorescence detector with 296 nm excitation, and 340 nm emission.

### Mortality and behavior

Adult male Sprague-Dawley rats weighing 380-420 g were used to study the protective effect of sesamin extract. Rats were fed with sesamin extract (30 mg/kg/day) for 3 days before the SE experiment. The control group was treated with the vehicle corn oil. SE was induced with kainic acid (12 mg/kg, in PBS, s.c.). Each behavioral seizure was recorded according to a modified classification from Racine [30]: 0, immobility or exploring; 1, facial clonus; 2, head nodding; 3, unilateral forelimb clonus; 4, bilateral forelimb clonus and rearing; 5, falling; 6, repeated falling; 7, bouncing; 8, generalized tonus. Four behavioral patterns of SE could be recognized: immobile (class 0), exploratory (class 0), masticatory (class 1-2) and clonic (class 3-8) [31]. Diazepam, 25 mg/kg i.p., was given to stop seizures at 5 h of SE and the 10-h mortality rate was recorded.

## Cell culture
Rat pheochromacytoma (PC12) cells and murine microglial BV-2 cells were maintained in Dulbecco's modified Eagle's medium (DMEM) supplemented with 10% fetal bovine serum (FBS), 5% heat-inactivated horse serum, 100 U/ml penicillin and 100 µg/ml streptomycin at 37°C in a humidified incubator under 5% $CO_2$. Confluent cultures were passaged by trypsinization. For experiments, cells were washed twice with warm DMEM (without phenol red), then treated in serum-free medium. In all experiments, cells were treated with and without sesamin and/or KA-stress for the indicated times.

## Cell viability
Cell viability was measured with blue formazan that was metabolized from colorless 3-(4,5-dimethyl-thiazol-2-yl)-2,5-diphenyl tetrazolium bromide (MTT) by mitochondrial dehydrogenases, which are active only in live cells. PC12 cells were pre-incubated in 24-well plates at a density of $5 \times 10^5$ cells per well for 24 h, and then washed with PBS. Cells with various concentrations of sesamin were treated with 150 mM KA for 24 h, and grown in 0.5 mg/ml MTT at 37°C. One hour later, 200 µl of solubilization solution was added to each well and absorption values read at 540 nm on an automated spectraMAX 340 (Molecular Devices, Sunnyvale, CA, USA) microtiter plate reader. Data were expressed as the mean percent of viable cells vs. control.

## Lactate dehydrogenase (LDH) release assay
Cytotoxicity was determined by measuring the release of LDH. PC12 cells or BV-2 cells with various concentrations of sesamin were treated with 150 mM KA for 24 h and the supernatant was used to assay LDH activity. The reaction was initiated by mixing 0.1 ml of cell-free supernatant with potassium phosphate buffer containing nicotinamide adenine dinucleotide (NADH) and sodium pyruvate in a final volume of 0.2 ml to 96-well plate. The rate of absorbance was read at 490/630 nm on a spectraMAX 340 instrument. Data were expressed as the mean percent of viable cells vs. 150 mM KA control.

## Calcium release
PC12 cells or BV-2 cells with various concentrations of sesamin were treated with 150 mM KA for 24 h and the supernatant was used to assay the release of $Ca^{2+}$. The 10 µl supernatant was added to 1 ml $Ca^{2+}$ reagent (Diagnostic Systems, Holzheim, Germany) and mixed well, stood for 5 min, then transferred the 100 µl aliquot to 96 well. The calcium concentration was determined using a microplate reader with a 620 nm absorbance and quantified with a 10 mg/ml $Ca^{2+}$ standard solution.

## Reactive oxygen species generation
Intracellular accumulation of ROS was determined with $H_2$ DCF-DA. This nonfluorescent compound accumulates within cells upon deacetylation. $H_2$ DCF then reacts with ROS to form fluorescent dichlorofluorescein (DCF). PC12 cells or BV-2 cells were plated in 96-well plates and grown for 24 h before addition of DMEM plus 10 µM $H_2$ DCF-DA, incubation for 60 min at 37°C, and treatment with 150 µM KA for 60 or 120 min. Cells were then washed twice with room temperature Hank's balanced salt solution (HBSS without phenol red). Cellular fluorescence was monitored on a Fluoroskan Ascent fluorometer (Labsystems Oy, Helsinki, Finland) using an excitation wavelength of 485 nm and emission wavelength of 538 nm.

## Measurement of lipid peroxidation
Lipid peroxidation is quantified by measuring malondialdehyde (MDA) of PC12 cells by lipid peroxidation (LPO) assay kit (Cayman Chemical, Ann Arbor, MI, USA). This kit works on the principle of condensation of one molecule of either MDA or 4-hydroxyalkenals with two molecules of N-methyl-2-phenylindole to yield a stable chromophore. MDA levels were assayed by measuring the amount expressed in $5 \times 10^5$ cells and the absorbance at 500 nm was determined using an ELISA reader (spectraMAX 340).

## Preparation of cell extracts
Test medium was removed from culture dishes and cells were washed twice with ice-cold PBS, scraped off with a rubber policeman, and centrifuged at $200 \times g$ for 10 min at 4°C. The cell pellets were resuspended in an appropriate volume ($\sim 4 \times 10^7$ cells/ml) of lysis buffer containing 20 mM Tris-HCl, pH 7.5, 137 mM NaCl, 1 mM phenyl-methylsulfonylfluoride, 10 µg/ml aprotinin, 10 µg/ml leupeptin, and 5 µg/ml pepstain A. The suspension was then sonicated. Protein concentration of samples was determined by Bradford assay (Bio-Rad, Hemel, Hempstead, UK) and samples equilibrated to 2 mg/ml with lysis buffer.

## Western blotting
Protein samples from PC12 cells or BV-2 cells containing 50 µg of protein were separated on 12% sodium dodecyl sulfate-polyacrylamide gels and transferred to immobile polyvinylidene difluoride membranes (Millipore, Bedford, MA). Membranes were incubated for 1 h with 5% dry skim milk in TBST buffer (0.1 M Tris-HCl, pH 7.4, 0.9% NaCl, 0.1% Tween-20) to block nonspecific binding, and then incubated with rabbit anti-COX-2, Rho A (1:1000; Cayman chemical; Cell Signaling, USA),

and anti-phospho-MAPKs. Subsequently, membranes were incubated with secondary antibody streptavidin-horseradish peroxidase conjugated affinity goat anti-rabbit IgG (Jackson, West Grove, PA, USA).

### Statistical analysis

Data were expressed as the mean ± SD and mean ± SE, in vivo and in vitro experiments, respectively. For single variable comparisons, Student's test was used. For multiple variable comparisons, data were analyzed by one-way analysis of variance (ANOVA) followed by Scheffe's test or the least significant differences post-hoc test. Categorical variables were analyzed by use of Fisher's exact test, two-tailed Pearson's chi-square test. Kendall's tau-c was used for testing a trend. P values less than 0.05 were considered significant.

## Results

### In vivo effect of sesamin extract on the KA-induced oxidative stress

Treatment with sesamin extract (30 mg/kg) significantly increased 50% and 55.8% of plasma α-tocopherol levels from rats without and with KA treatment, compared to the baseline level, respectively. In contrast, the plasma α-tocopherol level did not change in vehicle control rats. The TBARS level of the vehicle control group was 145% of the naïve control animals. The TBARS level of the sesamin (S-30) group was 117% of the naïve control and significantly different from that of the vehicle control (V-30) (p = 0.017). The sesamin treatment in SE mice increased the SOD activity from 55% of the vehicle control mice to 81% of sesamin-treated mice, respectively to the normal levels. (p = 0.013). However at 15 mg/kg dosage of sesamin treatment, neither TBARS nor SOD activity was different from the vehicle control (V-15) (p > 0.05, Table 1).

### Effect on mortality and behavior

Since the lower dosage of sesamin (15 mg/kg) did not have a good antioxidant effect, we used the higher

dosage for the next experiment. The result showed that treatment with sesamin extract (30 mg/kg) on the rats with KA-induced SE decreased the mortality rate from 22% of the vehicle (V-30) group to 0% (p = 0.049). However, sesamin extract did not significantly attenuate the maximal seizure classes or the predominant behavioral seizure patterns as compared with the vehicle (p > 0.05, Tables 2 and 3). Nevertheless, there was a trend of decreasing the clonic pattern of SE by sesamin treatment that 8/23 (35%) in the vehicle (V-30) group dropped to 3/22 (14%) in the sesamin (S-30) group (Table 3).

### In vitro protection of KA toxicity

KA can induce free radicals and damage neuronal cells, therefore the cell viability and LDH released from PC12 cells were measured using MTT and LDH ELISA assays [15]. As shown in Figure 1, PC12 cells were exposed to 150 μM KA for 24 h were protected by the presence of sesamin (0.1, 0.5, 1.0, or 2.0 μM). KA-induced LDH released was reduced and the cell viability was increased by sesamin treatment. Similarly, BV-2 cells were protected by sesamin under KA stimulation (data not shown).

### KA-induced calcium release

KA triggers neurons membrane depolarization by the release of calcium ions [18]. Our result showed that KA induced calcium release from both PC12 and BV-2 cells in a time-dependent manner and sesamin reduced the calcium release more prominently from BV-2 cells than from PC12 cells (Figure 2).

### KA-induced ROS and lipid peroxidation

KA-treated PC12 cells or BV-2 cells increased DCF fluorescence nearly one-fold after 120 min as compared with the control cells. Sesamin protected cells against KA-cytotoxicity by decreasing the ROS accumulation (DCF signals) in both cells (Figure 3). Marked increase

**Table 1 Effects of sesamin extract on TBARS (nmol/mg protein) and SOD (units/mg protein) in the mice with 2-h KA-induced SE**

| Variable | Vehicle | Sesamin extract | Naive | P-value[a] | P-value[b] | | |
|---|---|---|---|---|---|---|---|
| | M ± SD | M ± SD | M ± SD | | (V, S) | (V, N) | (S, N) |
| 15 mg/kg | | | | | | | |
| TBARS | 0.96 ± 0.22 | 0.85 ± 0.10 | 0.57 ± 0.04 | 0.001** | 0.225 | 0.0002** | 0.004** |
| SOD | 4.18 ± 1.01 | 5.27 ± 2.01 | 8.79 ± 1.22 | 0.005** | 0.686 | 0.003** | 0.006** |
| 30 mg/kg | | | | | | | |
| TBARS | 0.86 ± 0.14 | 0.69 ± 0.14 | 0.59 ± 0.06 | 0.003** | 0.017* | 0.001** | 0.126 |
| SOD | 5.17 ± 1.90 | 7.54 ± 2.10 | 9.48 ± 1.17 | 0.0004** | 0.013* | 0.0001** | 0.049* |

M ± SD: mean ± standard deviation. N: naïve. S: sesamin extract. V: vehicle.
[a] One-way ANOVA test.
[b] Least significant differences post-hoc test. *P < 0.05, **P < 0.01.

**Table 2 Effects of sesamin extract on the maximal seizure class (MSC) and mortality rate of the rats with 5-h KA-induced SE**

| Variables | Control (V-30) n (%) | Sesamin (S-30) n (%) | P-value |
|---|---|---|---|
| Mortality | 5 (22) | 0 (0) | 0.049[a] |
| MSC | | | |
| 1-2 | 2 (9) | 1 (4) | 0.797[b] |
| 3-6 | 17 (74) | 16 (73) | 0.530[c] |
| 7-8 | 4 (17) | 5 (23) | |

[a] Fisher's exact test.
[b] Pearson's chi-square test: all seizure classes were taken together.
[c] Kendall's tau-c: all seizure classes were taken together.
S-30: sesamin extract (30 mg/kg). V-30: vehicle.

in MDA level was observed in KA-exposed cells as compared with the control cells (Figures 4-5). Treatment with sesamin significantly reduced MDA levels as compared to the KA-treated control ($p < 0.01$,).

## Caspase-3 activation
Apoptotic signaling pathways were investigated in KA-treated PC12 cells and BV-2 cells. The results showed that KA increased Caspase-3 activation but sesamin reduced the Caspase-3 expression dose-dependently in both cells (Figure 6 and **data not shown**).

## COX-2 and MAPK activation
Seizures, inflammation and apoptosis in neuronal cells are known to be initiated with several signaling pathways such as MAPKs and Rho kinases [19-21]. Therefore, the KA induced the activation of signaling pathways were studied in PC12 cells and BV-2 cells for MAP kinases (JNK, ERK, p38), RhoA, and COX-2 (Figure 6). We evaluated the effect of sesamin on KA-induced pathways in PC12 cells at 10, 30, and 60 min and in BV-2 cells 30, 60, 120 min by Western blot. Western blot analysis revealed that sesamin (50 μM) significantly reduced ERK1/2, p38 MAPKs and COX-2 expression in both cells and RhoA expression in BV-2 cells as compared to KA controls.

**Table 3 The effect of sesamin extract on the predominant behavior patterns of the rats with 5-h KA-induced SE**

| Behavior Pattern | Control (V-30) n (%) | Sesamin (S-30) n (%) | P-value |
|---|---|---|---|
| Immobile or Exploratory | 11 (48) | 12 (54) | 0.211[a] |
| Masticatory | 4 (17) | 7 (32) | 0.323[b] |
| Clonic | 8 (35) | 3 (14) | |

[a] Pearson's chi-square test: all behavioral patterns were taken together.
[b] Kendall's tau-c: all behavioral patterns were taken together.
S-30: sesamin extract (30 mg/kg). V-30: vehicle.

## PGE₂ production
## PGE$_2$ production
We further evaluated whether the KA-induced COX-2 change would affect PGE$_2$ production. The result showed that sesamin reduced the PGE$_2$ production in both KA-induced PC12 cells and BV-2 cells as predicted (Figure 7).

## Discussion
The present result showed that sesamin protected animals from KA-induced brain injury. MDA and mortality were significantly reduced as compared with the non-treated one. The decreased mortality in the sesamin-treated animals could also be confirmed by the sesamin effect in vitro that showed a decreased LDH release and Caspase-3 activation and increased cell viability in KA-stimulated PC12 cells.

The neuroprotective effect of sesamin on KA-induced injury was mainly due to its antioxidant effect on reducing of MDA, the product of lipid peroxidation both in vivo and in vitro. The antioxidant effect on reducing of MDA could be attributed to the increased plasma α-tocopherol level from the supplementation with sesamin extract (Table 1). This is consistent with a study that reports consumption of sesame seed powder over five weeks increases plasma α-tocopherol levels in healthy human volunteers [32]. KA administration is associated with a depletion of ATP levels and accumulation of $[Ca^{2+}]_i$. PC12 cells treated with KA for 24 h reduced cell viability dose-dependently by MTT assay. This was not caused by changes in pH or osmotic pressure because the inert mannitol at the concentration of 150 mM, did not affect cell viability (data not shown). The increase in $[Ca^{2+}]_i$ may trigger $Ca^{2+}$-activated free radicals formation [33]. Sesamin decreased ROS and calcium release from KA-treated PC12 cells and BV-2 cells. This agrees with the earlier reports that antioxidants can protect brain from KA-induced calcium ions and ROS release [24-26]. It is also consistent with the sesamin antioxidant effect that protects hypoxia-or $H_2O_2$-induced PC12 cell injury [22]. A study with defatted sesame seeds extract (30, 100 and 300 mg/kg) given twice orally at 0 h and 2 h after onset of ischemia shows the reduction of brain infarct volume dose-dependently and improves sensory-motor function [34]. Thus, suppression of KA-induced ROS and $Ca^{2+}$ release by sesamin was consistent with these notions. Since seizure can be triggered by the KA-induced calcium ions release, the decreased severity of seizure behavior could be partially attributed to the sesamin antioxidative effect, although it was not statistically significant due to the small sample sizes

Since microglial activation as one mechanism by which early-life seizures contribute to increased vulnerability to neurologic insults in adulthood, therapies that

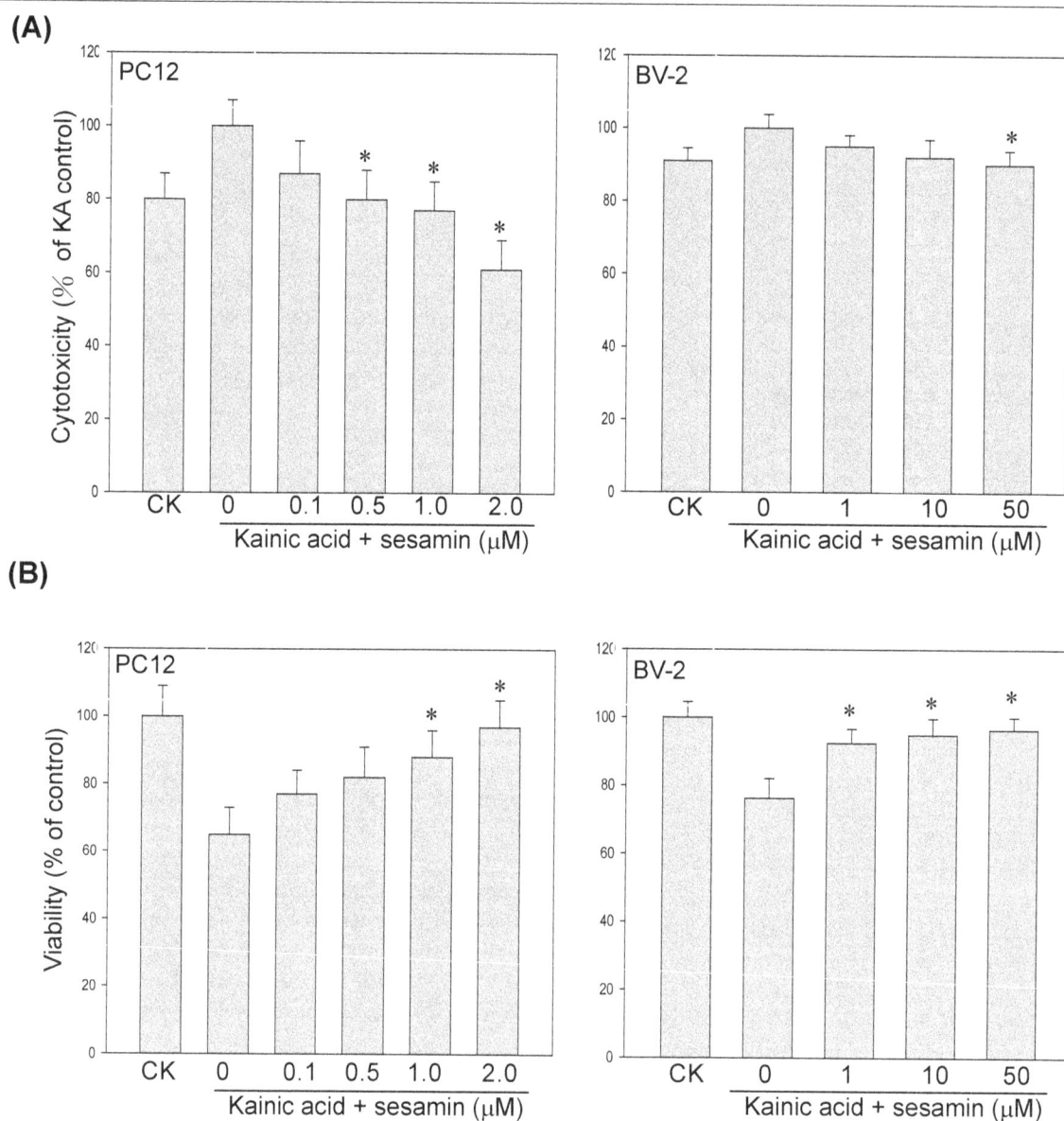

**Figure 1 Effect of sesamin on cell viability and cytotoxicity of kainic acid-stressed PC12 cells**. Cells were treated with KA (150 μM) alone or with various concentrations (0.1, 0.5, 1.0, 2.0 μM) of sesamin for 24 h. (A) LDH release was decreased and (B) cell viability increased by sesamin. $^*$ $P < 0.01$ as compared to KA control.

regulate of proinflammatory cytokines would be beneficial [35]. Present results showed that NO· production in KA-stimulated BV-2 cells was dose-dependently reduced by sesamin and $PGE_2$ production from both cells under KA stress was also significantly reduced. This agrees with other studies that sesamin protects PC12 cells from $MPP^+$-induced cellular death by increasing the SOD activity and inducible nitric oxide synthase protein (iNOS) expression and microglia from reducing interleukin-6 (IL-6) mRNA levels [23]. We have reported previously that sesamin or sesamolin inhibits NO, iNOS,

tumor necrosis factor-α and IL-6 production in LPS-stimulated BV-2 microglia [27]. In addition, sesamin and sesamolin also reduced LPS-activated cytokine, p38 MAPK and NF-κB activations [28].

The role of COX-2 mRNA and protein in KA-induced brain injury has been reported [36-38]. The KA-induced COX-2 expression parallels the appearance of neuronal apoptotic features [36] and involves with free radicals formation [39]. Several protease families are implicated in apoptosis, the most prominent being caspases [40]. We found that KA could

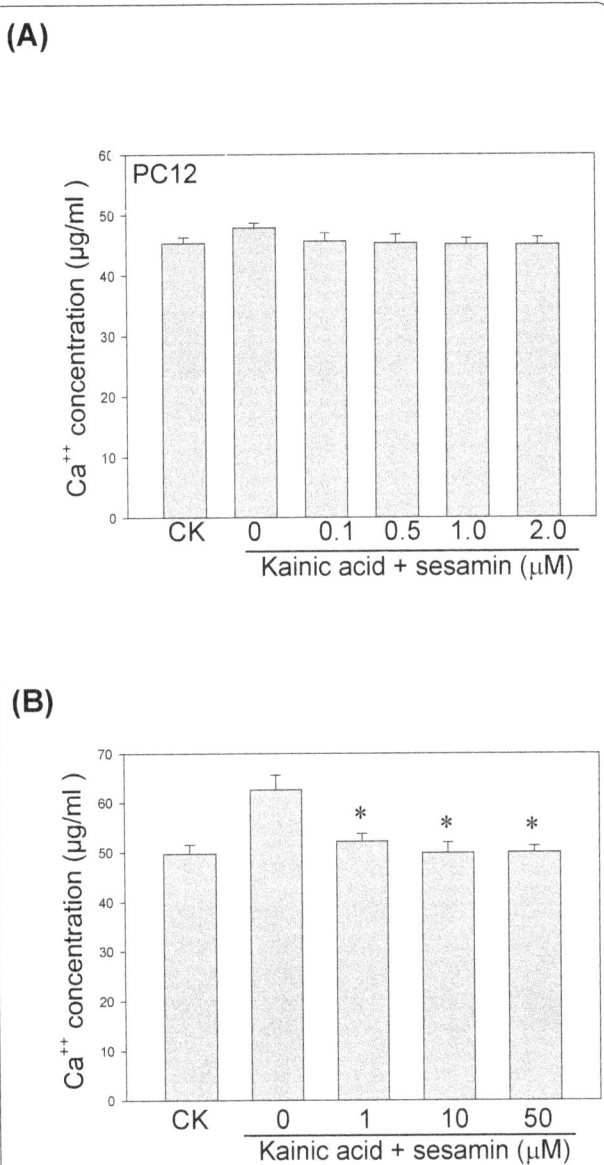

**(A)**

**(B)**

Figure 2 Effect of sesamin on $Ca^{2+}$ generation from KA-treated PC12 cells and BV-2 cells. Cells were treated with KA (150 μM) alone or with various sesamin concentrations (0.1-2.0 μM) of sesamin for 24 h. Treatment with sesamin effectively reduced the release of $Ca^{2+}$ under KA stress. * $P < 0.01$ as compared to the KA control.

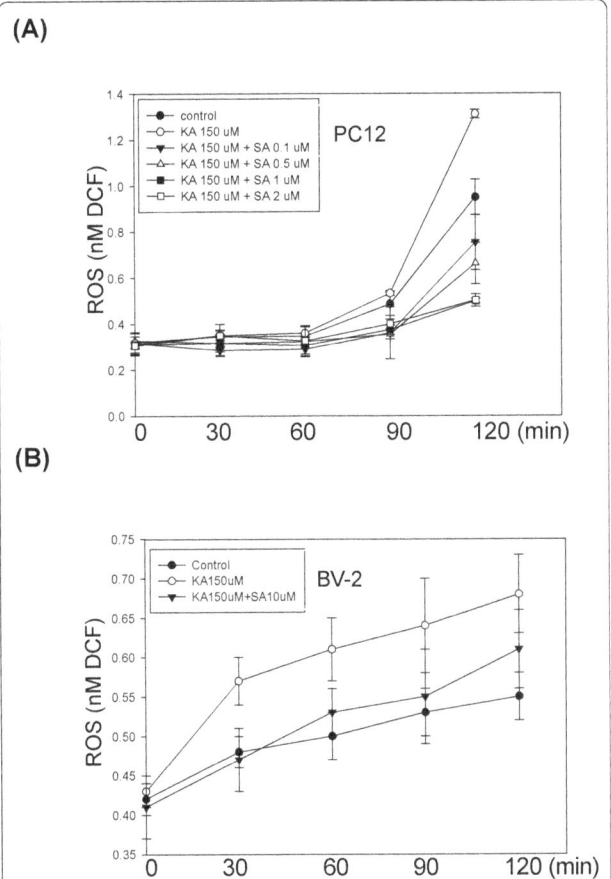

**(A)**

**(B)**

Figure 3 Effect of sesamin on ROS accumulation in PC12 cells and BV-2 cells under KA stress. Sesamin effectively reduced the ROS production from (PC12 cells induced by KA stress (150 μM) at 120-min. * $P < 0.01$ as compared to the KA control.

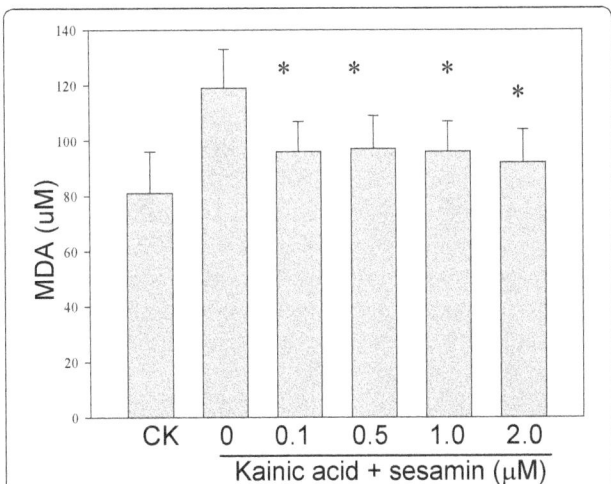

Figure 4 Effect of sesamin on lipid peroxidation of PC12 cells under KA stress. Lipid peroxidation (LPO) was determined by a LPO assay kit (Cayman Chemical, Ann Arbor, MI, USA). Malondialdehyde (MDA) of PC12 cells was induced by 24-h KA stress (150 μM) and effectively reduced by sesamin. * $P < 0.01$ as compared to the KA control.

affect the Caspase-3 activation in PC12 cells and BV-2 cells and sesamin could reduce both Caspase-3 expression. Since KA could induce the activation of MAP kinases (JNK, ERK, p38), RhoA and COX-2 in PC12 cells, we found that sesamin suppressed KA-induced COX-2, ERK, and p38 MAPK in PC12 cells and BV-2 cells. Our result is similar to a study of tea extract (TF3) treatment that shows TF3 reduces the gene and protein expression of COX-2 and iNOS, and NF-$\kappa$B activation from cerebral ischemia-reperfusion [41].

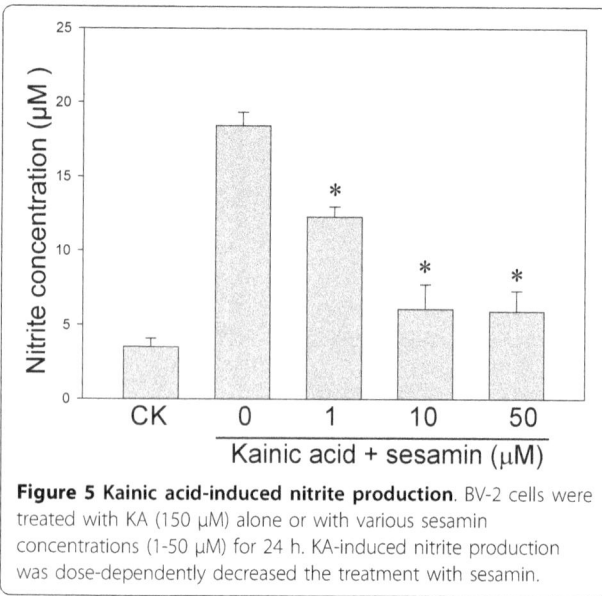

**Figure 5 Kainic acid-induced nitrite production**. BV-2 cells were treated with KA (150 μM) alone or with various sesamin concentrations (1-50 μM) for 24 h. KA-induced nitrite production was dose-dependently decreased the treatment with sesamin.

However, KA-induced RhoA pathway in BV-2 cells but not PC12 cells was reduced by sesamin.

Our data also showed that sesamin extract had the tendency to decrease the severity of seizure behavior. A recent study indicated the lack of effectiveness of antioxidants in the kainic acid SE model [42]. However, antioxidants had significant anticonvulsant activity against pilocarpine. This discrepancy could be explained by the fact that KA is a glutamate receptor agonist while pilocarpine is a muscarinic agonist [43]. Because of the small number of animals in our study, the ameliorating effect of sesamin extract on behavioral severity was not statistically significant. Further studies are needed to confirm whether sesamin has direct effects on the seizure behavior and the related molecular mechanism in this issue. The present results are consistent with previous reports that antioxidants such as resveratrol, vitamin-E, melatonin, and lipoic acids are also protective against various animal models of SE in terms of the oxidative stress or convulsions [44-51]. Particularly, resveratrol protects against KA-induced neuronal damage [7,10,14,49]. However, in the present study the concentrations of sesamin likely to be achieved in vivo were too low to act as chain-breaking antioxidants. Only higher dose (30 mg/kg) of sesamin supplementation significantly increased plasma α-tocopherol level and reduced the TBARS level as compared with the vehicle control rats. It is more likely that sesamin acts as a pharmacological antioxidant by blocking enzymes or pathways of neuroinflammation that would produce ROS/RNS.

Stopping the seizure activity earlier is the best way to prevent SE-induced free radicals and neuronal damage. However, clinical experience shows that SE can be

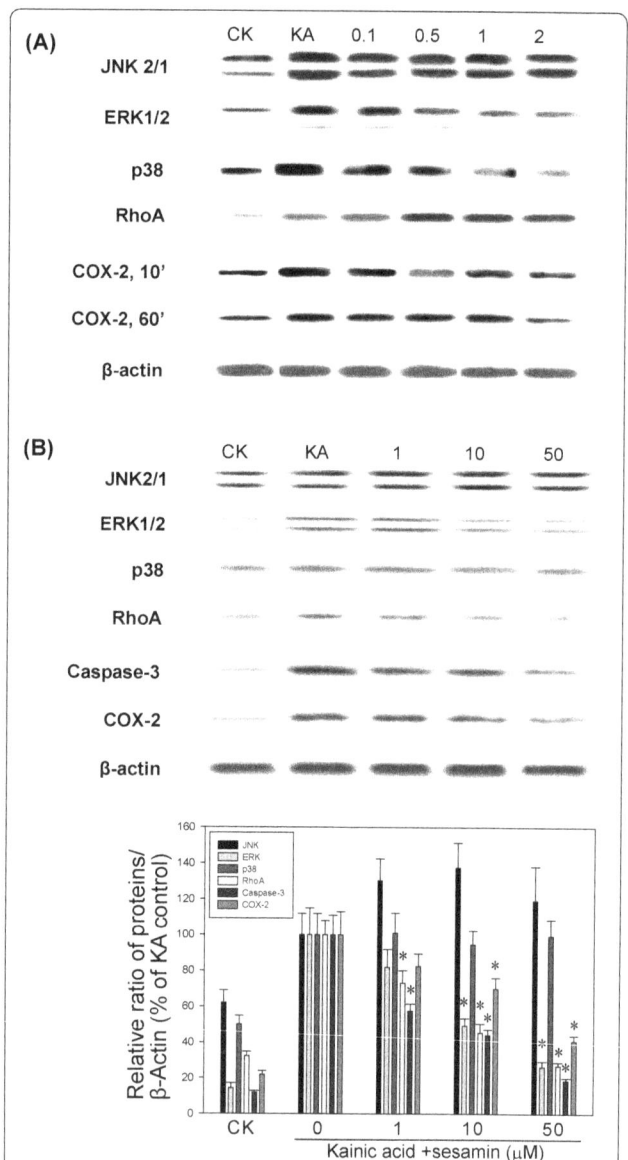

**Figure 6 Effect of sesamin on MAP kinases, RhoA and COX-2 activation in PC12 cells and BV-2 cells under KA stress**. The effect of sesamin (1-50 μM) on KA-activated cell signaling pathways was determined by Western blotting under KA stress, (A) PC12 cells for 10-min and 60-min and (B) BV-2 cells for 120 min. Sesamin effectively reduced the activation of COX-2, ERK, p38 MAP kinases. $P < 0.01$ as compared to the KA control. CK: normal control.

refractory to the commonly used medications. Therefore, intervention by antioxidants can be a potential beneficial approach in the treatment of SE.

## Conclusion

Sesamin ameliorates oxidative stress in KA-induced status epilepticus and warrants further study for the molecular mechanism.

**(A)**

**(B)**

**Figure 7 Effect of sesamin on PGE$_2$ production in PC12 cells and BV-2 cells**. Sesamin dose-dependently reduced KA-induced PGE$_2$ production in (A) PC12 cells and (B) BV-2 cells. PGE$_2$ concentration was determined by ELISA (R&D) assay. $^*$ $P < 0.01$ as compared to the KA control.

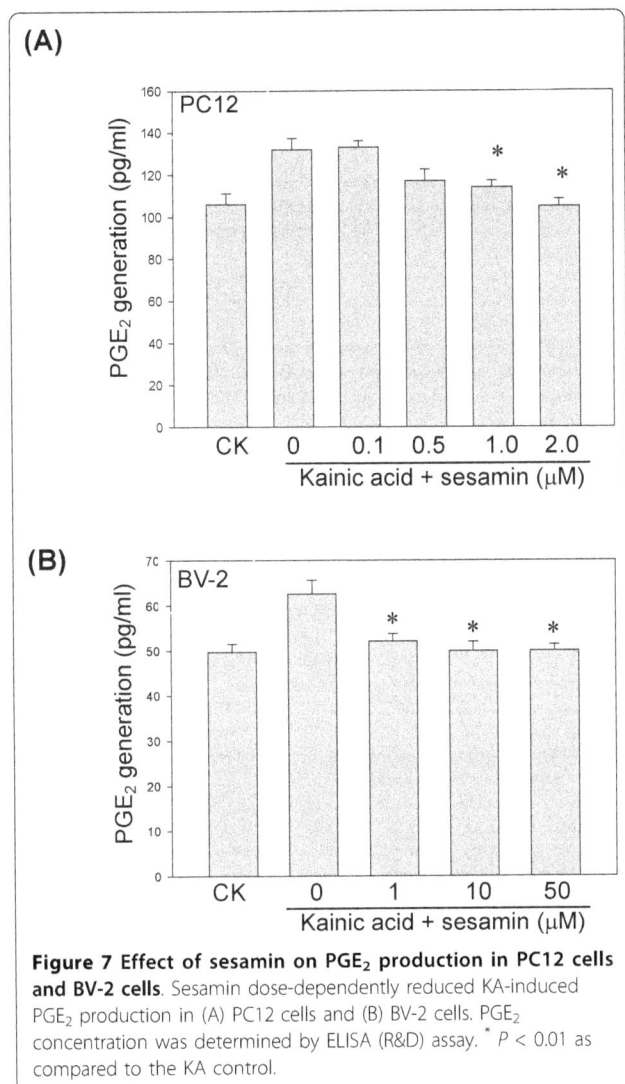

## List of abbreviations
(COX-2) Cyclooxygenase-2, (DCF) dichlorofluorescein, (DMEM) Dulbecco's modified Eagle's medium, (FBS) fetal bovine serum, (H$_2$ DCF-DA) 2',7'-dichlorodihydrofluorescein diacetate, (HBSS) Hank's balanced salt solution, (IL-6) interleukin-6, (iNOS) Inducible-nitric oxide synthase, (KA) Kainic acid, (LDH) Lactate dehydrogenase, (LPO) lipid peroxidation, (LPS) Lipopolysaccharide, (MDA) Malondialdehyde, (MAPKs) Mitogen-activated protein kinases, (MPP$^+$) 1-methyl-4-phenyl-pyridine, (MTT) 3-(4,5-dimethyl-thiazol-2-yl)-2,5-diphenyl tetrazolium bromide, (NADH) nicotinamide adenine dinucleotide, (NF-κB) Nuclear factor-κB, (NO) Nitric oxide, (PBS) Phosphate-buffered saline, (PC12 cells) Pheochromocytoma, (PGE$_2$) Prostaglandin E$_2$, (ROS) Reactive oxygen species, (SE) Status epilepticus, (SOD) Superoxide dismutase, (TBARS) thiobarbituric acid reacting substances.

## Acknowledgements
This work was supported by grants from the National Science Council, ROC (NSC 93-2314-B-075A-021, NSC 94-2314-B-075A-006) and Taichung Veterans General Hospital (TCVGH-943401A, TCVGH-983401A).

## Author details
[1]Division of Neurology, Taichung Veterans General Hospital, Taichung, Taiwan. [2]Graduate Institute of Biomedicine and Biomedical Technology, National Chi Nan University, Nantou, Taiwan. [3]Department of Biotechnology, Yuanpei University, Hsinchu, Taiwan. [4]Department of Physical Education Office, Yuanpei University, Hsinchu, Taiwan. [5]Department of Medical Research, Taichung Veterans General Hospital, Taichung, Taiwan.

## Authors' contributions
PFH and CWH participated in the design and Ms editing, in all treatment procedures, data elaboration and seizure and behavior studies. MS, CL, YC participated in all treatment procedures and daily control for animal food intake, weights and SOD and TBARS assay. SPW, YFP participated in all cell-treatment procedures, participated in ROS procedures and PWY, western blot and PGE$_2$ assay. KJ conceived the study and design, analyzed the data and prepared the manuscript. All authors read, discussed and approved the final manuscript.

## Competing interests
The authors declare that they have no competing interests.

## References
1. Wasterlain CG, Fujikawa DG, Penix L, Sankar R: Pathophysiological mechanisms of brain damage from status epilepticus. *Epilepsia* 1993, **34**: S37-S53.
2. Millikan D, Rice B, Silbergleit R: Emergency treatment of status epilepticus: current thinking. *Emerg Med Clin North Am* 2009, **27**:101-113.
3. Rocca WA, Sharbrough FW, Hauser WA, Annegers JF, Schoenberg BS: Risk factors for complex partial seizures: a population-based case-control study. *Ann Neurol* 1987, **21**:22-31.
4. Lee B, Cao R, Choi YS, Cho HY, Rhee AD, Hah CK, Hoyt KR, Obrietan K: The CREB/CRE transcriptional pathway: protection against oxidative stress-mediated neuronal cell death. *J Neurochem* 2009, **108**:1251-1265.
5. Penner MR, Pinaud R, Robertson HA: Rapid kindling of the hippocampus protects against neural damage resulting from status epilepticus. *Neuroreport* 2001, **12**:453-457.
6. Turski L, Ikonomidou C, Turski WA, Bortolotto ZA, Cavalheiro EA: Review: cholinergic mechanisms and epileptogenesis. The seizures induced by pilocarpine: a novel experimental model of intractable epilepsy. *Synapse* 1989, **3**:154-171.
7. Wang Q, Yu S, Simonyi A, Rottinghaus G, Sun GY, Sun AY: Resveratrol protects against neurotoxicity induced by kainic acid. *Neurochem Res* 2004, **29**:2105-2112.
8. Muller-Schwarze AB, Tandon P, Liu Z, Yang Y, Holmes GL, Stafstrom CE: Ketogenic diet reduces spontaneous seizures and mossy fiber sprouting in the kainic acid model. *Neuroreport* 1999, **10**:1517-1522.
9. Wasterlain CG, Shirasaka Y, Mazarati AM, Spigelman I: Chronic epilepsy with damage restricted to the hippocampus: possible mechanisms. *Epilepsy Res* 1996, **26**:255-265.
10. Gupta YK, Briyal S, Chaudhary G: Protective effect of trans-resveratrol gainst kainic acid-induced seizures and oxidative stress in rats. *Pharmacol Biochem Behav* 2002, **71**:245-249.
11. Miyamoto R, Shimakawa S, Suzuki S, Ogihara T, Tamai H: Edaravone prevents kainic acid-induced neuronal death. *Brain Res* 2008, **1209**:85-91.
12. Freitas RM, Sousa FC, Vasconcelos SM, Viana GS, Fonteles MM: Pilocarpine-induced status epilepticus in rats: lipid peroxidation level, nitrite formation, GABAergic and glutamatergic receptor alterations in the hippocampus, striatum and frontal cortex. *Pharmacol Biochem Behav* 2004, **78**:327-332.
13. Bashkatova V, Narkevich V, Vitskova G, Vanin A: The influence of anticonvulsant and antioxidant drugs on nitric oxide level and lipid peroxidation in the rat brain during penthylenetetrazole-induced epileptiform model seizures. *Prog Neuropsychopharmacol Biol Psychiatry* 2003, **27**:487-492.
14. Meyerhoff JL, Lee JK, Rittase BW, Tsang AY, Yourick DL: Lipoic acid pretreatment attenuates ferric chloride-induced seizures in the rat. *Brain Res* 2004, **1016**:139-144.
15. Sun AY, Cheng Y, Bu Q, Oldfield F: The biochemical mechanism of the excitotoxicity of kainic acid. *Mol Chem Neuropathol* 1992, **17**:51-63.
16. Bruce AJ, Baudry M: Oxygen free radicals in rat limbic structures after kainate-induced seizures. *Free Radical Biol Med* 1995, **18**:993-1002.

17. D'Antuono M, Benini R, Biagini G, D'Arcangelo G, Barbarosie M, Tancredi V, Avoli M: Limbic network interactions leading to hyperexcitability in a model of temporal lobe epilepsy. *J Neurophysiol* 2002, **87**:634-639.

18. Arispe N, Pollard HB, Rojas E: β-Amyloid $Ca^{2+}$ -channel hypothesis for neuronal death in Alzheimer disease. *Mol Cell Biochem* 1994, **140**:119-125.

19. Goodenough S, Davidson M, Chen M, Beckmann A, Pujic Z, Otsuki M, Matsumoto I: Immediate early gene expression and delayed cell death in limbic areas of the rat brain after kainic acid treatment and recovery in the cold. *Exp Neurol* 1997, **145**:451-461.

20. Dubreuil CI, Marklund N, Deschamps K, McIntosh TK, McKerracher L: Activation of Rho after traumatic brain injury and seizure in rats. *Exp Neurol* 2006, **198**:361-369.

21. Matagne V, Lebrethon MC, Gérard A, Bourguignon JP: Kainate/estrogen receptor involvement in rapid estradiol effects in vitro and intracellular signaling pathways. *Endocrinology* 2005, **146**:2313-2323.

22. Hou RC, Chen HL, Tzen JT, Jeng KC: Effect of sesame antioxidants on LPS-induced NO production by BV2 microglial cells. *Neuroreport* 2003, **14**:1815-1819.

23. Lahaie-Collins V, Bournival J, Plouffe M, Carange J, Martinoli MG: Sesamin modulates tyrosine hydroxylase, superoxide dismutase, catalase, inducible NO synthase and interleukin-6 expression in dopaminergic cells under MPP-induced oxidative stress. *Oxid Med Cell Longev* 2008, **1**:54-62.

24. Ma CJ, Kim SR, Kim J, Kim YC: Meso-dihydroguaiaretic acid and licarin A of Machilus thunbergii protect against glutamate-induced toxicity in primary cultures of a rat cortical cells. *Br J Pharmacol* 2005, **146**:752-759.

25. Kanada A, Nishimura J, Yamaguchi JY, Kobayashi M, Mishima K, Horimoto K, Kanemaru K, Oyama Y: Extract of Ginkgo biloba leaves attenuates kainate-induced increase in intracellular $Ca^{2+}$ concentration of rat cerebellar granule neurons. *Biol Pharm Bull* 2005, **28**:934-936.

26. Fukumoto LR, Mazza G: Assessing antioxidant and prooxidant activities and phenolic compounds. *J Agric Food Chem* 2000, **48**:3597-3604.

27. Hou RC, Huang HM, Tzen JT, Jeng KC: Protective effects of sesamin and sesamolin on hypoxic neuronal and PC12 cells. *J Neurosci Res* 2003, **74**:123-133.

28. Jeng KC, Hou RC, Wang JC, Ping LI: Sesamin inhibits lipopolysaccharide-induced cytokine production by suppression of p38 mitogen-activated protein kinase and nuclear factor-kappaB. *Immunol Lett* 2005, **97**:101-106.

29. Ohkawa H, Ohishi N, Yagi K: Assay for lipid peroxides in animal tissues by thiobarbituric acid reaction. *Anal Biochem* 1979, **95**:351-358.

30. Racine RJ: Modification of seizure activity by electrical stimulation. II. Motor seizure. *Electroencephalogr Clin Neurophysiol* 1972, **32**:281-294.

31. Handforth A, Ackermann RF: Functional $^{14}$ C 2-deoxyglucose mapping of progressive states of status epilepticus induced by amygdala stimulation in rat. *Brain Res* 1988, **460**:94-102.

32. Wu WH, Kang YP, Wang NH, Jou HJ, Wang TA: Sesame ingestion affects sex hormones, antioxidant status, and blood lipids in postmenopausal women. *J Nutr* 2006, **136**:1270-1275.

33. Dykens JA, Stern A, Trenkner E: Mechanisms of kainate toxicity to cerebellar neurons in vitro is analogous to reperfusion tissue injury. *J Neurochem* 1987, **49**:1222-1228.

34. Jamarkattel-Pandit N, Pandit NR, Kim MY, Park SH, Kim KS, Choi H, Kim H, Bu Y: Neuroprotective effect of defatted sesame seeds extract against in vitro and in vivo ischemic neuronal damage. *Planta Med* 2010, **76**:20-26.

35. Somera-Molina KC, Nair S, Van Eldik LJ, Watterson DM, Wainwright MS: Enhanced microglial activation and proinflammatory cytokine upregulation are linked to increased susceptibility to seizures and neurologic injury in a 'two-hit' seizure model. *Brain Res* 2009, **1282**:162-172.

36. Hashimoto K, Watanabe K, Nishimura T, Iyo M, Shirayama Y, Minabe Y: Behavioral changes and expression of heat shock protein HSP-70 mRNA, brain-derived neurotrophic factor mRNA, and cyclooxygenase-2 mRNA in rat brain following seizures induced by systemic administration of kainic acid. *Brain Res* 1998, **804**:212-223.

37. Sandhya TL, Ong WY, Horrocks LA, Farooqui AA: A light and electron microscopic study of cytoplasmic phospholipase A2 and cyclooxygenase-2 in the hippocampus after kainite lesions. *Brain Res* 1998, **788**:223-231.

38. Sanz O, Estrada A, Ferrer I, Planas AM: Differential cellular distribution and dynamics of HSP70, cyclooxygenase-2, and c-Fos in the rat brain after transient focal ischemia or kainic acid. *Neurosci* 1997, **80**:221-232.

39. Candelario-Jalil E, Ajamieh HH, Sam S, Martinez G, Leon OS: Nimesulide limits kainate-induced oxidative damage in the rat hippocampus. *Eur J Pharmacol* 2000, **390**:295-298.

40. Sarker KP, Nakata M, Kitajima I, Nakajima T, Maruyama I: Inhibition of caspase-3 activation by SB 203580, p38 mitogen-activated protein kinase inhibitor in nitric oxide-induced apoptosis of PC-12 cells. *J Mol Neurosci* 2000, **15**:243-250.

41. Cai C, Li J, Wu Q, Min C, Ouyang M, Zheng S, Ma W, Lin F: Modulation of the oxidative stress and nuclear factor kappaB activation by theaflavin 3,3'-gallate in the rats exposed to cerebral ischemia-reperfusion. *Folia Biol* 2007, **53**:164-172.

42. Xu K, Janet L, Stringer JL: Antioxidants and free radical scavengers do not consistently delay seizure onset in animal models of acute seizures. *Epilepsy & Behavior* 2008, **13**:77-82.

43. Turski L, Ikonomidou C, Turski WA, Bortolotto ZA, Cavalheiro EA: Cholinergic mechanisms and epileptogenesis. The seizures induced by pilocarpine: a novel experimental model of intractable epilepsy. *Synapse* 1989, **3**:154-171.

44. Ayyildiz M, Yildirim M, Agar E: The effects of vitamin E on penicillin-induced epileptiform activity in rats. *Exp Brain Res* 2006, **174**:109-113.

45. Milatovic D, Gupta RC, Dettbarn WD: Involvement of nitric oxide in kainic acid-induced excitotoxicity in rat brain. *Brain Res* 2002, **957**:330-337.

46. Tome AR, Feng D, Freitas RM: The effects of alpha-tocopherol on hippocampal oxidative stress prior to in pilocarpine-induced seizures. *Neurochem Res* 2010, **35**:580-587.

47. Champney TH, Champney JA: Novel anticonvulsant action of chronic melatonin in gerbils. *Neuroreport* 1992, **3**:1152-1154.

48. Yamamoto HA, Mohanan PV: Ganglioside GT1B and melatonin inhibit brain mitochondrial DNA damage and seizures induced by kainic acid in mice. *Brain Res* 2003, **964**:100-106.

49. Wu Z, Xu Q, Zhang L, Kong D, Ma R, Wang L: Protective effect of resveratrol against kainate-induced temporal lobe epilepsy in rats. *Neurochem Res* 2009, **34**:1393-1400.

50. Shin EJ, Jeong JH, Kim AY, Koh YH, Nah SY, Kim WK, Ko KH, Kim HJ, Wie MB, Kwon YS, Yoneda Y, Kim HC: Protection against kainate neurotoxicity by ginsenosides: attenuation of convulsive behavior, mitochondrial dysfunction, and oxidative stress. *J Neurosci Res* 2009, **87**:710-722.

51. Miyamoto R, Shimakawa S, Suzuki S, Ogihara T, Tamai H: Edaravone prevents kainic acid-induced neuronal death. *Brain Res* 2008, **1209**:85-91.

# 2

# Systemic autoinflammation with intractable epilepsy managed with interleukin-1 blockade

Allen D. DeSena[1*], Thuy Do[2] and Grant S. Schulert[2*]

## Abstract

**Background:** Autoinflammatory disorders are distinguished by seemingly random episodes of systemic hyperinflammation, driven in particular by IL-1. Recent pre-clinical work has shown a key role for IL-1 in epilepsy in animal models, and therapies for autoinflammation including IL-1 blockade are proposed for refractory epilepsy.

**Case presentation:** Here, we report an adolescent female with signs of persistent systemic inflammation and epilepsy unresponsive to multiple anti-epileptic drugs (AED). She was diagnosed with generalized epilepsy with a normal brain MRI and an electroencephalogram (EEG) showing occasional generalized spike and slow wave discharges. Her diagnostic evaluation showed no signs of autoimmunity or genetic causes of epilepsy or periodic fever syndromes but persistently elevated serum inflammatory markers including S100 alarmin proteins. She experienced prompt clinical response to IL-1 blockade with first anakinra and then canakinumab, with near complete resolution of clinical seizures. Additionally, she displayed marked improvements in quality of life and social/academic functioning. Baseline gene expression studies on peripheral blood mononuclear cells (PBMC) from this patient showed significantly activated gene pathways suggesting systemic immune activation, including focal adhesion, platelet activation, and Rap1 signaling, which is an upstream regulator of IL-1β production by the NLRP3 inflammasome. It also showed activation of genes that characterize inflammasome-mediated autoinflammatory disorders and no signs of interferon activation. This gene expression signature was largely extinguished after anakinra treatment.

**Conclusions:** Together, these findings suggest that patients with epilepsy responsive to immune modulation may have distinct autoinflammatory features supporting IL-1 blockade. As such, IL-1 blockade may be highly efficacious adjunctive medication for certain refractory epilepsy syndromes.

**Keywords:** Seizures, IL-1beta, Anakinra, Canakinumab

## Background

Autoinflammatory disorders represent a heterogeneous collection of both monogenic and complex diseases, characterized by seemingly random or unprovoked inflammation [1]. In contrast to classic autoimmune diseases, AID typically lack high-titer autoantibodies or autoreactive lymphocytes but are rather characterized by defects in innate immune responses. The best characterized autoinflammatory disorders have been linked to defects in specific pattern recognition receptors in the inflammasome complex, leading to hyperproduction of proinflammatory cytokines particularly of the IL-1 family [2]. These include the cyropyrin-associated periodic syndromes (CAPS), with mutations in NLPR3, which encompasses a broad phenotypic spectrum, from cold-associated urticaria (FCAS) to disorders with significant neurologic involvement and epilepsy such as neonatal-onset multisystem inflammatory disease (NOMID) [3, 4]. Recent work has also highlighted a distinct family of autoinflammatory disorders with prominent over-activation of the type I interferon response including

* Correspondence: allen.desena@cchmc.org; grant.schulert@cchmc.org
[1]Division of Neurology, Department of Pediatrics, Cincinnati Children's Hospital Medical Center, University of Cincinnati College of Medicine, 3333 Burnet Ave, MLC 2015, Cincinnati, OH 45229, USA
[2]Division of Rheumatology, Department of Pediatrics, Children's Hospital Medical Center, University of Cincinnati College of Medicine, 3333 Burnet Ave, MLC 4010, Cincinnati, OH 45229, USA

Aicardi-Goutieres syndrome, which causes progressive encephalopathy [5, 6].

Inflammation and particularly pro-inflammatory cytokines such as IL-1 are also increasingly implicated in the pathogenesis of seizures and epilepsy [7, 8]. Indeed, in multiple distinct animal models of epileptogenesis, pharmacologic blockade of IL-1 through the use of the IL-1 receptor antagonist (IL-1RA) reduced seizures and signs of cellular injury [9–11], leading to the proposal that medications for peripheral autoinflammation could be beneficial for intractable epilepsy [12]. Here, we report an adolescent female with signs of systemic inflammation and epilepsy unresponsive to multiple anti-epileptic drugs (AED), with a profound clinical improvement in response to IL-1 blockade. Gene expression profiling demonstrated an inflammatory signature that is largely extinguished upon treatment, further suggesting immune correlates that could identify patients with epilepsy who could benefit from IL-1 blockade.

## Patient data and study approval

This study was approved by the Cincinnati Children's Hospital Institutional Review Board (IRB 2011-1517), and informed consent was obtained from all patients and/or their legal guardians. Data pertaining to this patient's clinical course, laboratory values, and treatment were collected from the electronic medical records. Peripheral blood mononuclear cells (PBMC) were obtained and RNA extracted as described [13].

## AmpliSeq transcriptome analysis

Gene expression profiles from PBMC of the patient and healthy controls were determined using the AmpliSeq Transcriptome Gene Expression Kit via the Ion Torrent S5 system (Thermo Fisher, Carlsbad, CA). Differential gene expression was visualized using the Morpheus platform and pathway analysis performed using DAVID Functional Annotation Tool. Full methodologic details are provided in the supplementary information.

## Case presentation

The patient is a 14-year-old female diagnosed with generalized epilepsy after presenting with early morning involuntary jerking of her upper extremities and an electroencephalogram (EEG) with occasional generalized spike and slow wave discharges. She later had frequent staring spells, suspected to be absence seizures, along with increasing memory loss and poor academic performance. Notably, she had no history of fevers, rash, arthritis, or serositis. Her brain MRI was normal aside from a single nonspecific dorsal thalamic T2 lesion that has remained stable. Over 2 years, she seized on average 4–15 times daily despite multiple AED. Upon presentation to our neuroimmunology clinic, she was treated with levetiracetam 1500 mg twice daily (later increased to 2000 mg twice daily), ethosuximide 250 mg in

the morning and 500 mg in the evening, lamotrigine 100 mg twice daily, and topiramate 100 mg twice daily; clonazepam 0.25 mg was later added also without dramatic reduction in seizure frequency. An extensive laboratory evaluation is summarized in Table 1. Notably, she had negative testing for all autoantibodies but had persistently elevated C-reactive protein and erythrocyte sedimentation rate (ESR) (Fig. 1). Serum levels of S100A8/A9 and S100A12 alarmin proteins, which serve to amplify innate immune

**Table 1** Summary of diagnostic evaluation

| Test | Results | Normal range |
|---|---|---|
| White blood cell count ($10^3/\mu$L) | 13.1 | 4.5–13.0 |
| Absolute neutrophil count ($10^3/\mu$L) | 10.2 | 1.8–8.0 |
| Hemoglobin (g/dL) | 13.1 | 12.0–16.0 |
| Platelet count ($10^3/\mu$L) | 300 | 135–466 |
| AST (U/L) | 9 | 5–26 |
| ALT (U/L) | 19 | 12–49 |
| Albumin (g/dL) | 3.7 | 3.3–4.8 |
| Total protein (g/dL) | 7.8 | 6.4–8.3 |
| TSH (mcIU/mL) | 1.39 | 0.43–4.00 |
| S100A8/A9 (ng/mL) | 5617 | 716–3004 |
| S100A12 (ng/mL) | 429 | 32–385 |
| Erythrocyte sedimentation rate (mm/h) | 30 | 0–20 |
| C-reactive protein (mg/dL) | 2.8 | < 0.30 |
| IgA (mg/dL) | 118 | 68–376 |
| IgG (mg/dL) | 1050 | 724–1611 |
| IgM (mg/dL) | 66 | 60–264 |
| Anti-nuclear antibody | Negative | < 1:80 |
| Extractable nuclear antigens (Jo-1, Ro, La, RNP, Sm) | Negative | |
| Anti-dsDNA | Negative | |
| Anti-phospholipid antibody panel | Negative | |
| c-ANCA (U/mL) | 0 | 0–19 |
| p-ANCA (U/mL) | 0 | 0–19 |
| Anti-ASMA | Negative | |
| Anti-LKM | Negative | |
| Endomysial antibody | < 1:10 | < 1:10 |
| Anti-thyroglobulin antibody (U/mL) | 10.1 | 10–114 |
| Anti-thyroid peroxidase antibody (U/mL) | 6.6 | 5–33 |
| Anti-ribosomal antibody (U/mL) | 0 | 0–40 |
| Intrinsic factor blocking antibody | Negative | |
| Anti-NMO antibody | Negative | |
| Anti-NMDA receptor ab | Negative | |
| Paraneoplastic panel | Negative | |
| CSF RBC count (per mm$^3$) | 29 | 0–4 |
| CSF WBC count (per mm$^3$) | 1 | 0–4 |
| CSF protein (mg/dL) | 37 | 15–45 |
| CSF glucose (mg/dL) | 43 | 40–70 |
| CSF oligoclonal bands | 0 | 0–4 |
| CSF index | 0.39 | 0.3–0.77 |

responses and inflammation, were also elevated (Table 1) [14]. Both epiSeek Infancy and Childhood Epilepsy Panel and Genetic Periodic Fever Syndromes Panel including *NLRP3* was negative. Cerebral spinal fluid studies showed no elevation in her white blood cells or protein, absent oligoclonal bands, and a normal IgG index and synthesis rate. Cytokine levels in the CSF showed only a mild elevation in IL-1β (25 pg/mL; normal ≤ 10 pg/mL); however, it is unknown how CSF sample processing could affect IL-1 levels. Serum IL-1β was within normal limits, but circulating IL-1 levels are frequently normal even in active systemic autoinflammatory disorders [15]. Finally, a PET scan showed no areas consistent with inflammatory foci.

Due to a suspected systemic inflammatory process related to her epilepsy, she was empirically treated with oral dexamethasone 120 mg daily for 5 days, leading to a dramatic but transient response, with no seizures for 1 week followed by regression to her baseline seizure frequency. After a lengthy discussion, treatment with the recombinant IL-1RA anakinra 100 mg daily was initiated, upon which she experienced a rapid approximately 80% reduction in seizure frequency to about four per week. She had rapid normalization in her inflammatory markers (Fig. 1). Anakinra was later increased to 100 mg twice daily, resulting in 2 months without clinically evident seizures. She also noted profound improvements in her fatigue, general malaise, quality of life, and academic performance, now allowing her to work and consider pursuing higher education. Repeat EEG testing showed occasional generalized spike and slow wave discharges with increased frequency in sleep. Repeat CSF examination was not performed. The patient was changed to the anti-IL-1β monoclonal antibody canakinumab 300 mg every 4 weeks, and she enjoyed long periods of being seizure-free, currently averaging one seizure per several months. She was weaned off lamotrigine and ethosuximide, and her clonazepam changed to clobazam.

## Peripheral blood gene expression profiles demonstrate features of autoinflammation

In order to define the systemic immune activation in this patient, PBMC gene expression profiles were determined both before and after initiation of anakinra treatment and compared to three healthy, age-matched controls using AmpliSeq Transcriptome [16]. Full sequencing details are shown in the supplemental information. Compared to the mean of healthy controls, pre-treatment patient PBMC showed 178 genes upregulated and 260 genes downregulated > 2-fold (Fig. 2a, Additional file 1: Table S3). Pathway analysis of the upregulated genes showed multiple significantly enriched gene pathways suggesting systemic immune activation, including focal adhesion ($p = 9.1 \times 10^{-5}$), platelet activation ($p = 0.0011$), Rap1 signaling ($p = 0.0028$), and cytokine-cytokine receptor interaction ($p = 0.018$). Of particular note, Rap1 signaling is an upstream regulator of IL-1β production and plays a key role in NLRP3 inflammasome activation [17]. In addition, 83% (148/178) of upregulated genes showed lower expression in patient PBMC after anakinra treatment, including 87.5% (7/8) of elevated Rap1 pathway genes (Additional file 1: Table S4). Regarding downregulated genes, the most significantly enriched GO term was type I interferon signaling pathways ($p = 8.8 \times 10^{-8}$), strongly supporting the absence of an interferon-induced gene signature in this patient. Indeed, full analysis of the interferon-induced signature described in autoinflammatory interferonopathies [6] shows no evidence of interferon activation before or after anakinra treatment (Fig. 2b).

To further examine for the presence of an autoinflammatory signature responsive to IL-1 blockade, we utilized well-characterized PBMC gene expression profiles that could clearly distinguish patients with CAPS, regardless of underlying disease activity [18]. As shown in Fig. 2c, this patient showed increased expression of a broad spectrum of immune response genes activated in CAPS

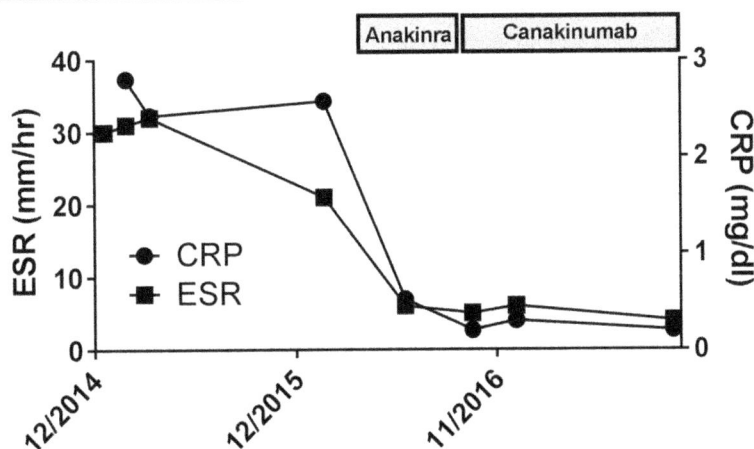

**Fig. 1** IL-1 blockade leading to resolution of systemic inflammation in patient with refractory epilepsy

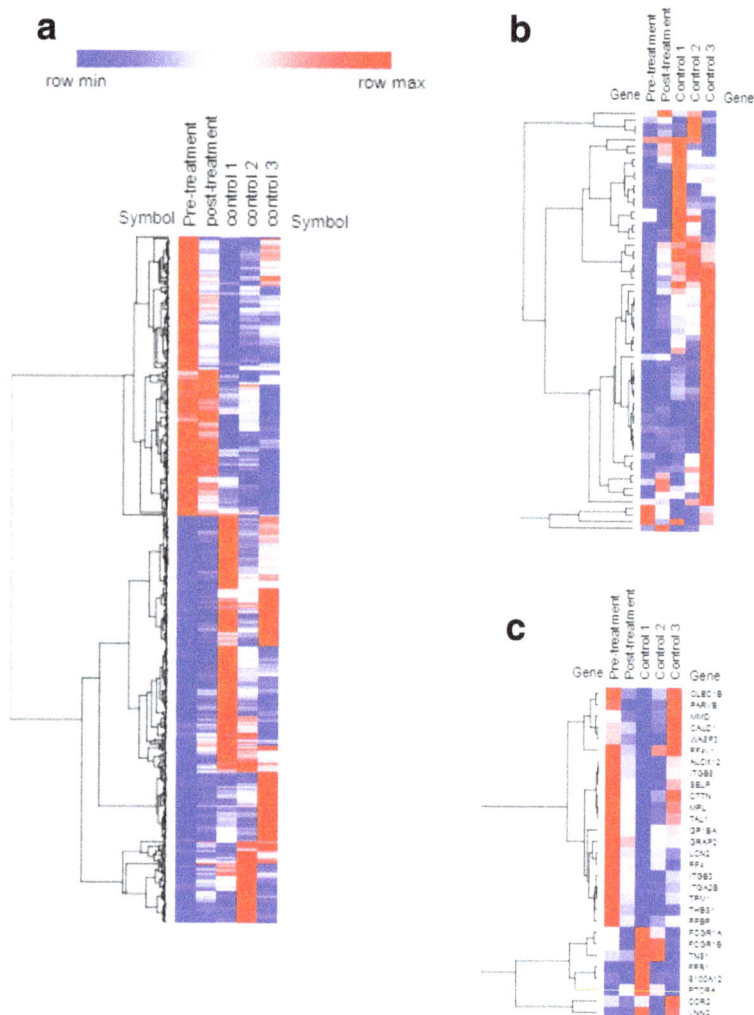

**Fig. 2** PBMC gene expression signatures before and after anakinra treatment. Gene expression was quantified using the AmpliSeq Transcriptome kit and the Ion Torrent S5 system as described. Heatmaps show hierarchical clustering of normalized log-2 RPKM from patient PBMC as well as three pediatric control samples. **a** Heatmap showing genes with > 2-fold difference between pre-treatment sample and mean of control samples. **b** Heatmap showing genes associated with autoinflammatory interferonopathies, as determined in [6]. **c** Heatmap showing immune response genes associated with the IL-1-driven autoinflammatory disorder CAPS [18]

patients, expression of which was largely extinguished with anakinra treatment. Taken together, these findings suggest that this patient displays features of IL-1-driven systemic autoinflammation, which were markedly reduced with anakinra treatment.

**Discussion and conclusion**

There is increasing evidence from animal models that inflammation, and in particular IL-1, is a key driver of epilepsy [7, 9–11]. IL-1 family cytokines are recognized as central to the pathogenesis of systemic autoinflammatory disorders such as CAPS, and blockade of IL-1 using anakinra or canakinumab leads to rapid and sustained clinical improvement in inflammatory symptoms [19]. Here, we describe a patient with refractory epilepsy and features of

systemic inflammation including elevated CRP, ESR, and S100 proteins, treated with IL-1 blockade. This patient showed a profound improvement in her symptoms likely related to a systemic inflammatory syndrome and a greater than 90% reduction in seizure frequency since starting anti-IL-1 immunotherapy. Although other changes were made to her AED regimen, sustained seizure reduction seemed to correlate best with initiation of anakinra or canakinumab. In conjunction with seizure reduction, the patient showed sustained normalization of inflammatory markers and marked improvement in quality of life and social/academic functioning.

Although genetic testing for well characterized, monogenetic autoinflammatory disorders was negative, this patient had significant signs of systemic autoinflammation.

Her ESR and CRP, while nonspecific, were persistently elevated and normalized in conjunction with seizure control. S100 proteins, which are also associated with systemic autoinflammation [14], were also elevated. She had no features of autoimmunity such as elevated total IgG or specific autoantibodies (Table 1). Most interestingly, PBMC gene expression profiling showed upregulation of numerous gene pathways suggesting systemic immune activation, including upstream regulators of the NLRP3 inflammasome [17], and genes associated with anakinra response [18] (Fig. 2). Indeed, the vast majority of this gene signature was diminished upon anakinra treatment. This suggests that patients with epilepsy responsive to immune modulation may have distinct inflammatory features supporting IL-1 blockade.

The potential utility of IL-1 blockade for seizures has been noted in multiple preclinical studies [7, 8] but to our knowledge has not been reported in patients with idiopathic epilepsy. There is one recent report of a patient with febrile infection-related epilepsy syndrome (FIRES), a rare but devastating encephalopathy occurring after a febrile illness, that had improvement with anakinra while in super-refractory status epilepticus [20]. The patient reported here thus represents the second patient with epilepsy treated with IL-1 blockade (and first treated non-emergently without status epilepticus), suggesting that in selected cases, this treatment might be a profoundly impactful adjunctive medication for certain refractory epilepsy syndromes.

## Acknowledgements
Not applicable

## Funding
Dr. Schulert was supported by a Scientist Development Award from the Rheumatology Research Foundation and Procter Scholar Award from the Cincinnati Children's Research Foundation.

## Authors' contributions
ADD and GSS conceived of the study, treated the patient, and wrote the manuscript. GSS and TD designed the experiments and analyzed the data. TD performed the experiments. All authors contributed to the drafting of the manuscript and approved the final version.

## Consent for publication
Consent for publication was obtained from all patients and/or their legal guardians.

## Competing interests
Dr. Schulert has received consulting fees from Novartis. The other authors declare that they have no competing interests.

## References
1. Masters SL, Simon A, Aksentijevich I, Kastner DL. Horror autoinflammaticus: the molecular pathophysiology of autoinflammatory disease. Annu Rev Immunol. 2009;27:621–68.
2. de Jesus AA, Canna SW, Liu Y, Goldbach-Mansky R. Molecular mechanisms in genetically defined autoinflammatory diseases: disorders of amplified danger signaling. Annu Rev Immunol. 2015;33:823–74.
3. Aksentijevich I, Nowak M, Mallah M, Chae JJ, Watford WT, Hofmann SR, et al. De novoCIAS1 mutations, cytokine activation, and evidence for genetic heterogeneity in patients with neonatal-onset multisystem inflammatory disease (NOMID): a new member of the expanding family of pyrin-associated autoinflammatory diseases. Arthritis Rheum. 2002;46:3340–8.
4. Prieur AM, Griscelli C, Lampert F, Truckenbrodt H, Guggenheim MA, Lovell DJ, et al. A chronic, infantile, neurological, cutaneous and articular (CINCA) syndrome. A specific entity analysed in 30 patients. Scand J Rheumatol Suppl. 1987;66:57–68.
5. Crow YJ. Type I interferonopathies: a novel set of inborn errors of immunity. Ann N Y Acad Sci. 2011;1238:91–8.
6. Liu Y, Jesus AA, Marrero B, Yang D, Ramsey SE, Montealegre Sanchez GA, et al. Activated STING in a vascular and pulmonary syndrome. N Engl J Med. 2014;371:507–18.
7. Kołosowska K, Maciejak P, Szyndler J, Turzyńska D, Sobolewska A, Płaźnik A. The role of IL-1β and glutamate in the effects of lipopolysaccharide on the hippocampal electrical kindling of seizures. J Neuroimmunol. 2016;298:146–52.
8. Arisi GM, Foresti ML, Katki K, Shapiro LA. Increased CCL2, CCL3, CCL5, and IL-1β cytokine concentration in piriform cortex, hippocampus, and neocortex after pilocarpine-induced seizures. J Neuroinflammation. 2015;12:129.
9. Marchi N, Fan Q, Ghosh C, Fazio V, Bertolini F, Betto G, et al. Antagonism of peripheral inflammation reduces the severity of status epilepticus. Neurobiol Dis. 2009;33:171–81.
10. Librizzi L, Noè F, Vezzani A, de Curtis M, Ravizza T. Seizure-induced brain-borne inflammation sustains seizure recurrence and blood-brain barrier damage. Ann Neurol. 2012;72:82–90.
11. Noe FM, Polascheck N, Frigerio F, Bankstahl M, Ravizza T, Marchini S, et al. Pharmacological blockade of IL-1β/IL-1 receptor type 1 axis during epileptogenesis provides neuroprotection in two rat models of temporal lobe epilepsy. Neurobiol Dis. 2013;59:183–93.
12. Terrone G, Salamone A, Vezzani A. Inflammation and epilepsy: preclinical findings and potential clinical translation. Curr Pharm Des. 2017;23
13. Sikora KA, Fall N, Thornton S, Grom AA. The limited role of interferon-gamma in systemic juvenile idiopathic arthritis cannot be explained by cellular hyporesponsiveness. Arthritis Rheum. 2012;64:3799–808.
14. Holzinger D, Kessel C, Omenetti A, Gattorno M. From bench to bedside and back again: translational research in autoinflammation. Nat Rev Rheumatol. 2015;11:573–85.
15. de Jager W, Hoppenreijs EPAH, Wulffraat NM, Wedderburn LR, Kuis W, Prakken BJ. Blood and synovial fluid cytokine signatures in patients with juvenile idiopathic arthritis: a cross-sectional study. Ann Rheum Dis. 2007;66:589–98.
16. Zhang JD, Schindler T, Küng E, Ebeling M, Certa U. Highly sensitive amplicon-based transcript quantification by semiconductor sequencing. BMC Genomics. 2014;15:565.
17. Liu H, Lo CM, OWH Y, Li CX, Liu XB, Qi X, et al. NLRP3 inflammasome induced liver graft injury through activation of telomere-independent RAP1/KC axis. J Pathol. 2017;242:284–96.
18. Balow JE, Ryan JG, Chae JJ, Booty MG, Bulua A, Stone D, et al. Microarray-based gene expression profiling in patients with cryopyrin-associated periodic syndromes defines a disease-related signature and IL-1-responsive transcripts. Ann Rheum Dis. 2013;72:1064–70.
19. Federici S, Martini A, Gattorno M. The central role of anti-IL-1 blockade in the treatment of monogenic and multi-factorial autoinflammatory diseases. Front Immunol. 2013;4:351.
20. Kenney-Jung DL, Vezzani A, Kahoud RJ, RG LF-C, Ho M-L, Muskardin TW, et al. Febrile infection-related epilepsy syndrome treated with anakinra. Ann Neurol. 2016;80:939–45.

# 3

# Mesial temporal lobe epilepsy with psychiatric comorbidities: a place for differential neuroinflammatory interplay

Ludmyla Kandratavicius[1,2†], Jose Eduardo Peixoto-Santos[1†], Mariana Raquel Monteiro[1], Renata Caldo Scandiuzzi[1], Carlos Gilberto Carlotti Jr[3], Joao Alberto Assirati Jr[3], Jaime Eduardo Hallak[1,2,4] and Joao Pereira Leite[1,2*]

## Abstract

**Background:** Despite the strong association between epilepsy and psychiatric comorbidities, few biological substrates are currently described. We have previously reported neuropathological alterations in mesial temporal lobe epilepsy (MTLE) patients with major depression and psychosis that suggest a morphological and neurochemical basis for psychopathological symptoms. Neuroinflammatory-related structures and molecules might be part of the altered neurochemical milieu underlying the association between epilepsy and psychiatric comorbidities, and such features have not been previously investigated in humans.

**Methods:** MTLE hippocampi of subjects without psychiatric history (MTLE_W), MTLE + major depression (MTLE + D), and MTLE + interictal psychosis (MTLE + P) derived from epilepsy surgery and control necropsies were investigated for reactive astrocytes (glial fibrillary acidic protein (GFAP)), activated microglia (human leukocyte antigen, MHC class II (HLA-DR)), glial metallothionein-I/II (MT-I/II), and aquaporin 4 (AQP4) immunohistochemistry.

**Results:** We found an increased GFAP immunoreactive area in the molecular layers, granule cell layer, and *cornus ammonis* region 2 (CA2) and *cornus ammonis* region 1 (CA1) of MTLE_W and MTLE + P, respectively, compared to MTLE + D. HLA-DR immunoreactive area was higher in *cornus ammonis* region 3 (CA3) of MTLE + P, compared to MTLE + D and MTLE_W, and in the hilus, when compared to MTLE_W. MTLE_W cases showed increased MT-I/II area in the granule cell layer and CA1, compared to MTLE + P, and in the parasubiculum, when compared to MTLE + D and MTLE + P. Differences between MTLE and control, such as astrogliosis, microgliosis, increased MT-I/II, and decreased perivascular AQP4 in the epileptogenic hippocampus, were in agreement to what is currently described in the literature.

**Conclusions:** Neuroinflammatory-related molecules in MTLE hippocampus show a distinct pattern of expression when patients present with a comorbid psychiatric diagnosis, similar to what is found in the pure forms of schizophrenia and major depression. Future studies focusing on inflammatory characteristics of MTLE with psychiatric comorbidities might help in the design of better therapeutic strategies.

**Keywords:** Temporal lobe epilepsy, Psychosis, Major depression, Astrocytes, Microglia, Aquaporin 4, Metallothionein

* Correspondence: jpleite@fmrp.usp.br
†Equal contributors
[1]Department of Neurosciences and Behavior, Ribeirao Preto Medical School, University of Sao Paulo (USP), Av Bandeirantes 3900, CEP 14049-900 Ribeirao Preto, SP, Brazil
[2]Center for Interdisciplinary Research on Applied Neurosciences (NAPNA), USP, Ribeirao Preto, Brazil
Full list of author information is available at the end of the article

# Background

Mesial temporal lobe epilepsy (MTLE) is the most common cause of intractable epilepsy in adults and is characterized by hippocampal sclerosis, neuronal loss, gliosis, and mossy fiber sprouting [1-4]. Psychiatric comorbidities are frequent in MTLE patients, and in population-based studies, epilepsy has been consistently associated with increased risk of schizophrenia [5]. However, the exact biological substrate behind the association of MTLE and psychiatric comorbidities is unknown [6,7]. We have recently shown neuropathological alterations in the hippocampus of patients with epilepsy and the history of major depression or interictal psychosis, which may indicate that structural changes and neurochemical dysfunctions may underlie psychiatric symptoms in MTLE [8-10].

Neuroinflammation-related abnormalities such as glial pathology, glutamate dysregulation, and blood-brain-barrier dysfunction are found not only in epilepsy, but also in schizophrenia and major depression [11]. Glial proteins, such as metallothionein I and II (MT-I/II), are able to quench free zinc and modulate glutamatergic neurotransmission [12], and aquaporin 4 (AQP4), found in astrocytic endfeets, is a regulator of water homeostasis that majorly controls edema formation and tissue excitability [13,14]. In schizophrenia, upregulation of MT-I/II and of astrocyte and microglia markers have been documented in several brain regions [15-17]. By contrast, neuropathological studies in specimens from major depression patients indicate reduction in hippocampal glial fibrillary acidic protein (GFAP)-positive astrocytes and of AQP4 and MT-I/II in the frontal cortex [18,19]. Protein expression and neuropathological features in MTLE with psychiatric comorbidities may resemble what is found in the pure form of the correspondent psychiatric illness [20]. Therefore, we hypothesized that expression of reactive astrocytes, activated microglia, glial MT-I/II, and AQP4 would be altered in the hippocampal formation of MTLE patients with major depression and interictal psychosis.

# Methods

## Patients

We analyzed the hippocampal formation from MTLE specimens freshly collected in the operating room and non-epileptic controls from necropsy, collected between 4 and 9 h after death. A <24-h postmortem time limit allows comparison of necropsy tissue with freshly collected surgical specimens for their protein levels, cell morphology, and tissue integrity [4,21,22]. Tissue collection and processing were conducted according to a protocol approved by our institution's Research Ethics Board (# 2634/2008 and # 9370/2003).

MTLE specimens were derived from 43 MTLE patients who underwent a standard *en bloc* anterior temporal resection (including 3 to 4 cm of the hippocampus) for medically intractable seizures. All had clinical neuropathological confirmation of hippocampal sclerosis (HS). They were divided into three groups: 17 MTLE patients without any history of psychiatric disorder (MTLE$_W$ group), 11 MTLE patients with interictal psychosis (MTLE + P group), and 15 MTLE patients with a diagnosis of major depression (MTLE + D group). For comparison purposes, 14 human non-epileptic control hippocampi from necropsies were processed and analyzed in the same manner as the surgical cases. Underlying diseases causing death were cardiomyopathy, sepsis, acute lymphoblastic leukemia, gastric adenocarcinoma, pulmonary infarct, or renal-hepatic failure, and patients had no history of hypoxic episodes during agony, seizures, or neurological diseases. Furthermore, there was no evidence of brain pathological abnormalities on clinical postmortem examination of the mesial temporal structures. MTLE and control specimens were collected between 1998 and 2008. A summary of clinical characteristics of all groups is depicted in Table 1.

## Clinical features of MTLE patients

All patients were referred for pre-surgical assessment due to drug-resistant seizures as defined in the literature [23]. Patients were evaluated at the Ribeirao Preto Epilepsy Surgery Program using standardized protocols approved by the institution's Ethics Committee and a written consent form was obtained from each patient. Pre-surgical investigation at the Epilepsy Monitoring Unit included detailed clinical history, neurological examination, interictal and ictal scalp/sphenoidal electroencephalography (EEG), neuropsychology evaluation, and intracarotid amobarbital procedure (Wada test) for memory and language lateralization whenever deemed clinically necessary.

Definition of MTLE followed Engel's criteria [24]: (I) seizure semiology consistent with MTLE, usually with epigastric/autonomic/psychic auras, followed by complex partial seizures; (II) pre-surgical investigation confirming the seizure onset zone in the temporal lobe; (III) anterior and mesial temporal interictal spikes on EEG; (IV) no lesions other than uni- or bilateral hippocampal atrophy on high-resolution magnetic resonance imaging scans (reduced hippocampal dimensions and increased T2 signal); (V) clinical histopathological examination compatible with HS; and (VI) no evidence of dual pathology identifiable by any of the assessment methods described (clinical, electrophysiology, neuroimaging, and histopathology). Exclusion criteria were as follows: (I) focal neurological abnormalities on physical examination, (II) generalized or extra-temporal EEG spikes, and (III) marked cognitive impairment indicating dysfunction

**Table 1 Demographic and clinical data**

| | MTLE$_W$ | MTLE + D | MTLE + P | Controls | Statistics |
|---|---|---|---|---|---|
| Male (n) | 10 | 5 | 8 | 11 | No difference |
| Female (n) | 7 | 10 | 3 | 3 | |
| IPI present (n) | 7 | 10 | 8 | n.a. | No difference |
| IPI absent (n) | 10 | 5 | 3 | n.a. | |
| Age of first seizure (years) | 3.8 ± 3.3 | 6.3 ± 7.5 | 7.4 ± 8.5 | n.a. | No difference |
| Age when seizures became recurrent or age of onset (years) | 10.0 ± 5.4 | 12.0 ± 9.7 | 13.5 ± 7.7 | n.a. | No difference |
| Seizure type: CPS (n) | 7 | 9 | 5 | n.a. | No difference |
| Seizure type: SGS (n) | 10 | 6 | 6 | n.a. | |
| Seizure frequency (monthly) | 14.3 ± 11.4 | 12.6 ± 8.9 | 16.4 ± 11.2 | n.a. | No difference |
| Right HS (n) | 12 | 9 | 5 | n.a. | No difference |
| Left HS (n) | 5 | 4 | 5 | n.a. | |
| Bilateral HS (n) | 0 | 2 | 1 | n.a. | |
| Right handedness (n) | 14 | 14 | 11 | n.a. | No difference |
| Left handedness (n) | 2 | 0 | 0 | n.a. | |
| Bilateral handedness (n) | 1 | 1 | 0 | n.a. | |
| Memory in verbal tasks: average or above (n) | 7 | 7 | 2 | n.a. | No difference |
| Memory in verbal tasks: below average (n) | 10 | 8 | 9 | n.a. | |
| Memory in non-verbal tasks: average or above (n) | 11 | 9 | 3 | n.a. | No difference |
| Memory in non-verbal tasks: below average (n) | 6 | 6 | 8 | n.a. | |
| Full-scale IQ | 85.9 ± 7.7 | 84.9 ± 9.3 | 83.4 ± 7.1 | n.a. | No difference |
| Years at school | 7.1 ± 3.5 | 5.5 ± 3.5 | 6.3 ± 4.1 | n.a. | No difference |
| Age at surgery (or at death for controls) (years) | 33.5 ± 8.0 | 37.6 ± 11.7 | 40.0 ± 5.9 | 42.6 ± 16.0 | No difference |
| Duration of epilepsy (years) | 23.9 ± 8.2 | 24.9 ± 13.6 | 26.4 ± 8.6 | n.a. | No difference |
| Collected side: right (n) | 12 | 11 | 6 | 6 | No difference |
| Collected side: left (n) | 5 | 4 | 5 | 8 | |
| Surgical outcome: complete remission (n) | 15 | 10 | 9 | n.a. | No difference |
| Surgical outcome: only auras and/or fewer seizures (n) | 2 | 5 | 2 | n.a. | |

Values indicated as mean ± standard deviation when applicable. CPS: Complex partial seizure; HS: Hippocampal sclerosis; IPI: Initial precipitant injury; MTLE: mesial temporal lobe epilepsy; MTLE + D: MTLE + major depression; MTLE + P: MTLE + interictal psychosis; MTLE$_W$: MTLE subjects without psychiatric history; n.a.: Not applicable; SGS: Secondarily generalized seizures.

beyond the temporal regions (intelligence quotient (IQ) < 69).

Information regarding antecedent of an initial precipitant injury, febrile seizures, seizure types, drug regimen, and estimated monthly seizure frequency (within the 2 years prior to surgery) were retrospectively collected from medical records for each patient. Psychiatric evaluations were conducted in all MTLE patients. Each diagnosis of major depression was independently established during the presurgical evaluation by two psychiatrists with experience in psychiatric disorders associated with epilepsy, using the guidelines of the Diagnostic and Statistical Manual of Mental Disorders, 4th edition. Once a consensus on the classification of psychotic syndromes associated with epilepsy was lacking at the time of collection, and neither DSM-IV nor ICD-10 has addressed this issue specifically (for a review, please see

[20]), the diagnosis of psychosis associated with MTLE was established according to Sachdev [25], meaning that patients with interictal psychosis did not experience the following: psychotic disorder temporally associated with seizures, changes in antiepileptic medications, epileptic status, delirium, and psychosis for paradoxical normalization (for review, please see [26]). This group was defined by a prolonged psychotic state that was not related to the epileptic seizures. Typically, the psychotic states closely resemble schizophrenia, with paranoid ideas which might become systematized, ideas of influence, and auditory hallucinations often of a menacing quality. The points of difference are as follows: common religious coloring of the paranoid ideas, tendency of the affect to remain warm and appropriate, and no typical deterioration to the hebephrenic state [27]. Patients had no history of previous psychiatric disorders (prior to seizure onset) or of substance dependence at any time.

Global IQ was calculated after neuropsychological tests (complete Wechsler Adult Intelligence Scale, version III (WAIS-III) or WAIS-R protocol).

## Tissue collection and immunohistochemical processing

Specimens were segmented into 1-cm blocks transversely oriented to the hippocampal long axis. Blocks were placed in buffered paraformaldehyde (Sigma, St Louis, MO, USA). After 48 to 96 h, specimens were paraffin embedded for immunohistochemistry.

Immunohistochemistry was performed with antibodies that identified immunoreactivity for reactive astrocytes (GFAP, 1:500 dilution; Dako, Glostrup, Denmark), activated microglia (human leukocyte antigen, MHC class II (HLA-DR), 1:100 dilution; Dako, Glostrup, Denmark), astroglial metallothionein I/II (MT-I/II, 1:500 dilution, Dako, Glostrup, Denmark), and perivascular aquaporin 4 (AQP4, 1:200 dilution; Santa Cruz Biotechnology, Santa Cruz, CA, USA). Antibodies specificity was verified, and immunohistochemistry was performed as described in Peixoto-Santos et al. [4]. Briefly, paraffin-embedded MTLE and control hippocampi were processed together for each antibody, with overnight incubation at room temperature, and developed simultaneously in 0.05% 3,3′-diaminobenzidine tetrahydrochloride (Pierce, Rockford, USA) and 0.01% hydrogen peroxide (Merck, Darmstadt, Germany). After sufficient colorization, reaction was halted by washing in several rinses of distilled water, dehydrated through graded ethanol to xylene (Merck, Darmstadt, Germany), and cover slipped with Krystalon (EM Science, Gibbstown, NJ, USA). Adjacent sections were hematoxilin-eosin stained (Laborclin, Pinhais, Brazil) and examined for tissue integrity. Control sections without the primary antisera did not reveal staining (data not shown).

## Semi-quantitative analysis of immunohistochemistry

MTLE and control hippocampi were compared for immunoreactivity in several hippocampal formation subfields using Lorente de No's classification [28], which included fascia dentata granular cells and hilar neurons, as well as pyramidal cells in the *cornus ammonis* region 4 (CA4), *cornus ammonis* region 3 (CA3), *cornus ammonis* region 2 (CA2), *cornus ammonis* region 1 (CA1), prosubiculum, subiculum, parasubiculum, and entorhinal cortex layer III. Immunoreactivity were estimated in 8-μm Neu-N stained slices at × 200 magnification as previously described and well established in the literature for surgical hippocampal fragments [1,3,4,29,30].

Images of each hippocampal formation subfield from all specimens were collected and digitized with a high-resolution CCD monochrome camera attached to an Olympus microscope. Uniform luminance was maintained and checked every ten measurements using an optical density standard and a gray value scale ranging

from 0 (white) to 255 (black). In brief, all digitized images were analyzed with Image J software, following the same criteria: (I) the software identifies the gray value distribution of a subfield's digital image; (II) the immunoreactive area is selected (that is, positive stained pixels), limited to a threshold range; and (III) the threshold range is pre-settled based on control group sections, to exclude the low-intensity gray value of background staining from the analysis. For GFAP, the threshold selected allowed the quantification of positive staining present in the soma, branches, and also of the fine and characteristic astroglial meshwork. For HLA-DR, the threshold selected allowed the quantification of proteins present in the soma and branches of the immunostained cells, whereas the MT-I/II threshold allowed the quantifications of proteins in the soma and proximal branches of astrocytes. As for AQP4, we selected a higher threshold, in order to quantify only AQP4 present in the endfeets of astrocytes (that is, perivascular AQP4). A similar approach was used by our group elsewhere [3,4]. Analyses were conducted blind to hippocampal pathology and group classification.

## Data analysis

Data were analyzed using the statistical program PASW (version 18.0) and SigmaPlot (version 11.0). Groups were compared using analysis of variance (ANOVA one way, with Bonferroni *post hoc* test) or unpaired *t* test for variables with normal distribution and Kruskal-Wallis One Way Analysis of Variance on Ranks (with Dunn *post hoc* test) or Mann-Whitney Rank Sum Test for variables without normal distribution. The Fisher Exact test was applied for comparison of relative frequencies of clinical variables between groups. Statistical significance was set at $P < 0.05$ and values presented as mean ± standard deviation (SD).

## Results
### Clinical profiles

The four patient groups did not show significant differences in gender, age, or collected side (Table 1). Clinical variables such as presence of an initial precipitant injury, age of first seizure and seizure onset, seizure frequency, type and outcome, epilepsy duration, HS side, handedness, IQ, years at school, and performance in neuropsychological tests were homogeneously distributed among MTLE groups.

All epileptic patients were on antiepileptic drugs (carbamazepine, oxcarbazepine, phenobarbital, and/or phenytoin). In addition, patients were also taking benzodiazepines (MTLE$_W$ group: 11 of 17; MTLE + D group: 10 of 15; MTLE + P group: 8 of 11), fluoxetine (MTLE + D group: 5 of 15), and haloperidol (MTLE + P group: 6 of 11). No differences in neuropsychological tests between patients taking or not taking benzodiazepines, fluoxetine, or haloperidol were seen. No significant influence of fluoxetine or haloperidol was seen on hippocampal GFAP, HLA-DR, or AQP4 expression. Haloperidol influence on MT-I/II expression will be described below.

## Reactive astrocytes

Immunohistochemistry for GFAP, a marker of reactive astrocytes, showed a higher number of immunopositive cells and astrocytic processes in MTLE patients (Figure 1A, B,C), compared to staining in the controls (Figure 1D). Evaluation of the immunopositive area fraction (Figure 2A) revealed a higher GFAP area in all MTLE groups in the outer molecular layer, inner molecular layer, granule cell layer, hilus, CA4, CA3, CA1, prosubiculum, subiculum, and parasubiculum ($P \leq 0.024$) when compared to controls.

MTLE$_W$ and MTLE + P had also increased immunopositive area in the inner molecular layer, granule cell layer, and CA2 ($P \leq 0.049$) compared to MTLE + D. In CA1, MTLE$_W$ had a higher immunopositive area than MTLE + D ($P < 0.001$). In the outer molecular layer, MTLE + P had a higher GFAP immunopositive area than MTLE + D ($P = 0.013$). In the entorhinal cortex, only the groups with psychiatric comorbidities (that is, MTLE + D and MTLE + P) had increased GFAP immunopositive area when compared to controls ($P \leq 0.032$).

## Activated microglia

Activated microglia, evaluated with antibody against HLA-DR, was observed in MTLE patients as small, highly branched cells, well defined and spaced from each other (Figure 1E,F,G). In control specimens, activated

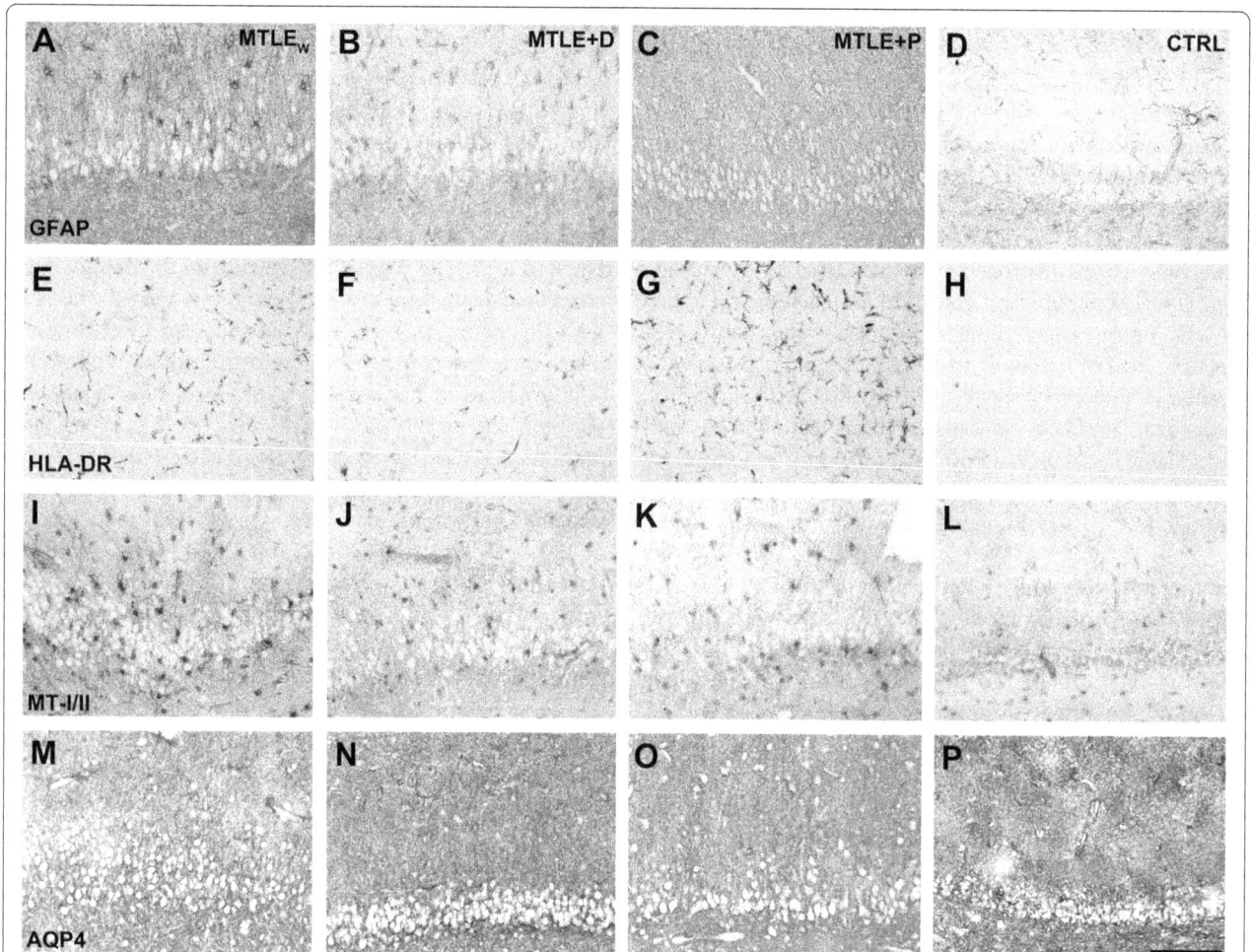

**Figure 1** Representative images of *fascia dentata* immunostained for GFAP (A, B, C, D), HLA-DR (E, F, G, H), MT-I/II (I, J, K, L), and AQP4 (M, N, O, P) from patients with MTLE$_W$ (A, E, I, M), MTLE + D (B, F, J, N), MTLE + P (C, G, K, O) and autopsy controls (D, H, L, P). Observe the increased astroglial reaction (A, B, C), microglial activation (E, F, G), MT-I/II immunopositive astrocytes (I, J, K), and reduced perivascular aquaporin 4 (M, N, O) in MTLE groups (MTLE$_W$, MTLE + D, and MTLE + P), when compared to the respective staining pattern of the CTRL group (D, H, L, P). Bar in (P) indicates 150 μm. AQP4 = aquaporin 4; CTRL = control; GFAP = glial fibrillary acidic protein; HLA-DR = human leukocyte antigen, MHC class II; MT-I/II = metallothionein-I/II; MTLE = mesial temporal lobe epilepsy; MTLE + D = MTLE + major depression; MTLE + P = MTLE + interictal psychosis; MTLE$_W$ = MTLE subjects without psychiatric history.

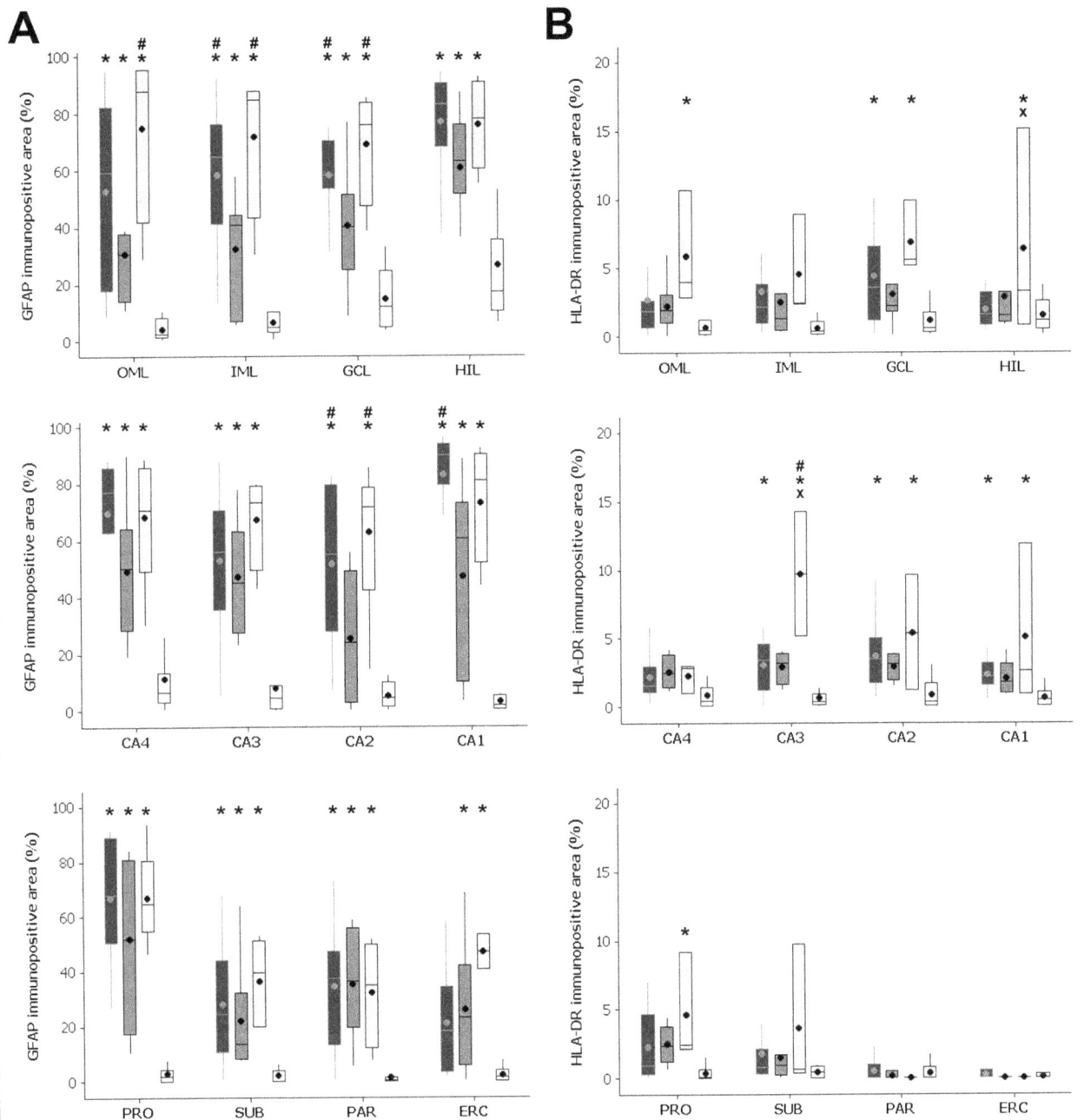

**Figure 2** Immunopositive area fraction of GFAP (A) and HLA-DR (B) in the hippocampal subfields of MTLE_W (black boxplots), MTLE + D (dark gray boxplots), MTLE + P (light gray boxplots), and CTRL group (white boxplots). **(A)** All MTLE groups showed higher GFAP immunopositive area in OML, IML, GCL, HIL, CA4, CA3, CA1, PRO, SUB, and PAR (compared to CTRL). MTLE_W and MTLE + P had increased GFAP area in IML, GCL, and CA2 (compared to MTLE + D). MTLE + D and MTLE + P had increased GFAP area in the ERC (compared to CTRL). MTLE_W had increased GFAP immunopositive area in CA1, and MTLE + P had higher GFAP immunopositive area in the OML (compared to MTLE + D). **(B)** MTLE + P had increased immunopositive HLA-DR area in CA3 (when compared to all other groups), in the HIL (compared to MTLE and CTRL), and OML, GCL, CA2, CA1, and PRO (compared to CTRL). MTLE patients had increased HLA-DR immunopositive area in GCL, CA3, and CA2 (compared to CTRL). CA1 = cornus ammonis region 1; CA2 = cornus ammonis region 2; CA3 = cornus ammonis region 3; CA4 = cornus ammonis region 4; CTRL = control; ERC = entorhinal cortex; GCL = granule cell layer; GFAP = glial fibrillary acidic protein; HLA-DR = human leukocyte antigen, MHC class II; HIL = hilus; IML = inner molecular layer; MTLE = mesial temporal lobe epilepsy; MTLE + D = MTLE + major depression; MTLE + P = MTLE + interictal psychosis; MTLE_W = MTLE subjects without psychiatric history; OML = outer molecular layer; PAR = parasubiculum; PRO = prosubiculum; SUB = subiculum. *Indicates difference from CTRL; #indicates difference from MTLE + D; and ×indicates difference from MTLE_W.

microglia were rarely seen and, when present, were in much smaller number than in MTLE cases (Figure 1H). Quantitative evaluation of activated microglia (Figure 2B) revealed increased immunopositivity in the outer molecular layer, granule cell layer, hilus, CA3, CA2, CA1, and prosubiculum of MTLE + P when compared to the control ($P \leq 0.047$). Patients of the MTLE + P group had also a higher immunopositive area in the hilus when compared to MTLE$_W$ ($P = 0.04$), and in CA3 when compared to MTLE$_W$ and MTLE + D ($P \leq 0.002$). MTLE patients had an increased HLA-DR immunopositive area in the granule cell layer, CA3, CA2, and CA1 when compared to the control ($P \leq 0.038$).

### Metallothioneins I/II

The immunopositive staining for MT-I/II was observed in cells with astroglial morphology (see Figure 1I,J,K,L). Although only patients from the MTLE$_W$ group had significant increase in MT-I/II immunopositive cells, qualitatively, all MTLE groups present a higher number of MT-I/II positivity in comparison to the control group (compare the micrography L with the micrographies I to K in Figure 1). Higher immunopositive staining (Figure 3A) was observed in the inner molecular layer, CA2, CA1, parasubiculum, and entorhinal cortex of MTLE$_W$ when compared to the control group ($P \leq 0.015$). Compared to MTLE + P, higher immunopositive area was observed in the granule cell layer, the CA1, and the parasubiculum of MTLE$_W$ cases ($P \leq 0.019$). In the parasubiculum, the group MTLE$_W$ had a higher area fraction than the group MTLE + D ($P < 0.001$).

MT-I/II expression was increased in the inner molecular layer of the MTLE + P patients taking haloperidol when compared to those not taking it (with haloperidol, mean area fraction = $7.5 \pm 3.5$; without haloperidol, mean area fraction = $1.7 \pm 2.2$; $t$ (9) = 2.885; $P = 0.02$). Also, we found a trend of increased CA2 MT-I/II expression in patients who achieved complete seizure remission after surgery (remission, mean area fraction = $20.3 \pm 24.6$; no-remission, mean area fraction = $9.1 \pm 6.2$; $t$ (38) = $-1.946$; $P = 0.06$).

### Aquaporin 4

AQP4 immunohistochemistry revealed a reduction in the perivascular staining intensity in MTLE specimens, when compared to controls (compare micrography P with micrographies M to O in Figure 1). Compared to the control, all MTLE groups had decreased perivascular AQP4 area fraction in the hilus ($P \leq 0.015$), whereas in CA4, only MTLE + P showed significant decrease ($P = 0.026$), and in the subiculum, MTLE$_W$ and MTLE + P had reduced immunopositive area ($P \leq 0.015$). A direct correlation was seen between IQ and AQP4 expression in the CA1 ($R = 0.530$; $P = 0.006$) and in the prosubiculum

($R = 0.529$; $P = 0.008$) of MTLE patients. Also, we found a trend to increased AQP4 expression in the CA2 of those patients who achieved complete seizure remission after surgery (remission, mean area fraction = $9.9 \pm 9.0$; no-remission, mean area fraction = $5.3 \pm 2.9$; $t$ (38) = $-1.930$; $P = 0.07$).

### Discussion

In the present study, we investigated the expression of glial proteins GFAP, HLA-DR, MT-I/II, and perivascular AQP4 in the hippocampal formation of MTLE with and without psychiatric comorbidities and in non-epileptic controls. Comparing the MTLE groups, we found in specific hippocampal subfields an increased immunoreactive area of GFAP and HLA-DR and decreased MT-I/II and AQP4 in specimens from the MTLE patients with psychosis; while in specimens from patients with MTLE and major depression, GFAP and MT-I/II were decreased. Differences between MTLE and controls, in astrogliosis, microgliosis, increased MT-I/II, and decreased perivascular AQP4 in the epileptogenic hippocampus, were similar to what is currently described in the literature [4,31]. Given that differences between epileptogenic and control hippocampi are already well established in the literature, our discussion will focus mainly on psychiatric subgroups and their differences when compared to MTLE without psychiatric comorbidities, unless otherwise specified.

Studies in humans and animal models of epilepsy have shown upregulation of several inflammatory molecules [32,33]. However, only a few experimental studies have focused on inflammatory changes in correlates of major depression comorbid with epilepsy. For example, rats injected with pilocarpine exhibit behavioral equivalents of anhedonia and despair and alterations in inflammatory molecules as found in human major depression [34,35]. No information regarding neuroinflammatory mechanisms in psychosis of epilepsy is available to date.

Astrogliosis and microgliosis are part of a common response to injury. Although the reactive astrocyte expression profile may depend on the type of inducing injury, increased inflammatory-related molecules are always found in reactive astrocytes [36]. Interleukins 1b (IL-1beta) and 6 (IL-6) are among the molecules released after injury that can lead to glial reaction [37]. In fact, the crosstalk between activated microglia and reactive astrocytes seems crucial to the maintenance of chronic gliosis [38]. Increased astrocytic GFAP expression, a marker of reactive astrogliosis, is a common finding in the hippocampus of MTLE patients [3,4]. Likewise, we detected an increased GFAP immunoreactive area in all hippocampal subfields of MTLE patients. In patients with MTLE + D, GFAP expression levels were intermediary between the controls and MTLE$_W$ or MTLE + P.

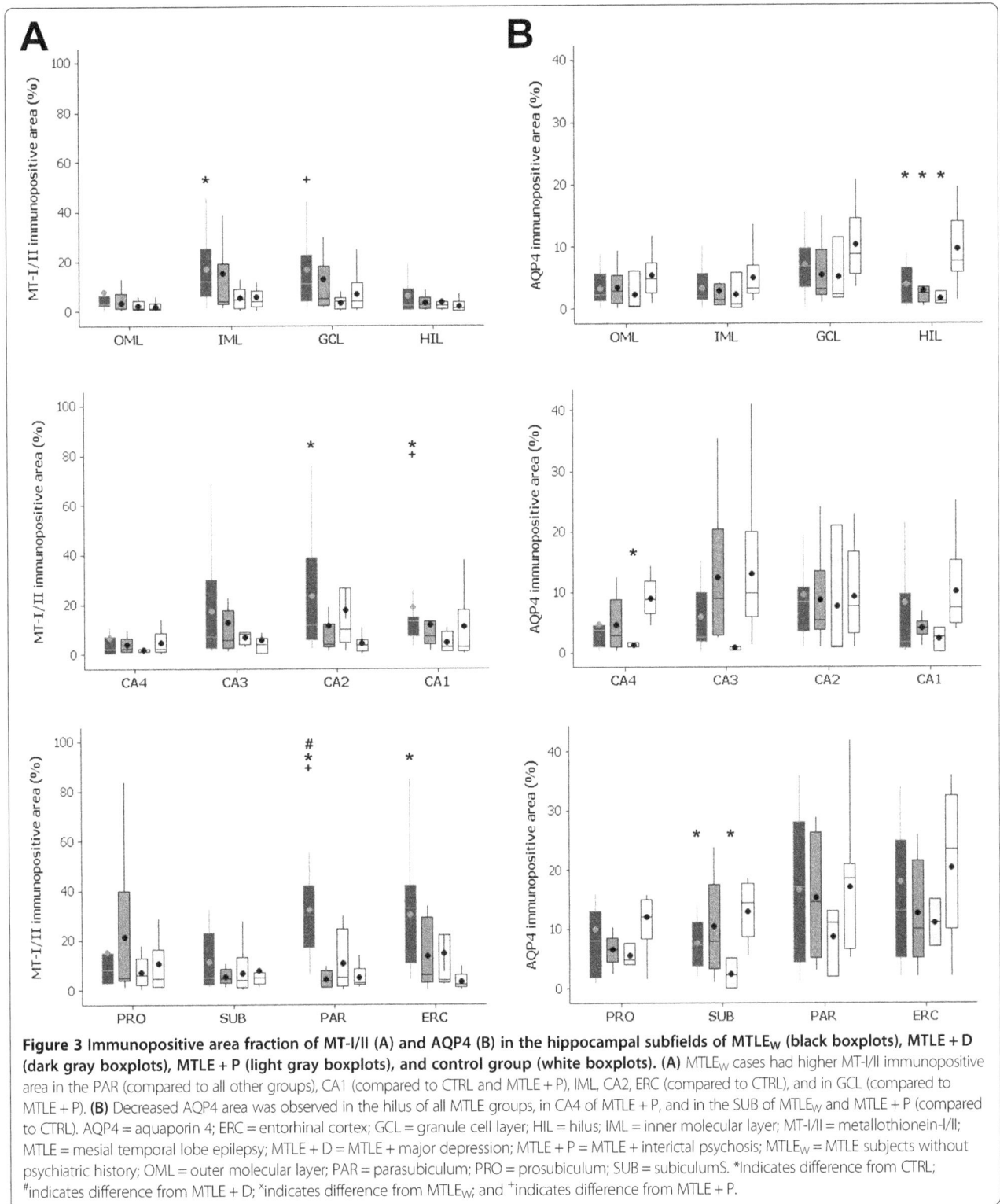

**Figure 3** Immunopositive area fraction of MT-I/II (A) and AQP4 (B) in the hippocampal subfields of MTLE$_W$ (black boxplots), MTLE + D (dark gray boxplots), MTLE + P (light gray boxplots), and control group (white boxplots). (A) MTLE$_W$ cases had higher MT-I/II immunopositive area in the PAR (compared to all other groups), CA1 (compared to CTRL and MTLE + P), IML, CA2, ERC (compared to CTRL), and in GCL (compared to MTLE + P). (B) Decreased AQP4 area was observed in the hilus of all MTLE groups, in CA4 of MTLE + P, and in the SUB of MTLE$_W$ and MTLE + P (compared to CTRL). AQP4 = aquaporin 4; ERC = entorhinal cortex; GCL = granule cell layer; HIL = hilus; IML = inner molecular layer; MT-I/II = metallothionein-I/II; MTLE = mesial temporal lobe epilepsy; MTLE + D = MTLE + major depression; MTLE + P = MTLE + interictal psychosis; MTLE$_W$ = MTLE subjects without psychiatric history; OML = outer molecular layer; PAR = parasubiculum; PRO = prosubiculum; SUB = subiculumS. *Indicates difference from CTRL; #indicates difference from MTLE + D; ×indicates difference from MTLE$_W$; and +indicates difference from MTLE + P.

Since studies have shown that patients with major depression have reduced GFAP expression [18,39], it is possible that the mechanisms underlying the decreased GFAP expression observed in major depression counterbalance the increase found in epilepsy, resulting in the intermediary values observed in our MTLE + D cases. In schizophrenia, a study showed that increased GFAP expression in the prefrontal cortex of patients with schizophrenia is increased [16], but other cortical areas and the hippocampus have shown inconclusive results [17,40,41]. In MTLE patients with interictal psychosis, we found increased GFAP expression, especially when compared to the MTLE + D cases, in agreement with a recent hypothesis that astrocyte pathology may be associated with psychotic symptoms, although the exact nature of this change remains unclear [16]. In particular, increased GFAP in schizophrenia/psychotic symptoms could be closely related to increased neuroinflammatory markers [42], as well as to increased IL-1beta and IL-6 serum levels [43]. A recent study comparing MTLE hippocampi from patients with and without *de novo* psychosis (postoperative psychosis) analyzed GFAP expression and found no qualitative differences between groups [44]. In our present series, quantitative differences in GFAP between MTLE$_W$ and MTLE + P were also subtle, and major differences were seen in respect to the MTLE + D group.

Increased cortical and hippocampal HLA-DR+ microglia has been described in schizophrenia [17,45], in accordance to our findings in several hippocampal subfields of MTLE patients with interictal psychosis. Of note, increased hippocampal HLA-DR was particularly associated with paranoid schizophrenia [45], a core symptom especially represented in interictal psychosis [20]. HLA-DR levels in MTLE specimens from patients without psychiatric comorbidities and in those with major depression were similar and higher than in the controls, although statistically significant differences were detected only in the granule cell layer and CA3-1 of MTLE$_W$ versus control. Microglia is an important source of inflammatory molecules [32], and a high expression of pro-inflammatory cytokines is observed in major depression [46]. Similar apparent microglial activation in MTLE$_W$ and MTLE + D could partially explain why patients with epilepsy frequently develop mood disorders, an association still incompletely understood [47]. However, the levels of microglial-related inflammatory molecules such as cytokines remain to be evaluated in human epilepsy with and without major depression.

Metallothioneins are regulators of free zinc levels, an important modulator of glutamatergic neurotransmission [12]. Besides metals, oxidative stress agents and inflammatory molecules can induce MT-I/II expression [12]. Knockout mice for IL-6 have low microglial activation and low expression of MT-I/II, indicating a crucial role of inflammation in MT-I/II expression [48]. In fact, mice overexpressing MT-I/II show reduced microgliosis and reduced levels of interleukins following kainic acid *status epilepticus* [49]. In psychiatric diseases, MT-I/II gene expression in the prefrontal cortex has been found increased in schizophrenia [15] and decreased in major depression [19]. No reports are available regarding the hippocampus, but in our series, we found decreased values in cases with psychosis and in those with major depression when compared to MTLE without psychiatric

comorbidities in several hippocampal subfields. Interestingly, we have found in other series of patients decreased mossy fiber sprouting in MTLE + P and increased in MTLE + D [8,9]. Since mossy fibers are zinc enriched and MT-I/II chelates zinc, cadmium, and copper, it would be expected that hippocampi from MTLE + D have a deficient metal homeostasis and likely zinc excess in neurons and glial cells and in the neuropile. A possible mechanism would be through zinc overflow from serum to brain [50] due to an inefficient blood-brain barrier in major depression [51]. In fact, low-serum zinc is a hallmark of major depressive disorders [52]. Our results of decreased hippocampal MT-I/II in MTLE associated to psychosis can be related to decreased hippocampal zinc levels/mossy fibers in interictal psychosis [8,9], as well as in schizophrenia [53,54]. Interestingly, MTLE + P patients taking haloperidol showed increased expression of MT-I/II in the inner molecular layer. In the amphetamine animal model of schizophrenia, zinc administration is able to revert behavioral equivalents of positive symptoms [55], but it is unknown if systemic zinc administration alters hippocampal zinc and/or MT-I/II expression. In fact, zinc is a ligand of the haloperidol-sensitive sigma 2 receptor in the mossy fiber of rats [56], suggesting that an increased MT-I/II expression in the mossy fiber of MTLE + P patients would facilitate zinc chelation and proper haloperidol binding. We also found a trend to increased MT-I/II in the CA2 of patients who achieved complete seizure remission after surgery, in agreement to the MT-I/II role in the control of excitability [57]. Likewise, other recent evidences indicate that hippocampal expression of proteins used as markers of full-blown epileptogenesis might be able to predict seizure outcome [58,59].

AQP4 is the main water channel in the central nervous system and presents with multifaceted functions. In inflammatory conditions, microglia can release IL-1beta, which in turn induces AQP4 expression in astrocytes [60]. AQP4 is able to regulate brain response to insults or injury, and also to influence synaptic plasticity and behavior [61]. In the AQP4 knockout mouse, memory is impaired [62]. In accordance, our results showed a direct correlation between perivascular AQP4 expression in the Sommer sector and IQ scores. AQP4 participation in synaptic plasticity and cognition occurs together with neurotrophin (NT) receptors [62]. Of note, NTs and NT receptors are differentially regulated in MTLE with psychiatric comorbidities [9,58], which could further change how AQP4 modulates plasticity. For instance, the brain-derived neurotrophic factor (BDNF) is increased in MTLE$_W$ but decreased in MTLE + P [9]. In addition, tyrosine kinase receptor type 2 (TrkB) (a BDNF receptor) is increased in MTLE + P but not in MTLE$_W$ [58]. Given that low levels of AQP4 associated with increased BDNF and TrkB or p75 neurotrophin receptor (p75NTR) may result in increased excitability, AQP4 levels near to control levels could be more efficient in controlling excessive excitatory activation trough a BDNF-TrkB or p75NTR loop [62,63]. In fact, we found a trend to increased AQP4 in cases with complete seizure remission, thus reinforcing the role of AQP4 in neuron activity. In addition, AQP4 has an important role in K$^+$ homeostasis [13,64], and AQP4 knockout mice have higher seizure threshold but longer seizure duration [13].

## Conclusion

In summary, we described hippocampal neuroinflammatory-related molecules that show a distinct pattern of expression when MTLE patients present with a comorbid psychiatric diagnosis of interictal psychosis or major depression. Studies have reported successful treatment of patients with seizures, schizophrenia, and major depression using drugs with anti-inflammatory effect as an add-on therapy [65-68]. Given the differential expression of neuroinflammatory-related molecules in MTLE with psychiatric comorbidities, these patients could also benefit from a more targeted treatment. Further research is needed to expand and validate these findings and to better investigate possible causal mechanisms.

### Abbreviations
AQP4: aquaporin 4; BDNF: brain-derived neurotrophic factor; CA1: *cornus ammonis* region 1; CA2: *cornus ammonis* region 2; CA3: *cornus ammonis* region 3; CA4: *cornus ammonis* region 4; EEG: electroencephalogram; GFAP: glial fibrillary acidic protein; HLA-DR: human leukocyte antigen, MHC class II; HS: hippocampal sclerosis; IQ: intelligence quotient; MT-I/II: metallothionein I and II; MTLE: mesial temporal lobe epilepsy; MTLE + D: MTLE + major depression; MTLE + P: MTLE + interictal psychosis; NT: neurotrophin; p75NTR: p75 neurotrophin receptor; SD: standard deviation; TrkB: tyrosine kinase receptor, type 2; WAIS-III: Wechsler Adult Intelligence Scale, version III.

### Competing interests
The authors declare that they have no competing interests.

### Authors' contributions
Conception and design of research (LK); performed research (LK, JEPS, MRM, RCS); analyzed data (JEPS); contributed with reagents/analytic tools and/or important intellectual input (JAA, CGC, JEH); wrote the manuscript (LK, JEPS, JPL). All authors read and approved the final manuscript.

### Acknowledgements
This work was supported by Fundacao de Apoio a Pesquisa do Estado de Sao Paulo - Fapesp (CInAPCe Project 05/56447-7, to JPL; *PhD fellowship* 2010/51515-2, to JEPS; *PhD fellowship* 2011/23691-3, to MRM), Conselho Nacional de Desenvolvimento Cientifico e Tecnologico - CNPq, and Coordenacao de Aperfeicoamento de Pessoal de Nivel Superior - CAPES (*postdoc fellowship* A034-2013, to LK).

### Disclosures
The funders had no role in study design, data collection and analysis, decision to publish, or preparation of the manuscript.

### Author details
[1]Department of Neurosciences and Behavior, Ribeirao Preto Medical School, University of Sao Paulo (USP), Av Bandeirantes 3900, CEP 14049-900 Ribeirao Preto, SP, Brazil. [2]Center for Interdisciplinary Research on Applied Neurosciences (NAPNA), USP, Ribeirao Preto, Brazil. Department of Surgery, Ribeirao Preto Medical School, USP, Ribeirao Preto, Brazil. [4]National Institute of Science and Technology in Translational Medicine (INCT-TM - CNPq), Ribeirao Preto, Brazil.

### References
1. Mathern GW, Babb TL, Pretorius JK, Leite JP. Reactive synaptogenesis and neuron densities for neuropeptide Y, somatostatin, and glutamate decarboxylase immunoreactivity in the epileptogenic human fascia dentata. J Neurosci. 1995;15:3990–4004.
2. Babb TL, Kupfer WR, Pretorius JK, Crandall PH, Levesque MF. Synaptic reorganization by mossy fibers in human epileptic fascia dentata. Neuroscience. 1991;42:351–63.
3. Kandratavicius L, Rosa-Neto P, Monteiro MR, Guiot MC, Assirati Jr JA, Carlotti Jr CG, et al. Distinct increased metabotropic glutamate receptor type 5 (mGluR5) in temporal lobe epilepsy with and without hippocampal sclerosis. Hippocampus. 2013;23:1212–30.
4. Peixoto-Santos JE, Galvis-Alonso OY, Velasco TR, Kandratavicius L, Assirati JA, Carlotti CG, et al. Increased metallothionein I/II expression in patients with temporal lobe epilepsy. PLoS One. 2012;7:e44709.
5. Qin P, Xu H, Laursen TM, Vestergaard M, Mortensen PB. Risk for schizophrenia and schizophrenia-like psychosis among patients with epilepsy: population based cohort study. BMJ. 2005;331:23.
6. Kandratavicius L, Lopes-Aguiar C, Bueno-Junior LS, Romcy-Pereira RN, Hallak JE, Leite JP. Psychiatric comorbidities in temporal lobe epilepsy: possible relationships between psychotic disorders and involvement of limbic circuits. Rev Bras Psiquiatr. 2012;34:454–66.
7. Kandratavicius L, Ruggiero RN, Hallak JE, Garcia-Cairasco N, Leite JP. Pathophysiology of mood disorders in temporal lobe epilepsy. Rev Bras Psiquiatr. 2012;34 Suppl 2:S233–45.
8. Kandratavicius L, Hallak JE, Young LT, Assirati JA, Carlotti Jr CG, Leite JP. Differential aberrant sprouting in temporal lobe epilepsy with psychiatric co-morbidities. Psychiatry Res. 2012;195:144–50.
9. Kandratavicius L, Monteiro MR, Assirati Jr JA, Carlotti Jr CG, Hallak JE, Leite JP. Neurotrophins in mesial temporal lobe epilepsy with and without psychiatric comorbidities. J Neuropathol Exp Neurol. 2013;72:1029–42.
10. Kandratavicius L, Monteiro MR, Hallak JE, Carlotti Jr CG, Assirati Jr JA, Leite JP. Microtubule-associated proteins in mesial temporal lobe epilepsy with and without psychiatric comorbidities and their relation with granular cell layer dispersion. Biomed Res Int. 2013;2013:960126.
11. Najjar S, Pearlman DM, Alper K, Najjar A, Devinsky O. Neuroinflammation and psychiatric illness. J Neuroinflammation. 2013;10:43.
12. Ebadi M, Iversen PL, Hao R, Cerutis DR, Rojas P, Happe HK, et al. Expression and regulation of brain metallothionein. Neurochem Int. 1995;27:1–22.
13. Binder DK, Yao X, Zador Z, Sick TJ, Verkman AS, Manley GT. Increased seizure duration and slowed potassium kinetics in mice lacking aquaporin-4 water channels. Glia. 2006;53:631–6.
14. Jukkola P, Guerrero T, Gray V, Gu C. Astrocytes differentially respond to inflammatory autoimmune insults and imbalances of neural activity. Acta Neuropathol Commun. 2013;1:70–89.
15. Choi KH, Elashoff M, Higgs BW, Song J, Kim S, Sabunciyan S, et al. Putative psychosis genes in the prefrontal cortex: combined analysis of gene expression microarrays. BMC Psychiatry. 2008;8:87.
16. Feresten AH, Barakauskas V, Ypsilanti A, Barr AM, Beasley CL. Increased expression of glial fibrillary acidic protein in prefrontal cortex in psychotic illness. Schizophr Res. 2013;150:252–7.
17. Radewicz K, Garey LJ, Gentleman SM, Reynolds R. Increase in HLA-DR immunoreactive microglia in frontal and temporal cortex of chronic schizophrenics. J Neuropathol Exp Neurol. 2000;59:137–50.
18. Rajkowska G, Stockmeier CA. Astrocyte pathology in major depressive disorder: insights from human postmortem brain tissue. Curr Drug Targets. 2013;14:1225–36.
19. Shelton RC, Claiborne J, Sidoryk-Wegrzynowicz M, Reddy R, Aschner M, Lewis DA, et al. Altered expression of genes involved in inflammation and apoptosis in frontal cortex in major depression. Mol Psychiatry. 2011;16:751–62.
20. Kandratavicius L, Hallak JE, Leite JP. What are the similarities and differences between schizophrenia and schizophrenia-like psychosis of epilepsy? A neuropathological approach to the understanding of schizophrenia spectrum and epilepsy. Epilepsy Behav. 2014;38C:143–7.

21. Gittins R, Harrison PJ. Neuronal density, size and shape in the human anterior cingulate cortex: a comparison of Nissl and NeuN staining. Brain Res Bull. 2004;63:155–60.

22. Stan AD, Ghose S, Gao XM, Roberts RC, Lewis-Amezcua K, Hatanpaa KJ, et al. Human postmortem tissue: what quality markers matter? Brain Res. 2006;1123:1–11.

23. Berg AT. Identification of pharmacoresistant epilepsy. Neurol Clin. 2009;27:1003–13.

24. Engel Jr J. Surgery for seizures. N Engl J Med. 1996;334:647–52.

25. Sachdev P. Schizophrenia-like psychosis and epilepsy: the status of the association. Am J Psychiatry. 1998;155:325–36.

26. Elliott B, Joyce E, Shorvon S. Delusions, illusions and hallucinations in epilepsy: 2. Complex phenomena and psychosis. Epilepsy Res. 2009;85:172–86.

27. Beard AW, Slater E. The schizophrenic-like psychoses of epilepsy. Proc R Soc Med. 1962;55:311–6.

28. LorentedeNo R. Studies on the structure of the cerebral cortex II: continuation of study of the ammonic system. J Psychol Neurol. 1934;46:113–77.

29. Mathern GW, Mendoza D, Lozada A, Pretorius JK, Dehnes Y, Danbolt NC, et al. Hippocampal GABA and glutamate transporter immunoreactivity in patients with temporal lobe epilepsy. Neurology. 1999;52:453–72.

30. Mathern GW, Pretorius JK, Kornblum HI, Mendoza D, Lozada A, Leite JP, et al. Human hippocampal AMPA and NMDA mRNA levels in temporal lobe epilepsy patients. Brain. 1997;120(Pt 11):1937–59.

31. Eid T, Lee TS, Thomas MJ, Amiry-Moghaddam M, Bjornsen LP, Spencer DD, et al. Loss of perivascular aquaporin 4 may underlie deficient water and K+ homeostasis in the human epileptogenic hippocampus. Proc Natl Acad Sci U S A. 2005;102:1193–8.

32. Arisi GM. Nervous and immune systems signals and connections: cytokines in hippocampus physiology and pathology. Epilepsy Behav. 2014;38C:43–7.

33. Vezzani A, Ravizza T, Balosso S, Aronica E. Glia as a source of cytokines: implications for neuronal excitability and survival. Epilepsia. 2008;49 Suppl 2:24–32.

34. Pineda E, Shin D, Sankar R, Mazarati AM. Comorbidity between epilepsy and depression: experimental evidence for the involvement of serotonergic, glucocorticoid, and neuroinflammatory mechanisms. Epilepsia. 2010;51 Suppl 3:110–4.

35. Xie W, Cai L, Yu Y, Gao L, Xiao L, He Q, et al. Activation of brain indoleamine 2,3-dioxygenase contributes to epilepsy-associated depressive-like behavior in rats with chronic temporal lobe epilepsy. J Neuroinflammation. 2014;11:41.

36. Zamanian JL, Xu L, Foo LC, Nouri N, Zhou L, Giffard RG, et al. Genomic analysis of reactive astrogliosis. J Neurosci. 2012;32:6391–410.

37. Hostenbach S, Cambron M, D'Haeseleer M, Kooijman R, De Keyser J. Astrocyte loss and astrogliosis in neuroinflammatory disorders. Neurosci Lett. 2014;565:39–41.

38. Liu W, Tang Y, Feng J. Cross talk between activation of microglia and astrocytes in pathological conditions in the central nervous system. Life Sci. 2011;89:141–6.

39. Muller MB, Lucassen PJ, Yassouridis A, Hoogendijk WJ, Holsboer F, Swaab DF. Neither major depression nor glucocorticoid treatment affects the cellular integrity of the human hippocampus. Eur J Neurosci. 2001;14:1603–12.

40. Steffek AE, McCullumsmith RE, Haroutunian V, Meador-Woodruff JH. Cortical expression of glial fibrillary acidic protein and glutamine synthetase is decreased in schizophrenia. Schizophr Res. 2008;103:71–82.

41. Webster MJ, Knable MB, Johnston-Wilson N, Nagata K, Inagaki M, Yolken RH. Immunohistochemical localization of phosphorylated glial fibrillary acidic protein in the prefrontal cortex and hippocampus from patients with schizophrenia, bipolar disorder, and depression. Brain Behav Immun. 2001;15:388–400.

42. Catts VS, Wong J, Fillman SG, Fung SJ, Weickert CS. Increased expression of astrocyte markers in schizophrenia: association with neuroinflammation. Aust N Z J Psychiatry. 2014;48:722–34.

43. Song X, Fan X, Song X, Zhang J, Zhang W, Li X, et al. Elevated levels of adiponectin and other cytokines in drug naive, first episode schizophrenia patients with normal weight. Schizophr Res. 2013;150:269–73.

44. Thom M, Kensche M, Maynard J, Liu J, Reeves C, Goc J, et al. Interictal psychosis following temporal lobe surgery: dentate gyrus pathology. Psychol Med. 2014;44:3037–49.

45. Busse S, Busse M, Schiltz K, Bielau H, Gos T, Brisch R, et al. Different distribution patterns of lymphocytes and microglia in the hippocampus of patients with residual versus paranoid schizophrenia: further evidence for disease course-related immune alterations? Brain Behav Immun. 2012;26:1273–9.

46. Rosenblat JD, Cha DS, Mansur RB, McIntyre RS. Inflamed moods: a review of the interactions between inflammation and mood disorders. Prog Neuropsychopharmacol Biol Psychiatry. 2014;53C:23–34.

47. Kanner AM. Can neurobiological pathogenic mechanisms of depression facilitate the development of seizure disorders? Lancet Neurol. 2012;11:1093–102.

48. Penkowa M, Molinero A, Carrasco J, Hidalgo J. Interleukin-6 deficiency reduces the brain inflammatory response and increases oxidative stress and neurodegeneration after kainic acid-induced seizures. Neuroscience. 2001;102:805–18.

49. Penkowa M, Florit S, Giralt M, Quintana A, Molinero A, Carrasco J, et al. Metallothionein reduces central nervous system inflammation, neurodegeneration, and cell death following kainic acid-induced epileptic seizures. J Neurosci Res. 2005;79:522–34.

50. Takeda A. Movement of zinc and its functional significance in the brain. Brain Res Brain Res Rev. 2000;34:137–48.

51. Najjar S, Pearlman DM, Devinsky O, Najjar A, Zagzag D. Neurovascular unit dysfunction with blood–brain barrier hyperpermeability contributes to major depressive disorder: a review of clinical and experimental evidence. J Neuroinflammation. 2013;10:142.

52. Szewczyk B, Kubera M, Nowak G. The role of zinc in neurodegenerative inflammatory pathways in depression. Prog Neuropsychopharmacol Biol Psychiatry. 2011;35:693–701.

53. Goldsmith SK, Joyce JN. Alterations in hippocampal mossy fiber pathway in schizophrenia and Alzheimer's disease. Biol Psychiatry. 1995;37:122–6.

54. Kolomeets NS, Orlovskaya DD, Uranova NA. Decreased numerical density of CA3 hippocampal mossy fiber synapses in schizophrenia. Synapse. 2007;61:615–21.

55. Joshi M, Akhtar M, Najmi AK, Khuroo AH, Goswami D. Effect of zinc in animal models of anxiety, depression and psychosis. Hum Exp Toxicol. 2012;31:1237–43.

56. Connor MA, Chavkin C. Ionic zinc may function as an endogenous ligand for the haloperidol-sensitive sigma 2 receptor in rat brain. Mol Pharmacol. 1992;42:471–9.

57. Carrasco J, Penkowa M, Hadberg H, Molinero A, Hidalgo J. Enhanced seizures and hippocampal neurodegeneration following kainic acid-induced seizures in metallothionein-I + II-deficient mice. Eur J Neurosci. 2000;12:2311–22.

58. Kandratavicius L, Hallak JE, Carlotti CG, Assirati JA, Leite JP. Neurotrophin receptors expression in mesial temporal lobe epilepsy with and without psychiatric comorbidities and their relation with seizure type and surgical outcome. Acta Neuropathol Commun. 2014;2:81–98.

59. Kandratavicius L, Hallak JE, Carlotti CG, Assirati JA, Leite JP. Hippocampal expression of heat shock proteins in mesial temporal lobe epilepsy with psychiatric comorbidities and their relation to seizure outcome. Epilepsia. 2014;55:1834–43.

60. Ohnishi M, Monda A, Takemoto R, Fujimoto Y, Sugitani M, Iwamura T, et al. High-mobility group box 1 up-regulates aquaporin 4 expression via microglia-astrocyte interaction. Neurochem Int. 2014;75:32–8.

61. Scharfman HE, Binder DK. Aquaporin-4 water channels and synaptic plasticity in the hippocampus. Neurochem Int. 2013;63:702–11.

62. Skucas VA, Mathews IB, Yang J, Cheng Q, Treister A, Duffy AM, et al. Impairment of select forms of spatial memory and neurotrophin-dependent synaptic plasticity by deletion of glial aquaporin-4. J Neurosci. 2011;31:6392–7.

63. Zhang Z, Fan J, Ren Y, Zhou W, Yin G. The release of glutamate from cortical neurons regulated by BDNF via the TrkB/Src/PLC-gamma1 pathway. J Cell Biochem. 2013;114:144–51.

64. Amiry-Moghaddam M, Williamson A, Palomba M, Eid T, de Lanerolle NC, Nagelhus EA, et al. Delayed K+ clearance associated with aquaporin-4 mislocalization: phenotypic defects in brains of alpha-syntrophin-null mice. Proc Natl Acad Sci U S A. 2003;100:13615–20.

65. Krogias C, Hoepner R, Muller A, Schneider-Gold C, Schroder A, Gold R. Successful treatment of anti-Caspr2 syndrome by interleukin 6 receptor blockade through tocilizumab. JAMA Neurol. 2013;70:1056–9.

66. Chaudhry IB, Hallak J, Husain N, Minhas F, Stirling J, Richardson P, et al. Minocycline benefits negative symptoms in early schizophrenia: a randomised double-blind placebo-controlled clinical trial in patients on standard treatment. J Psychopharmacol. 2012;26:1185–93.
67. Muller N, Schwarz MJ, Dehning S, Douhe A, Cerovecki A, Goldstein-Muller B, et al. The cyclooxygenase-2 inhibitor celecoxib has therapeutic effects in major depression: results of a double-blind, randomized, placebo controlled, add-on pilot study to reboxetine. Mol Psychiatry. 2006;11:680–4.
68. Devinsky O, Vezzani A, Najjar S, De Lanerolle NC, Rogawski MA. Glia and epilepsy: excitability and inflammation. Trends Neurosci. 2013;36:174–84.

# 4

# Immune response in the eye following epileptic seizures

Matilda Ahl[1,2], Una Avdic[1,2], Cecilia Skoug[3], Idrish Ali[1,2], Deepti Chugh[1,2], Ulrica Englund Johansson[3] and Christine T Ekdahl[1,2]*

**Abstract**

**Background:** Epileptic seizures are associated with an immune response in the brain. However, it is not known whether it can extend to remote areas of the brain, such as the eyes. Hence, we investigated whether epileptic seizures induce inflammation in the retina.

**Methods:** Adult rats underwent electrically induced temporal status epilepticus, and the eyes were studied 6 h, 1, and 7 weeks later with biochemical and immunohistochemical analyses. An additional group of animals received CX3CR1 antibody intracerebroventricularly for 6 weeks after status epilepticus.

**Results:** Biochemical analyses and immunohistochemistry revealed no increased cell death and unaltered expression of several immune-related cytokines and chemokines as well as no microglial activation, 6 h post-status epilepticus compared to non-stimulated controls. At 1 week, again, retinal cytoarchitecture appeared normal and there was no cell death or micro- or macroglial reaction, apart from a small decrease in interleukin-10. However, at 7 weeks, even if the cytoarchitecture remained normal and no ongoing cell death was detected, the numbers of microglia were increased ipsi- and contralateral to the epileptic focus. The microglia remained within the synaptic layers but often in clusters and with more processes extending into the outer nuclear layer. Morphological analyses revealed a decrease in surveying and an increase in activated microglia. In addition, increased levels of the chemokine KC/GRO and cytokine interleukin-1β were found. Furthermore, macroglial activation was noted in the inner retina. No alterations in numbers of phagocytic cells, infiltrating macrophages, or vascular pericytes were observed. Post-synaptic density-95 cluster intensity was reduced in the outer nuclear layer, reflecting seizure-induced synaptic changes without disrupted cytoarchitecture in areas with increased microglial activation. The retinal gliosis was decreased by a CX3CR1 immune modulation known to reduce gliosis within epileptic foci, suggesting a common immunological reaction.

**Conclusions:** Our results are the first evidence that epileptic seizures induce an immune response in the retina. It has a potential to become a novel non-invasive tool for detecting brain inflammation through the eyes.

**Keywords:** Inflammation, Microglia, Astrocytes, Epilepsy, Retina, Brain

* Correspondence: Christine.Ekdahl_Clementson@med.lu.se
Matilda Ahl, Una Avdic, Ulrica Englund Johansson, and Christine T Ekdahl shared first and last authorship, respectively.
[1]Inflammation and Stem Cell Therapy Group, Division of Clinical Neurophysiology, Lund University, BMC A11, Sölvegatan 17, SE-221 84 Lund, Sweden
[2]Lund Epilepsy Center, Lund University, SE-221 85 Lund, Sweden
Full list of author information is available at the end of the article

# Background

Epilepsy is a neurological disorder characterized by spontaneous seizures, affecting almost 1 % of the population worldwide [1]. An epileptic seizure is an abrupt abnormal synchronized activity affecting the entire—or parts, of the brain. When a seizure engages the entire brain, called a generalized seizure, the patients experience disturbed consciousness and often tonic-clonic muscle movements. Seizures initiated in parts of the brain are named focal seizures and may induce a plethora of symptoms often correlated to the function or lack of function of that particular brain region. The etiology of epilepsy varies. It may arise due to a brain infection, trauma, ischemia, tumor, neurodegenerative disease, or genetic predisposition. A large proportion is cryptogenic. Almost 40 % of epilepsy patients are resistant to current anti-epileptic therapy, which makes investigation of new therapeutic targets and biomarkers for patient stratification warranted.

Pathological hallmarks in the brain associated with epilepsy include imbalance in synaptic transmission, neuronal damage, and an exaggerated immune response [2–6]. During the acute innate immune response in the brain following seizures, microglia release pro- and anti-inflammatory mediators [7], undergo phenotypic changes, and migrate towards the epileptic foci where they phagocytize cell debris [8, 9]. Moreover, astrocytes change their activity state and exhibit disturbed buffering capacity of ions and glutamate uptake [10]. In addition to the innate immune reaction, seizures may cause blood-brain barrier dysfunction and activation of vascular-associated and blood-derived immune cells [5]. Hitherto, a seizure-induced immune response has primarily been described within the epileptic foci of the brain, such as in hippocampal sclerosis in medial temporal lobe epilepsy, the most common form of epilepsy [4]. However, recent findings support the idea that seizures may be viewed as a disturbance of entire brain networks, including subcortical nodes for seizure propagation [11]. More remote areas of the brain, such as the retina, have not yet been investigated at all. Recently, we reported microglial activation in both cortical and subcortical brain areas even before behavioral seizures had developed in a genetic mouse model of epilepsy [12]. Therefore, the relationship between brain inflammation and epileptogenesis may also be further understood by studying the immune response in remote areas to the epileptic foci that are not known to either generate or propagate seizures.

In the present study, we therefore decided to explore whether a post-seizure immune response can extend beyond an epileptic focus within the temporal lobes and, hence, be detected as far as the retina of adult rats. The retina lines the back of the eyeball and constitutes a remote extension of the brain, so far not considered to exhibit seizure-induced pathology. It is a light-sensitive neural structure with several layers of strictly interconnected neurons [13]. The innate and adaptive immune response of the retina involves, similar to other brain regions, the activation of microglia and macroglial cells (i.e., astrocytes and Müller cells), vascular pericytes, and leucocytes that cross the blood-retina barrier (BRB) [14–16]. Since the retinal immune response is more accessible than the cerebral immune response for non-invasive investigations, it may become an attractive biomarker of brain inflammation if it reflects the immune response in the rest of the brain. Here, we evaluated micro- and macroglial activation, leukocyte infiltration, and number of vascular pericytes in the retina, acutely and late after electrically induced temporal status epilepticus. We also investigated whether a seizure-induced retinal immune response may be modulated by intracerebroventricular infusion of an antibody (Ab) against the chemokine receptor CX3CR1.

# Methods

## Animals

Adult male Sprague Dawley rats ($n = 78$) weighing between 200 and 250 g were procured from Charles River (Germany). The animals were housed in a 12-h light/dark cycle with ad libitum food and water. All experimental procedures followed the guidelines set by the Malmö-Lund Ethical Committee in Sweden for the use and care of laboratory animals, and the ARVO statement for the use of animals in ophthalmic and vision research.

## Group assignment

Animals were divided into three survival groups following electrically induced temporal status epilepticus (SE) and corresponding non-stimulated controls (NSC): 6 h (SE $n = 4$ and NSC $n = 5$ were perfused, SE $n = 4$ and NSC $n = 4$ were homogenized), 1 week (SE $n = 9$ and NSC $n = 8$ were perfused, SE $n = 6$ and NSC $n = 6$ were homogenized), and 7 weeks (SE $n = 6$, SE + CX3CR1 antibody $n = 7$ and NSC + saline infusion $n = 9$ were perfused SE $n = 5$ and NSC $n = 5$ were homogenized).

## Surgeries, drug infusions, and electrically induced temporal status epilepticus

Animals were anesthetized with 2 % isofluorane and implanted with a bipolar-insulated stainless steel electrode (Plastics One, Roanoke, VA) into the right ventral CA1/CA3 region of the hippocampus (coordinates 4.8 mm posterior and 5.2 mm lateral from the bregma and 6.3 mm ventral from the dura, tooth bar set at −3.0 mm) for stimulation and recording. A unipolar electrode was placed between the skull and adjacent muscle to serve as ground electrode. In addition, a subset of animals were implanted with intracerebroventricular cannulae (Brain Infusion Kit 1, ALZET, USA): coordinates 1.0 mm posterior and 1.5 mm lateral to the bregma and 3.5 mm ventral to the flat skull position (with the bregma as reference) ipsilateral to the electrode placement for continuous saline or CX3CR1 antibody infusion (20 µg/ml; Abcam, UK) from a subcutaneously implanted osmotic pump (ALZET) during either 1 week after SE or during 6 weeks starting 1 week after SE. Following a week of recovery after surgery, rats were subjected to electrically induced temporal SE according to previously described protocol [17]. Electrode- and cannulae-implanted non-stimulated rats served as controls (NSC). Only rats that displayed self-sustained ictal electroencephalographic (EEG) activity for 2 h (Fig. 1) in the temporal lobe and mainly partial seizure semiology according to previous description [17], e.g., oralfacial twitches, nodding, drooling, and unilateral forelimb clonus, according to Racine's scale, were included in this study [18]. Behavioral symptoms and ictal EEG activity were completely interrupted after 2 h of self-sustained SE by the administration of pentobarbital (65 mg/kg, intraperitoneal injection) (Fig. 1a).

### Tissue preparation

For biochemical analyses, rats were decapitated and the eyes, excluding the lenses, were immediately collected, frozen on dry ice, and stored in –80 °C. For immunohistochemistry, rats were perfused with ice-cold 0.9 % saline and paraformaldehyde (PFA) (4 % in 0.1 M phosphate-buffered saline (PBS), pH 7.4). The eyes were enucleated and post-fixed in PFA for 4 h, rinsed in

PBS, incubated in 10 % sucrose (16 h) and 25 % sucrose (16 h), consecutively embedded in a Yazulla medium (30 % egg albumin, 3 % gelatin), and finally cut in 20 µm-thick sagittal cryosections (Microm HM 560, US) and stored at –20 °C.

### Multiplex enzyme-linked immunosorbent assay (ELISA)

Samples were homogenized on ice in buffer (pH 7.6) containing (in millimolars) 50.0 Tris-HCl, 150 NaCl, 5.0 CaCl$_2$, 0.02 % NaN$_3$, and 1 % Triton X-100, and then centrifuged at 17,000$g$ for 30 min at 4 °C. The supernatant was collected into a microcentrifuge tube, where the total protein concentration was determined by BCA protein assay (BCA, Pierce, Rockford, IL) as per manufacturer's instructions. Levels of interleukin (IL)-1β, tumor necrosis factor (TNF)-α, interferon (IFN)-γ, IL-4, IL-5, IL-6, IL-10, IL-13, and keratinocyte chemoattractant/growth-related oncogene (KC/GRO) were measured by sandwich immunoassay methods using commercially available electrochemiluminescent detection system, plates, and reagents (V-PLEX Proinflammatory Panel 2 (rat) kit, Meso Scale Discovery (MSD), Gaithersburg, MD, USA) as per manufacturer's instructions with minor modifications. Briefly, 100 µg (50 µl) of the protein sample was loaded per well in the MSD plate. The samples were incubated overnight at 4 °C with shaking. For each assay, samples were analyzed in duplicates and compared with known concentrations of protein standards. Plates were analyzed using the SECTOR Imager 2400.

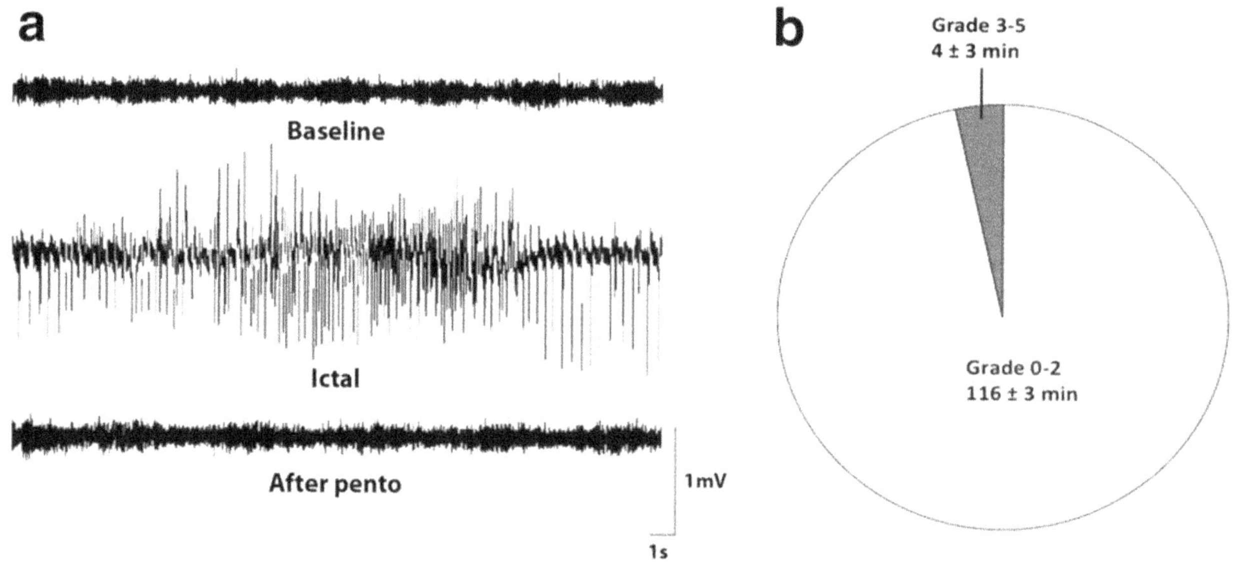

**Fig. 1** Electroencephalographic recordings from intrahippocampal electrodes before, during, and after electrically induced temporal status epilepticus (SE). **a** Representative baseline activity in rats before stimulations (*top*), high-frequency epileptiform activity during the 2 h of self-sustained SE (*middle*), and baseline activity after SE was terminated with pentobarbital injection (*bottom*). **b** Pie chart showing the relative distribution of different seizure semiology during the 2-h SE period. The semiology is based on the Racine's scale [18], where stages 0–2 and 3–5 represent partial and generalized seizure semiology, respectively. Each segment depicts the mean percentage of time spent exhibiting the behavior

## Western blot analysis

Western blot analyses were performed as previously described [19]. The following primary Abs were used: mouse monoclonal anti-β actin (1:10,000; Sigma-Aldrich, MO, US), rabbit monoclonal anti-glyceraldehyde 3-phosphate dehydrogenase (GAPDH) (1:2000; Cell Signaling Technologies, CA, USA), rabbit polyclonal anti-CX3CR1 (1:500; Abcam, Cambridge, UK), and mouse monoclonal anti-postsynaptic density-95 (PSD-95) (1:200, Abcam). Secondary Abs used were either horseradish peroxidase-conjugated anti-mouse or anti-rabbit (both 1:5000; Sigma-Aldrich). Band intensities were quantified using ImageJ software (NIH, USA), and β-actin or GAPDH was used as a loading control.

## Fluoro-Jade staining

Sections were washed with potassium PBS, hydrated, and pretreated with 0.06 % potassium permanganate for 15 min, rinsed with distilled water, and treated with 0.001 % Fluoro-Jade (Histo-Chem, Jefferson, AR, USA) for 30 min. They were then washed with distilled water, dehydrated by treatment with ethanol and xylene, and coverslipped with PERTEX mounting medium.

## Immunohistochemistry and hematoxylin-eosin staining

Immunohistochemistry was performed as previously described [20]. The following primary Abs were used: rabbit polyclonal anti-Iba1 (1:1000; Wako, Japan), mouse anti-rat CD68/ED1 (1:200; AbD Serotec, NC, USA), rabbit anti-CD-45 (1:100; Santa Cruz Biotechnology, TX, USA), mouse anti-neuron glial antigen 2 (NG2) (1:200; Millipore, MA, USA), mouse anti-glial fibrillary acidic protein (GFAP) (1:400; Sigma-Aldrich), goat anti-Iba1 (1:250; AbD Serotec), mouse anti-PSD-95 (1:500; Abcam), rabbit anti- IL-6 (1:400; Abcam), rabbit anti-IL-4 (1:100, Abcam), and goat anti-IL-1β (1:100; Santa Cruz Biotechnology). Sections were incubated with appropriate primary Abs overnight at 4 °C and secondary antibody for 1 h at room temperature. For each immunohistochemical assessment, some eye sections went through the entire protocol without primary Abs incubation to serve as the negative controls. The following secondary Abs were used: Cy3-conjugated donkey anti-mouse/rabbit/goat (1:200; Jackson ImmunoResearch, UK), Alexa-488 conjugated donkey anti-mouse/rabbit (1:200; Invitrogen, NY, USA), and Cy2-conjugated donkey anti-rabbit (1:200; Jackson ImmunoResearch). For counterstaining of nuclei, the sections were coverslipped using 496-diamidino-2-phenylindole (DAPI)-containing VECTASHIELD mounting medium (Vector Laboratories, Burlingame, CA, USA) and stored in −20 °C until cell quantification. For gross morphological analyses, sections were stained with hematoxylin-eosin (Htx-eosin) for 1 min, dehydrated, and coverslipped using PERTEX mounting medium (HistoLab, Sweden).

## Morphological analyses, cell countings, and intensity measurements

First, an overall gross morphological analysis of retinal lamination was performed throughout the entire retina using light microscopy, in four sections from ipsi- and contralateral eyes, respectively. Second, detailed analyses were performed with regard to nuclear layer morphology using the ranking system 0–2 (0 = normal nuclear layer morphology and the presence of 0–10 pyknotic (shrunken) nuclei; 1 = islands of disseminated nuclear layers without nuclei (typically the size of 1–2 cells) and 11–20 pyknotic nuclei; 2 = completely disseminated nuclear layers and >20 pyknotic nuclei) as described previously [21].

Quantifications of Iba1, ED1, CD45, and NG2-positive cells were performed in 8–12 regions of interest (ROIs) within 4–6 sections/eye, located in the peripheral retina, approximately 500 μm from the ora serrata (the junction between the retina and the ciliary body), using an Olympus BX61 epifluorescence microscope. The data is presented as the number of cells per ROI, which constituted an area of $16 \times 10^4$ μm$^2$ in the Iba1, ED1, NG2, and CD45 stainings. Each ROI included the following retinal layers: inner limiting membrane (ILM), nerve fiber layer (NFL), ganglion cell layer (GCL), inner plexiform layer (IPL), inner nuclear layer (INL), outer plexiform layer (OPL), and outer nuclear layer (ONL) (Fig. 2). For morphological analyses of microglia phenotypes in the same regions, a total number of 240 (6 h) and 120 (1 and 7 weeks) Iba1$^+$ cells were analyzed per eye for three different subtypes: ramified (small soma and extensive dendritic tree), intermediate (larger soma and less extensive dendritic tree), and round/amoeboid (no processes), according to previously described definitions [12, 19]. The relative occurrence of each subtype was expressed as the mean percentage of Iba1$^+$ cells per eye. The morphological assessments were further confirmed by quantifications of the length of the most extended process per Iba1$^+$ cell, and Iba1$^+$ cell soma diameter in ten Iba1$^+$ cells per retina, from the same ROIs in the peripheral ipsilateral retina as the morphological evaluations, using Cell Sense Olympus software and Olympus BX61 epifluorescence microscope.

Semi-quantitative analysis of GFAP expression was performed in 12 representative images from four sections/eye, using Olympus BX61 epifluorescence microscope. The density of GFAP$^+$ radial Müller cell processes was graded according to a 0–5 scale in IPL (0 = none, 1 = 1–5, 2 = 6–10, 3 = 11–20, 4 = 21–50, 5 = >50 processes) and a 0–3 scale in INL + OPL and ONL, respectively (0 = none, 1 = 1–5, 2 = 6–10, 3 = >10 processes). In addition, number of GFAP$^+$ retinal astrocytes was manually quantified in 12 representative images of the inner retina from four sections/eye.

Intensity measurements of GFAP expression in the GCL, NFL, and ILM were performed in fluorescence

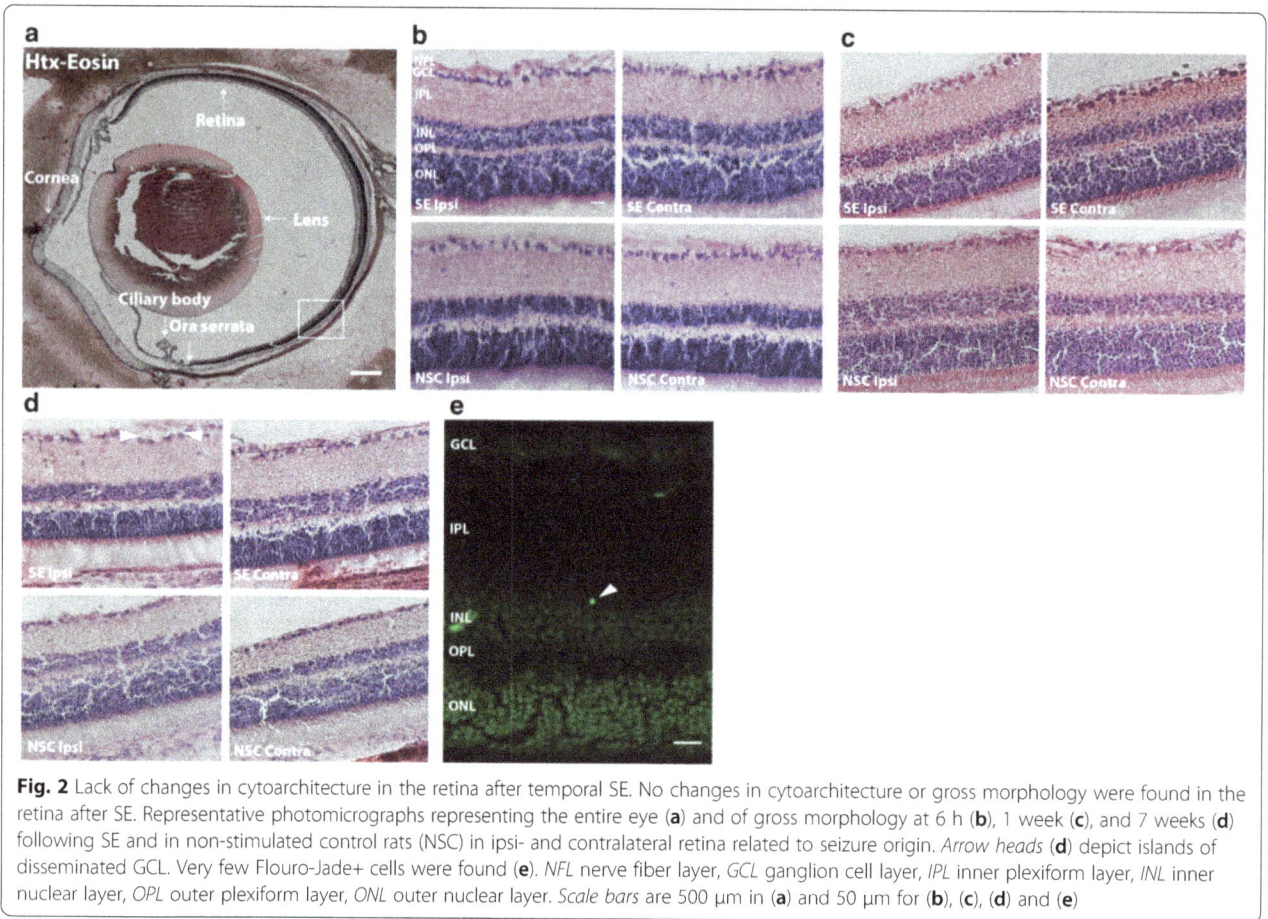

**Fig. 2** Lack of changes in cytoarchitecture in the retina after temporal SE. No changes in cytoarchitecture or gross morphology were found in the retina after SE. Representative photomicrographs representing the entire eye (**a**) and of gross morphology at 6 h (**b**), 1 week (**c**), and 7 weeks (**d**) following SE and in non-stimulated control rats (NSC) in ipsi- and contralateral retina related to seizure origin. *Arrow heads* (**d**) depict islands of disseminated GCL. Very few Flouro-Jade+ cells were found (**e**). *NFL* nerve fiber layer, *GCL* ganglion cell layer, *IPL* inner plexiform layer, *INL* inner nuclear layer, *OPL* outer plexiform layer, *ONL* outer nuclear layer. *Scale bars* are 500 μm in (**a**) and 50 μm for (**b**), (**c**), (**d**) and (**e**)

images from 12 sections/eye (each image corresponding to $13 \times 10^3$ $\mu m^2$), using an Olympus BX61 epifluorescence microscope (Leica, Germany). Intensity measurements of PSD-95 expression in IPL, INL, OPL, and ONL, respectively, were performed with confocal laser scanning microscope (Zeiss, Germany) with a 561-nm excitation filter, ×63 oil-immersion objective, and ×5 zoom. Intensity measurements of IL-6, IL-4, and IL-1β expression in IPL, INL, OPL, and ONL, respectively, were carried out with a 488-nm and 561-nm excitation filter, ×40 oil-immersion objective, and ×5 digital zoom. Images were taken from three representative areas from each animal. Each image was acquired in a z-stack at an interval of 0.2 μm, on average 50 slices per z-stack. The images were analyzed in ImageJ software and the brightness and contrast corrected and noise reduced using the built-in ImageJ functions. Background intensity was measured in every image and subsequently subtracted from the mean gray value from each image in order to obtain a background-corrected mean gray value per animal.

To ensure the lack of bias, all analyses were conducted by an observer blind to the treatment conditions.

## Statistics

Statistical analyses were performed with the unpaired Student's *t* test when comparing two groups, using GraphPad Prism software, except for analyses of gross morphology and grading of GFAP+ processes where Mann-Whitney's rank sum test for non-parametric variables was applied. Microglial morphology was analyzed with two-way analysis of variance (ANOVA) followed by a Bonferroni post hoc test. Data are presented as means ± SEM, apart from gross morphology and GFAP+ process evaluations, which are presented as median ± range with upper quartile range. Differences were considered statistically significant at $p \leq 0.05$.

## Results

### Lack of acute changes in the expression of immune mediators, glial activation, and cell death in the eyes after temporal status epilepticus

We performed cytoarchitectural analyses of the eye tissue. However, in the retina at the time point 6 h post-SE, no obvious pathological signs were found at the gross cytoarchitectural level, when assessed using Htx-eosin staining (Fig. 2a), with the retina showing well-defined and homogenous nuclear and synaptic layers and nerve fiber layer. Detailed morphological analysis of the retina revealed no differences between SE and NSC group in the ipsi- and contralateral eyes, with both retinas displaying well-preserved nuclear layer morphology and no pyknotic cells and disseminated GCL at 6 h (ipsilateral SE 0 $u = 0$ vs NSC 0 $u = 0$ and contralateral SE 0 $u = 0$ vs NSC 0 $u = 0$; Fig. 2b). Less than three Fluoro-Jade[+] cells were observed in total per animal in both SE and NSC groups (Fig. 2e), which made statistical analyses inadequate. In order to detect an acute immune response in the eye, we first performed immunohistochemical evaluations of number of Iba1[+] cells and the morphology of the microglia, including ramified, intermediate, and round/amoeboid phenotypes. However, no differences in Iba1[+] cell number (Fig. 3a) or microglial morphology (Fig. 3b) could be detected. Seizure-induced microglial activation is also associated with a more phagocytic profile [6] and we therefore double-stained Iba1[+] cells with the phagocytic marker ED1. Though, the number of Iba1[+]/ED1[+] cells was too low to be adequately analyzed (rarely more than 1–2 cells per retina in both NSC and SE group).

Next, biochemical analyses of pro- and anti-inflammatory mediators in the protein homogenates from the eye tissue excluding the lens at 6 h following SE were evaluated. At this time point, several immune factors are upregulated in the epileptic focus of the hippocampus (Avdic U, Ahl M, Ekdahl CT, unpublished

observation). However, even though the chemokine KC/GRO, chemokine receptor CX3CR1, and the cytokines IL-6, IL-5, and IL-1β were detectable in the eyes, the levels were unaltered compared to the NSC group, both ipsi- and contralateral to the epileptic focus (Fig. 3d, e).

### Lack of subacute changes in the expression of immune mediators, glial activation, and cell death in the eyes after temporal status epilepticus

We next performed cytoarchitectural analyses of the eye tissue 1 week post-SE. At this time point, neuronal necrosis and apoptotic cell death are readily observed in varying degree within temporal structures, including the hippocampus [17, 22]. However, in the retina, again, no obvious pathological signs were found at the gross cytoarchitectural level. Detailed morphological analysis of the retina showed no differences between SE and NSC group in the ipsi- and contralateral eyes, with both retinas displaying well-preserved nuclear layer morphology and only occasional pyknotic cells and disseminated GCL (ipsilateral SE 0.25 $u = 0.875$ vs NSC 0.5 $u = 0.5$ and contralateral SE 0 $u = 0.75$ vs NSC 0.25 $u = 0.458$ score) (Fig. 2c). Less than three Fluoro-Jade[+] cells per animal were observed in both groups.

Furthermore, no differences in Iba1[+] cell number (Fig. 4a) or microglial morphology (Fig. 4b) could be detected. The number of Iba1[+]/ED1[+] cells was less than

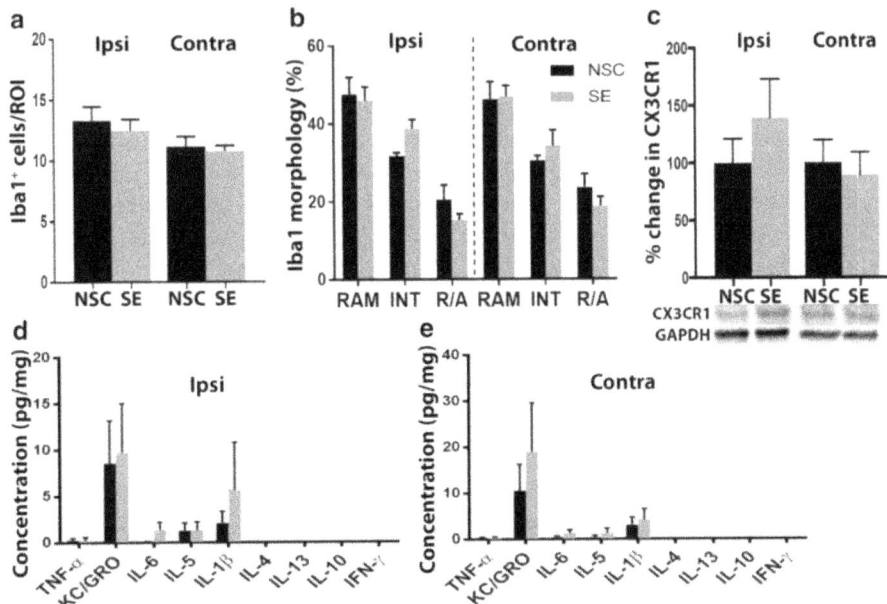

Fig. 3 No changes in microglial activation or cytokine and chemokine protein expression in the eyes 6 h after temporal SE. No changes were observed in number of Iba1+ cells (a) or in Iba1+ cell morphology (b) between NSC and SE. Representative Western blot and quantification of CX3CR1 protein (~50 kDa) relative to NSC in the ipsilateral and contralateral eye 6 h post SE (c). Quantification of cytokine and chemokine protein expression, using mesoscale multiplex ELISA, in ipsilateral (d) and contralateral (e) eye homogenates 6 h after SE showed no differences compared to NSC. Data are presented as mean ± SEM, $n = 5$ NSC and $n = 4$ SE for WB and ELISA, $n = 4$ NSC and $n = 4$ SE for cell count and morphology. *$p \leq 0.05$, unpaired $t$ test in (a) and (c–e) two-way ANOVA in (b)

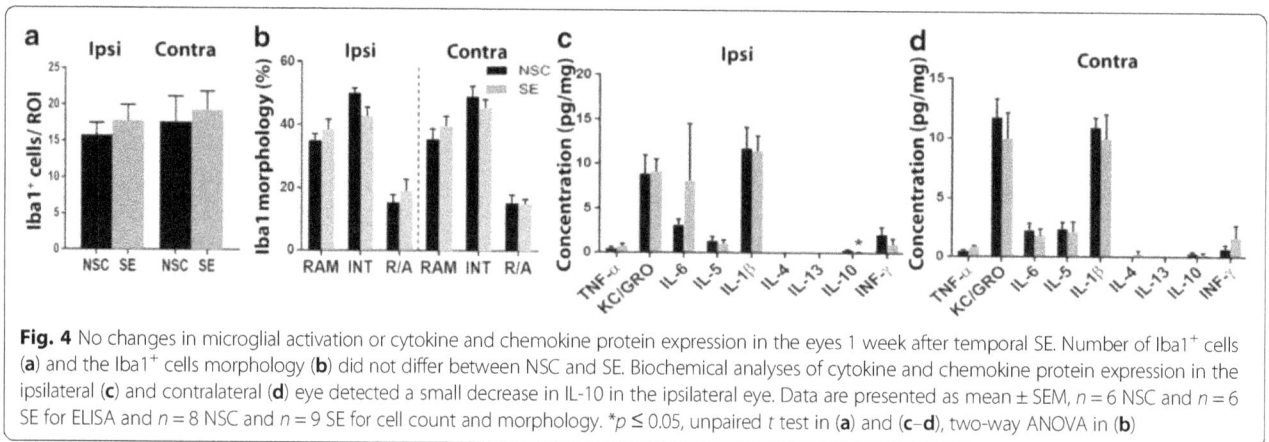

**Fig. 4** No changes in microglial activation or cytokine and chemokine protein expression in the eyes 1 week after temporal SE. Number of Iba1$^+$ cells (**a**) and the Iba1$^+$ cells morphology (**b**) did not differ between NSC and SE. Biochemical analyses of cytokine and chemokine protein expression in the ipsilateral (**c**) and contralateral (**d**) eye detected a small decrease in IL-10 in the ipsilateral eye. Data are presented as mean ± SEM, $n = 6$ NSC and $n = 6$ SE for ELISA and $n = 8$ NSC and $n = 9$ SE for cell count and morphology. *$p \leq 0.05$, unpaired $t$ test in (**a**) and (**c–d**), two-way ANOVA in (**b**)

2–3 cells per retina in both groups. The expression of immune mediators was unaltered, apart from a small decrease in IL-10 in the ipsilateral eye (Fig. 4c, d).

### Delayed glial activation in the retina after temporal status epilepticus

We hypothesized that a seizure-induced tissue injury may be delayed in the retina compared to other brain structures and, therefore, we extended our analyses to a later time point, i.e., 7 weeks after SE. Again, no changes in retinal laminar organization or significant changes in the cytoarchitecture (ipsilateral SE 1.0 $u = 1$ vs NSC 0.5 $u = 0.75$ and contralateral SE 0.25 $u = 0.375$ vs NSC 0.333 $u = 0.50$ score) could be detected (Fig. 2d). The quantification of Fluoro-Jade$^+$ cells in the retina never exceeded three cells per eye.

The immune response in epileptic foci is often characterized by a prominent activation of microglial cells, which can be detected both acutely and chronically after SE [6, 23]. In the retina of both the NSC and 7 weeks post-SE group, the Iba1$^+$ microglial cells were primarily located in the synaptic layers (OPL and IPL) and the GCL (Fig. 5a, b). The morphology of the microglia included again ramified, intermediate, and round/amoeboid phenotypes (Fig. 5c). Interestingly, the number of Iba1$^+$ cells was increased bilaterally (Fig. 5d), with a few aberrant cell clusters in the INL and the occurrence of processes in the ONL (Fig. 5b). Accordingly, the morphology of the Iba1$^+$ cells significantly changed. The SE group showed a relative decrease in ramified and an increase in round/amoeboid microglial phenotype with a significant interaction between groups and morphology in both the ipsi- and contralateral retina (Fig. 5e). The morphological differences were further confirmed in a subset of animals ($n = 3 + 3$, NSC and 7 weeks post-SE group, respectively) with larger Iba1$^+$ cell soma diameter (SE 13.59 ± 0.71 vs NSC 9.57 ± 0.27 μm) and less extended processes per Iba1$^+$ cell (SE 28.18 ± 2.11 vs NSC

38.78 ± 2.73 μm) in the ipsilateral retina of SE rats. Biochemical analyses of eye homogenates showed increased KC/GRO levels in the ipsilateral eye (Fig. 5f, g). Intensity measurement of immonohistochemical stainings for three pro- and anti-inflammatory markers, showed regional alterations in Il-1β levels, with an increase in IPL (Fig. 5h) in the ipsilateral eye, while the intensity of IL-6 or IL-4 remained unaltered (Fig. 5i, j). No changes in Il-1β, IL-6, and IL-4 intensity could be detected in other retinal layers including INL, OPL, and ONL (data not shown).

Less than 1–2 single-labeled ED1$^+$ cells and Iba1$^+$/ED1$^+$ cells per retina were detected at 7 weeks post-SE (data not shown). The cells were uniformly distributed among the retinal layers (Fig. 5k). In order to evaluate a possible systemic contribution of leukocytes to the immune response in the retina after SE, numbers of CD45$^+$ cells were evaluated at 7 weeks, but again, very low cell numbers were found with no differences between the two groups (ipsilateral SE 0.38 ± 0.13 vs NSC 0.97 ± 0.22, contralateral SE 0.88 ± 0.38 vs NSC 1.53 ± 0.34). At both 1 and 7 weeks, CD45$^+$ cells were primarily located in the subretinal layers, not overlapping with the Iba1 staining (Fig. 5l).

In an attempt to define whether the immune response in the retina was associated with a subtle microvascular disturbance, we also analyzed the numbers of vascular NG2-expressing pericytes [16]. NG2$^+$ cells were found in the same retinal layers as the Iba1$^+$ cells, but their expressions did not overlap (Fig. 5m). Often, the NG2$^+$ cells were aligned in a cluster of 2–3 cells, as if embracing a microvessel (Fig. 5m inset). However, the cell numbers did not differ between SE and NSC group neither 1 nor 7 weeks post-SE (1 week ipsilateral SE 9.64 ± 0.40 vs NSC 8.76 ± 0.62 and contralateral SE 8.67 ± 0.29 vs NSC 9.60 ± 0.51; 7 weeks ipsilateral SE 7.97 ± 0.64 vs NSC 8.38 ± 0.31, contralateral SE 7.47 ± 0.51 vs NSC 8.16 ± 0.76).

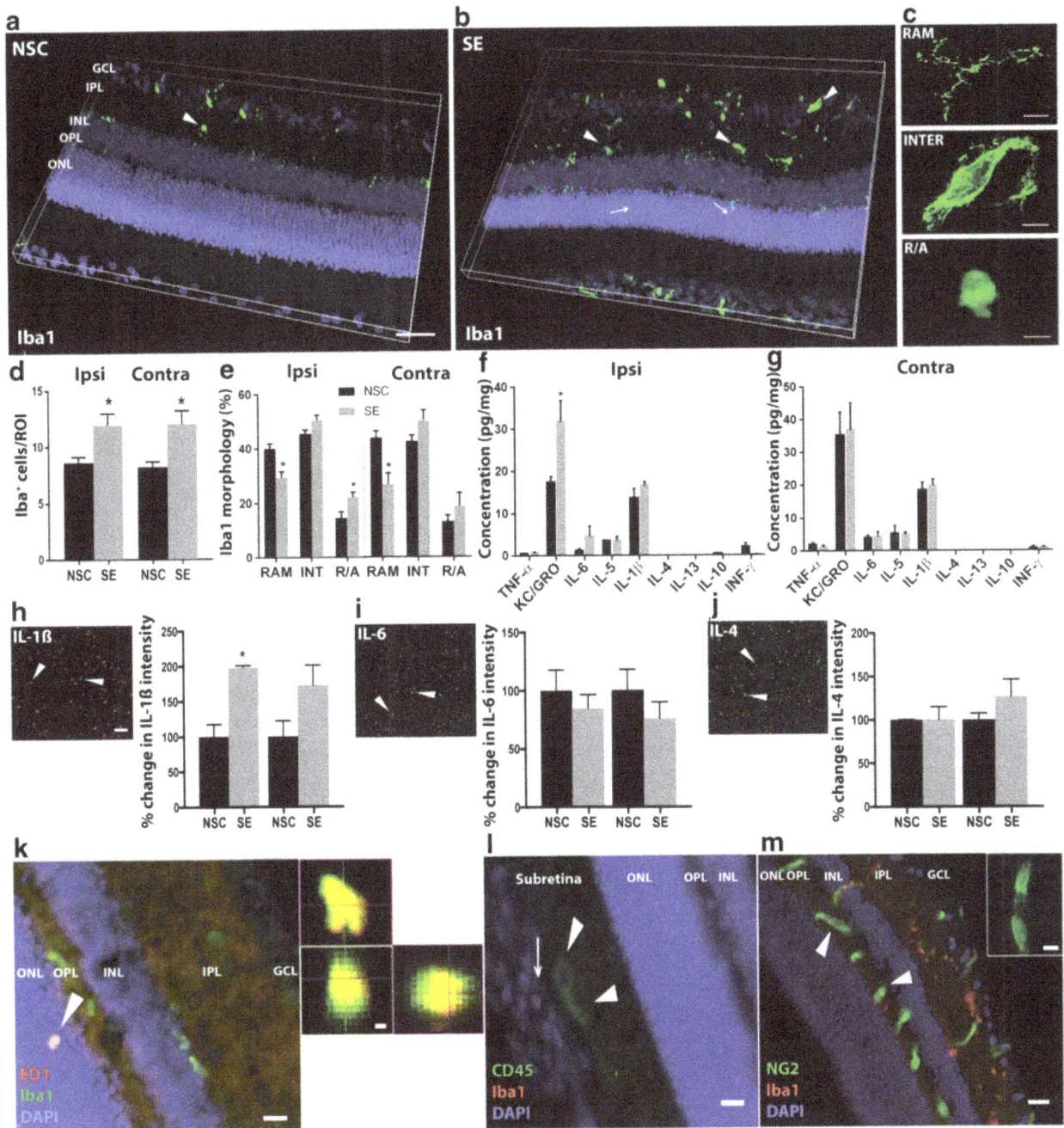

**Fig. 5** Delayed microglial activation in the retina 7 weeks after temporal SE. Representative confocal photomicrographs of microglial activation in non-stimulated controls NSC (**a**) and 7 weeks after SE (**b**). *Arrow heads* in (**a**) and (**b**) depict Iba1[+] cells in IPL and GCL. *Arrows* in **B** mark Iba1[+] processes in the ONL. Representative images of different Iba1[+] cell morphologies, including ramified (RAM), intermediate (INT), and round/amoeboid (R/A) (**c**). Note the elongated cell soma and thicker proximal processes in INT compared the RAM cells. Quantification of numbers of Iba1[+] cells in the ipsi- and contralateral retina 7 weeks following SE compared to NSC showed an increase after SE (**d**). Quantification of the relative percentage of microglia with the three different morphologies revealed a relative reduction in ramified and an increase in amoeboid morphology in the SE group (**e**). Biochemical analysis detected a SE-induced increase in chemokine KC/GRO levels in ipsilateral retina (**f**), but no changes in the contralateral eye (**g**). Representative pictures and intensity measurements in the IPL of cytokine IL-1β (**h**), IL-6 (**i**), and IL-4 (**j**) immune staining showed increased levels of IL-1β only. Confocal images of Iba1 and ED1 immunostaining of the retina (*left*) and orthogonal projection of an Iba1[+] ED1[+] cell (*right*) (**k**), Iba1 and CD45 immunostaining of the retina (**l**), and Iba1 and NG2 immunostaining of the retina with NG2[+] cells in higher magnification in *inset* (**m**). Data are presented as means ± SEM, $n = 5$ NSC and $n = 5$ SE for ELISA, $n = 9$ NSC and $n = 6$ SE for cell quantification and evaluation. *$p \leq 0.05$ un-paired $t$ test in (**d**) and (**i–j**), 2-way ANOVA in (**e**). Scale bars are 500 μm for (**a**) and (**b**), 10 μm for (**c**) 5 μm for (**h-j**), 25 μm for (**k–m**), and insets 3 μm for (**k**) and 5 μm for (**m**)

Apart from microglial activation, seizure-induced gliosis in the brain is also associated with a strong astrocytic reaction, which is readily evaluated by the typical upregulation of GFAP [24, 25]. In the retina, Müller cells and retinal astrocytes, together referred to as macroglia, are responsible for injury-induced gliosis [26]. In NSC rats at 7 weeks post-SE, only weakly labeled GFAP$^+$ Müller cell end feet/processes and astrocytes were found in ILM and GCL (Fig. 6a, arrows). We graded the number of GFAP$^+$ Müller cell processes in the IPL, INL + OPL, and ONL, respectively, and found extensive GFAP$^+$ staining in the ILM and GCL and, occasionally, also in the Müller cell end feet in the outer limiting membrane outside the ONL. It was significantly increased in the IPL contralaterally and there was a trend towards an increase ($p = 0.07$) ipsilaterally to the epileptic focus (Fig. 6a, b). The increase was also significant in the INL and OPL on the contralateral side (ipsilateral SE 0 $u = 1.56$ vs NSC 0 $u = 0$, contralateral SE 0.13 $u = 1.04$ vs NSC 0 $u = 0$). No differences were found in the ONL (data not shown). The high variation in glial activation in the SE group did not correlate to SE severity (total time a rat exhibited generalized tonic-clonic seizures during the 2 h of SE (regression analysis $p = 0.7$, $r$-value = $-0.12$), as previously seen for microglial activation in the brain [6]). This increase in number of GFAP$^+$ processes at 7 weeks was not evident at either 6 h or 1 week post-SE (data not shown). However, at these acute and sub-acute time points, high variation within both the NSC and SE group made statistical analyses uncertain. At 6 h post-SE, we even detected a small decrease in GFAP$^+$ processes in the IPL contralateral to the epileptic focus (ipsilateral SE 1.083 $u = 1.21$ vs NSC 1.694 $u = 2.93$, contralateral SE 1 $u = 1.04$ vs NSC 1.74 $u = 3.48$) compared to NSC. In addition, the overall intensity of GFAP

immunostaining was measured in the ILM, NFL, and GCL but showed no differences either 6 h, 1, or 7 weeks post-SE compared to NSC group (6 h ipsilateral SE 19.6 $\pm 3.3$ vs NSC $16.7 \pm 2.7$, contralateral SE $23.5 \pm 2.7$ vs NSC $21.5 \pm 1.0$; 1 week ipsilateral SE $26.94 \pm 2.10$ vs NSC $24.31 \pm 2.05$, contralateral SE $24.62 \pm 2.70$ vs NSC $25.48 \pm 2.06$; 7 weeks ipsilateral SE $18.61 \pm 1.53$ vs NSC $19.09 \pm 0.89$, contralateral SE $19.93 \pm 1.62$ vs NSC $18.73 \pm 0.60$). At all time points, in both the NSC and SE group, small cell bodies of GFAP$^+$ retinal astrocytes with relatively thin processes were found also in the IPL (Fig. 6a, arrow heads). However, the number of GFAP$^+$ retinal astrocytes in the IPL did not differ at 7 weeks (ipsilateral SE $0.14 \pm 0.06$ vs NSC $0.07 \pm 0.06$, contralateral SE $0.03 \pm 0.02$ vs NSC $0.05 \pm 0.03$).

### Altered synaptic protein expression in the retina after temporal status epilepticus

Even if the epileptic seizures did not induce a prominent cell loss with changes in the cytoarchitecture of the retina, it may still induce a more subtle imbalance in synaptic transmission between neurons. The activation of micro- and macroglia may indicate such an ongoing synaptic/neuronal dysfunction. We have previously shown that levels of the scaffolding protein PSD-95, expressed primarily in excitatory synapses, may change due to an immune response in the brain [20]. Here, we measured the protein levels of PSD-95 in the eye 6 h post-SE but found no differences (ipsilateral SE $135.40 \pm 44.07$ $n = 3$ vs NSC $100.00 \pm 50.44$ $n = 4$, contralateral SE $172.20 \pm 57.34$ $n = 3$ vs NSC $100.00 \pm 27.92$ $n = 5$). However, intensity measurements of PSD-95 clusters 1 and 7 weeks post-SE in the different retinal layers revealed a small decrease in the ONL at 7 weeks in the retina ipsilateral to the epileptic focus (Fig. 7a–c).

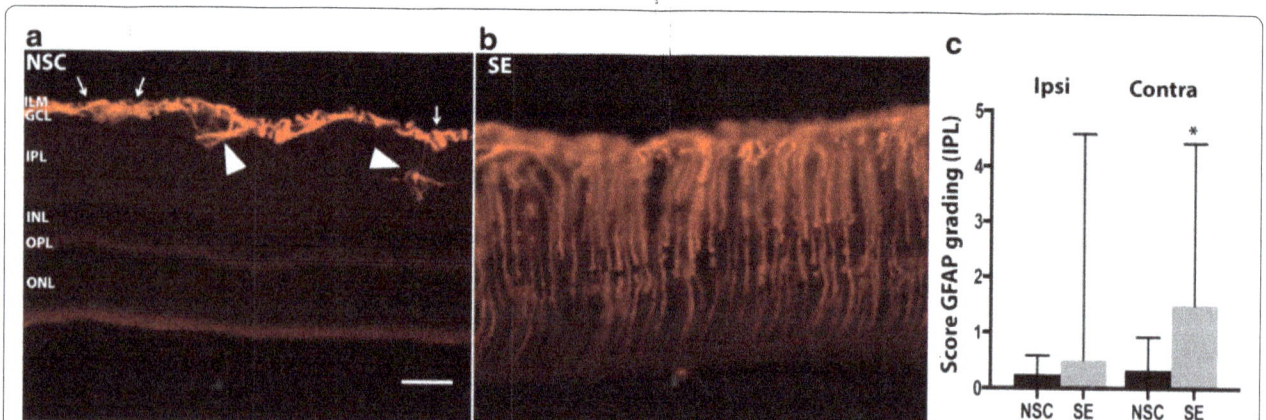

**Fig. 6** Delayed macroglial activation in the retina after temporal SE. Representative photomicrographs of GFAP expression on macroglia in the retina of NSC (**a**) and 7 weeks post-SE (**b**). The extension of GFAP$^+$ processes and their end feet in different retinal layers are *visualized in* (**b**). *Arrows* depict GFAP$^+$ end feet of Müller cells in ILM and *arrow heads* mark GFAP$^+$ retinal astrocytes. Quantification of GFAP$^+$ Müller cell processes in the IPL showed increased expression after SE (**c**). Data are presented as median range with upper quartile range, $n = 9$ NSC and $n = 6$ SE group (**c**). *$p \leq 0.05$ Mann-Whitney's rank sum test. Scale bar is 50 μm for (**a**) and (**b**)

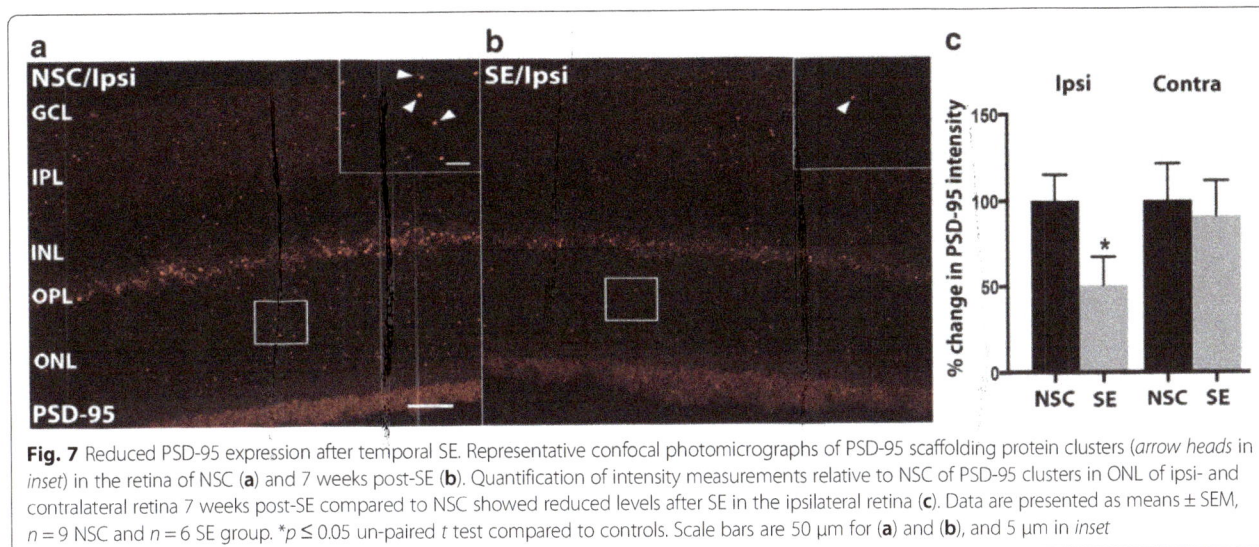

**Fig. 7** Reduced PSD-95 expression after temporal SE. Representative confocal photomicrographs of PSD-95 scaffolding protein clusters (*arrow heads* in *inset*) in the retina of NSC (**a**) and 7 weeks post-SE (**b**). Quantification of intensity measurements relative to NSC of PSD-95 clusters in ONL of ipsi- and contralateral retina 7 weeks post-SE compared to NSC showed reduced levels after SE in the ipsilateral retina (**c**). Data are presented as means ± SEM, $n = 9$ NSC and $n = 6$ SE group. *$p \leq 0.05$ un-paired $t$ test compared to controls. Scale bars are 50 μm for (**a**) and (**b**), and 5 μm in *inset*

## Intracerebroventricular CX3CR1 antibody infusion decreases micro- and macroglial activation in the retina after temporal status epilepticus

In order to evaluate possible similarities between the immune reaction in the retina and within the epileptic focus, an antibody (Ab) against the chemokine receptor CX3CR1 was infused intracerebroventricularly during 6 weeks starting 1 week after SE. The CX3CR1 is expressed on the microglia in the brain, including the retina, and can be upregulated both before and after seizures. Its ligand, fractalkine, is expressed by neurons and glial cells [27, 28]. Recently, we showed that inhibition of CX3CR1 with the same CX3CR1 Ab decreases microglial activation within the temporal epileptic foci [19]. Then, micro- and macroglial activation was evaluated in the retina 7 weeks post-SE. We observed an almost 25 % significant decrease in the number of Iba1$^+$ cells in the contralateral retina in the SE group treated with CX3CR1 Ab, compared to the SE group with saline infusion, and there was a trend towards a decrease ($p = 0.07$) in the ipsilateral retina (Fig. 8a–c). The morphology of Iba1$^+$ cells was also changed with a higher percentage of ramified and less intermediate and round phenotypes in the CX3CR1 Ab-treated SE group on both the ipsi- and contralateral side (Fig. 8d). In addition, the number of GFAP$^+$ Müller cell processes was decreased in the CX3CR1 Ab-treated group, with fewer processes in the IPL in both ipsilateral and contralateral retina (Fig. 8e–g). However, the decrease did not reach significance in the INL and OPL on either sides (data not shown). The decrease in the IPL was not due to the differences in seizure severity during the SE (data not shown).

## Discussion

Here, we provide the first evidence that epileptic seizures arising within the temporal lobes of the adult rat brain lead to glial activation in the retina. The activation includes both micro- and macroglia and is delayed in the retina compared to the epileptic focus. The seizures originated from one hemisphere, but the retinal glial activation occurred both ipsi- and contralaterally. Furthermore, we show that the seizure-induced retinal glial activation can be significantly reduced with intracerebroventricular infusion of the same CX3CR1Ab as we have previously demonstrated to reduce microglial activation within the epileptic focus. This suggests common immunological features in the retina and the epileptic focus.

Although the retina exhibited a pronounced glial reaction, retinal neurodegeneration was subtle compared to the pathology within the epileptic focus [5, 17, 19, 23]. We found no evidence for prominent retinal neuronal death in terms of disseminated retinal lamination, increased numbers of pyknotic cells, or Fluoro-Jade-positive cells at the time points studied. Still, the increased number of activated microglia, often in clusters, disarranged the normally very strict territorial distribution of the retinal microglia [29], and is most likely reflecting alterations in their normal function as regulators of synaptogenesis and synaptic transmission [30, 31]. Similarly, the decreased levels of the excitatory synaptic scaffolding protein PSD-95 in the ONL, where we observed seizure-induced aberrant microglia processes, may indicate a homeostatic imbalance in excitatory transmission. The technique for intensity measurements was not sensitive enough for detecting minor differences in high intensity regions, which may explain why we did not detect changes in synaptic plexiform layers with strong PSD-95 expression [32]. Future electrophysiological recordings of retinal neuronal networks will be important for validating synaptic transmission and functional deficiencies.

Interestingly, other neurological diseases have also recently been described to induce retinal inflammation but

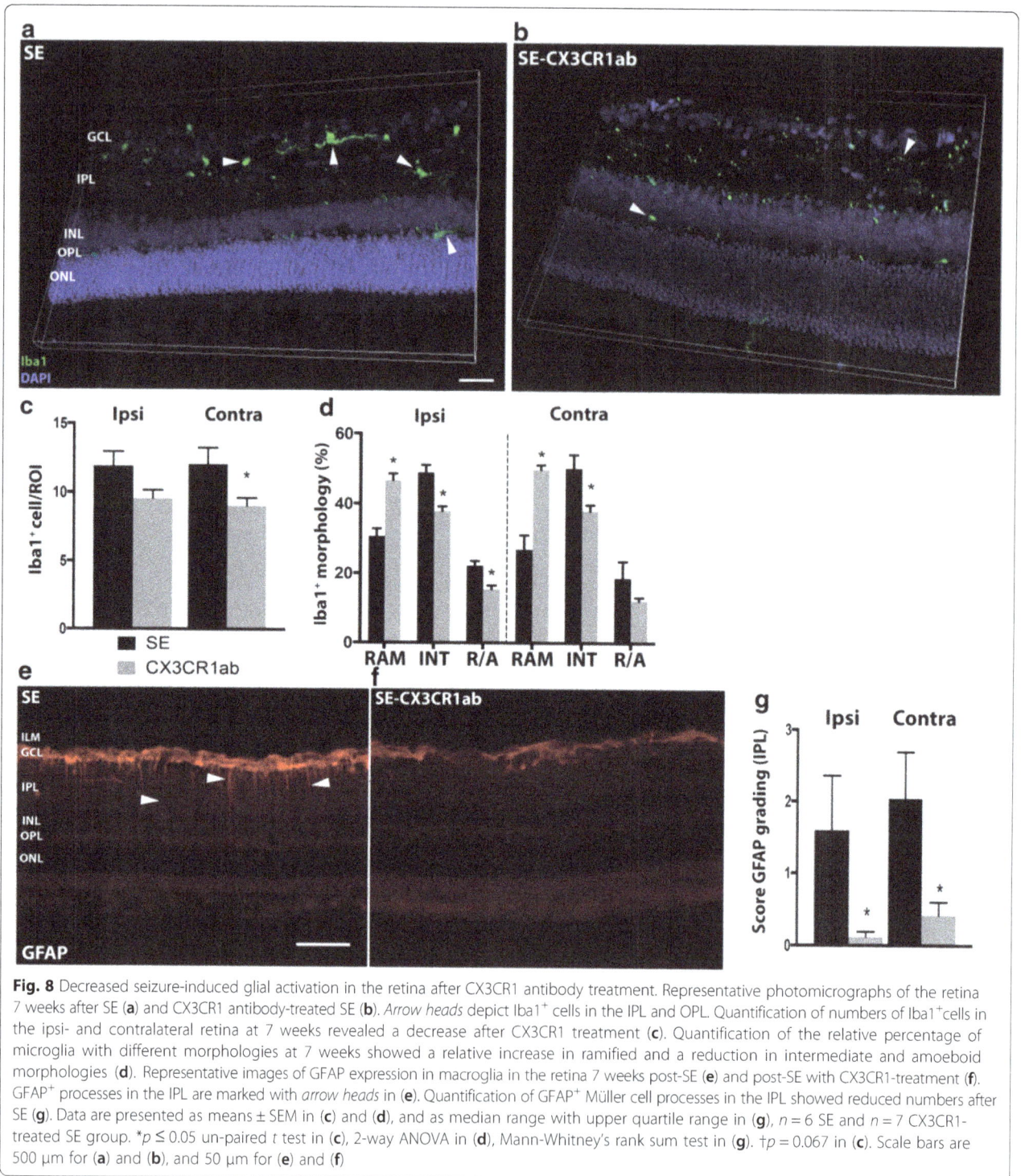

**Fig. 8** Decreased seizure-induced glial activation in the retina after CX3CR1 antibody treatment. Representative photomicrographs of the retina 7 weeks after SE (**a**) and CX3CR1 antibody-treated SE (**b**). *Arrow heads* depict Iba1$^+$ cells in the IPL and OPL. Quantification of numbers of Iba1$^+$cells in the ipsi- and contralateral retina at 7 weeks revealed a decrease after CX3CR1 treatment (**c**). Quantification of the relative percentage of microglia with different morphologies at 7 weeks showed a relative increase in ramified and a reduction in intermediate and amoeboid morphologies (**d**). Representative images of GFAP expression in macroglia in the retina 7 weeks post-SE (**e**) and post-SE with CX3CR1-treatment (**f**). GFAP$^+$ processes in the IPL are marked with *arrow heads* in (**e**). Quantification of GFAP$^+$ Müller cell processes in the IPL showed reduced numbers after SE (**g**). Data are presented as means ± SEM in (**c**) and (**d**), and as median range with upper quartile range in (**g**), $n = 6$ SE and $n = 7$ CX3CR1-treated SE group. *$p \leq 0.05$ un-paired $t$ test in (**c**), 2-way ANOVA in (**d**), Mann-Whitney's rank sum test in (**g**). †$p = 0.067$ in (**c**). Scale bars are 500 μm for (**a**) and (**b**), and 50 μm for (**e**) and (**f**)

with more pronounced neurodegeneration. In experimental and clinical studies on stroke, Parkinson's, Huntingtons', and Alzheimer's diseases, reduced retinal ganglion cell numbers, and nerve fiber layer thinning are evident, causing visual disturbances [33]. Activation of micro- and macroglia, mononuclear infiltrations, and microvascular abnormalities have also been reported [33–39]. In addition,

demyelinating diseases like multiple sclerosis show optic disc and nerve dysfunction [33]. Notably, experimental AD studies linked increased retinal glial activation to astrocyte changes in the brain [37]. However, since the presented delayed upregulation of GFAP in macroglia after SE is an early indicator of reactive gliosis [40], we cannot rule out that the pathology may progress beyond 7 weeks post-SE and with additional seizures. Conversely, since there was a high variation in retinal GFAP expression within both the SE and NSC group 6 h and 1 week after SE, we cannot rule out that there may be changes occurring acutely that were not detected with our analyses. The significance of the small decrease in GFAP at 6 h after SE also remains to be clarified.

Another important distinction between the current and previous studies on stroke and neurodegenerative diseases is the fact that the temporal seizures were initiated from implanted electrodes within a very localized area of an initially healthy brain, without genetic susceptibility or systemic immunological/vascular deficiencies. Hence, the retinal changes could only have occurred as a result of the SE insult, the SE-induced spontaneous seizures, and/or SE-induced epileptogenesis and not due to an underlying disease, which is otherwise often the case in epilepsy. Future correlation studies of seizure numbers and degree of retinal inflammation as well as studies on retinal inflammation in other models of epilepsy may give more answers to what extent retinal inflammation is a biomarker of epileptogenesis or merely a reaction to seizures per se.

There are at least four possible scenarios that may explain the underlying mechanisms of the seizure-induced retinal immune response. First, temporal seizures initiate an acute systemic immune response which may spread through the BRB. Common inflammatory mediators are upregulated in both the hippocampus and enthorinal cortex 24 h after SE [41]. However, when evaluating the same immune factors at an earlier time point in eye homogenates, no such increase was found. Instead, subtle changes in cytokine/chemokine levels were observed with a delay. A systemic immune response may also trigger a delayed infiltration of leukocytes from the retinal vessels in the subretinal or retinal layers. Though, we did not observe such an adaptive response, it may still occur at other time points. We also did not find changes in numbers of vascular pericytes, as in, i.e., diabetic retinopathy [42, 43]. Vascular pericytes are situated along endothelial cells in the wall of small blood vessels [44, 45] and sense microvascular dysfunction [46, 47]. Here, we cannot rule out that seizures lead to altered BRB function and a more subtle microvascular reorganization. Moreover, there are studies describing retinal microglial activation without prominent infiltrating leukocytes during a systemic inflammation and viral infections [14].

Secondly, the seizures may change the intracranial pressure (ICP) and influence the intraocular pressure (IOP) within the eyes. An imbalance between the anterior IOP and posterior ICP fluid pressures on the optic nerve may lead to abnormal function and nerve damage in GCL and ONL due to changes in axonal transport or altered blood flow, as seen in glaucoma [48, 49]. Initial signs of increased IOP may include altered PSD-95 expression and gliosis [50, 51].

Thirdly, the immune response in the epileptic focus may spread to other brain areas involved in the temporal seizure networks, including subcortical structures, and via the visual pathways initiate changes as far as the retina. It is likely that such a scenario would induce a stronger immune response close to the entrance of the optic nerve and inner part of the retina. Accordingly, we found macroglia activation primarily in the inner retina. However, the microglial cells did not gather within the inner layers but were evenly distributed within synaptic layers and aberrantly in the ONL. Detailed investigations of the nerve fiber tract and optic disc may reveal more subtle local changes in favor of a direct rostral cerebrum-to-retina signaling. In support, studies in AD patients suggest that inflammation may, through soluble pathogenic factors such as small nucleic acids, spread from the limbic structures both into the visual cortex, optic nerve, and the retina [39, 52].

Fourthly, an epileptic seizure may induce a retrograde current through the optic nerve, initiating an imbalance in excitatory/inhibitory transmission in the retinal network and thereby a glial activation. Whether the retinal neurons may have the properties to exhibit abnormal synchronized firing similar to a seizure among cortical neurons is to our knowledge not known. Activated Müller cell processes in the inner retina may perhaps contribute to epileptic discharges, as suggested for astrocytes in the rest of the brain [10].

The seizure-induced glial activation was evident in the retina both ipsi- and contralateral to the temporal epileptic focus. A previous case report on Rasmussen's encephalitis, a severe inflammatory epileptic encephalopathy engaging only one brain hemisphere, described an ipsilateral ocular inflammation in the patient [53]. The authors speculated to what extent an immune reaction in the eye after focal seizures may also be associated with clinical manifestations. However, apart from small alterations in cytokine/chemokine levels in the ipsilateral retina only, we could not find significant differences between the two retinas after focal temporal seizures helping in determining whether the rat exhibited left or right temporal lobe seizures. In the current study, we did not differentiate between lateral and medial parts of the retina; and therefore, we cannot define whether the retinal inflammation may be correlated to the left or right hemisphere-innervated visual field. This will be important to analyze in future studies.

A reduced glial activation both in the retina and within epileptic foci following intracerebroventricular CX3CR1 Ab treatment suggests that the two immune responses, despite being remotely located, share similar activated signaling pathways. The fractalkine-CX3CR1 pathway is involved in the activation and migration of immune cells [27, 54, 55], and an increased expression of CX3CR1 in the epileptic focus suggests a dysfunctional neuron-glial cross talk [19, 56, 57]. Thus, a reduced immune response in the eye after CX3CR1 Ab treatment may be due to a reduced propagation of the immune response from the epileptic focus/network, which could be a result of both a reduced microglia activation and neurodegeneration within the epileptic focus and a direct inhibition of the migratory capacity of the immune cells. However, CX3CR1 deficiency has been associated with eye-related disorders [58–60]; thus, we do not know the functional consequences of inhibiting seizure-induced retinal immune response with CX3CR1 Ab. During healthy conditions, the glial cells are important for keeping the homeostasis. The seizure-induced retinal immune response or the remaining immune response after CX3CR1 Ab treatment may be dysfunctional. As for the immune response in the rest of the brain, the retinal immune response is likely to both contribute to and restore pathology [61]. However, we believe that the mere existence of a retinal glial activation may turn out to be a potential novel biomarker of seizure-induced or epileptogenesis-associated brain inflammation. The fact that the retina is more accessible than many other parts of the brain makes it more attractive for diagnostic purposes. Studying the immune reaction in the eyes of epilepsy patients and correlating it to the seizure semiology, development, and prognosis may turn out to be clinically relevant.

To what extent a visual dysfunction in patients with temporal epilepsy exists and correlates to a glial activation in the retina and brain remains to be shown. Patients with epilepsy do not commonly describe visual disturbances, except for those with visual cortical involvements or drug-induced side effects. Therefore, we do not currently know if patients have retinal inflammation and visual disturbances subclinically. In the present study, we have also not addressed the question as to what extent rodents with temporal epileptic seizures suffer from functional retinal deficiencies. Future studies with pattern evoked electroretinography and multielectrode array analysis of retinal physiology will be highly relevant [62, 63].

## Conclusions

These are the first evidence that epileptic seizures lead to an immune response in the retina. The finding has a potential to become a novel non-invasive tool for detecting brain inflammation through the eyes.

## Abbreviations

Ab, antibody; AD, Alzheimer's disease; BRB, blood-retina barriers; DAPI, 496-diamidino-2-phenylindole; EEG, electroencephalographic; ELISA, enzyme-linked immunosorbent assay; GAPDH, glyceraldehyde 3-phosphate dehydrogenase; GCL, ganglion cell layer; GFAP, glial fibrially acidic protein; Htx-eosin, hematoxylin-eosin; ICP, intracranial pressure; IFN-γ, interferon gamma; IL-1β, 4–6, 10, 13, interleukin 1beta, 4-6, 10, 13; IML, inner limiting membrane; INL, inner nuclear layer; IOP, intraocular pressure; IPL, inner plexiform layer; KC/GRO, keratinocyte chemoattractant/growth-related oncogene; MSD, Meso-Scale Discovery; NFL, nerve fiber layer; NG2, neuron glial antigen 2; NSC, non-stimulated control; ONL, outer nuclear layer; OPL, outer plexiform layer; PBS, phosphate-buffered saline; PFA, paraformaldehyde; PSD-95, postsynaptic density-95; SE, status epilepticus; TNF-α, tumor necrosis factor alpha

## Acknowledgements

This work was supported by the Swedish Research Council, ALF Grant for funding medical training and research, Zoega's Foundation, Tore Nilson's Foundation, and Åhlens' Foundation. The research leading to these results has received funding from the European Union's Seventh Framework Programme (FP7/2007-2013) under grant agreement no. 602102 (EPITARGET). We thank biomedical analysts Susanne Jonsson, Hodan Abdshill, and Birgitta Stenström for technical support.

## Funding

This work (including data collection, analysis, interpretation, and writing of paper) was supported by the Swedish Research Council, ALF Grant for funding medical training and research, Zoega's Foundation, Tore Nilson's Foundation, and Åhlens Foundation. The research leading to these results has also received funding from the European Union's Seventh Framework Programme (FP7/2007-2013) under grant agreement no. 602102 (EPITARGET).

## Authors' contributions

MA partly acquired data shown in Figs. 2, 3, 4, 5, and 8. UA contributed with data shown in Figs. 6 and 7 and partly Figs. 3, 4, 5, and 8. UA, IA, and DC provided the animal material in the study. CS contributed with the data shown in Fig. 2. UEJ and CE provided the experimental design and most of the writing. All authors reviewed the results, took part in the writing, and approved the final version of the manuscript.

## Competing interests

The authors declare that they have no competing interests.

## Consent for publication

Not applicable

## Author details

[1]Inflammation and Stem Cell Therapy Group, Division of Clinical Neurophysiology, Lund University, BMC A11, Sölvegatan 17, SE-221 84 Lund, Sweden. [2]Lund Epilepsy Center, Lund University, SE-221 85 Lund, Sweden. [3]Division of Ophthalmology, Department of Clinical Sciences, Lund University, SE-221 85 Lund, Sweden.

## References

1.  Savage N. Epidemiology: the complexities of epilepsy. Nature. 2014;511:S2–3.
2.  Kan AA, de Jager W, de Wit M, Heijnen C, van Zuiden M, Ferrier C, van Rijen P, Gosselaar P, Hessel E, van Nieuwenhuizen O, de Graan PN. Protein expression profiling of inflammatory mediators in human temporal lobe epilepsy reveals co-activation of multiple chemokines and cytokines. J Neuroinflammation. 2012;9:207.
3.  Ravizza T, Balosso S, Vezzani A. Inflammation and prevention of epileptogenesis. Neurosci Lett. 2011;497:223–30.
4.  Crespel A, Coubes P, Rousset MC, Brana C, Rougier A, Rondouin G, Bockaert J, Baldy-Moulinier M, Lerner-Natoli M. Inflammatory reactions in human medial temporal lobe epilepsy with hippocampal sclerosis. Brain Res. 2002;952:159–69.

5. Legido A, Katsetos CD. Experimental studies in epilepsy: immunologic and inflammatory mechanisms. Semin Pediatr Neurol. 2014;21:197–206.

6. Ekdahl CT, Claasen JH, Bonde S, Kokaia Z, Lindvall O. Inflammation is detrimental for neurogenesis in adult brain. Proc Natl Acad Sci U S A. 2003;100:13632–7.

7. Pernhorst K, Herms S, Hoffmann P, Cichon S, Schulz H, Sander T, Schoch S, Becker AJ, Grote A. TLR4, ATF-3 and IL8 inflammation mediator expression correlates with seizure frequency in human epileptic brain tissue. Seizure. 2013;22:675–8.

8. Kettenmann H, Hanisch UK, Noda M, Verkhratsky A. Physiology of microglia. Physiol Rev. 2011;91:461–553.

9. Ekdahl CT, Kokaia Z, Lindvall O. Brain inflammation and adult neurogenesis: the dual role of microglia. Neuroscience. 2009;158:1021–9.

10. Crunelli V, Carmignoto G, Steinhauser C. Novel astrocyte targets: new avenues for the therapeutic treatment of epilepsy. Neuroscientist. 2015;21:62–83.

11. Pittau F, Megevand P, Sheybani L, Abela E, Grouiller F, Spinelli L, Michel CM, Seeck M, Vulliemoz S. Mapping epileptic activity: sources or networks for the clinicians? Front Neurol. 2014;5:218.

12. Chugh D, Ali I, Bakochi A, Bahonjic E, Etholm L, Ekdahl CT. Alterations in brain inflammation, synaptic proteins, and adult hippocampal neurogenesis during epileptogenesis in mice lacking synapsin2. PLoS One. 2015;10:e0132366.

13. Kolb H, Nelson R, Fernandez E, Jones B. The organization of the retina and visual systems. In: Anatomy and Physiology of the retina. University of Utah Health Science Center: Webvision; 2013.

14. Karlstetter M, Scholz R, Rutar M, Wong WT, Provis JM, Langmann T. Retinal microglia: just bystander or target for therapy? Prog Retin Eye Res. 2014;45:30-57.

15. Pfister F, Przybyt E, Harmsen MC, Hammes HP. Pericytes in the eye. Pflugers Arch. 2013;465:789–96.

16. Liu G, Meng C, Pan M, Chen M, Deng R, Lin L, Zhao L, Liu X. Isolation, purification, and cultivation of primary retinal microvascular pericytes: a novel model using rats. Microcirculation. 2014;21:478–89.

17. Mohapel P, Ekdahl CT, Lindvall O. Status epilepticus severity influences the long-term outcome of neurogenesis in the adult dentate gyrus. Neurobiol Dis. 2004;15:196–205.

18. Racine RJ. Modification of seizure activity by electrical stimulation. II. Motor seizure. Electroencephalogr Clin Neurophysiol. 1972;32:281–94.

19. Ali I, Chugh D, Ekdahl CT. Role of fractalkine-CX3CR1 pathway in seizure-induced microglial activation, neurodegeneration, and neuroblast production in the adult rat brain. Neurobiol Dis. 2015;74:194–203.

20. Chugh D, Nilsson P, Afjei SA, Bakochi A, Ekdahl CT. Brain inflammation induces post-synaptic changes during early synapse formation in adult-born hippocampal neurons. Exp Neurol. 2013;250:176–88.

21. Soderstjerna E, Bauer P, Cedervall T, Abdshill H, Johansson F, Johansson UE. Silver and gold nanoparticles exposure to in vitro cultured retina—studies on nanoparticle internalization, apoptosis, oxidative stress, glial- and microglial activity. PLoS One. 2014;9:e105359.

22. Ekdahl CT, Zhu C, Bonde S, Bahr BA, Blomgren K, Lindvall O. Death mechanisms in status epilepticus-generated neurons and effects of additional seizures on their survival. Neurobiol Dis. 2003;14:513–23.

23. Bonde S, Ekdahl CT, Lindvall O. Long-term neuronal replacement in adult rat hippocampus after status epilepticus despite chronic inflammation. Eur J Neurosci. 2006;23:965–74.

24. Eng LF. Glial fibrillary acidic protein (GFAP): the major protein of glial intermediate filaments in differentiated astrocytes. J Neuroimmunol. 1985;8:203–14.

25. Eng LF, Ghirnikar RS. GFAP and astrogliosis. Brain Pathol. 1994;4:229–37.

26. Norton WT, Aquino DA, Hozumi I, Chiu FC, Brosnan CF. Quantitative aspects of reactive gliosis: a review. Neurochem Res. 1992;17:877–85.

27. Harrison JK, Jiang Y, Chen S, Xia Y, Maciejewski D, McNamara RK, Streit WJ, Salafranca MN, Adhikari S, Thompson DA, et al. Role for neuronally derived fractalkine in mediating interactions between neurons and CX3CR1-expressing microglia. Proc Natl Acad Sci U S A. 1998;95:10896–901.

28. Sheridan GK, Murphy KJ. Neuron-glia crosstalk in health and disease: fractalkine and CX3CR1 take centre stage. Open Biol. 2013;3:130181.

29. Thanos S. Sick photoreceptors attract activated microglia from the ganglion cell layer: a model to study the inflammatory cascades in rats with inherited retinal dystrophy. Brain Res. 1992;588:21–8.

30. Paolicelli RC, Bolasco G, Pagani F, Maggi L, Scianni M, Panzanelli P, Giustetto M, Ferreira TA, Guiducci E, Dumas L, et al. Synaptic pruning by microglia is necessary for normal brain development. Science. 2011;333:1456–8.

31. Roumier A, Bechade C, Poncer JC, Smalla KH, Tomasello E, Vivier E, Gundelfinger ED, Triller A, Bessis A. Impaired synaptic function in the microglial KARAP/DAP12-deficient mouse. J Neurosci. 2004;24:11421–8.

32. Koulen P, Fletcher EL, Craven SE, Bredt DS, Wassle H. Immunocytochemical localization of the postsynaptic density protein PSD-95 in the mammalian retina. J Neurosci. 1998;18:10136–49.

33. London A, Benhar I, Schwartz M. The retina as a window to the brain-from eye research to CNS disorders. Nat Rev Neurol. 2013;9:44–53.

34. Cheung N, Mosley T, Islam A, Kawasaki R, Sharrett AR, Klein R, Coker LH, Knopman DS, Shibata DK, Catellier D, Wong TY. Retinal microvascular abnormalities and subclinical magnetic resonance imaging brain infarct: a prospective study. Brain. 2010;133:1987–93.

35. Kaur M, Saxena R, Singh D, Behari M, Sharma P, Menon V. Correlation between structural and functional retinal changes in Parkinson disease. J Neuroophthalmol. 2015;35:254-258.

36. Ragauskas S, Leinonen H, Puranen J, Ronkko S, Nymark S, Gurevicius K, Lipponen A, Kontkanen O, Puolivali J, Tanila H, Kalesnykas G. Early retinal function deficit without prominent morphological changes in the R6/2 mouse model of Huntington's disease. PLoS One. 2014;9:e113317.

37. Edwards MM, Rodriguez JJ, Gutierrez-Lanza R, Yates J, Verkhratsky A, Lutty GA. Retinal macroglia changes in a triple transgenic mouse model of Alzheimer's disease. Exp Eye Res. 2014;127:252–60.

38. Blanks JC, Schmidt SY, Torigoe Y, Porrello KV, Hinton DR, Blanks RH. Retinal pathology in Alzheimer's disease. II. Regional neuron loss and glial changes in GCL. Neurobiol Aging. 1996;17:385–95.

39. Hill JM, Dua P, Clement C, Lukiw WJ. An evaluation of progressive amyloidogenic and pro-inflammatory change in the primary visual cortex and retina in Alzheimer's disease (AD). Front Neurosci. 2014;8:347.

40. Taylor L, Arner K, Ghosh F. First responders: dynamics of pre-gliotic Muller cell responses in the isolated adult rat retina. Curr Eye Res. 2014;40:1-16.

41. Gorter JA, van Vliet EA, Aronica E, Breit T, Rauwerda H, da Silva FH, Wadman WJ. Potential new antiepileptogenic targets indicated by microarray analysis in a rat model for temporal lobe epilepsy. J Neurosci. 2006;26:11083–110.

42. Motiejunaite R, Kazlauskas A. Pericytes and ocular diseases. Exp Eye Res. 2008;86:171–7.

43. Makita J, Hosoya K, Zhang P, Kador PF. Response of rat retinal capillary pericytes and endothelial cells to glucose. J Ocul Pharmacol Ther. 2011;27:7–15.

44. Sims DE. The pericyte—a review. Tissue Cell. 1986;18:153–74.

45. Buzney SM, Massicotte SJ, Hetu N, Zetter BR. Retinal vascular endothelial cells and pericytes. Differential growth characteristics in vitro. Invest Ophthalmol Vis Sci. 1983;24:470–80.

46. von Tell D, Armulik A, Betsholtz C. Pericytes and vascular stability. Exp Cell Res. 2006;312:623–9.

47. Yamagishi S, Imaizumi T. Pericyte biology and diseases. Int J Tissue React. 2005;27:125–35.

48. Berdahl JP, Fautsch MP, Stinnett SS, Allingham RR. Intracranial pressure in primary open angle glaucoma, normal tension glaucoma, and ocular hypertension: a case-control study. Invest Ophthalmol Vis Sci. 2008;49:5412–8.

49. Weinreb RN, Aung T, Medeiros FA. The pathophysiology and treatment of glaucoma: a review. Jama. 2014;311:1901–11.

50. Pang JJ, Frankfort BJ, Gross RL, Wu SM. Elevated intraocular pressure decreases response sensitivity of inner retinal neurons in experimental glaucoma mice. Proc Natl Acad Sci U S A. 2015;112:2593–8.

51. Park HY, Kim JH, Park CK. Alterations of the synapse of the inner retinal layers after chronic intraocular pressure elevation in glaucoma animal model. Mol Brain. 2014;7:53.

52. Pogue AI, Hill JM, Lukiw WJ. MicroRNA (miRNA): sequence and stability, viroid-like properties, and disease association in the CNS. Brain Res. 2014;1584:73–9.

53. Fukuda T, Oguni H, Yanagaki S, Fukuyama Y, Kogure M, Shimizu H, Oda M. Chronic localized encephalitis (Rasmussen's syndrome) preceded by ipsilateral uveitis: a case report. Epilepsia. 1994;35:1328–31.

54. Fuhrmann M, Bittner T, Jung CK, Burgold S, Page RM, Mitteregger G, Haass C, LaFerla FM, Kretzschmar H, Herms J. Microglial Cx3cr1 knockout prevents neuron loss in a mouse model of Alzheimer's disease. Nat Neurosci. 2010;13:411–3.

55. Noda M, Doi Y, Liang J, Kawanokuchi J, Sonobe Y, Takeuchi H, Mizuno T, Suzumura A. Fractalkine attenuates excito-neurotoxicity via microglial clearance of damaged neurons and antioxidant enzyme heme oxygenase-1 expression. J Biol Chem. 2011;286:2308–19.

56. Yeo SI, Kim JE, Ryu HJ, Seo CH, Lee BC, Choi IG, Kim DS, Kang TC. The roles of fractalkine/CX3CR1 system in neuronal death following pilocarpine-induced status epilepticus. J Neuroimmunol. 2011;234:93–102.

57. Roseti C, Fucile S, Lauro C, Martinello K, Bertollini C, Esposito V, Mascia A, Catalano M, Aronica E, Limatola C, Palma E Fractalkine/CX3CL1 modulates GABAA currents in human temporal lobe epilepsy. Epilepsia. 2013;54:1834–44.

58. Combadiere C, Feumi C, Raoul W, Keller N, Rodero M, Pezard A, Lavalette S, Houssier M, Jonet L, Picard E, et al. CX3CR1-dependent subretinal microglia cell accumulation is associated with cardinal features of age-related macular degeneration. J Clin Invest. 2007;117:2920–8.

59. Bosco A, Romero CO, Breen KT, Chagovetz AA, Steele MR, Ambati BK, Vetter ML. Neurodegeneration severity can be predicted from early microglia alterations monitored in vivo in a mouse model of chronic glaucoma. Dis Model Mech. 2015;8:443–55.

60. Wang K, Peng B, Lin B. Fractalkine receptor regulates microglial neurotoxicity in an experimental mouse glaucoma model. Glia. 2014;62:1943–54.

61. Ekdahl CT. Microglial activation—tuning and pruning adult neurogenesis. Front Pharmacol. 2012;3:41.

62. Dutca LM, Stasheff SF, Hedberg-Buenz A, Rudd DS, Batra N, Blodi FR, Yorek MS, Yin T, Shankar M, Herlein JA, et al. Early detection of subclinical visual damage after blast-mediated TBI enables prevention of chronic visual deficit by treatment with P7C3-S243. Invest Ophthalmol Vis Sci. 2014;55:8330–41.

63. Thompson S, Blodi FR, Lee S, Welder CR, Mullins RF, Tucker BA, Stasheff SF, Stone EM. Photoreceptor cells with profound structural deficits can support useful vision in mice. Invest Ophthalmol Vis Sci. 2014;55:1859–66.

# 5

# Everolimus is better than rapamycin in attenuating neuroinflammation in kainic acid-induced seizures

Ming-Tao Yang[1,2†], Yi-Chin Lin[3,4†], Whae-Hong Ho[3], Chao-Lin Liu[5,6] and Wang-Tso Lee[3,4*]

## Abstract

**Background:** Microglia is responsible for neuroinflammation, which may aggravate brain injury in diseases like epilepsy. Mammalian target of rapamycin (mTOR) kinase is related to microglial activation with subsequent neuroinflammation. In the present study, rapamycin and everolimus, both as mTOR inhibitors, were investigated in models of kainic acid (KA)-induced seizure and lipopolysaccharide (LPS)-induced neuroinflammation.

**Methods:** In vitro, we treated BV2 cells with KA and LPS. In vivo, KA was used to induce seizures on postnatal day 25 in B6.129P-Cx3cr1[tm1Litt]/J mice. Rapamycin and everolimus were evaluated in their modulation of neuroinflammation detected by real-time PCR, Western blotting, and immunostaining.

**Results:** Everolimus was significantly more effective than rapamycin in inhibiting iNOS and mTOR signaling pathways in both models of neuroinflammation (LPS) and seizure (KA). Everolimus significantly attenuated the mRNA expression of iNOS by LPS and nitrite production by KA and LPS than that by rapamycin. Only everolimus attenuated the mRNA expression of mTOR by LPS and KA treatment. In the present study, we also found that the modulation of mTOR under LPS and KA treatment was not mediated by Akt pathway but was primarily mediated by ERK phosphorylation, which was more significantly attenuated by everolimus. This inhibition of ERK phosphorylation and microglial activation in the hippocampus by everolimus was also confirmed in KA-treated mice.

**Conclusions:** Rapamycin and everolimus can block the activation of inflammation-related molecules and attenuated the microglial activation. Everolimus had better efficacy than rapamycin, possibly mediated by the inhibition of ERK phosphorylation. Taken together, mTOR inhibitor can be a potential pharmacological target of anti-inflammation and seizure treatment.

**Keywords:** Epilepsy, ERK, Everolimus, Kainic acid, mTOR, Neuroinflammation, Rapamycin

## Background

Seizure is the clinical manifestation of abnormal, excessive, hypersynchronous discharges of a population of cortical neurons, while epilepsy is a chronic disorder characterized by recurrent unprovoked seizures [1]. Seizure could be initiated by neuronal abnormality as well as by glial activation [2, 3]. Kainic acid (KA), an agonist of kainate glutamate receptors, can cause overstimulation of glutamate receptors and subsequent neuronal excitotoxicity and neuronal death [4]. KA-induced seizure model is one of the most commonly used animal models of seizures [5].

Both clinical and experimental findings have demonstrated that inflammation may play a role in the generation and modulation of seizures and epilepsies, and using anti-inflammatory drugs, such as IL-1β blockers, has been proposed as a potential strategy for seizure therapy [6, 7]. KA administration could induce microglial activation and cytokines production, such as TNF-α, IL-1β, IL-12, and IL-18 [4]. The nucleotide-binding oligomerization domain-like receptor family pyrin domain-containing 3 (NLRP3) inflammasome triggers the transformation of procaspase-1 to caspase-1, as well as the production and

* Correspondence: leeped@hotmail.com
†Equal contributors
3Department of Pediatric Neurology, National Taiwan University Children's Hospital, No. 7 Chung-Shan South Road, Taipei 100, Taiwan
4Graduate Institute of Brain and Mind Science, National Taiwan University, Taipei, Taiwan
Full list of author information is available at the end of the article

secretion of mature IL-1β and IL-18 [8]. IL-1β and NLRP3 levels increased after amygdala kindling-induced status epilepticus, and inhibition of NLRP3 provided neuroprotection in rats following status epilepticus [9].

In addition to inflammation, nitric oxide (NO) plays an essential role in the epileptogenesis and excitotoxicity in the brain [10, 11]. Nitric oxide synthase (NOS) activation and NO production were observed in animal models of seizure, including the KA model [10–12]. Aminoguanidine, a selective inducible NOS (iNOS) inhibitor, attenuated KA-induced neuronal death [13], which proves the relationship between iNOS and KA-induced excitotoxicity.

The mammalian target of rapamycin (mTOR), a protein kinase, is part of two larger signaling complexes, mTORC1 and mTORC2. mTORC1, sensitive to the inhibition by rapamycin, is regulated by the upstream Akt pathway in anabolic states and by the AMPK pathway in catabolic states [14]. mTOR signaling pathway has been found to influence the immune response [15], tumorigenesis [16], brain development [17], and epilepsy [14]. Regarding immune response, mTOR is implicated in the regulation of both innate and adaptive immune responses [15]. Rapamycin (or sirolimus), the prototype mTOR inhibitor, enhanced the anti-inflammatory activities of regulatory T cells, decreased the production of proinflammatory cytokines and chemokines by macrophages and microglia, and thus attenuated secondary injury after focal ischemia in rats [18]. Several animal and human studies have shown that mTOR activation resulted in neuroexcitability, seizure, and epilepsy [14, 19], which encouraged researchers to use mTOR inhibitors in seizure therapy [14, 19, 20]. Everolimus is a second-generation rapamycin derivative. Although having a similar structure, the two drugs exhibit significant differences in their pharmacokinetic, pharmacodynamic, and toxicodynamic properties, resulting in distinct clinical profiles [21, 22]. Everolimus and rapamycin share a central macrolide structure and differ in the functional groups added at C40 [22]. The functional groups added at C40 affect their pharmacokinetics, e.g., bioavailability, half-life, and distribution [22]. Everolimus has higher potency of interacting with the mTORC 2 than rapamycin [21]. Everolimus demonstrated better ability than rapamycin in treating subependymal giant cell astrocytomas and other tuberous sclerosis (TSC) manifestations, based on more robust clinical trial experience [22]. However, to our knowledge, their efficacy in seizure treatment had never been investigated.

In this study, we used BV2 microglial cell line and B6.129P-Cx3cr1[tm1Litt]/J mice to investigate the in vitro and in vivo effects of rapamycin and everolimus on neuroinflammation. We hypothesize that their different effects on neuroinflammation may contribute to their different anti-seizure efficacies.

## Methods

### BV2 microglial cell line

BV2 cell line is the most frequently used substitute for primary microglia and has been used in studies related to neurodegenerative disorders [23]. In the present study, BV2 cells were cultured in DMEM (Corning, Manassas, VA, USA), supplemented with 10% fetal bovine serum, 1% non-essential amino acids, and 1% antibiotics (penicillin 100 U/mL, streptomycin 100 μg/mL), and were kept in an incubator at 37 °C, 5% $CO_2$, and 95% relative humidity.

### Animals

B6.129P-Cx3cr1[tm1Litt]/J mice (The Jackson laboratory) possess microglia with a fluorescent protein, which expresses fluorescence when the microglia are activated by stimuli such as inflammation and damage. The mice were raised in the National Laboratory Animal Center (NLAC) in Taiwan and housed and maintained on a 12-h-on/12-h-off light/dark cycle. All of the animals were allowed free access to food and water. The maintenance of the mice and the experiments were conducted in accordance with the Guide for the Care and Use of Laboratory Animals [24] and the study was approved by the animal ethical committee of Medical College of National Taiwan University.

### Chemicals and drugs

Lipopolysaccharide (LPS), KA, minocycline, everolimus, and rapamycin were purchased from Sigma-Aldrich (St. Louis, MO, USA). The primary antibodies Akt and GAPDH used for Western blotting were purchased from Santa Cruz Biotechnology (Dallas, TX, USA) and Genetex (Irvine, CA, USA), respectively. The other primary antibodies, including ERK and phosphor-ERK, used for Western blotting were purchased from Cell Signaling (Danvers, MA, USA).

### MTT assay for cell viability

Before the nitrite assay and the qPCR assay, the MTT (3-(4,5-dimethylthiazol-2-yl)-2,5-diphenyltetrazolium bromide) assay was performed to assess whether the drugs and the combination of drugs at the specific concentrations we used affect the cell viability. BV2 cells at a concentration of $1.5 \times 10^5$ cells/well were seeded into 24-well plates overnight. After treatment with different drugs for 24 h, MTT (Sigma-Aldrich, St. Louis, MO, USA) was added to each well at the final concentration of 0.5 mg/mL. After 3 h of incubation, the medium was removed and 500 μL of DMSO was added to each well. After 15 min of shaking for thorough mixing of DMSO and formazan, 200 μL of the mixture from each well was collected and placed into 96-well plates. The optical density was measured at 570 nm using a spectrophotometer. The amount of formazan formed directly correlates well with the number of live cells in the culture.

## Nitrite assay

Nitrite is a metabolite of NO, and NO production can be measured through quantification analysis of nitrite production [25]. BV2 cells at a concentration of $1.5 \times 10^5$ cells/well were seeded into 24-well plates overnight. After treatment with different drugs for 24 h, 100 µL of medium from each well was collected and placed into 96-well plates, mixed with 100 µL of Griess reagent (Sigma-Aldrich, St. Louis, MO, USA) and shaken for 15 min to measure the nitrite amount. The optical density was measured at 562 nm using a spectrophotometer. The amount of nitrite in medium correlates well with the NO production by the cells.

## Real-time PCR

BV2 cells at a concentration of $4.5 \times 10^5$ cells/3 mL were seeded into 40-mm dishes overnight. After treatment with different drugs for 24 h, total RNA was extracted by TRIZOL, and reverse transcribed to cDNA using the RevertAid H Minus First Strand cDNA Synthesis Kit (Thermo Scientific, Waltham, MA, USA). For real-time PCR, Maxima SYBR Green qPCR Master Mix (Thermo Scientific, Waltham, MA, USA) was used. For detecting iNOS, mTOR, NLRP3, and IL-1β level, we used the following primer sequences: iNOS, forward 5′-CTG CAT GGA ACA GTA TAA GGC AAA C-3′ and reverse 5′-CAG ACA GTT TCT GGT CGA TGT CAT GA-3′; mTOR, forward 5′-ACT GAG GAG GGA GAA CAG CA-3′ and reverse 5′-TGG CTC CAT CTG CTA GTG TG-3′; NLRP3, forward 5′-AGA GCC TAC AGT TGG GTG AAA TG-3′ and reverse 5′-CCA CGC CTA CCA GGA AAT CTC-3′; IL-1β, forward 5′-CCC TGC AGC TGG AGA GTG TGG A-3′ and reverse 5′-TGT GCT CTG CTT GTG AGG TGC TG-3′; and β-actin, forward 5′-CTA AGG CCA ACC GTG AAA AG-3′ and reverse 5′-ACC AGA GGC ATA CAG GGA CA-3′. Relative amounts of the indicated mRNA levels were determined by the $2^{-\Delta\Delta CT}$ method, normalizing with β-actin levels.

## KA-induced seizures and the two-hit seizure model

The severity of seizures induced by KA can be distinguished using the modified Racine's scale based on the abnormal behavior of mice as follows: stage I—chewing; stage II—head nodding; stage III—unilateral forelimb clonus; stage IV—bilateral forelimb clonus; stage V—bilateral forelimb clonus and falling; stage VI—running or bouncing seizure; stage VII—tonic hindlimb extension; and stage VIII—tonic hindlimb extension culminating in death [26–28]. The behavior from stage III to stage VIII can be recognized in the present mouse model.

The rearing and falling behavior of stage V can be easily demonstrated in mice. Mice exhibiting at least stage V were included in this study due to microglial activation and neuronal loss in this stage [28–32]. The latency was recorded when mice first showed rearing behavior of stage V in this study. Koh et al. [33] developed a two-hit seizure model, demonstrating that "an early-life seizure permanently decreases seizure threshold and increases the susceptibility to seizure-induced cell death in adulthood". In addition, they showed that anti-inflammatory therapy with minocycline after the initial status epilepticus blocked the epileptogenic process and mitigated the long-term damaging effects of early-life seizures [34].

Based on the 7-day protocol of Koh et al. with some modification, in this study, the postnatal day 25 (P25) mice received intra-peritoneal injection of KA 25 mg/kg on days 1 and 7. The durations from injection to stage V seizures on days 1 and 7, which were defined as latency 1 and 2, respectively, were recorded. Three hours after the seizure onset on day 1 and the following days until day 6, mice were injected with everolimus or PBS as control q.d. intraperitoneally. Mice were divided into the following three groups: KpK group, KA injection on days 1 and 7 and PBS from day 1 to day 6; KeK group, KA injection on days 1 and 7 and everolimus from day 1 to day 6; and PpP group as controls, PBS injection throughout the experiment. A 14-day protocol was followed with the same procedures: the first and second KA injection on days 1 and 14 and everolimus or PBS from day 1 to day 13.

## Quantification of microglial activation

Five to six mice were analyzed per group. Mice were sacrificed and perfused with PBS and 4% paraformaldehyde/0.1 M sodium phosphate buffer. The brains were harvested and kept in 4% paraformaldehyde/0.1 M sodium phosphate buffer for post-fixation. Before slicing the brains, they were kept in 30% sucrose/4% paraformaldehyde solution. Then the brains were cut into 30-µm horizontal slices until the hippocampus was revealed. The slices were then collected every six slices, and at least six slices were gathered for each brain. Images of the hippocampus CA1 and CA3 regions were taken by a fluorescence microscope and a camera under ×10 objective. All images were captured under identical settings. The activated microglial cells exhibited fluorescence. The number of activated microglial cells in each slice was counted within the CA1 and CA3 regions in each animal. The mean number of activated microglial cells was calculated by the Image J software. Data were expressed as the mean of activated microglial cells in CA1 or CA3 regions per slice in each animal.

## Western blotting

For in vitro experiment, the BV2 cells were seeded at a concentration of $1.5 \times 10^6$ cells/10 mL into 100-mm dishes overnight. After treatment with different drugs for 24 h, the cell lysates were collected for protein analysis. For in vivo experiment, 5 to 11 mice were sacrificed 24 h after KA injection on day 7, and the hippocampi were resected and stored in liquid nitrogen. After homogenization, protein expression was analyzed by Western blotting. After electrophoresis and transfer to nitrocellulose membranes, the membranes were blocked with 5% bovine serum albumin (BSA) in PBST (PBS and 0.05% tween-20) for 30 min, incubated with primary antibodies in 5% BSA solution overnight, and then incubated with secondary antibodies in 5% BSA solution for 1 h. Signals were visualized using the ECL reagent and a chemiluminescence and fluorescence image analyzer. ImageJ software was used to subtract background and to perform densitometry.

## Statistical analysis

For in vitro and in vivo experiments, one-way ANOVA test was used to analyze cell viability, nitrite production, mRNA levels, and protein phosphorylation among the different treatment groups, with post hoc comparison by LSD test. Seizure severity at days 1 and 7 was compared using chi-square test. All data were analyzed using IBM® SPSS® Statistics software version 19.0 (IBM Inc., Somers, NY, USA). A $p$ value <0.05 was considered to be statistically significant.

## Results

### No effect on cell viability under LPS and KA treatment for different drugs in BV2 cell line

The BV2 cells were treated with KA (150 μM), LPS (500 ng/mL), minocycline (1 ng/mL), everolimus (1 nM), rapamycin (1 nM), KA with minocycline, KA with everolimus, KA with rapamycin, LPS with minocycline, LPS with everolimus, and LPS with rapamycin. After 24 h of treatment, all combinations of the drugs showed no effect on the viability of BV2 cells.

### Reduction of nitrite production by everolimus under both LPS and KA treatment, while by rapamycin only under KA treatment in BV2 cell line

As mentioned above, NO plays an essential role in the epileptogenesis and excitotoxicity in the brain [10, 11]. We therefore measured nitrite, a metabolite of NO. Previous studies have shown that both LPS and KA increased nitrite production in microglia [11, 35]. Similarly, LPS and KA significantly increased nitrite production in BV2 cell line in this study ($p < 0.001$ and $p = 0.040$, respectively) (Fig. 1). Minocycline and everolimus significantly attenuated nitrite production under

both LPS and KA treatment ($p < 0.05$ and $p < 0.001$, respectively). However, rapamycin inhibited nitrite production only under KA treatment ($p = 0.001$) and did not attenuate the increased nitrite production stimulated by LPS in the BV2 cell line.

### Inhibition of iNOS mRNA production under both LPS and KA treatment by minocycline, everolimus, and rapamycin in BV2 cell line

Both everolimus and rapamycin attenuated nitrite production under KA treatment, while only everolimus attenuated nitrite production under LPS treatment. We further investigated their effects on the mRNA levels of IL-1β, NLRP3, mTOR, and iNOS. LPS, a component of the outer membrane of Gram-negative bacteria, can elicit a strong immune response and has been commonly used in animal experiments of inflammation. LPS significantly increased the mRNA expression levels of IL-1β, NLRP3, and iNOS ($p < 0.001$), and marginally increased expression of mTOR mRNA ($p = 0.058$) (Fig. 2). Under LPS treatment, minocycline, rapamycin, and everolimus, all inhibited the mRNA expression of iNOS (Fig. 2d), and the inhibition by everolimus was significantly better compared to that by rapamycin ($p < 0.001$). KA alone significantly increased the mRNA expression of mTOR and iNOS ($p = 0.047$ and $p < 0.001$, respectively). The elevated mRNA expression of iNOS

**Fig. 1** Minocycline and everolimus reduced nitrite production under both LPS and kainic acid treatment, while rapamycin only reduced nitrite production under kainic acid treatment in BV2 cell line. After treatment with different drugs for 24 hours, nitrite was assayed. Both LPS ($n = 10$) and kainic acid (KA, $n = 4$) increased nitrite production significantly. Minocycline (LM and KM groups, $n = 5$ and 4, respectively) and everolimus (LE and KE groups, $n = 10$ and 5, respectively) attenuated the increased nitrite levels under both LPS and KA treatment,. Rapamycin, however, attenuated the elevated nitrite level only under KA treatment (KR group, $n = 5$), and it had no effect on the nitrite level under LPS treatment (LR group, $n = 5$). ***$p < 0.001$; *$p < 0.05$, compared with the control group (Ctl, $n = 17$). ###$p < 0.001$; ##$p < 0.01$; #$p < 0.05$, compared with the LPS and KA groups, respectively. Data are presented as mean ± SEM. *Ctl* control, *Eve/E* everolimus, *KA/K* kainic acid, *LPS/L* lipopolysaccharide, *Min/M* minocycline, *Rap/R* rapamycin

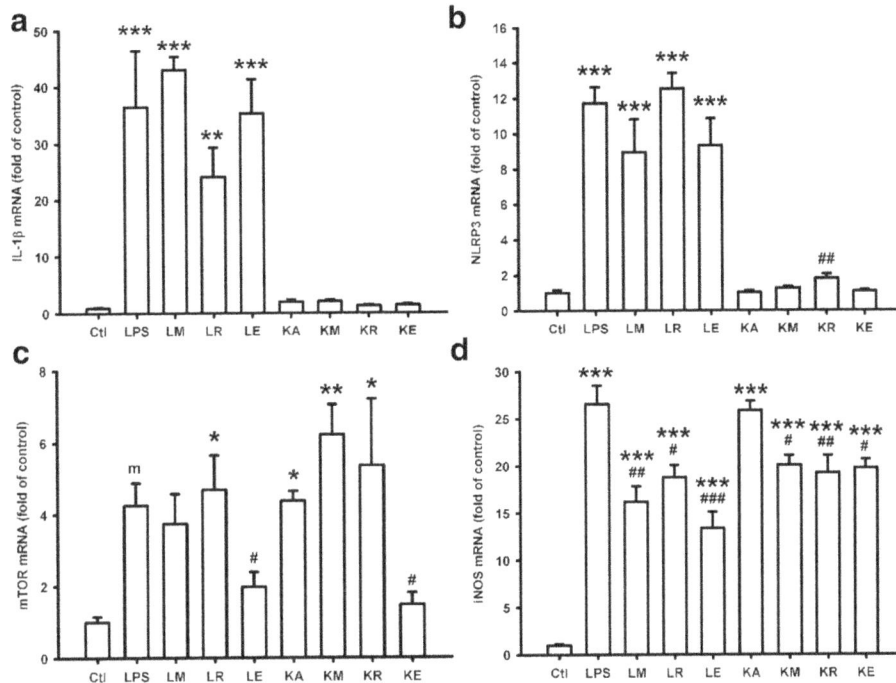

**Fig. 2** Inhibition of inflammation-related mRNAs and iNOS mRNA production under both LPS and kainic acid treatment by minocycline, everolimus, and rapamycin in BV2 cell line. Lipopolysaccharide (LPS) increased IL-1β, NLRP3, mTOR, and iNOS mRNA production (**a–d**), and kainic acid (KA) increased only mTOR and iNOS mRNA production (**c, d**). **a** Minocyclin, rapamycin, and everolimus had no effect on IL-1β mRNA production under both LPS and KA treatment. **b** Rapamycin increased NLRP3 mRNA production under KA treatment significantly, but not under LPS treatment. Minocyclin and everolimus had no effect on NLRP3 mRNA production. **c** Everolimus decreased mTOR mRNA production under both LPS and KA treatment, while minocyclin and rapamycin had no effect on it. **d** Minocyclin, rapamycin, and everolimus all attenuated iNOS mRNA production under both LPS and KA treatment. $n = 4$ for each group. ***$p < 0.001$; **$p < 0.01$; *$p < 0.05$; m: $p < 0.1$, compared with the control group (Ctl). ###$p < 0.001$; ##$p < 0.01$; #$p < 0.05$, compared with the LPS and KA groups. Data are presented as mean ± SEM. *Ctl* control, *E* everolimus, *KA/K* kainic acid, *LPS/L* lipopolysaccharide, *M* minocycline, *R* rapamycin

stimulated by KA was significantly attenuated by minocycline, rapamycin, and everolimus. However, only everolimus attenuated the mRNA expression of mTOR under both LPS and KA treatment (Fig. 2c, $p = 0.021$ and $p = 0.034$, respectively), and rapamycin did not inhibit mRNA expression of mTOR under both LPS and KA treatment. However, both drugs had no effect on IL-1β expression, and rapamycin increased the mRNA expression of NLRP3 under KA treatment (Fig. 2b, $p = 0.009$), which may aggravate the neuroinflammation.

### Decreased ERK phosphorylation, but not Akt phosphorylation by everolimus under both LPS and KA treatment, while that by minocycline and rapamycin only under LPS treatment in BV2 cell line

Rapamycin and its analogs, e.g., everolimus, bind to FK506-binding protein 12 (FKBP12), form a ternary complex with mTORC1, and thus allosterically inhibit the functioning and downstream signaling of mTOR [36]. Interestingly, everolimus inhibited the mRNA expression of mTOR under both LPS and KA treatment in the present study, while rapamycin did not. mTOR expression is regulated by the upstream Akt pathway in

anabolic states and by the AMPK pathway in catabolic states [14]. Therefore, we further investigated the influence of Akt and ERK phosphorylation by rapamycin and everolimus in the BV2 cell line. As shown in Fig 3, there was no statistically significant effect of rapamycin or everolimus treatment on Akt phosphorylation. In contrast, monotherapy with everolimus, minocycline, or rapamycin inhibited ERK phosphorylation under both LPS and KA treatment, and the effect of everolimus on the inhibition was most significant compared to those of minocycline and rapamycin (Fig. 3a, $p < 0.001$).

### Change of seizure latency after treatment with KA and everolimus

To investigate the effect of KA and everolimus treatment on the seizure latency, B6.129P-Cx3cr1[tm1Litt]/J mice, which express fluorescence when the microglial cells are activated, were used in this study. KA was administered at days 1 and 7 for the KpK group. For the KeK group, everolimus (1 mg/kg/day) was also injected daily for 7 days. The seizure staging for all mice were recorded after injection. All mice in KpK group at most reached stage V in days 1 and 7. In contrast, 4 of 12 mice in KeK

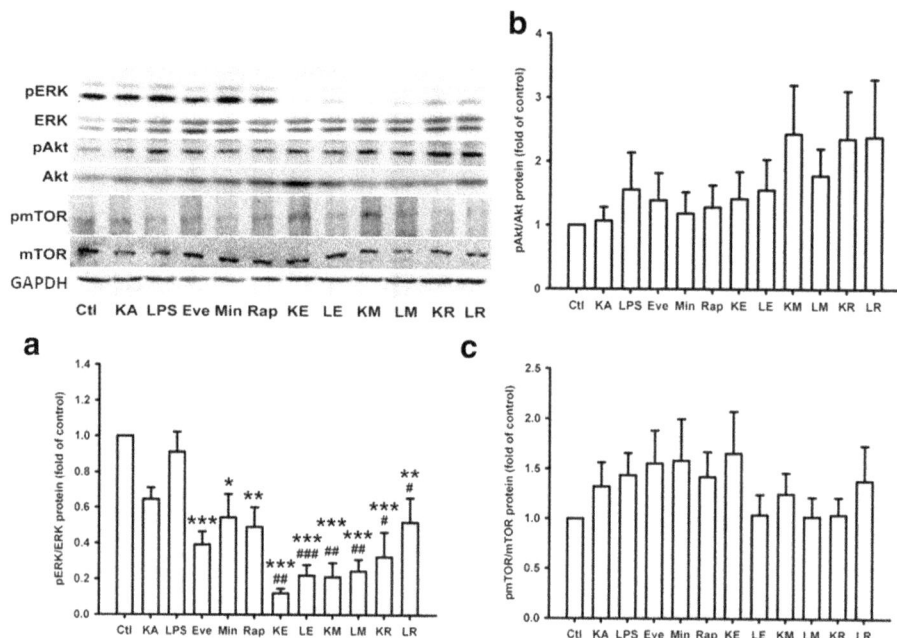

**Fig. 3** Decreased ERK phosphorylation by everolimus, minocyclin, and rapamycin under both LPS and kainic acid treatment in BV2 cell line. **a** After both LPS and kainic acid (KA) treatment for 24 h, ERK phosphorylation was attenuated significantly by everolimus (LE and KE groups), minocycline (LM and KM groups), and rapamycin (LR and KR groups), while everolimus performed best. **b, c** No effect on Akt and mTOR phosphorylation by everolimus, minocycline, and rapamycin was noted. $n = 5$ for each group. ***$p < 0.001$; **$p < 0.01$;*$p < 0.05$, compared with the control group (Ctl). ##$p < 0.01$; #$p < 0.05$, compared with the LPS and KA groups. Data are presented as mean ± SEM. *Ctl* control, *Eve/E* everolimus, *KA/K* kainic acid, *LPS/L* lipopolysaccharide, *Min/M* minocycline, *Rap/R* rapamycin

group reached stage VI at day 1, while no mice in KeK group reached stage VI at day 7 ($p = 0.047$). The seizure latency to stage V after the first dose and second dose of KA was $2200 \pm 874$ s and $1940 \pm 450$ s in the KpK group ($n = 9$), and $1909 \pm 363$ s and $2287 \pm 706$ s in the KeK group ($n = 12$), respectively ($p = 0.077$) (Fig. 4). Although there was no statistical significance in seizure latency, treatment with everolimus tended to prolong

the seizure latency to stage V and attenuated seizure severity.

### Significantly decreased ERK phosphorylation by everolimus in the animal model of KA-induced seizures

To support our in vitro finding, we investigated the effect of everolimus on Akt and ERK phosphorylation by applying the two-hit seizure model of KA in mice [33].

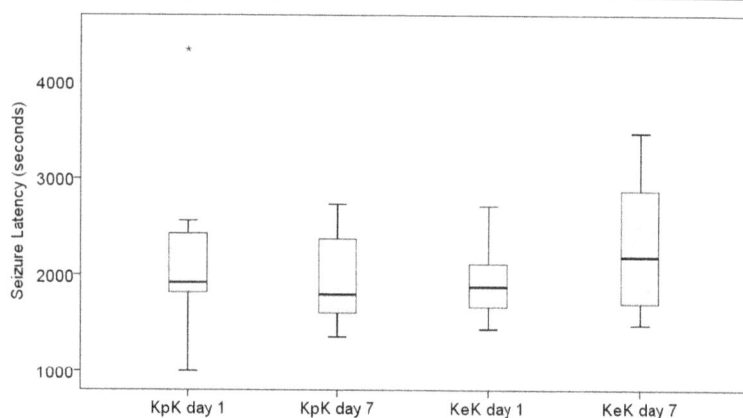

**Fig. 4** Boxplots of seizure latency to stage V in days 1 and 7 for KpK and KeK groups, showing the relative prolonged seizure latency to stage V in day 7 for KeK group

The two-hit seizure model of KA i.p. injection at days 1 and 7 significantly increased ERK phosphorylation ($p = 0.004$) and mTOR phosphorylation ($p = 0.034$) in the hippocampus of mice in the KpK group (Fig. 5 a, c). Compared with the KpK group, everolimus significantly inhibited ERK phosphorylation similar to the results of the in vitro studies (Fig. 5a, KeK group, $p = 0.048$). However, there was no significant difference in ERK phosphorylation in control group and KeK group ($p = 0.167$). In contrast, the two-hit seizure model of KA injection did not increase Akt phosphorylation significantly (Fig. 5b, $p = 0.135$).

### Treatment with everolimus decreased the microglial activation in the hippocampus under KA treatment

To investigate the effect of everolimus treatment on microglial activation in the hippocampus (both CA1 and CA3 regions), we further counted the activated microglial cells in the KpK and KeK groups at day 15 after treatment with KA for two times. We found that the number of activated microglial cells in the CA1 and CA3 regions was statistically significantly higher in the KpK groups than in the KeK group. The mean number of activated microglial cells in CA1 and CA3 regions per slice in the KpK and KeK groups was $51.8 \pm 22.1$ vs.

$15.1 \pm 5.1$ in CA1 ($p = 0.009$) and $35.7 \pm 6.2$ vs. $9.5 \pm 2.2$ in CA3 regions, respectively ($p < 0.001$). This result indicated that everolimus can significantly downregulate the activation of microglial cells in the hippocampus of mice with KA-induced seizures.

### Discussion

Several animal and human studies have demonstrated that mTOR activation can result in neuroexcitability, seizure, and epilepsy [14, 19]. Therefore, mTOR inhibitors have been applied in seizure therapy. Although both rapamycin and everolimus are mTOR inhibitors, the present study showed that both drugs had differential effects on nitrite production, mRNA expression of iNOS and mTOR, and ERK phosphorylation (Fig. 6). Both drugs had no effect on IL-1$\beta$ expression while rapamycin increased NLRP3 expression, which may aggravate the neuroinflammation. Everolimus was significantly more effective than rapamycin in inhibiting iNOS and mTOR signaling pathways in both models of neuroinflammation (LPS) and seizure (KA). In the iNOS pathway, everolimus attenuated the iNOS mRNA expression stimulated by LPS and nitrite production by KA and LPS more significantly than rapamycin. In the mTOR pathway, only everolimus attenuated the mTOR mRNA expression

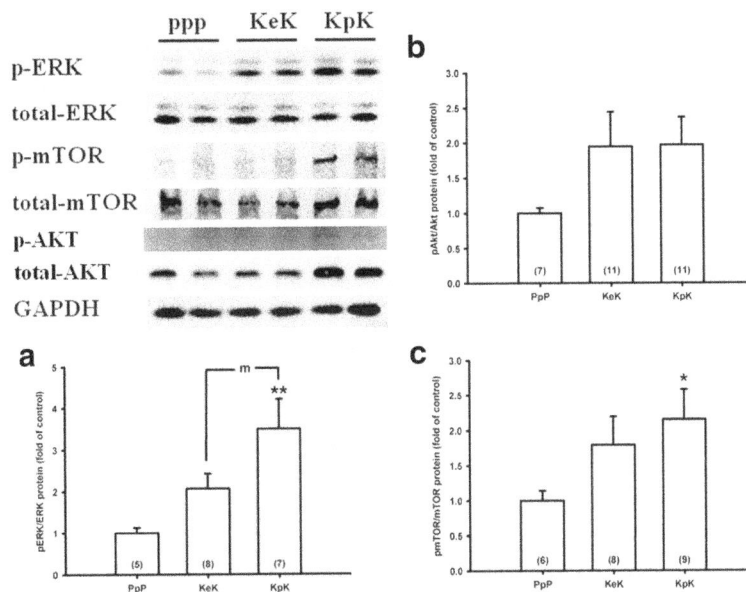

**Fig. 5** Decreased ERK phosphorylation by everolimus significantly in the animal model of kainic acid-induced seizures. B6.129P-Cx3cr1[tm1Litt]/J mice received kainic acid (KA) i.p. injection on day 1 and day 7 (two-hit seizure model), and received i.p. injection of PBS (KpK group) or everolimus (KeK group) during day 1 to day 6. Sham mice received PBS during day 1 to day 7 (PpP group). Twenty-four hours after KA injection on day 7, mice were sacrificed, the hippocampus was resected, and the protein expression was analyzed by Western blotting. **a** KA injection twice significantly increased ERK phosphorylation, which was attenuated by everolimus. **b, c** Everolimus did not decrease Akt and mTOR phosphorylation after repeated KA injection. Bars depict mean ± S.E.M. The number of mice used in each experiment was shown in the bottom of each bar figure. *$p = 0.034$ and **$p = 0.004$, compared with the sham group; m: $p = 0.048$, compared between KeK and KpK groups

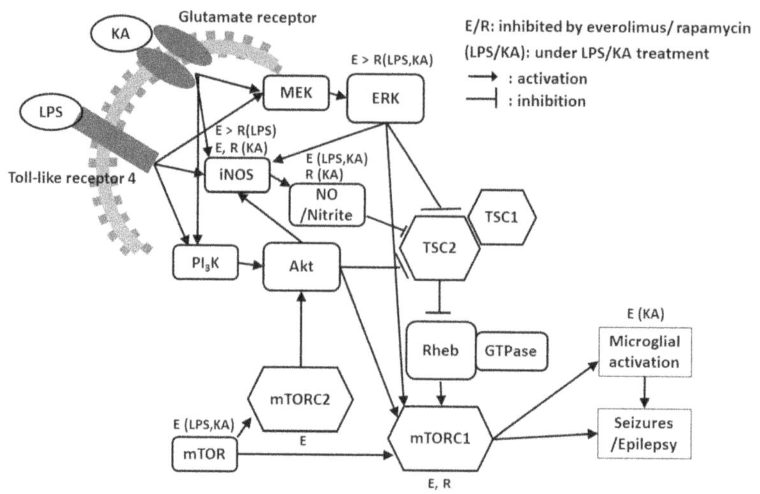

**Fig. 6** A summary of the effects of rapamycin and everolimus on signaling pathways involved in neuroinflammation and seizure. The direct inhibition of mTORC1 and mTORC2 by rapamycin and everolimus is from previous studies. The other effects of rapamycin and everolimus depicted in this figure are based on this study. *E* everolimus, *ERK* extracellular signal-regulated kinases, *iNOS* inducible nitric oxide synthase, *KA* kainic acid, *LPS* lipopolysaccharide, *mTORC1/2* mechanistic target of rapamycin complex 1/2, *NO* nitric oxide, *R* rapamycin, *Rheb* Ras homolog-enriched in brain, *TSC1/2* tuberous sclerosis complex 1/2

induced by LPS and KA treatment. We also found that the modulation of mTOR under LPS and KA treatment was not mediated by Akt pathway but may be primarily mediated by ERK phosphorylation, which was attenuated more significantly by everolimus. Everolimus was also shown to inhibit ERK phosphorylation and microglial activation in the hippocampus of KA-treated mice.

Although not involved in regulating KA seizure generation and propagation, NO has been shown to be involved in status epilepticus-induced neuronal degeneration [11]. Rapamycin has been shown to reduce the mRNA levels of iNOS in the astrocytes under treatment with cytokines or LPS plus INFg [37]. Everolimus has also been shown to affect NOS activity and NOS2 expression, thereby reducing microglial proliferation [38]. The present study demonstrated that both rapamycin and everolimus can decrease iNOS mRNA and nitrite production after LPS or KA treatment in the microglia, suggesting that the neuroprotective role of mTOR inhibitors may partially arise from iNOS inhibition. However, our data also showed that everolimus was significantly more effective than rapamycin in the inhibition of iNOS and nitrite production.

The reason why rapamycin increased NLRP3 mRNA in the present study was not clear. NO has been reported to suppress NLRP3 inflammasome activation under LPS treatment [39]. In our study under KA treatment, rapamycin inhibited iNOS mRNA and NO/nitrite production, which may contribute to the increase of NLRP3 mRNA (Fig. 2). However, everolimus also inhibited iNOS mRNA and NO/nitrite production without increase of NLRP3 mRNA, which needs further investigation.

mTOR is part of two larger signaling complexes, mTORC1 and mTORC2. The primary pharmacodynamic effect of mTOR inhibitors is selective binding to FKBP12 and subsequent association with and inhibition of mTORC 1 [22]. Everolimus exhibited higher potency of interacting with mTORC 2 than rapamycin [21] and was shown to be better than rapamycin in treating subependymal giant cell astrocytomas and other TSC manifestations [22]. Interestingly, our study also showed that everolimus decreased the mRNA levels of mTOR under LPS and KA treatment compared with rapamycin. This finding may explain the higher potency of everolimus in inhibiting mTORC2 than that of rapamycin.

mTOR is regulated by the upstream Akt pathway and the AMPK pathway [14]. Inhibition of ERK phosphorylation by everolimus observed in the present study is consistent with an earlier study [40]. In a previous study of anti-HLA antibody-mediated endothelial cell signaling, everolimus was shown to be more effective in inhibiting mTORC2 and thus more effective in preventing Akt phosphorylation and ERK phosphorylation, an ability that rapamycin lacked [40]. ERK pathway plays a well-known role in neuroinflammation and neurodegeneration [41]. Therefore, everolimus may play a protective role in neuroinflammation via inhibiting ERK phosphorylation. Interestingly, in *N*-methyl-D-aspartic acid-induced retinal neurotoxicity in rats, the protective effect of everolimus was mediated partially by the activation of ERK pathway [42]. Nevertheless, both anti-inflammation and neuroprotection by everolimus are beneficial.

Our study showed that everolimus reduced neuroinflammation more effectively than rapamycin. mTORC1 and mTORC2 play different roles in inflammation [43, 44]. mTORC2 exerts a pro-inflammatory effect, while mTORC1 exerts some anti-inflammatory effect [44]. Therefore, everolimus, by inhibiting mTORC2, may be more effective than rapamycin in inhibiting neuroinflammation. Similarly, a recent study showed that a dual mTORC1 and mTORC2 inhibitor was more effective against neuroinflammation than rapamycin [45]. In addition, as shown in the present study and previous studies, everolimus, but not rapamycin, can inhibit ERK phosphorylation [21]. This inhibition of ERK pathway may augment the anti-inflammatory activity of everolimus.

Other mechanisms except for attenuating neuroinflammation may also play a role in anti-seizure activity of mTOR inhibitors. Activation of the mTOR pathway may trigger several downstream cellular and molecular events in brain leading to increased neuronal excitability and seizure generation. mTOR pathway is also implicated in epileptogenesis, especially mossy fiber sprouting [46]. Furthermore, the mTOR pathway may be involved in anti-seizure effects of the ketogenic diet and has a close link with nutrient signaling [47]. Therefore, the anti-seizure effect of mTOR inhibitors may arise from multiple mechanisms, and attenuation of neuroinflammation is one of the important mechanisms.

In this study, we also found that mice treated with everolimus following the initial seizure tended to prolong the seizure latency at second KA-induced seizure. Microglial activation with production of proinflammatory cytokines plays important roles in seizure generation [48, 49]. Previous study had shown that KA-induced exaggerated microglial response may increase the susceptibility to the second seizure later in life and produce CNS injury [34, 48, 49]. Therefore, the inhibition of seizure-induced microglial activation may prolong the seizure latency and attenuate the seizure-related CNS damage [50, 51].

## Conclusions
In this study, a direct comparison of rapamycin and everolimus in both cell and animal models of neuroinflammation and seizure was made. Everolimus showed greater inhibition of iNOS mRNA production, nitrite production, and mTOR mRNA production than rapamycin, which may partly arise from the inhibition of ERK phosphorylation. mTOR as a target of anti-epileptic therapy may be a potential pharmacological target of reducing neuroinflammation and deserves more application in the future.

## Abbreviations
BSA: Bovine serum albumin; KA: Kainic acid; LPS: Lipopolysaccharide; mTOR: Mammalian target of rapamycin; NLRP-3: Nucleotide binding and oligomerization domain-like receptor family pyrin domain-containing 3; NO: Nitric oxide; NOS: Nitric oxide synthase

## Funding
The study was supported by Far Eastern Memorial Hospital National Taiwan University Hospital Joint Research Program (Grant No: 103-FTN09 and 104-FTN23).

## Authors' contributions
MT and YC draft the manuscript and performed parts of the data analysis. YC and WH carried out the molecular and other related studies. CL participated in data analysis and manuscript revision. WT designed the experiments, participated in data analysis, draft the manuscript, and revised the manuscript. All authors read and approved the final manuscript.

## Competing interests
The authors declare that they have no competing interests.

## Consent for publication
Not applicable.

## Author details
[1]Department of Pediatrics, Far Eastern Memorial Hospital, New Taipei City, Taiwan. [2]Department of Chemical Engineering and Materials Science, Yuan Ze University, Taoyuan, Taiwan. [3]Department of Pediatric Neurology, National Taiwan University Children's Hospital, No. 7 Chung-Shan South Road, Taipei 100, Taiwan. [4]Graduate Institute of Brain and Mind Science, National Taiwan University, Taipei, Taiwan. [5]Department of Chemical Engineering, Ming Chi University of Technology, New Taipei City, Taiwan. [6]College of Engineering, Chang Gung University, Taoyuan, Taiwan.

## References
1. Wei SH, Lee WT. Comorbidity of childhood epilepsy. J Formos Med Assoc. 2015;114:1031–8.
2. Shapiro LA, Wang L, Ribak CE. Rapid astrocyte and microglial activation following pilocarpine-induced seizures in rats. Epilepsia. 2008;49 Suppl 2:33–41.
3. Wetherington J, Serrano G, Dingledine R. Astrocytes in the epileptic brain. Neuron. 2008;58:168–78.
4. Zhang XM, Zhu J. Kainic Acid-induced neurotoxicity: targeting glial responses and glia-derived cytokines. Curr Neuropharmacol. 2011;9:388–98.
5. Reddy DS, Kuruba R. Experimental models of status epilepticus and neuronal injury for evaluation of therapeutic interventions. Int J Mol Sci. 2013;14:18284–318.
6. Shimada T, Takemiya T, Sugiura H, Yamagata K. Role of inflammatory mediators in the pathogenesis of epilepsy. Mediators Inflamm. 2014;2014:901902.
7. Vezzani A, Friedman A, Dingledine RJ. The role of inflammation in epileptogenesis. Neuropharmacology. 2013;69:16–24.
8. Shao B-Z, Xu Z-q, Han B-Z, Su D-F, Liu C. NLRP3 inflammasome and its inhibitors: a review. Front Pharmacol. 2015;6:262.
9. Meng XF, Tan L, Tan MS, Jiang T, Tan CC, Li MM, Wang HF, Yu JT. Inhibition of the NLRP3 inflammasome provides neuroprotection in rats following amygdala kindling-induced status epilepticus. J Neuroinflammation. 2014;11:212.
10. Murashima YL, Yoshii M, Suzuki J. Role of nitric oxide in the epileptogenesis of EL mice. Epilepsia. 2000;41 Suppl 6:S195–199.
11. Milatovic D, Gupta RC, Dettbarn W-D. Involvement of nitric oxide in kainic acid-induced excitotoxicity in rat brain. Brain Res. 2002;957:330–7.
12. Swamy M, Yusof WR, Sirajudeen KN, Mustapha Z, Govindasamy C. Decreased glutamine synthetase, increased citrulline-nitric oxide cycle activities, and oxidative stress in different regions of brain in epilepsy rat model. J Physiol Biochem. 2011;67:105–13.
13. Byun J-S, Lee S-H, Jeon S-H, Kwon Y-S, Lee HJ, Kim S-S, Kim Y-M, Kim M-J, Chun W. Kainic acid-induced neuronal death is attenuated by

aminoguanidine but aggravated by L-NAME in mouse hippocampus. Korean J Physiol Pharmacol. 2009;13:265–71.

14. Ostendorf A, Wong M. mTOR inhibition in epilepsy: rationale and clinical perspectives. CNS Drugs. 2015;29:91–9.

15. Soliman GA. The role of mechanistic target of rapamycin (mTOR) complexes signaling in the immune responses. Nutrients. 2013;5:2231–57.

16. Xu K, Liu P, Wei W. mTOR signaling in tumorigenesis. Biochim Biophys Acta. 2014;1846:638–54.

17. Takei N, Nawa H. mTOR signaling and its roles in normal and abnormal brain development. Front Mol Neurosci. 2014;7:28.

18. Xie L, Sun F, Wang J, Mao X, Xie L, Yang SH, Su DM, Simpkins JW, Greenberg DA, Jin K. mTOR signaling inhibition modulates macrophage/microglia-mediated neuroinflammation and secondary injury via regulatory T cells after focal ischemia. J Immunol. 2014;192:6009–19.

19. Curatolo P. Mechanistic target of rapamycin (mTOR) in tuberous sclerosis complex-associated epilepsy. Pediatr Neurol. 2015;52:281–9.

20. Sadowski K, Kotulska-Jozwiak K, Jozwiak S. Role of mTOR inhibitors in epilepsy treatment. Pharmacol Rep. 2015;67:636–46.

21. Klawitter J, Nashan B, Christians U. Everolimus and sirolimus in transplantation-related but different. Expert Opin Drug Saf. 2015;14:1055–70.

22. MacKeigan JP, Krueger DA. Differentiating the mTOR inhibitors everolimus and sirolimus in the treatment of tuberous sclerosis complex. Neuro Oncol. 2015;17:1550–9.

23. Stansley B, Post J, Hensley K. A comparative review of cell culture systems for the study of microglial biology in Alzheimer's disease. J Neuroinflammation. 2012;9:115.

24. NRC. Guide for the Care and Use of Laboratory Animals. Washington, D.C: National Academies Press; 2011.

25. Tsikas D. Methods of quantitative analysis of the nitric oxide metabolites nitrite and nitrate in human biological fluids. Free Radic Res. 2005;39:797–815.

26. Racine RJ. Modification of seizure activity by electrical stimulation. II. Motor seizure. Electroencephalogr Clin Neurophysiol. 1972;32:281–94.

27. Phelan KD, Shwe UT, Williams DK, Greenfield LJ, Zheng F. Pilocarpine-induced status epilepticus in mice: a comparison of spectral analysis of electroencephalogram and behavioral grading using the Racine scale. Epilepsy Res. 2015;117:90–6.

28. Butler LS, Silva AJ, Abeliovich A, Watanabe Y, Tonegawa S, McNamara JO. Limbic epilepsy in transgenic mice carrying a Ca2+/calmodulin-dependent kinase II alpha-subunit mutation. Proc Natl Acad Sci U S A. 1995;92:6852–5.

29. Santoro B, Lee JY, Englot DJ, Gildersleeve S, Piskorowski RA, Siegelbaum SA, Winawer MR, Blumenfeld H. Increased seizure severity and seizure-related death in mice lacking HCN1 channels. Epilepsia. 2010;51:1624–7.

30. Cavazos JE, Das I, Sutula TP. Neuronal loss induced in limbic pathways by kindling: evidence for induction of hippocampal sclerosis by repeated brief seizures. J Neurosci. 1994;14:3106–21.

31. Schauwecker PE. Susceptibility to seizure-induced excitotoxic cell death is regulated by an epistatic interaction between Chr 18 (Sicd1) and Chr 15 (Sicd2) loci in mice. PLoS One. 2014;9:e110515.

32. Avignone E, Ulmann L, Levavasseur F, Rassendren F, Audinat E. Status epilepticus induces a particular microglial activation state characterized by enhanced purinergic signaling. J Neurosci. 2008;28:9133–44.

33. Koh S, Storey TW, Santos TC, Mian AY, Cole AJ. Early-life seizures in rats increase susceptibility to seizure-induced brain injury in adulthood. Neurology. 1999;53:915–21.

34. Abraham J, Fox PD, Condello C, Bartolini A, Koh S. Minocycline attenuates microglia activation and blocks the long-term epileptogenic effects of early-life seizures. Neurobiol Dis. 2012;46:425–30.

35. Landry RP, Jacobs VL, Romero-Sandoval EA, DeLeo JA. Propentofylline, a CNS glial modulator does not decrease pain in post-herpetic neuralgia patients: in vitro evidence for differential responses in human and rodent microglia and macrophages. Exp Neurol. 2012;234:340–50.

36. Yang H, Rudge DG, Koos JD, Vaidialingam B, Yang HJ, Pavletich NP. mTOR kinase structure, mechanism and regulation. Nature. 2013;497:217–23.

37. Lisi L, Navarra P, Feinstein DL, Dello Russo C. The mTOR kinase inhibitor rapamycin decreases iNOS mRNA stability in astrocytes. J Neuroinflammation. 2011;8:1.

38. Dello Russo C, Lisi L, Tringali G, Navarra P. Involvement of mTOR kinase in cytokine-dependent microglial activation and cell proliferation. Biochem Pharmacol. 2009;78:1242–51.

39. Mao K, Chen S, Chen M, Ma Y, Wang Y, Huang B, He Z, Zeng Y, Hu Y, Sun S, et al. Nitric oxide suppresses NLRP3 inflammasome activation and protects against LPS-induced septic shock. Cell Res. 2013;23:201–12.

40. Jin YP, Valenzuela NM, Ziegler ME, Rozengurt E, Reed EF. Everolimus inhibits anti-HLA I antibody-mediated endothelial cell signaling, migration and proliferation more potently than sirolimus. Am J Transplant. 2014;14:806–19.

41. Kim EK, Choi E-J. Compromised MAPK signaling in human diseases: an update. Arch Toxicol. 2015;89:867–82.

42. Hayashi I, Aoki Y, Asano D, Ushikubo H, Mori A, Sakamoto K, Nakahara T, Ishii K. Protective effects of everolimus against N-Methyl-D-aspartic acid-induced retinal damage in rats. Biol Pharm Bull. 2015;38:1765–71.

43. Fan W, Cheng K, Qin X, Narsinh KH, Wang S, Hu S, Wang Y, Chen Y, Wu JC, Xiong L, Cao F. mTORC1 and mTORC2 play different roles in the functional survival of transplanted adipose-derived stromal cells in hind limb ischemic mice via regulating inflammation in vivo. Stem Cells. 2013;31:203–14.

44. Perl A. Activation of mTOR (mechanistic target of rapamycin) in rheumatic diseases. Nat Rev Rheumatol. 2016;12:169–82.

45. Cordaro M, Paterniti I, Siracusa R, Impellizzeri D, Esposito E, Cuzzocrea S. KU0063794, a Dual mTORC1 and mTORC2 inhibitor, reduces neural tissue damage and locomotor impairment after spinal cord injury in mice. Mol Neurobiol. 2016. doi:10.1007/s12035-016-9827-0.

46. Buckmaster PS, Ingram EA, Wen X. Inhibition of the mammalian target of rapamycin signaling pathway suppresses dentate granule cell axon sprouting in a rodent model of temporal lobe epilepsy. J Neurosci. 2009;29:8259–69.

47. McDaniel SS, Rensing NR, Thio LL, Yamada KA, Wong M. The ketogenic diet inhibits the mammalian target of rapamycin (mTOR) pathway. Epilepsia. 2011;52:e7–e11.

48. Lehnardt S. Innate immunity and neuroinflammation in the CNS: the role of microglia in Toll-like receptor-mediated neuronal injury. Glia. 2010;58:253–63.

49. Avignone E, Lepleux M, Angibaud J, Nägerl UV. Altered morphological dynamics of activated microglia after induction of status epilepticus. J Neuroinflammation. 2015;12:202.

50. Lin TY, Lu CW, Wang SJ, Huang SK. Protective effect of hispidulin on kainic acid-induced seizures and neurotoxicity in rats. Eur J Pharmacol. 2015;755:6–15.

51. Chiu KM, Wu CC, Wang MJ, Lee MY, Wang SJ. Protective effects of bupivacaine against kainic acid-induced seizure and neuronal cell death in the rat hippocampus. Biol Pharm Bull. 2015;38:522–30.

# 6

# Peroxisome proliferator-activated receptors γ/mitochondrial uncoupling protein 2 signaling protects against seizure-induced neuronal cell death in the hippocampus following experimental status epilepticus

Yao-Chung Chuang[1,2*], Tsu-Kung Lin[1], Hsuan-Ying Huang[3], Wen-Neng Chang[1], Chia-Wei Liou[1], Shang-Der Chen[1,2*], Alice YW Chang[2] and Samuel HH Chan[2]

## Abstract

**Background:** Status epilepticus induces subcellular changes that may lead to neuronal cell death in the hippocampus. However, the mechanism of seizure-induced neuronal cell death remains unclear. The mitochondrial uncoupling protein 2 (UCP2) is expressed in selected regions of the brain and is emerged as an endogenous neuroprotective molecule in many neurological disorders. We evaluated the neuroprotective role of UCP2 against seizure-induced hippocampal neuronal cell death under experimental status epilepticus.

**Methods:** In Sprague–Dawley rats, kainic acid (KA) was microinjected unilaterally into the hippocampal CA3 subfield to induce prolonged bilateral seizure activity. Oxidized protein level, translocation of Bcl-2, Bax and cytochrome $c$ between cytosol and mitochondria, and expression of peroxisome proliferator-activated receptors γ (PPARγ) and UCP2 were examined in the hippocampal CA3 subfield following KA-induced status epilepticus. The effects of microinjection bilaterally into CA3 area of a PPARγ agonist, rosiglitazone or a PPARγ antagonist, GW9662 on UCP2 expression, induced superoxide anion ($O_2^-$) production, oxidized protein level, mitochondrial respiratory chain enzyme activities, translocation of Bcl-2, Bax and cytochrome $c$, and DNA fragmentation in bilateral CA3 subfields were examined.

**Results:** Increased oxidized proteins and mitochondrial or cytosol translocation of Bax or cytochrome $c$ in the hippocampal CA3 subfield was observed 3–48 h after experimental status epilepticus. Expression of PPARγ and UCP2 increased 12–48 h after KA-induced status epilepticus. Pretreatment with rosiglitazone increased UCP2 expression, reduced protein oxidation, $O_2^-$ overproduction and dysfunction of mitochondrial Complex I, hindered the translocation of Bax and cytochrome $c$, and reduced DNA fragmentation in the CA3 subfield. Pretreatment with GW9662 produced opposite effects.

* Correspondence: ycchuang@adm.cgmh.org.tw; chensd@adm.cgmh.org.tw
[1]Department of Neurology, Kaohsiung Chang Gung Memorial Hospital and Chang Gung University College of Medicine, Kaohsiung 83301, Taiwan
[2]Center for Translational Research in Biomedical Sciences, Kaohsiung Chang Gung Memorial Hospital and Chang Gung University College of Medicine, Kaohsiung 83301, Taiwan
Full list of author information is available at the end of the article

**Conclusions:** Activation of PPARγ upregulated mitochondrial UCP2 expression, which decreased overproduction of reactive oxygen species, improved mitochondrial Complex I dysfunction, inhibited mitochondrial translocation of Bax and prevented cytosolic release of cytochrome *c* by stabilizing the mitochondrial transmembrane potential, leading to amelioration of apoptotic neuronal cell death in the hippocampus following status epilepticus.

**Keywords:** Status epilepticus, Mitochondrial uncoupling protein 2, Peroxisome proliferator-activated receptors γ, Hippocampal neuronal cell death, Oxidative stress

## Background

Epileptic seizure is a major form of acute brain damage that could lead to a large number of changes at the cellular level, including oxidative stress, cytokine activation, changes in plasticity or activation of some late cell death pathways [1,2]. In particular, prolonged and continuous epileptic seizures (status epilepticus) results in significant cerebral damage and increases the risk of subsequent epileptic episodes, along with a characteristic pattern of preferential neuronal cell loss in the hippocampus that is accompanied by long-term behavioral changes and cognitive decline [3,4]. It follows that prevention of seizure-induced hippocampal neuronal damage is also an important goal for treatment of status epilepticus. However, the cellular and molecular mechanisms via which status epilepticus induces neuronal cell death in the hippocampus remain to be fully understood.

Animal [5-8] and human [9] studies suggest that mitochondrial dysfunction occur as a consequence of prolonged epileptic seizures and may play a pivotal role in seizure-induced brain damage. Prolonged seizures affect selectively complex I in the respiratory chain; the induced oxidative and nitrosative stress precede neuronal cell death in the hippocampus and cause subsequent epileptogenesis [2,10]. Therefore, the mitochondria can be considered a target for potential neuroprotective strategies in epilepsy.

The uncoupling proteins (UCPs) have emerged as important natural antioxidants in the maintenance of reactive oxygen species (ROS) homeostasis [11]. UCPs belong to a superfamily of mitochondrial anion transporters that uncouple ATP synthesis from oxidative phosphorylation by causing proton leakage across the mitochondrial inner membrane, leading to energy dissipation and heat production [12]. More importantly, the resultant decrease in proton electrochemical gradient across the inner mitochondrial membrane elicited by the UCPs mitigates mitochondrial ROS production [11,13]. In mammals, five homologues, *UCP1* to *UCP5*, have so far been cloned [13]. Among them, accumulating evidence suggests that an increase in *UCP2* gene expression is related to the decline of mitochondrial ROS production [14,15]. UCP2 has been widely studied in the context of obesity, diabetes mellitus

and inflammatory responses [14,16]; an absence of UCP2 potentially promotes ROS accumulation and induces oxidative damages and inflammatory response. In the central nervous system (CNS), UCP2 has been shown to be upregulated by stress signals such as kainate administration, injury or ischemia, and overexpression of UCP2 has been reported to be neuroprotective against oxidative stress *in vivo* and *in vitro* [13,17,18]. However, the exact mechanism has not been fully established.

We have shown previously that dysfunction of complex I respiratory chain enzyme and mitochondrial ultrastructural damage in the hippocampus are associated with prolonged seizure during experimental temporal lobe status epilepticus [5]. Based on this animal model, our recent studies [19-22] demonstrated that an excessive production of nitric oxide (NO) generated by the upregulated NO synthase II (NOS II), accompanied by an increase in superoxide anion ($O_2^-$) production and peroxynitrite formation, followed by a reduction in mitochondrial complex I activity and release of cytochrome *c* from mitochondria to the cytosol, which triggers the caspase cascades that lead to apoptotic cell death in the hippocampus. In addition to this detrimental chain reaction under status epilepticus, it is conceivable that cellular responses that counteract these detrimental effects may be activated as an endogenous protective mechanism. In this regard, we have demonstrated previously that rosiglitazone, a peroxisome proliferator-activated receptor γ (PPARγ) agonist, enhances UCP2 expression after cerebral ischemia to protect against neuronal cell death in the hippocampus [23,24]. It follows that as an antioxidant, UCP2 may be activated during experimental status epilepticus, leading to decreased ROS production, reduced mitochondrial dysfunction, impeded apoptotic pathway and retarded neuronal injury in the hippocampus. Results from the present study validated this hypothesis.

## Methods

All experimental procedures were carried out in compliance with the guidelines for the care and use of experimental animals endorsed by our institutional animal care committee. All efforts were made to reduce the number of animals used and to minimize animal suffering during the experiment.

## Animals

Experiments were carried out in specific pathogen-free adult male Sprague–Dawley rats (260 to 300 g) that were obtained from the Experimental Animal Center of the National Science Council, Taiwan, Republic of China. They were housed in an animal room under temperature control (24 to 25°C) and a 12-h light–dark (08:00 to 20:00 h) cycle. Standard laboratory rat chow and tap water were available *ad libitum*.

## Experimental temporal lobe status epilepticus

An experimental model of temporal lobe status epilepticus established previously by us [5,19-21] was used. This model entails microinjection unilaterally of kainic acid (KA) into the hippocampal CA3 subfield that results in a progressive buildup of bilateral seizure-like hippocampal electroencephalographic (hEEG) activity. The head of the animal was fixed to a stereotaxic headholder (Kopf, Tujunga, CA, USA) after intraperitoneal (ip) administration of chloral hydrate (400 mg/kg) to induce anesthesia, and the rest of the body was placed on a heating pad to maintain body temperature at 37°C. KA (0.5 nmol; Tocris Cookson, Bristol, UK) dissolved in 0.1 M PBS, pH 7.4, was microinjected stereotaxically (3.3 to 3.6 mm posterior to the bregma, 2.4 to 2.7 mm from the midline, and 3.4 to 3.8 mm below the cortical surface) into the CA3 subfield of the hippocampus on the left side. The volume of microinjection of KA was restricted to 50 nL and was delivered using a 27-gauge needle connected to a 0.5-µL Hamilton microsyringe (Reno, NV, USA). This consistently resulted in progressive and concomitant increase in both root mean square and mean power frequency values of hEEG signals recorded from the CA3 subfield on the right side [5,20,21]. As a routine, these experimental manifestations of continuous seizure activity were followed by hEEG for 60 minutes, followed by ip administration of diazepam (30 mg/kg) to terminate seizures [5,20,21]. The wound was then closed in layers, and sodium penicillin (10,000 IU; YF Chemical Corporation, Taipei, Taiwan) was given intramuscularly to prevent postoperative infection. Animals were returned to the animal room for recovery in individual cages. Rats that received unilateral microinjection of 50 nL of PBS and did not exhibit seizure-like hEEG activities served as our vehicle controls. Animals that received choral hydrate anesthesia and surgical preparations without additional experimental manipulations served as sham-controls.

## Pharmacological pretreatments

In experiments that involved pharmacological pretreatments, test agents were microinjected bilaterally and sequentially into the CA3 subfield of the hippocampus, at a volume of 150 nL on each side. Test agents used included an activator of PPARγ [24,25], rosiglitazone (Cayman Chemical, Ann Arbor, MI, USA) and a PPARγ antagonist [25,26], GW9662 (Cayman Chemical). The doses of test agents used were 6 nmol for rosiglitazone, and 500 ng for GW9662 [24,26]. Microinjection of 3% dimethyl sulfoxide (DMSO) solvent served as the vehicle and volume control. To avoid the confounding effects of drug interaction, each animal received only one single pharmacological pretreatment, followed 30 minutes later by microinjection of KA (0.5 nmol) or PBS into the left hippocampal CA3 subfield.

## Collection of tissue samples from the hippocampus

At predetermined time intervals (3, 6, 12, 24 or 48 h; or 7 days) after microinjection of KA or PBS into the hippocampus, rats were again anesthetized by ip administration of chloral hydrate (400 mg/kg,) and were perfused intracardially with 50 mL of warm (37°C) saline that contained heparin (100 U/mL). As we reported previously [5,19-21], the brain was rapidly removed under visual inspection and placed on a piece of gauze moistened with ice-cold 0.9% saline. We routinely collected tissues from the ipsilateral (injection side for KA) and the contralateral (recording side for hEEG) hippocampal CA3 subfield [5,19-21]. Hippocampal samples were stored at −80°C until biochemical analysis. In experiments involving immunofluorescence staining, brains were post-fixed in 4% paraformaldehyde for 48 h at 4°C followed by cryoprotection with 30% sucrose solution. The concentration of total proteins extracted from tissue samples was determined by the bicinchoninic acid (BCA) protein assay (Pierce, Rockford, IL, USA). In some experiments, proteins from the nuclear or cytosolic fraction of the hippocampal samples were extracted by a commercial kit (Active Motif, Carlsbad, CA, USA).

## Measurement of protein oxidation

Oxidized protein was determined using a protein oxidation detection kit (OxyBlot, Chemicon, Temecula, CA, USA). This kit provides reagents for sensitive immunodetection of the carbonyl group, which is a hallmark of the oxidation status of proteins [27,28]. Total proteins extracted from the hippocampal CA3 subfield were reacted with 2,4-dinitrophenylhydrazine and derivatized to 2,4-dinitrophenylhydrazone (DNP-hydrazone) [29]. The DNP-derivatized protein samples were separated on a 15% SDS-polyacrylamide gel followed by western blot. The blot was incubated with a rabbit anti-DNP antibody, followed by incubation with a horseradish peroxidase-conjugated goat anti-rabbit IgG according to manufacturers' instructions.

## Western blot analysis

Western blot analysis for UCP2, PPARγ, Bcl-2, Bax, cytochrome *c* or β-actin was carried out on proteins extracted from nuclear fractions or from mitochondrial or cytosolic fractions of hippocampal samples. The purity of the mitochondrial fraction was verified by the selective expression of the mitochondrial inner membrane-specific protein, cytochrome $c$ oxidase subunit IV (COX IV). Protein concentration was determined by the BCA Protein Assay (Pierce). The primary antisera used included rabbit polyclonal antiserum against Bax and COX IV (Cell Signaling, Danvers, MA, USA), goat polyclonal antiserum against UCP2 (Santa Cruz Biotechnology, Santa Cruz, CA, USA), mouse monoclonal antiserum against Bcl-2, cytochrome $c$ and PPARγ (Santa Cruz Biotechnology) or β-actin (Chemicon, Temecula, CA, USA). β-actin was used for internal control of total protein or proteins in the cytosolic fraction, and COX IV for proteins in the mitochondrial fraction. . The secondary antisera used included horseradish peroxidase-conjugated sheep anti-mouse IgG (Amersham Biosciences, Little Chalfont, UK) for Bcl-2, cytochrome $c$, PPARγ and β-actin; donkey anti-goat IgG (Chemicon) for UCP2, or donkey anti-rabbit IgG (Amersham Biosciences) for Bax, and COX IV. Specific antibody-antigen complex was detected by an enhanced chemiluminescence western blot detection system (NEN, Boston, MA, USA). The amount of protein was quantified by ImageMaster software (Amersham Pharmacia Biotech, Piscataway, NJ, USA), and was expressed as the ratio relative to β-actin protein (for analysis of total protein or proteins in the cytosolic fraction) or COX IV (for analysis of proteins in the mitochondrial fraction).

### RNA isolation and reverse transcription real-time polymerase chain reaction

For quantitative analysis of *Ucp2* mRNA expression in the hippocampal CA3, at 3, 6, 12 h or 24 h after microinjection of KA or PBS into the hippocampus, the brain was rapidly removed and total RNA from the hippocampal CA3 was isolated with TRIzol reagent (Invitrogen) according to the manufacturer's protocol. All RNA isolated was quantified by spectrophotometry and the optical density 260/280 nm ratio was determined. RT reaction was performed using a SuperScript Preamplification System (Invitrogen) for the first-strand cDNA synthesis [25,30]. Real-time PCR for amplification of cDNA was performed using a LightCycler (Roche Diagnostics, Mannheim, Germany). PCR for each sample was carried out in duplicate for all cDNAs and for the glyceraldehyde-3-phosphate dehydrogenase (GAPDH) control [25,30]. The PCR mixture (total volume 20 μl), which was prepared with nuclease-free water, contained 2 μL of LightCycler FastStart DNA Master SYBR Green 1 (Roche Diagnostics), 3 mM MgCl2, and 5 μM each primer, together with 5 μL of purified DNA or negative control. The primer pairs for amplifi-cation of *Ucp2* cDNA (GenBank: U69135) were 5′-TCCCCTGTTGATGTGGTCAA-3′ for the forward primer, and 5′-CAGTGACCTGCGCTGTGGTA-3′ for the

reverse [25]. Primer pairs for GAPDH cDNA (GenBank: NM017008) were 5′-GCCAAAAGGGTCATCATCTC-3′ for the forward primer, and 5′-GGCCATCCACAGTCTTCT-3′ for the reverse [25]. The amplification protocol for cDNA was a 10-minute denaturation step at 95℃ for polymerase activation; a so-called touchdown PCR step of 10 cycles consisting of 10 s at 95℃, 10s at 65℃, and 30s at 72℃; followed by 40 cycles consisting of 10 s at 95℃, 10 s at 55℃, and 30s at 72℃. After slow heating (0.1℃ per second) of the amplified product from 65 to 95℃ to generate a melting temperature curve, which serves as a specificity control, the PCR samples were cooled to 40℃. The PCR products were subsequently subjected to agarose gel electrophoresis for further confirmation of amplification specificity. Fluorescence signals from the amplified products were quantitatively assessed using the LightCycler software program (version 3.5). Second derivative maximum mode was chosen with baseline adjustment set in the arithmetic mode. The relative change in *Ucp2* mRNA expression was determined by the fold-change analysis [25], in which:

$$\text{Fold change} = 2^{-(\Delta\Delta Ct)}$$

where:

$$\Delta\Delta Ct = (Ct_{UCP2} - Ct_{GAPDH})_{\text{pharmacological treatment}}$$
$$-(Ct_{UCP2} - Ct_{GAPDH})_{\text{control}})$$

Note that $Ct$ value is the cycle number at which the fluorescence signal crosses the threshold.

### Double immunofluorescence staining and laser confocal microscopy

Free-floating sections of the hippocampus (35 μm) were processed for double immunofluorescence staining by procedures we reported previously [19-21]. Double immunofluorescence staining was carried out using a rabbit polyclonal antiserum against UCP2 (Bioss, Woburn, MA, USA) or against a marker for astrocytes, glial fibrillary acidic protein (GFAP; Abcam, Cambridge, UK); or rabbit polyclonal antiserum against a mitochondrial membrane protein, COX IV (Cell Signaling). The secondary antisera included a goat anti-rabbit IgG conjugated with AlexaFluor 488 and a goat anti-mouse IgG conjugated with Alexa Fluor 568 or a goat anti-rabbit IgG conjugated with AlexaFluor 546 (Molecular Probes, Eugene, OR, USA). Hippocampal CA3b area was viewed under a Fluorview FV10i laser scanning confocal microscope (Olympus, Tokyo, Japan), and immunoreactivity for NeuN, COX IV or GFAP exhibited red fluorescence and UCP2 manifested green fluorescence. The exhibition of yellow fluorescence on merged images indicated the presence of UCP2 immunoreactivity in neurons, mitochondria or astrocytes.

## Measurement of superoxide anion production

Measurement of $O_2^-$ production was determined by lucigenin-enhanced chemiluminescence [21,31]. Fresh samples from the hippocampal CA3 subfield were homogenized in 20 mM sodium phosphate buffer, pH 7.4, containing 0.01 mM EDTA by a glass-to-glass homogenizer. The homogenate was subject to centrifugation at $1000\,g$ for 10 minutes at 4 °C to remove nuclei and unbroken cell debris. The pellet was discarded and the supernatant was obtained immediately for $O_2^-$ measurement. Background chemiluminescence in buffer (2 mL) containing lucigenin (5 μM) was measured for 5 minutes. An aliquot of 100 μl of supernatant was then added, and the chemiluminescence measured for 30 minutes at room temperature with a Sirius luminometer (Berthold, Germany) [21]. $O_2^-$ production was calculated and expressed as mean light units per minute per mg protein. Specificity for $O_2^-$ was determined by adding superoxide dismutase (SOD) (350 U/mL) into the incubation medium.

## Assays for activity of mitochondrial respiratory enzymes

Isolation of rat mitochondria from the hippocampal samples was carried out according to our previous report [5,21] and modification [32]. Hippocampal tissues were suspended in wash buffer and homogenized in an ice-cold mitochondrial isolation buffer kit (MS850, MitoSciences, Eugene, OR, USA) using a loose-fit 2 mL glass homogenizer (Kontes, Vineland, NJ, USA). The homogenate was centrifuged at $1000\,g$ for 10 minutes at 4°C, and the supernatant obtained was further centrifuged at $12000\,g$ for 15 minutes. The pellet was resuspended in isolation buffer and protease inhibitor was added, and then centrifuged at 12000 g for 15 minutes. The final mitochondrial pellet was suspended in a minimal amount of isolation buffer and protease inhibitor and stored at −80°C until measurement of mitochondrial respiratory enzyme activity, which was undertaken within 3 days. Total protein in the mitochondrial suspension was determined by the BCA Protein Assay (Pierce, Rockford, IL, USA), using bovine serum albumin as a standard.

The activity of complex I (nicotinamide adenine dinucleotide (NADH) ubiquinone oxidoreductase) and complex IV (cytochrome $c$ oxidase) of mitochondrial respiratory enzymes were analyzed by enzyme activity immunocapture assays [32,33]. A 96-well plate coated with monoclonal antibodies against the oxidative phosphorylation complex I (MS141, MitoSciences) and IV (MS444, MitoSciences) were used according to manufacturers'

instructions. Complex I activity was measured by adding an assay solution and the oxidation of NADH was monitored by measuring its decrease in absorbance at 450 nm in kinetic mode at 30°C for 2 h. Complex IV activity was measured by adding an assay solution and the oxidation of reduced cytochrome $c$ was monitored by measuring its decrease in absorbance at 550 nm in kinetic mode at room temperature for 30 minutes. Assays for mitochondrial respiratory enzyme activity were performed using a Multiskan Spectrum reader (Thermo Scientific, Miami, USA). At least duplicate determination was carried out on each tissue sample.

## Qualitative and quantitative analysis of DNA fragmentation

Tissue samples from the hippocampal CA3 subfield were subject to qualitative and quantitative analysis of DNA fragmentation. After extraction of total DNA from hippocampal tissues, nucleosomal DNA ladders were amplified by a PCR kit for DNA ladder assay (Maxim Biotech, San Francisco, CA, USA) to enhance the detection sensitivity, and were separated by electrophoresis on 1% agarose gel [19-21]. To quantify apoptosis-related DNA fragmentation, a cell death ELISA (Roche Molecular Biochemicals, Mannheim, Germany) that detects apoptotic but not necrotic cell death [34] was used to assay the level of histone-associated DNA fragments in the cytoplasm [35]. Proteins from the cytosolic fraction of hippocampal samples were used as the antigen source, together with primary anti-histone antibody and secondary anti-DNA antibody coupled to peroxidase. The amount of nucleosomes in the cytoplasm was quantitatively determined using 2,2′-azino-di-[3-ethylbenzthiazoline] sulfonate as the substrate. Absorbance was measured at 405 nm and referenced at 490 nm using a microtiter plate reader (Anthros Labtec).

## Statistical analysis

One-way analysis of variance (ANOVA) was used, as appropriate, to assess group means, followed by the Scheffé multiple-range test for post hoc assessment of individual means. All values are expressed as mean ± standard error of the mean (SEM). A $P$-value $< 0.05$ was taken to indicate statistical significance.

## Results

### Strategies for biochemical analyses and pharmacological treatments

As in our previous studies [5,19-22], we routinely carried out biochemical analysis separately on tissues collected from the ipsilateral (injection side for KA) and the contralateral (recording side for hEEG) hippocampal CA3 subfield. This allowed us to ascertain that results from those analyses were consequential directly to experimental temporal lobe status epilepticus and not indirectly to KA excitotoxicity. Since seizure activity was activated bilaterally, test agents were also routinely microinjected into the bilateral hippocampal CA3 subfield to confirm that parallel results were obtained from CA3 areas on both sides.

### Temporal changes in protein oxidation in the hippocampal CA3 subfield following experimental temporal lobe status epilepticus

We reported recently [21] that a significant surge in $O_2^-$ production took place as early as 3 h after the induction of experimental temporal lobe status epilepticus, which gradually declined over 24 h. Our first series of experiments therefore, established that oxidative stress damages occurred in hippocampal CA3 neural cells following experimental lobe status epilepticus. We observed a significantly heightened content of oxidized proteins in the ipsilateral hippocampal CA3 subfield as early as 3 h, followed by a progressive reduction over 24 h after unilateral microinjection of KA (0.5 nmol) into the left CA3 area (Figure 1). We also observed a significant increase in oxidized proteins in the contralateral CA3 subfield over the same time intervals after local application of KA into the left hippocampal CA3 subfield. Importantly, the temporal changes of protein

oxidations in the bilateral hippocampal CA3 subfield paralleled the time course of $O_2^-$ production after experimental status epilepticus [21].

### Temporal course of Bax and cytochrome c translocation in the hippocampal CA3 subfield following experimental temporal lobe status epilepticus

Our second series of experiments investigated whether the Bcl-2, Bax and cytochrome c signaling cascades are associated with excessive ROS production in the hippocampal CA3 subfield following experimental temporal lobe status epilepticus. Western blot analysis revealed that Bcl-2 was not discernibly altered in either the mitochondrial or cytosolic fraction of samples obtained from the hippocampal CA3 subfield. However, there was a significant decrease of Bax level and increase of cytochrome c level in the cytosolic fraction (Figure 2A) of samples from the bilateral hippocampal CA3 subfield after unilateral microinjection of KA (0.5 nmol) into the left CA3 region, accompanied by a corresponding increase of Bax level and decrease of cytochrome c level in the mitochondrial fraction (Figure 2B). Of note is that this induced mitochondria-bound translocation of Bax from the cytosol and cytosol-bound translocation of cytochrome c from the mitochondria followed a time frame that started from 3 h in the ipsilateral and 6 h in the contralateral CA3 area, and was sustained 48 h after the induction of experimental temporal lobe status epilepticus.

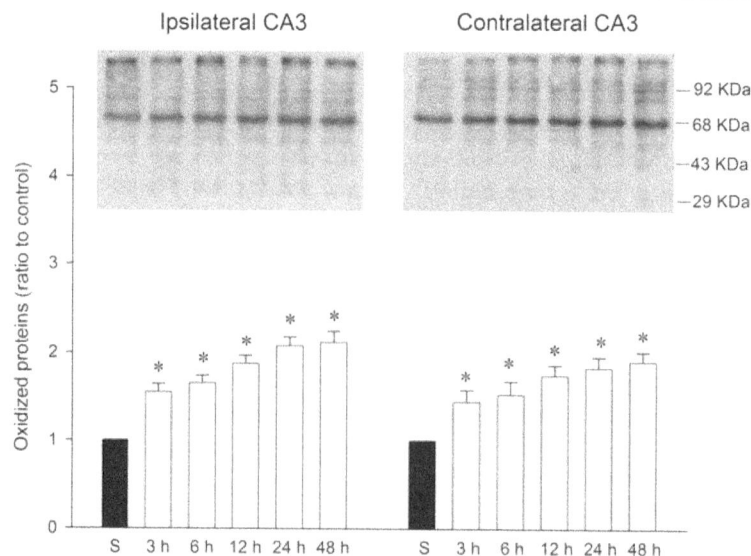

**Figure 1** Representative gels (inset) or temporal changes of protein oxidation detected in samples collected from the CA3 subfield of the hippocampus at 3, 6, 12, 24 and 48 h after microinjection of 0.5 nmol kainic acid (KA) or PBS into the left hippocampal CA3 subfield. Total proteins were extracted from the hippocampal CA3 subfield at the indicted times or from sham-operated controls followed by immunoblot analysis for the extent of protein oxidation. Values in the lower panel are fold changes with reference to sham-control (S) and are mean ± standard error of the mean (SEM) of four animals per experimental group. *$P < 0.05$ versus sham-control group in the Scheffé multiple-range test.

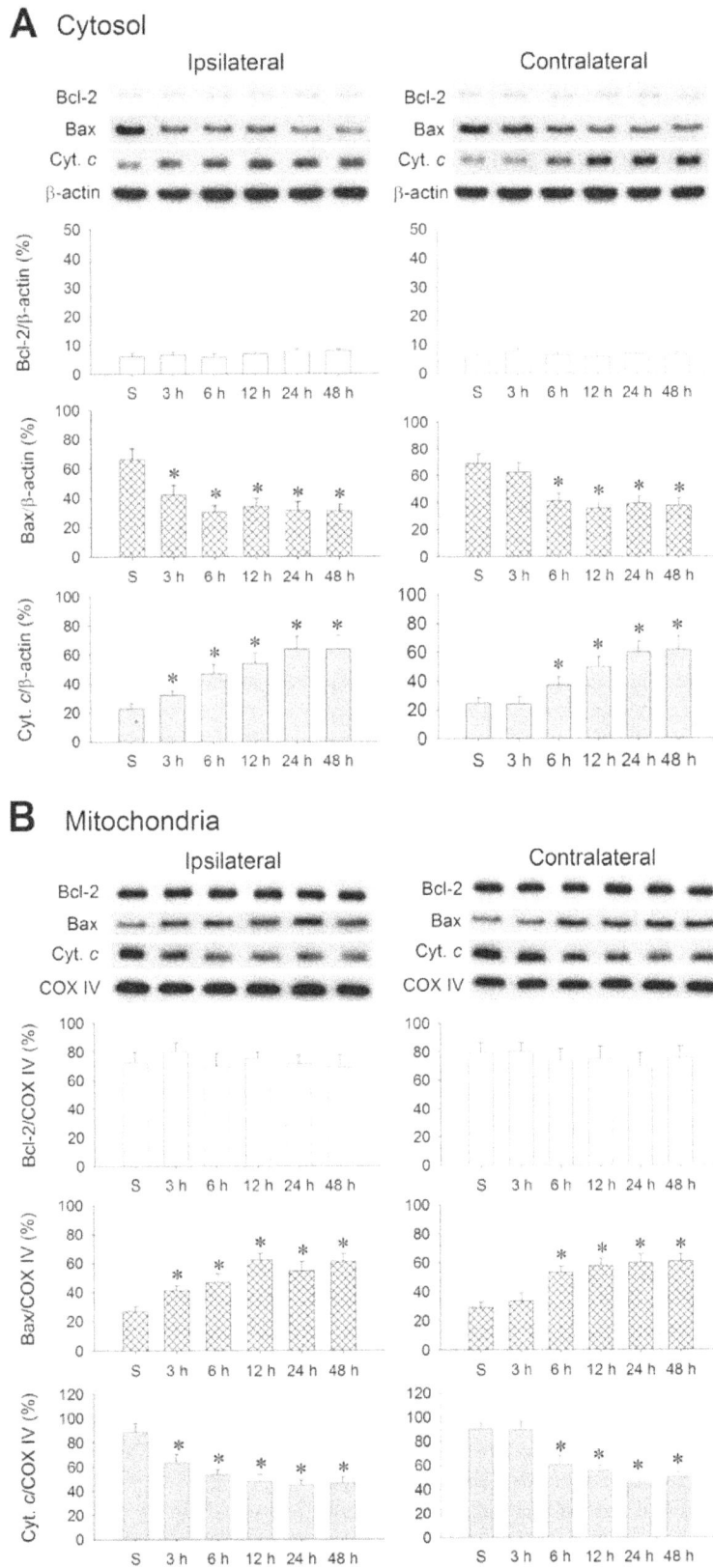

**Figure 2** (See legend on next page.)

(See figure on previous page.)
**Figure 2** Representative gels (inset) or temporal changes in Bcl-2, Bax or cytochrome *c* relative to β-actin protein detected in the cytosolic fraction or relative to cytochrome *c* oxidase subunit IV (COX-IV) in the mitochondrial fraction of samples collected from the CA3 subfield of the hippocampus after microinjection of kainic acid (KA) or PBS. **(A)** Cytosolic fraction and **(B)** mitochondrial fraction of samples collected 3, 6, 12, 24 and 48 h after microinjection of KA (0.5 nmol) or PBS into the left hippocampal CA3 subfield. β-actin or COX-IV was used as the internal loading control for the cytosolic or mitochondrial fraction. Values are mean ± standard error of the mean (SEM) of the ratio of Bcl-2, Bax or cytochrome *c* to the loading controls, and are quadruplicate analyses from six animals per experimental group. *$P < 0.05$ versus sham-control (S) group in the Scheffé multiple-range test.

### Temporal changes of PPARγ and UCP2 expression in the hippocampal CA3 subfield following experimental temporal lobe status epilepticus

Our third series of experiments examined whether PPARγ and UCP2 in the hippocampal CA3 subfield exhibit changes in expression level following experimental temporal lobe status epilepticus. After unilateral microinjection of KA into the left CA3 region, western blot analysis revealed a slight decrease of PPARγ 6 h after ipsilateral KA treatment, followed by a significant increase of expression from 12 to 48 h in the bilateral hippocampal CA3 subfields (Figure 3A). More intriguingly, real-time PCR analysis (Figure 3B) revealed that *Ucp2* mRNA underwent a significant increase in the bilateral hippocampal CA3 area that peaked at 6 h after the elicitation of sustained hippocampal seizure discharges. Also, western blot analysis showed a significant increase of UCP2 protein expression from 12 to 48 h in both hippocampal CA3 subfields (Figure 3C) that paralleled the augmented expression of PPARγ.

### Effects of rosiglitazone and GW9662 on UCP2 expression in hippocampal CA3 neurons following experimental temporal lobe status epilepticus

Our fourth series of experiments further explored a causal role for PPARγ and UCP2 in experimental temporal lobe status epilepticus. Bilateral microinjection of the PPARγ agonist, rosiglitazone (6 nmol) into the hippocampal CA3 region significantly increased the expression of UCP2 in the mitochondrial fraction (Figure 4) from the CA3 subfield 24 h after the elicitation of sustained hippocampal seizure discharges. On the other hand, bilateral microinjection of the PPARγ antagonist, GW9662 (500 ng) reduced the elicited UCP2 expression (Figure 4). Similar observations were obtained from double immunofluorescence staining coupled with laser scanning confocal microscopy. Compared to sham-control (Figure 5A), there was an increase in UCP2 immunoreactivity in neurons from the hippocampal CA3 subfield on the right side (Figure 5B) 24 h after KA-induced status epilepticus. Moreover, whereas pretreatment with rosiglitazone (6 nmol) increased (Figure 5C), GW9662 (500 ng) pretreatment decreased (Figure 5D) UCP2 immunoreactivity in the hippocampal CA3 neurons.

We also verified the localization of UCP2 immunoreactivity in mitochondria by co-immunofluorescence staining with the mitochondrial membrane protein, COX IV (Figure 5E-H) of hippocampal CA3 neurons on the right side (Figure 5F), 24 h after KA-induced status epilepticus compared with sham-control (Figure 5E). Additionally, pretreatment with rosiglitazone (6 nmol) increased (Figure 5G), and GW9662 (500 ng) pretreatment decreased (Figure 5H) UCP2 immunoreactivity in the mitochondria of hippocampal CA3 neurons. However, the immunoreactivity for UCP2 was not significantly changed in hippocampal cells that were immunoreactive to the astrocyte marker GFAP 24 h following experimental status epilepticus (Figure 5I-L).

### Effects of rosiglitazone and GW9662 on superoxide production and oxidized protein expression in the hippocampal CA3 subfield following experimental temporal lobe status epilepticus

To strengthen a pivotal role of the PPARγ/UCP2 signaling pathway in oxidative stress damage in the hippocampus following experimental status epilepticus, we observed that bilateral microinjection of rosiglitazone into the hippocampal CA3 region, at a dose (6 nmol) that enhanced UCP2 expression, also decreased the levels of $O_2^-$ ((Figure 6A) or oxidized protein (Figure 6B) in the CA3 subfield 24 h after KA-induced experimental status epilepticus. On the other hand, pretreatment with GW9662 (500 ng) increased the levels of $O_2^-$ (Figure 6A) or oxidized protein (Figure 6B).

### Effects of rosiglitazone and GW9662 on the activity of mitochondrial respiratory enzymes in the hippocampal CA3 subfield following experimental temporal lobe status epilepticus

Our laboratory reported previously [5,21] that depression of mitochondrial complex I and preservation of complex IV enzyme activity in the hippocampus takes place in our experimental model of temporal lobe status epilepticus. Our next series of experiments examined whether the induced mitochondrial dysfunction is causally related to upregulation of UCP2. We found that the significantly reduced complex I respiratory enzyme activity in the bilateral hippocampal CA3 subfield 3 and 24 after local application of KA into the left CA3 subfield was significantly

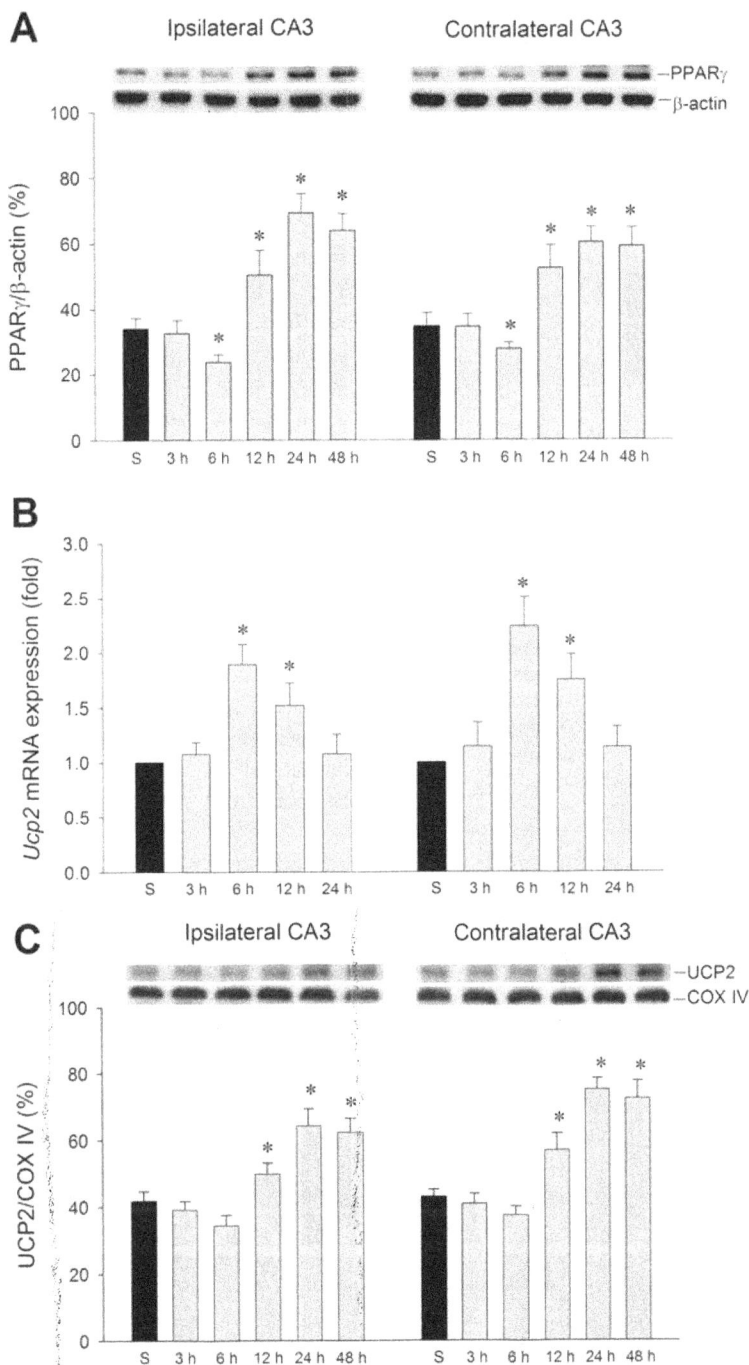

**Figure 3** Temporal changes in peroxisome proliferator-activated receptor γ (PPARγ) protein relative to β-actin protein and UCP2 protein relative to cytochrome c oxidase subunit IV (COX-IV), and real-time PCR analysis showing fold changes in uncoupling protein 2 (*Ucp2*) mRNA expression relative to glyceraldehyde-3-phosphate dehydrogenase after microinjection of kainic acid or PBS into the left hippocampal CA3 subfield. **(A)** Changes in PPARγ protein relative to β-actin protein. **(B)** Fold changes in *Ucp2* mRNA expression relative to glyceraldehyde-3-phosphate dehydrogenase. **(C)** Changes in UCP2 protein relative to COX-IV. Changes were detected in samples collected from the CA3 subfield of the hippocampus at 3, 6, 12, 24 or 48 h after microinjection of 0.5 nmol kainic acid or PBS into the left hippocampal CA3 subfield. Values are mean ± standard error of the mean (SEM) of quadruplicate analyses from six animals per experimental group. *$P < 0.05$ versus sham-control group (S) in the Scheffé multiple-range test.

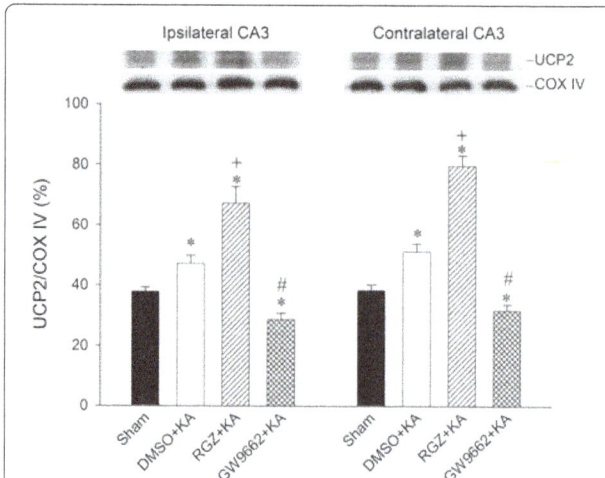

**Figure 4** Representative gels (inset) or changes in uncoupling protein (UCP)-2 relative to cytochrome *c* oxidase subunit IV (COX-IV), detected in the mitochondrial fraction of samples collected from the CA3 subfield of the hippocampus 24 h after microinjection of 0.5 nmol kainic acid or PBS into the left hippocampal CA3 subfield after pretreatment with 3% dimethyl sulfoxide (DMSO), rosiglitazone (RGZ, 6 nmol) or 500 ng GW9662 applied to the bilateral CA3 subfield. Values are mean ± standard error of the mean (SEM) of quadruplicate analyses from six animals per experimental group. *$P < 0.05$ versus sham-control group, +$P < 0.05$ versus sham-control, DMSO + KA or GW9662 + KA group, and #$P < 0.05$ versus sham-control, DMSO + KA or RGZ + KA group in the Scheffé multiple-range test.

blunted by pretreatment with rosiglitazone (6 nmol) (Figure 7A). However, the induced dysfunction of complex I was aggravated by pretreatment with GW9662 (500 ng) (Figure 7A). On the other hand, there was a lack of discernible changes in complex IV activities 3 and 24 h after experimental status epilepticus in animals pretreated with rosiglitazone or GW9662 (Figure 7B).

### Effects of rosiglitazone and GW9662 on apoptotic cell death in the hippocampal CA3 subfield following experimental temporal lobe status epilepticus

We have shown previously that an excessive oxidative and nitrosative stress followed by the release of cytochrome *c* to the cytosol that triggers the caspase cascades, leads to apoptotic cell death in the hippocampus during experimental status epilepticus [20,21]. Our final series of experiments explored whether the upregulated PPARγ/UCP2 signaling pathway plays a significant role in ameliorating this process. We found that whereas pretreatment with rosiglitazone (6 nmol) significantly reduced, the extent of Bax translocation from cytosol to mitochondria and cytochrome *c* translocation from mitochondria to cytosol in the CA3 areas 24 h after experimental temporal lobe status epilepticus, GW9662 (500 ng) significantly augmented it (Figure 8). Comparable results were obtained from qualitative (Figure 9A) and quantitative

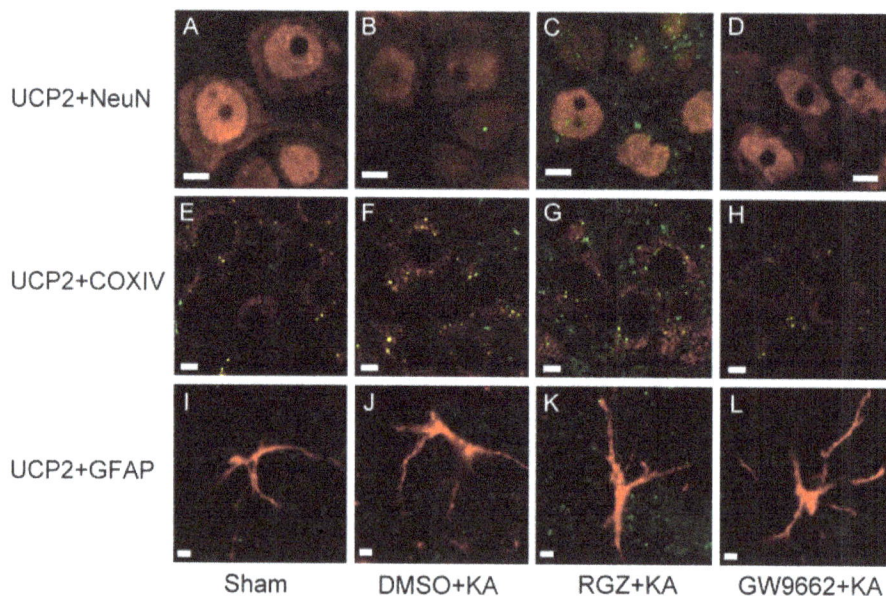

**Figure 5** Laser scanning confocal microscopic images of the right CA3b subregion of hippocampus showing cells that were immunoreactive to a neuronal marker, a mitochondrial protein marker, or a marker for astrocytes, and additionally stained for uncoupling protein (UCP)-2. Scanning was performed 24 h after microinjection of 0.5 nmol kainic acid (KA) or PBS into the left hippocampal CA3 subfield in animals that received pretreatment with application into the bilateral CA3 subfield of 3% dimethyl sulfoxide (DMSO), 6 nmol rosiglitazone (RGZ) or 500 ng GW9662. **(A-D)** Neuronal marker, NeuN (red fluorescence). **(E-H)** Mitochondrial protein marker, cytochrome *c* oxidase subunit IV (COX IV) (red fluorescence). **(I-L)** Marker for astrocytes, glial fibrillary acidic protein (GFAP) (red fluorescence). Cells were additionally stained for UCP2 (green fluorescence). Note that double-labeled neurons, mitochondria or astrocytes displayed yellow fluorescence. These results are typical of three animals from each experimental group. Scale bar, 5 μm in 5A-H; 2 μm in 5I-L.

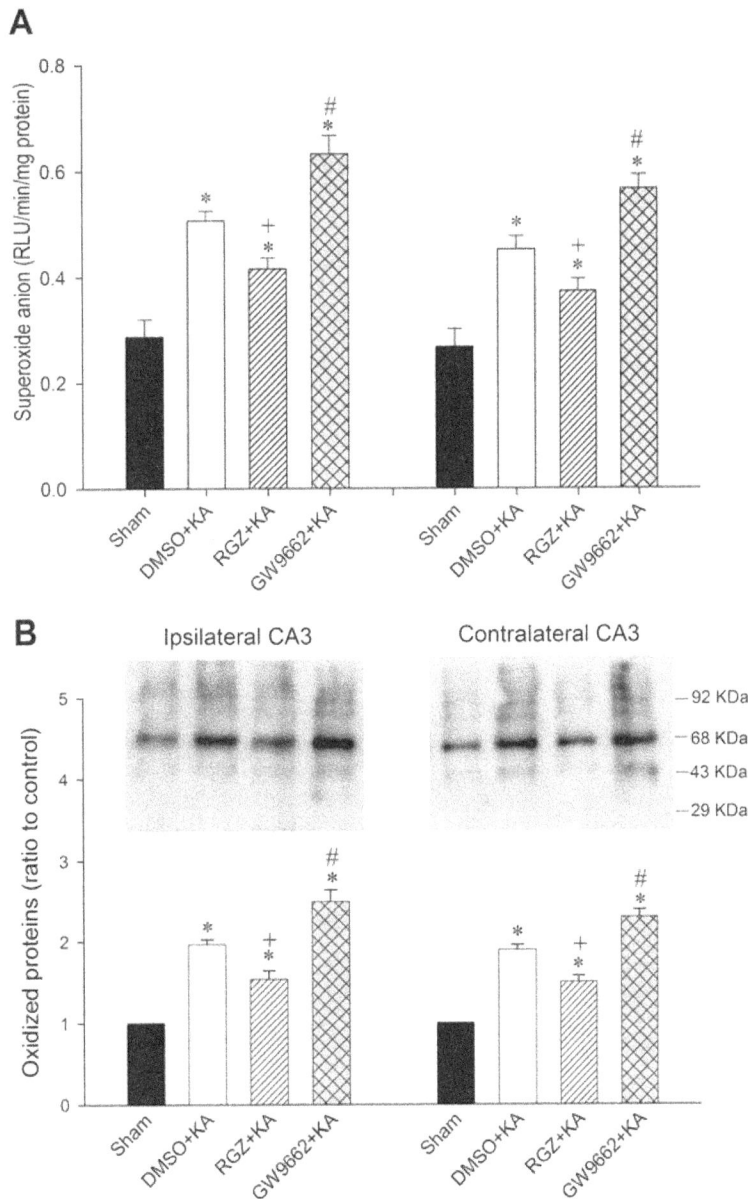

**Figure 6** Representative changes in superoxide anion (O$_2^{\bullet-}$) production and protein oxidation in the bilateral CA3 subfield of the hippocampus 24 h after microinjection of kainic acid (KA) (0.5 nmol) or PBS into the left hippocampal CA3 subfield in animals that received pretreatment with application into the bilateral CA3 subfield of 3% dimethyl sulfoxide (DMSO), 6 nmol rosiglitazone (RGZ) or 500 ng GW9662. **(A)** Changes in O$_2^{\bullet-}$ production. **(B)** Changes in protein oxidation. Values are mean ± standard error of the mean (SEM) of quadruplicate analyses from four animals per experimental group. *$P < 0.05$ versus sham-control group, +$P < 0.05$ versus sham-control, DMSO + KA or GW9662 + KA group, and #$P < 0.05$ versus sham-control, DMSO + KA or RGZ + KA group in the Scheffé multiple-range test.

(Figure 9B) analysis of DNA fragmentation as another index for apoptosis, 7 days after the induction of status epilepticus.

## Discussion

Based on a clinically relevant animal model, the present study provided novel evidence to support an antioxidant role for UCP2 in temporal lobe status epilepticus.

Specifically, our results revealed that upregulation of UCP2 expression induced by experimental status epileptics decreased oxidative stress, reduced mitochondrial dysfunction, blunted mitochondrial intrinsic apoptotic cell death pathway and protected against neuronal cell death in the hippocampal CA3 subfield.

PPARs are known to modulate the inflammatory and oxidative response [36]. The beneficial effects of PPARs

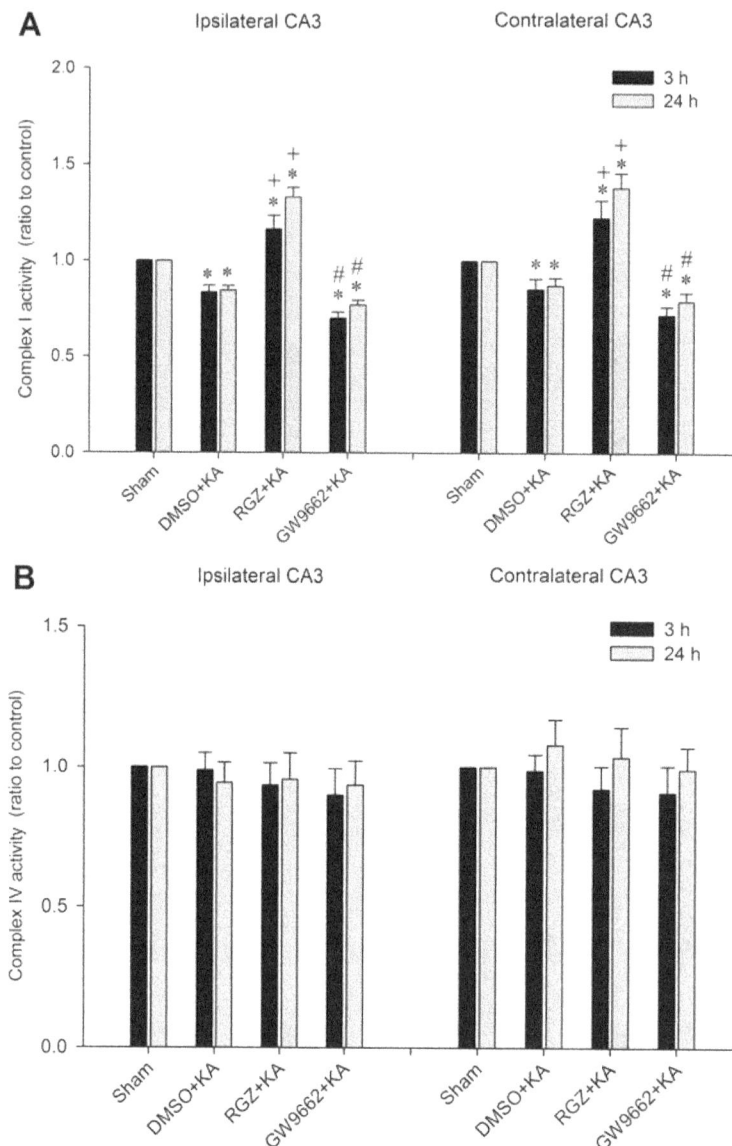

**Figure 7** Enzyme assay for the activity of complex I or complex IV in mitochondria isolated from the CA3 subfield of the hippocampus 3 h and 24 h after microinjection of kainic acid (KA) (0.5 nmol) or PBS into the left hippocampal CA3 subfield, in animals that received pretreatment with application into the bilateral CA3 subfield of 3% dimethyl sulfoxide (DMSO), 6 nmol rosiglitazone (RGZ) or 500 ng GW9662. **(A)** Complex I. **(B)** Complex IV. Values are fold changes with reference to sham-control and are mean ± standard error of the mean (SEM) of four animals per experimental group. *$P < 0.05$ versus sham-control group, +$P < 0.05$ versus sham-control, DMSO + KA or GW9662 + KA group, and #$P < 0.05$ versus sham-control, DMSO + KA or RGZ + KA group in the Scheffé multiple-range test.

in inflammatory diseases are exerted through regulation of cytokine production and adhesion molecule expression by interfering with transcription factors, including nuclear factor-κB (NF-κB), activator protein-1 (AP-1), signal transducers and activators of transcription (STATs) [36-38]. Treatments with PPARγ agonists increase the expression of UCP2 in both animal and cell studies [25,39,40], suggesting that UCP2 may be regulated by PPARγ activity. We have demonstrated previously [23,24] that the PPARγ agonist, rosiglitazone

enhances UCP2 expression in the hippocampal neurons, leading to protection against oxidative stress and neuronal cell death associated with cerebral ischemia. We also showed previously [25] that gene knockdown of UCP2 by antisense oligonucleotide or pharmacological pretreatment with PPARγ agonist and antagonist also pointed to an antioxidative role for UCP2 in the brain stem against neurogenic hypertension. Moreover, in mice overexpressing human UCP-2 gene, brain damage was diminished after experimental stroke and traumatic

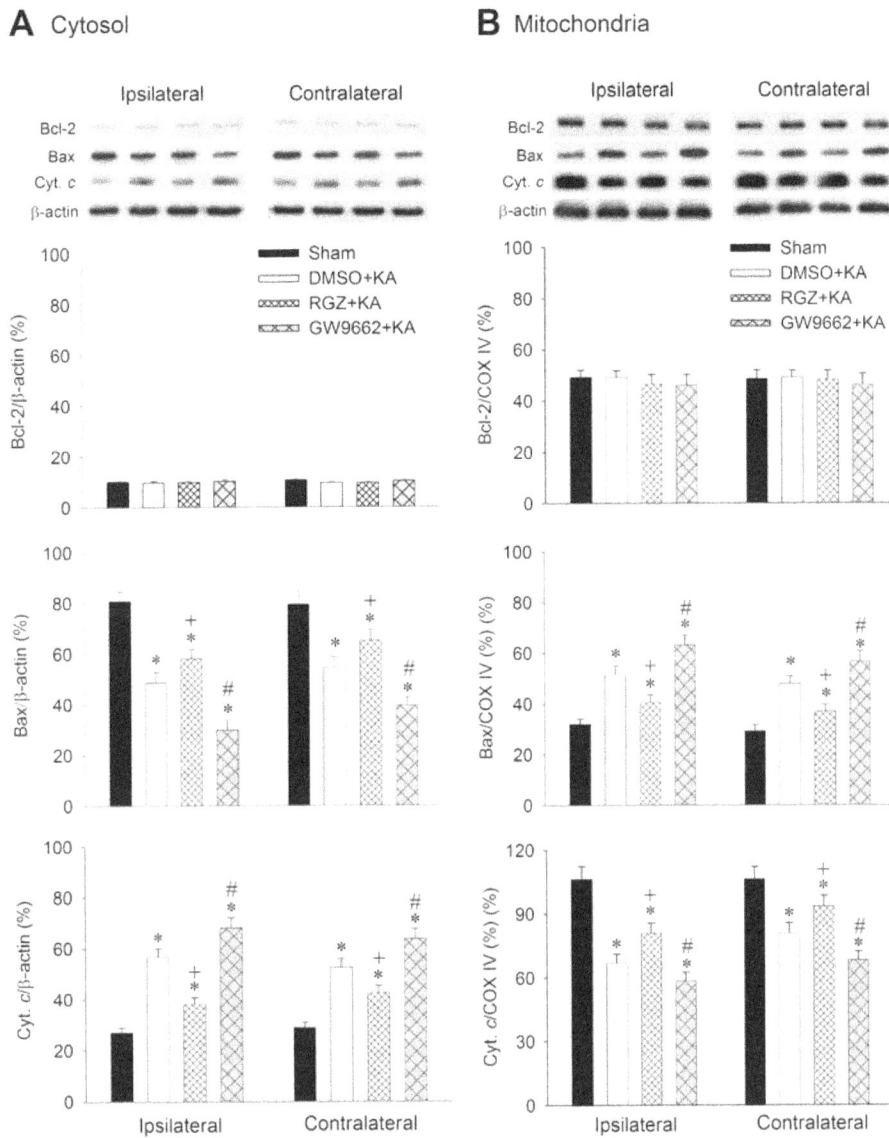

**Figure 8** Representative gels (inset) or temporal changes in Bcl-2, Bax or cytochrome *c* relative to β-actin protein detected in the cytosolic or relative to cytochrome *c* oxidase subunit IV (COX-IV) in the mitochondrial fraction of samples collected from the CA3 subfield of the hippocampus 24 h after microinjection of kainic acid (KA) (0.5 nmol) or PBS into the left hippocampal CA3 subfield, in animals that received pretreatment with application into the bilateral CA3 subfield of 3% dimethyl sulfoxide (DMSO), 6 nmol rosiglitazone (RGZ) or 500 ng GW9662. **(A)** Cytosolic fraction and **(B)** mitochondrial fraction of samples. Values are mean ± standard error of the mean (SEM) of quadruplicate analyses from six animals per experimental group. *$P < 0.05$ versus sham-control group, +$P < 0.05$ versus sham-control, DMSO + KA or GW9662 + KA group, and #$P < 0.05$ versus sham-control, DMSO + KA or RGZ + KA group in the Scheffé multiple-range test.

brain injury, and neurological recovery was enhanced [18]. In rat cultured cortical neurons, overexpression of UCP-2 gene reduced cell death and inhibited caspase-3 activation induced by oxygen and glucose deprivation [18]. It is intriguing that results from the present study also showed that pretreatment with rosiglitazone increased mitochondrial UCP2 expression, reduced the extent of protein oxidation, $O_2^-$ overproduction and dysfunction of mitochondrial respiratory enzyme complex I, hindered the translocation of Bax or cytochrome *c*

between cytosol and mitochondria and reduced neuronal damage in the hippocampal CA3 subfield elicited by experimental status epilepticus. In contrast, treatment with the PPARγ antagonist, GW9662 exerted opposite effects. Thus, the present study provided a novel demonstration of an antioxidant role for the PPARγ/UCP2 signaling pathway against oxidative stress and mitochondrial dysfunctions that reduced neuronal cell injury in the hippocampal CA3 subfield after the experimental model of temporal lobe status epilepticus.

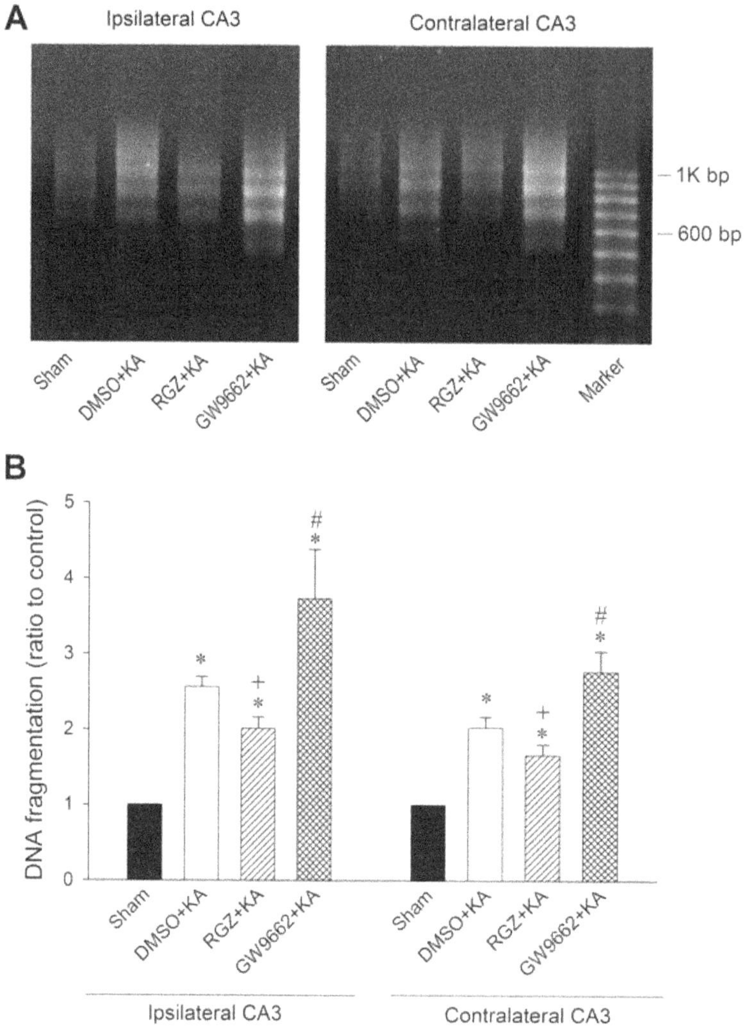

**Figure 9** Analysis of DNA fragmentation detected in samples collected from the CA3 subfield of the hippocampus 7 days after microinjection of kainic acid (KA) (0.5 nmol) or PBS into the left hippocampal CA3 subfield in animals that received pretreatment with application into the bilateral CA3 subfield of 3% dimethyl sulfoxide (DMSO), 6 nmol rosiglitazone (RGZ) or 500 ng GW9662. (A) Qualitative analysis. (B) Quantitative analysis. Values in panel B are fold changes with reference to sham-control and are mean ± standard error of the mean (SEM) of four animals per experimental group. $*P < 0.05$ versus sham-control group, $+P < 0.05$ versus sham-control, DMSO + KA or GW9662 + KA group, and $\#P < 0.05$ versus sham-control, DMSO + KA or RGZ + KA group in the Scheffé multiple-range test.

Neuroprotection following prolonged seizures, such as status epilepticus should encompass not only the prevention of neuronal cell death, but also preservation of neuronal and network function. Less well studied are the protective mechanisms elicited by seizure activity especially under status epilepticus. Except for the detrimental chain reaction under status epilepticus, acute response protein to counteract these detrimental effects may be elicited as an endogenous protective mechanism. Endogenous neuronal survival mechanisms following prolonged seizure insult are those that have been evolutionarily conserved and may trigger a number of signaling pathways to exert the protective effect and therefore be strong candidates to imply as therapeutic

strategies [41]. In animal studies with status epilepticus, several endogenous protective mechanisms to lessen neuronal damage were proposed, including activation ERK1/2, epileptic tolerance, vascular endothelial growth factor, activation of adenosine A1 receptors, erythropoietin receptor [41-45]. Based on real-time PCR and western blot analyses, we demonstrated a significant increase in UCP2 mRNA in the hippocampal CA3 subfield after KA-elicited status epilepticus, followed by augmented UCP2 protein levels. In addition, immunofluorescence staining demonstrated that the activated UCP2 was mainly in the mitochondria of hippocampal CA3 neurons. Thus, our results suggested that mitochondrial UCP2 may play an endogenous neuroprotective role against hippocampal neuronal cell damage under the stress of prolonged epileptic seizures.

Several antioxidant systems are present in the cell to counteract oxidative stress and to restore redox balance, and may be considered endogenous protective mechanisms under pathological conditions. In addition to the documented ROS-detoxifying enzymes and low molecular weight antioxidants, whether mitochondrial UCP functions as a natural antioxidant defense mechanism against oxidative stress is still debatable. Mitochondrial UCPs control the leakage of protons across the inner mitochondrial membrane and have emerged as an important modulator for oxidative stress [17,46]. As UCP2 are most prevalent in the nervous system, and a majority of the neurodegenerative disorders engages free radical production [13,17,46], it is reasonable to propose that UCP2 induction will be involved in these neurological disorders, including status epilepticus. Although the physiological role of UCP2 is still not clear, emerging evidence suggests that UCP2 may be related to the regulation of mitochondrial membrane potential, regulation of ROS production, preservation of calcium homeostasis, modulation of neuronal activity, and inhibition of cellular damage and inflammation [17,46,47]. Several recent studies stressed the role of protective effects of UCP2 against the neuronal cell damage after cerebral ischemia and brain trauma [18,24,46-49]; limited studies explored the role of UCP2 in epileptic seizures. In transgenic mice that express UCP2 constitutively in the hippocampus, there is an attenuation of seizure-induced neuronal death and an increase in mitochondrial number and ATP levels, alongside a parallel decrease in free radical-induced damage [50]. Modulation of UCP2 expression and function by dietary fat protects neonatal rats against seizure-induced brain damage associated with oxidative stress and mitochondrial dysfunction [51]. In the present study, we found that mitochondrial UCP2 was significantly upregulated in the hippocampal CA3 region 12 to 48 h after the induction of experimental status epilepticus, at a time-point that lagged behind the increase in protein carbonylation and $O_2^-$ These results indicate that the endogenous activation of mitochondrial UCP2 in hippocampal CA3 neurons under prolonged epileptic seizures may be a consequence of the increase in ROS production.

Mitochondrial dysfunction has been implicated as an important factor in the pathogenesis of seizure-induced neuronal cell death [2,10,52]. As the cellular powerhouse, the primary function of mitochondria is the production of cellular energy in the form of ATP by way of oxidative phosphorylation through the mitochondrial respiratory chain [53]. However, mitochondrial metabolism is also responsible for a majority of ROS production in cells and complex I of the mitochondrial electron transport chain is noticeably more susceptible to both oxidative and nitrosative stress than other respiratory chain complexes [54]. Dysfunction of complex I may lead to incomplete mitochondrial electron transport and reduced ATP production. We reported previously [5,19-21] that activation of NF-κB in hippocampal CA3 neurons upregulates NOS II gene expression, accompanied by an increase in $O_2^-$ production and peroxynitrite formation, followed by reduction in mitochondrial complex I activity, leading to apoptotic neuronal cell death in the hippocampus via the intrinsic mitochondrial apoptotic pathway. Therefore, the dysfunction of complex I may be an important biochemical hallmark of seizure-induced neuronal cell death in the hippocampus and may play a crucial role in the mechanism of epileptogenesis [2,10]. It follows that our demonstration of an increase or decrease in mitochondrial UCP2 expression induced by rosiglitazone or GW9662 underlying the attenuation or exacerbation of seizure-induced mitochondrial complex I dysfunction, suggests that another cellular role for UCP2 induced by experimental status epilepticus is amelioration of bioenergetics inefficiency in the hippocampus. Thus, UCP-2 may be an inducible protein that provides a neuroprotective effect by activating cellular redox signaling as well as by inducing mild mitochondrial uncoupling [18].

One of the decisive steps of the apoptotic cascade is permeabilization of the outer mitochondrial membrane [55], which leads to the release of cytochrome $c$ from the intermediate space, followed by the activation of caspase-dependent apoptotic signaling. It is generally contended that the anti-apoptotic members of the Bcl-2 family work to prevent cytochrome $c$ release by stabilizing the mitochondrial membrane barrier function and the pro-apoptotic members tend to induce cytochrome $c$ release by permeabilizing the mitochondrial membrane [55,56]. Translocation of Bax from the cytosol to mitochondria is induced during apoptosis, and this process is inhibited by Bcl-2 [30,57]. The evidence of Bcl-2 family involvement in seizure-induced neuronal cell death has been demonstrated in recent studies, and both pro-apoptotic and anti-apoptotic Bcl-2 family proteins were found to be activated by seizures [1,58]. However, conflicting results on the expressional regulation of Bcl-2 family proteins in seizure-induced neuronal cell death have emerged [1,58]. The reason for the discrepancy is currently not well elucidated, but may be related to the severity and duration of the disease conditions, or differences in the experimental methods employed. Increased Bax translocation from cytosol to mitochondria in the hippocampus has been reported in an animal model of KA-induced epileptic seizures [59]. Bax has been detected in clusters and accumulations on the outer surface of mitochondria in the hippocampal neurons after intra-amygdala KA-induced seizures [60]. In the present study, we observed that the progressive translocation of cytosolic Bax to the mitochondria, alongside an increase in cytosolic presence of cytochrome $c$, are indicative of an interplay between Bax and cytochrome c-dependent apoptotic cell death in the hippocampus following status epilepticus. Whereas Bcl-2 is reported to be upregulated during seizure-induced neuronal cell death [58], the expression of Bcl-2 did not show significant changes in our present study. This discrepancy may be related to the highly specific functions and subcellular locations of Bax and Bcl-2; Bax protein is found in both cytoplasmic and mitochondrial compartments, and Bcl-2 protein is largely mitochondrial [1,55,56]. The present study also provided novel results to suggest that upregulation of UCP2 in the hippocampus following experimental status epilepticus exerts its anti-apoptotic action by interacting with Bax mitochondrial translocation and downstream cytochrome c-dependent apoptotic cascades. Overexpression of UCP2 in transgenic mice ameliorated ischemia-induced Bcl-2 suppression in the brain [47]. In skin cancer cells, upregulation of UCP2 blocked p53 mitochondrial translocation, which regulates the pro-apoptotic effector Bax and reduced apoptosis during early tumor promotion [61]. Therefore, we suggest that the upregulated UCP2 in the hippocampus may prevent the mitochondrial translocation of Bax by stabilizing the inner mitochondrial membrane potential, resulting in an antagonism against the downstream apoptotic events under prolonged epileptic challenges.

Considerable controversy exists among reported models of seizure-induced damage with regards to the distribution, magnitude or form of neuronal cell death [1,2,22,62]. The nature of hippocampal neuronal cell death following prolonged seizure was reported to be either apoptotic, necrotic or both [1,22,62,63]. Programmed cell death mechanisms associated with cellular apoptosis have been shown to be activated after experimental status epilepticus [1,63]. Whereas CA3 neurons in the ipsilateral hippocampus exhibited a mild degree of necrosis or the intermediate forms of neuronal damage [22] that may be directly related to KA excitatotoxicity, our experimental model revealed that seizure-induced apoptotic cell death via cytochrome c/caspase-3-dependent signaling cascade was detected in the vulnerable CA3 neurons after a low dose of intrahippocampal administration of KA. We found that the degree of dysfunction of complex I respiratory chain enzyme was similar at 3 h and 24 h after experimental status epilepticus. This implied that the complex I dysfunction did not progress beyond 24 h in this animal model. In addition, our previous study found that preserved mitochondrial ultrastructural integrity and maintained energy metabolism 3 to 7 days following experimental status epilepticus is associated specifically with apoptotic, not necrotic, cell death in hippocampal CA3 neurons [22]. It follows that differences in animal models of seizures, variations in duration and intensity of the induced seizure activity, and metabolic disturbances after seizures are all contributing factors that determine the level of energy production in the mitochondria, leading eventually to diverse neuronal cell death fate in vulnerable regions of the hippocampus.

Our results showed a temporal decrease in PPARγ expression 6 h after experimental status epilepticus, followed by a significant increase of expression from 12 to 48 h in the hippocampal CA3 subfield. Whereas the design of the present study did not allow us to address the underlying mechanism, we are aware that a transient decrease in the expression of PPARγ protein under pathological conditions such as hypoxia, cerebral ischemia and interferon-γ or nerve growth factor treatment have been reported in neuronal and non-neuronal cells [38,64-66]. This effect may be attributed to the activation of ubiquitin-proteasome pathway or cytokines and inflammatory responses [38,64,67]. At the same time, transcription factors such as NF-κB, AP-1 and STATs are known to regulate cytokine gene expression and inflammatory response [68]. We have demonstrated previously [19] that significantly augmented nucleus-bound translocation of NF-κB and DNA binding activity of NF-κB in hippocampal CA3 neurons and glial cells occurs as early as 30 minutes after the elicitation of sustained seizure activity. Therefore, the transient decrease of PPARγ expression in the hippocampus during experimental status epilepticus may be related to activation of NF-κB and other inflammatory responses. However, the interrelationship between NF-κB and PPARγ in this experimental paradigm warrants further exploration.

## Conclusions

We demonstrated that activation of PPARγ upregulated mitochondrial UCP2 expression, which decreased overproduction of ROS, improved mitochondrial complex I dysfunction, inhibited mitochondrial translocation of Bax and prevented cytosolic release of cytochrome c by stabilizing the mitochondrial transmembrane potential, leading to amelioration of apoptotic neuronal cell death in the hippocampus following status epilepticus. These findings may offer a new vista in the development of more effective strategies to enhance this endogenous protective mechanism and reduce brain damage caused by status epilepticus.

### Abbreviations
ANOVA: one-way analysis of variance; AP-1: activator protein-1; BCA: bicinchoninic acid; CNS: central nervous system; COX IV: cytochrome c oxidase subunit IV; DMSO: dimethyl sulfoxide; DNP-hydrazone: 2,4-dinitrophenylhydrazone; ELISA: enzyme-linked immunosorbent assay; GAPDH: glyceraldehyde-3-phosphate dehydrogenase; GFAP: glial fibrillary acidic protein; hEEG: hippocampal electroencephalography; ip: intraperitoneal; KA: kainic acid; NADH: nicotinamide adenine dinucleotide; NF-κB: nuclear factor-κB; NO: nitric oxide; NOS II: nitric oxide synthase II; O$_2$: superoxide anion; PBS: phosphate buffered saline; PCR: polymerase chain reaction; PPARγ: peroxisome proliferator-activated receptor γ; RT: reverse transcriptase; ROS: reactive oxygen species; SOD: superoxide dismutase; STATs: signal transducers and activators of transcription; UCP: uncoupling protein.

### Competing interest
The authors have no competing interests to declare in relation to this study.

## Authors' contributions
YCC, SDC, AYWC and SHHC conceived and designed the experiments. YCC, TKL, SDC, HYH and CWL performed the experiments. YCC, HYH, SDC, AYWC and SHHC analyzed the data. YCC, TKL, SDC and SHHC wrote the paper. YCC, SDC and SHHC supervised the research. YCC, TKL, HYH, WNC, SDC and CWL collected data. All authors have read and approved the final version of this manuscript.

## Authors' informations
YCC is Professor of Neurology and Head of the Division of Epilepsy in Kaohsiung Chang Gung Memorial Hospital. TKL, WNC, CWL and SDC are Associate Professors of Neurology in Kaohsiung Chang Gung Memorial Hospital. HYH is Professor of Pathology and Head of Pathology in Kaohsiung Chang Gung Memorial Hospital. AYWC is Professor of the Center in Translational Research in Biomedical Sciences in Kaohsiung Chang Gung Memorial Hospital. SHHC is the National Chair Professor in Neuroscience, awarded by the Ministry of Education, Taiwan. He is also a Distinguished Chair Professor of Translational Medicine, and the founding and current director of the Center in Translational Research in Biomedical Sciences in Kaohsiung Chang Gung Memorial Hospital. SHHC is currently the President of the Federation of Asian and Pacific Pharmacological Societies.

## Acknowledgements
This study was supported in part by research grants 98-2321-B-182A-002 and 99-2321-B-182A-002 to YCC from the National Science Council, and CMRPG880851 and 880852 to YCC from Chang Gung Memorial Hospital-Kaohsiung, Taiwan. We confirm that we have read the Journal's position on issues involved in ethical publication and affirm that this report is consistent with those guidelines.

## Author details
[1]Department of Neurology, Kaohsiung Chang Gung Memorial Hospital and Chang Gung University College of Medicine, Kaohsiung 83301, Taiwan. [2]Center for Translational Research in Biomedical Sciences, Kaohsiung Chang Gung Memorial Hospital and Chang Gung University College of Medicine, Kaohsiung 83301, Taiwan. [3]Department of Pathology, Kaohsiung Chang Gung Memorial Hospital and Chang Gung University College of Medicine, Kaohsiung 83301, Taiwan.

## References
1. Henshall DC, Simon RP: Epilepsy and apoptosis pathways. J Cereb Blood Flow Metab 2005, 25:1557–1572.
2. Chen SD, Chang AYW, Chuang YC: The potential role of mitochondrial dysfunction in seizure-associated cell death in the hippocampus and epileptogenesis. J Bioenerg Biomembr 2010, 42:461–465.
3. Cendes F: Progressive hippocampal and extrahippocampal atrophy in drug resistant epilepsy. Curr Opin Neurol 2005, 18:173–177.
4. Bouilleret V, Nehlig A, Marescaux C, Namer IJ: Magnetic resonance imaging follow-up of progressive hippocampal changes in a mouse model of mesial temporal lobe epilepsy. Epilepsia 2000, 41:642–650.
5. Chuang YC, Chang AYW, Lin JW, Hsu SP, Chan SHH: Mitochondrial dysfunction and ultrastructural damage in the hippocampus during kainic acid-induced status epilepticus in the rat. Epilepsia 2004, 45:1202–1209.
6. Cock HR, Tong X, Hargreaves IP, Heales SJ, Clark JB, Patsalos PN, Thom M, Groves M, Schapira AH, Shorvon SD, Walker MC: Mitochondrial dysfunction associated with neuronal death following status epilepticus in rat. Epilepsy Res 2002, 48:157–168.
7. Folbergrová J, Ješina P, Haugvicová R, Lisý V, Houštěk J: Sustained deficiency of mitochondrial complex I activity during long periods of survival after seizures induced in immature rats by homocysteic acid. Neurochem Int 2010, 56:394–403.
8. Kudin AP, Kudina TA, Seyfried J, Vielhaber S, Beck H, Elger CE, Kunz WS: Seizure-dependent modulation of mitochondrial oxidative phosphorylation in rat hippocampus. Eur J Neurosci 2002, 15:1105–1114.
9. Kunz WS, Kudin AP, Vielhaber S, Blumcke I, Zuschratter W, Schramm J, Beck H, Elger CE: Mitochondrial complex I deficiency in the epileptic focus of patients with temporal lobe epilepsy. Ann Neurol 2000, 48:766–773.
10. Kudin AP, Zsurka G, Elger CE, Kunz WS: Mitochondrial involvement in temporal lobe epilepsy. Exp Neurol 2009, 218:326–332.
11. Cannon B, Shabalina IG, Kramarova TV, Petrovic N, Nedergaard J: Uncoupling proteins: a role in protection against reactive oxygen species–or not? Biochim Biophys Acta 2006, 1757:449–458.
12. Echtay KS: Mitochondrial uncoupling proteins–what is their physiological role? Free Radic Biol Med 2007, 43:1351–1371.
13. Kim-Han JS, Dugan LL: Mitochondrial uncoupling proteins in the central nervous system. Antioxid Redox Signal 2005, 7:1173–1181.
14. Nègre-Salvayre A, Hirtz C, Carrera G, Cazenave R, Troly M, Salvayre R, Pénicaud L, Casteilla L: A role for uncoupling protein-2 as a regulator of mitochondrial hydrogen peroxide generation. FASEB J 1997, 11:809–815.
15. Teshima Y, Akao M, Jones SP, Marbán E: Uncoupling protein-2 overexpression inhibits mitochondrial death pathway in cardiomyocytes. Circ Res 2003, 93:192–200.
16. Rousset S, Alves-Guerra MC, Mozo J, Miroux B, Cassard-Doulcier AM, Bouillaud F, Ricquier D: The biology of mitochondrial uncoupling proteins. Diabetes 2004, 53(Suppl 1):S130–S135.
17. Andrews ZB, Diano S, Horvath TL: Mitochondrial uncoupling proteins in the CNS: in support of function and survival. Nat Rev Neurosci 2005, 6:829–840.
18. Mattiasson G, Shamloo M, Gido G, Mathi K, Tomasevic G, Yi S, Warden CH, Castilho RF, Melcher T, Gonzalez-Zulueta M, Nikolich K, Wieloch T: Uncoupling protein-2 prevents neuronal death and diminishes brain dysfunction after stroke and brain trauma. Nat Med 2003, 9:1062–1068.
19. Chuang YC, Chen SD, Lin TK, Chang WN, Lu CH, Liou CW, Chan SHH, Chang AYW: Transcriptional upregulation of nitric oxide synthase II by nuclear factor-κB promotes apoptotic neuronal cell death in the hippocampus following experimental status epilepticus. J Neurosci Res 2010, 88:1898–1907.
20. Chuang YC, Chen SD, Lin TK, Liou CW, Chang WN, Chan SHH, Chang AYW: Upregulation of nitric oxide synthase II contributes to apoptotic cell death in the hippocampal CA3 subfield via a cytochrome c/caspase-3 signaling cascade following induction of experimental temporal lobe status epilepticus in the rat. Neuropharmacology 2007, 52:1263–1273.
21. Chuang YC, Chen SD, Liou CW, Lin TK, Chang WN, Chan SHH, Chang AYW: Contribution of nitric oxide, superoxide anion, and peroxynitrite to activation of mitochondrial apoptotic signaling in hippocampal CA3 subfield following experimental temporal lobe status epilepticus. Epilepsia 2009, 50:731–746.
22. Chuang YC, Lin JW, Chen SD, Lin TK, Liou CW, Lu CH, Chang WN: Preservation of mitochondrial integrity and energy metabolism during experimental status epilepticus leads to neuronal apoptotic cell death in the hippocampus of the rat. Seizure 2009, 18:420–428.
23. Chen SD, Lin TK, Lin JW, Yang DI, Lee SY, Shaw FZ, Liou CW, Chuang YC: Activation of calcium/calmodulin-dependent protein kinase IV and peroxisome proliferator-activated receptor γ coactivator-1α signaling pathway protects against neuronal injury and promotes mitochondrial biogenesis in the hippocampal CA1 subfield after transient global ischemia. J Neurosci Res 2010, 88:3144–3154.
24. Chen SD, Wu HY, Yang DI, Lee SY, Shaw FZ, Lin TK, Liou CW, Chuang YC: Effects of rosiglitazone on global ischemia-induced hippocampal injury and expression of mitochondrial uncoupling protein 2. Biochem Biophys Res Commun 2006, 351:198–203.
25. Chan SHH, Wu CA, Wu KL, Ho YH, Chang AYW, Chan JYH: Transcriptional upregulation of mitochondrial uncoupling protein 2 protects against oxidative stress-associated neurogenic hypertension. Circ Res 2009, 105:886–896.
26. Lin TN, Cheung WM, Wu JS, Chen JJ, Lin H, Chen JJ, Liou JY, Shyue SK, Wu KK: 15d-prostaglandin J2 protects brain from ischemia-reperfusion injury. Arterioscler Thromb Vasc Biol 2006, 26:481–487.
27. Singhal AB, Wang X, Sumii T, Mori T, Lo EH: Effects of normobaric hyperoxia in a rat model of focal cerebral ischemia-reperfusion. J Cereb Blood Flow Metab 2002, 22:861–868.
28. Chen SD, Lin TK, Yang DI, Lee SY, Shaw FZ, Liou CW, Chuang YC: Protective effects of peroxisome proliferator-activated receptors γ coactivator-1α against neuronal cell death in the hippocampal CA1 subfield after transient global ischemia. J Neurosci Res 2010, 88:605–613.
29. Smith CD, Carney JM, Starke-Reed PE, Oliver CN, Stadtman ER, Floyd RA, Markesbery WR: Excess brain protein oxidation and enzyme dysfunction

in normal aging and in Alzheimer disease. *Proc Natl Acad Sci USA* 1991, 88:10540–10543.

30. Chang AYW, Chan JYH, Chou JLJ, Li FCH, Dai KY, Chan SHH: Heat shock protein 60 in rostral ventrolateral medulla reduces cardiovascular fatality during endotoxaemia in the rat. *J Physiol* 2006, 574:547–564.

31. Chuang YC, Chan JYH, Chang AYW, Sikorska M, Borowy-Borowski H, Liou CW, Chan SHH: Neuroprotective effects of coenzyme Q$_{10}$ at rostral ventrolateral medulla against fatality during experimental endotoxemia in the rat. *Shock* 2003, 19:427–432.

32. Nadanaciva S, Dykens JA, Bernal A, Capaldi RA, Will Y: Mitochondrial impairment by PPAR agonists and statins identified via immunocaptured OXPHOS complex activities and respiration. *Toxicol Appl Pharmacol* 2007, 223:277–287.

33. Willis JH, Capaldi RA, Huigsloot M, Rodenburg RJ, Smeitink J, Marusich MF: Isolated deficiencies of OXPHOS complexes I and IV are identified accurately and quickly by simple enzyme activity immunocapture assays. *Biochim Biophys Acta* 2009, 1787:533–538.

34. Bonfoco E, Krainc D, Ankarcrona M, Nicotera P, Lipton SA: Apoptosis and necrosis: two distinct events induced, respectively, by mild and intense insults with N-methyl-`aspartate or nitric oxide/superoxide in cortical cell cultures. *Proc Natl Acad Sci USA* 1995, 92:7162–7166.

35. Saito A, Narasimhan P, Hayashi T, Okuno S, Ferrand-Drake M, Chan PH: Neuroprotective role of a proline-rich Akt substrate in apoptotic neuronal cell death after stroke: relationships with nerve growth factor. *J Neurosci* 2004, 24:1584–1593.

36. Straus DS, Glass CK: Anti-inflammatory actions of PPAR ligands: new insights on cellular and molecular mechanisms. *Trends Immunol* 2007, 28:551–558.

37. Swanson CR, Joers V, Bondarenko V, Brunner K, Simmons HA, Ziegler TE, Kemnitz JW, Johnson JA, Emborg ME: The PPAR-γ agonist pioglitazone modulates inflammation and induces neuroprotection in parkinsonian monkeys. *J Neuroinflammation* 2011, 8:91.

38. Zhao Y, Patzer A, Herdegen T, Gohlke P, Culman J: Activation of cerebral peroxisome proliferator-activated receptors gamma promotes neuroprotection by attenuation of neuronal cyclooxygenase-2 overexpression after focal cerebral ischemia in rats. *FASEB J* 2006, 20:1162–1175.

39. Hammarstedt A, Smith U: Thiazolidinediones (PPARγ ligands) increase IRS-1, UCP-2 and C/EBPα expression, but not transdifferentiation, in L6 muscle cells. *Diabetologia* 2003, 46:48–52.

40. Kelly LJ, Vicario PP, Thompson GM, Candelore MR, Doebber TW, Ventre J, Wu MS, Meurer R, Forrest MJ, Conner MW, Cascieri MA, Moller DE: Peroxisome proliferator-activated receptors γ and α mediate in vivo regulation of uncoupling protein (UCP-1, UCP-2, UCP-3) gene expression. *Endocrinology* 1998, 139:4920–4927.

41. Simon R, Henshall D, Stoehr S, Meller R: Endogenous mechanisms of neuroprotection. *Epilepsia* 2007, 48(Suppl 8):72–73.

42. Sanchez PE, Fares RP, Risso JJ, Bonnet C, Bouvard S, Le-Cavorsin M, Georges B, Moulin C, Belmeguenai A, Bodennec J, Morales A, Pequignot JM, Baulieu EE, Levine RA, Bezin L: Optimal neuroprotection by erythropoietin requires elevated expression of its receptor in neurons. *Proc Natl Acad Sci USA* 2009, 106:9848–9853.

43. Jimenez-Mateos EM, Mouri G, Conroy RM, Henshall DC: Epileptic tolerance is associated with enduring neuroprotection and uncoupling of the relationship between CA3 damage, neuropeptide Y rearrangement and spontaneous seizures following intra-amygdala kainic acid-induced status epilepticus in mice. *Neuroscience* 2010, 171:556–565.

44. Berkeley JL, Decker MJ, Levey AI: The role of muscarinic acetylcholine receptor-mediated activation of extracellular signal-regulated kinase 1/2 in pilocarpine-induced seizures. *J Neurochem* 2002, 82:192–201.

45. Nicoletti JN, Shah SK, McCloskey DP, Goodman JH, Elkady A, Atassi H, Hylton D, Rudge JS, Scharfman HE, Croll SD: Vascular endothelial growth factor is up-regulated after status epilepticus and protects against seizure-induced neuronal loss in hippocampus. *Neuroscience* 2008, 151:232–241.

46. Mehta SL, Li PA: Neuroprotective role of mitochondrial uncoupling protein 2 in cerebral stroke. *J Cereb Blood Flow Metab* 2009, 29:1069–1078.

47. Haines B, Li PA: Overexpression of mitochondrial uncoupling protein 2 inhibits inflammatory cytokines and activates cell survival factors after cerebral ischemia. *PLoS One* 2012, 7:e31739.

48. Haines BA, Mehta SL, Pratt SM, Warden CH, Li PA: Deletion of mitochondrial uncoupling protein-2 increases ischemic brain damage after transient focal ischemia by altering gene expression patterns and enhancing inflammatory cytokines. *J Cereb Blood Flow Metab* 2010, 30:1825–1833.

49. Deierborg T, Wieloch T, Diano S, Warden CH, Horvath TL, Mattiasson G: Overexpression of UCP2 protects thalamic neurons following global ischemia in the mouse. *J Cereb Blood Flow Metab* 2008, 28:1186–1195.

50. Diano S, Matthews RT, Patrylo P, Yang L, Beal MF, Barnstable CJ, Horvath TL: Uncoupling protein 2 prevents neuronal death including that occurring during seizures: a mechanism for preconditioning. *Endocrinology* 2003, 144:5014–5021.

51. Sullivan PG, Dube C, Dorenbos K, Steward O, Baram TZ: Mitochondrial uncoupling protein-2 protects the immature brain from excitotoxic neuronal death. *Ann Neurol* 2003, 53:711–717.

52. Waldbaum S, Patel M: Mitochondria, oxidative stress, and temporal lobe epilepsy. *Epilepsy Res* 2010, 88:23–45.

53. Hatefi Y: The mitochondrial electron transport and oxidative phosphorylation system. *Annu Rev Biochem* 1985, 54:1015–1069.

54. Carreras MC, Franco MC, Peralta JG, Poderoso JJ: Nitric oxide, complex I, and the modulation of mitochondrial reactive species in biology and disease. *Mol Aspects Med* 2004, 25:125–139.

55. Crompton M: Mitochondrial intermembrane junctional complexes and their role in cell death. *J Physiol* 2000, 529(Pt 1):11–21.

56. Kroemer G, Reed JC: Mitochondrial control of cell death. *Nat Med* 2000, 6:513–519.

57. Hou Q, Hsu YT: Bax translocates from cytosol to mitochondria in cardiac cells during apoptosis: development of a GFP-Bax-stable H9c2 cell line for apoptosis analysis. *Am J Physiol Heart Circ Physiol* 2005, 289:H477–H487.

58. Engel T, Henshall DC: Apoptosis, Bcl-2 family proteins and caspases: the ABCs of seizure-damage and epileptogenesis? *Int J Physiol Pathophysiol Pharmacol* 2009, 1:97–115.

59. Liu XM, Pei DS, Guan QH, Sun YF, Wang XT, Zhang QX, Zhang GY: Neuroprotection of Tat-GluR6-9c against neuronal death induced by kainate in rat hippocampus via nuclear and non-nuclear pathways. *J Biol Chem* 2006, 281:17432–17445.

60. Henshall DC, Araki T, Schindler CK, Lan JQ, Tiekoter KL, Taki W, Simon RP: Activation of Bcl-2-associated death protein and counter-response of Akt within cell populations during seizure-induced neuronal death. *J Neurosci* 2002, 22:8458–8465.

61. Wang F, Fu X, Chen X, Zhao Y: Mitochondrial uncoupling inhibits p53 mitochondrial translocation in TPA-challenged skin epidermal JB6 cells. *PLoS One* 2010, 5:e13459.

62. Fujikawa DG: Prolonged seizures and cellular injury: understanding the connection. *Epilepsy Behav* 2005, 7(Suppl 3):S3–S11.

63. Bengzon J, Mohapel P, Ekdahl CT, Lindvall O: Neuronal apoptosis after brief and prolonged seizures. *Prog Brain Res* 2002, 135:111–119.

64. Waite KJ, Floyd ZE, Arbour-Reily P, Stephens JM: Interferon-γ-induced regulation of peroxisome proliferator-activated receptor γ and STATs in adipocytes. *J Biol Chem* 2001, 276:7062–7068.

65. Fuenzalida KM, Aguilera MC, Piderit DG, Ramos PC, Contador D, Quinones V, Rigotti A, Bronfman FC, Bronfman M: Peroxisome proliferator-activated receptor γ is a novel target of the nerve growth factor signaling pathway in PC12 cells. *J Biol Chem* 2005, 280:9604–9609.

66. Gamboa JL, Andrade FH: Mitochondrial content and distribution changes specific to mouse diaphragm after chronic normobaric hypoxia. *Am J Physiol Regul Integr Comp Physiol* 2010, 298:R575–R583.

67. Bernardo A, Levi G, Minghetti L: Role of the peroxisome proliferator-activated receptor-γ (PPAR-γ) and its natural ligand 15-deoxy-Delta12, 14-prostaglandin J2 in the regulation of microglial functions. *Eur J Neurosci* 2000, 12:2215–2223.

68. Desvergne B, Wahli W: Peroxisome proliferator-activated receptors: nuclear control of metabolism. *Endocr Rev* 1999, 20:649–688.

# 7

# Effects of dexamethasone on the Li-pilocarpine model of epilepsy: protection against hippocampal inflammation and astrogliosis

Adriana Fernanda K. Vizuete[*] ⓘ, Fernanda Hansen, Elisa Negri, Marina Concli Leite, Diogo Losch de Oliveira and Carlos-Alberto Gonçalves

**Abstract**

**Background:** Temporal lobe epilepsy (TLE) is the most common form of partial epilepsy and is accompanied, in one third of cases, by resistance to antiepileptic drugs (AED). Most AED target neuronal activity modulated by ionic channels, and the steroid sensitivity of these channels has supported the use of corticosteroids as adjunctives to AED. Assuming the importance of astrocytes in neuronal activity, we investigated inflammatory and astroglial markers in the hippocampus, a key structure affected in TLE and in the Li-pilocarpine model of epilepsy.

**Methods:** Initially, hippocampal slices were obtained from sham rats and rats subjected to the Li-pilocarpine model of epilepsy, at 1, 14, and 56 days after *status epilepticus* (SE), which correspond to the acute, silent, and chronic phases. Dexamethasone was added to the incubation medium to evaluate the secretion of S100B, an astrocyte-derived protein widely used as a marker of brain injury. In the second set of experiments, we evaluated the in vivo effect of dexamethasone, administrated at 2 days after SE, on hippocampal inflammatory (COX-1/2, PGE2, and cytokines) and astroglial parameters: GFAP, S100B, glutamine synthetase (GS) and water (AQP-4), and K$^+$ (Kir 4.1) channels.

**Results:** Basal S100B secretion and S100B secretion in high-K$^+$ medium did not differ at 1, 14, and 56 days for the hippocampal slices from epileptic rats, in contrast to sham animal slices, where high-K$^+$ medium decreased S100B secretion. Dexamethasone addition to the incubation medium per se induced a decrease in S100B secretion in sham and epileptic rats (1 and 56 days after SE induction). Following in vivo dexamethasone administration, inflammatory improvements were observed, astrogliosis was prevented (based on GFAP and S100B content), and astroglial dysfunction was partially abrogated (based on Kir 4.1 protein and GSH content). The GS decrease was not prevented by dexamethasone, and AQP-4 was not altered in this epileptic model.

**Conclusions:** Changes in astroglial parameters emphasize the importance of these cells for understanding alterations and mechanisms of epileptic disorders in this model. In vivo dexamethasone administration prevented most of the parameters analyzed, reinforcing the importance of anti-inflammatory steroid therapy in the Li-pilocarpine model and possibly in other epileptic conditions in which neuroinflammation is present.

**Keywords:** Epilepsy, Dexamethasone, Neuroinflammation, Astrocytes, S100B

* Correspondence: adrianavizuete@gmail.com
Department of Biochemistry, Instituto de Ciências Básicas da Saúde,
Universidade Federal do Rio Grande do Sul, Ramiro Barcelos, 2600-Anexo,
Porto Alegre, RS 90035-003, Brazil

## Background

Epilepsy is a neuronal disorder characterized by recurrent and spontaneous seizures, resulting from excessive, abnormal, and hypersynchronous neuronal activity [1–3]. Approximately 50 million people worldwide suffer from this neuronal disorder, which normally affect mostly children and the elderly population [4]. Temporal lobe epilepsy (TLE) that affects the limbic system [5, 6] is the most common form of partial epilepsy and resistance to anticonvulsive drugs which develops in about 30% of cases [7, 8]. The Li-pilocarpine-induced model of epilepsy exhibits similar hippocampal alterations to those observed in TLE patients [9, 10] and is accompanied by drug resistance [11].

Brain tissue samples from patients and experimental models show specific astroglial changes, mainly in the levels of glial fibrillary acidic protein (GFAP) and S100B protein [12–16]. In fact, results from several studies suggest that epileptogenesis involves changes in the glial cells beyond neuronal alterations [17, 18]. Astrocytes are glial cells that interact with neurons and form tripartite synapses [19]. Some studies have strongly implicated astrocytes in the development of epileptic disorders [20–23]. Astrogliosis and neuroinflammation have been correlated to epileptogenesis, recurrent, and spontaneous seizures [24–29]. For this reason, specific astroglial targets (e.g., S100B, glutamine synthetase (GS), potassium channel Kir 4.1, and water channel AQP-4) have been investigated with a view to improving therapeutic approaches and the development of antiepileptic drugs [30].

The S100B protein is a glial protein that is a widely used marker for brain injury conditions, including epileptic disorders [31, 32], and indeed displays an augmented secretion during brain injury condition, working as a neurotrophic cytokine or simply as a damage-associated molecular pattern (DAMP) [33]. Moreover, S100B secretion is modulated by LPS [34] and anti-inflammatory drugs [35, 36]. Chronically elevated extracellular levels of S100B potentially lead to neurodegenerative processes [37, 38].

Therapy with corticosteroids, such as dexamethasone palmitate, has been used to treat refractory epilepsy in children [39]. Dexamethasone has been shown to reduce seizures in epileptic encephalopathy patients [40, 41]; while dexamethasone use has been evaluated in the Li-pilocarpine model of epilepsy [42, 43], its effect on astroglial targets has not been fully investigated. We hypothesized that dexamethasone mediates downregulation of S100B secretion and that this change could contribute to decrease neuroinflammation and astrogliosis during epileptogenesis. In fact, extracellular levels of S100B are elevated in Li-pilocarpine model of epilepsy [14].

Herein, we investigated the effect of dexamethasone on inflammatory and astroglial parameter in the Li-pilocarpine model of epilepsy. Firstly, we evaluated the

modulation of S100B secretion by dexamethasone in acute hippocampal slices at 1, 14, and 56 days after the induction of status epilepticus (SE) by Li-pilocarpine administration in young rats. In this experimental model, these times correspond approximately to the acute, silent, and chronic phases, respectively [44]. In the second set of experiments, we administered intraperitoneal dexamethasone 1 day after SE and analyzed inflammatory and hippocampal astroglial parameters (S100B, GFAP, GS, GSH, AQP-4, and Kir 4.1) at 1 and 56 days afterward. Cerebrospinal fluid (CSF) and serum S100B were also determined.

## Methods

### Animals

Male *Wistar* rats, at postnatal day 27, were used in this study. We focused this study on young (27-day-old) rats to characterize glial changes from an age corresponding to childhood in rats [45]. It is important to mention that, at this age, rats have developed and matured their blood-brain barrier [46], energetic metabolism [47], and GABAergic neurotransmission [48]. Animals were obtained from our breeding colony (Department of Biochemistry, UFRGS) and maintained under controlled light and environmental conditions (12 h light/12 h dark cycle at a constant temperature of $22 \pm 1$ °C). Procedures were in accordance with the National Institutes of Health Guide for the Care and Use of Laboratory Animals (NIH Publications No. 80-23) following the regulations of the local animal house authorities and Committee of Animal Use of UFRGS (project number 24472).

This study was divided into two parts. The first was to analyze the S100B secretion in the acute hippocampal slices in animals submitted to the Li-pilocarpine epileptic model. The second part was to observe the in vivo effects of dexamethasone on inflammatory and astroglial parameters in the model (Additional file 1).

### Epilepsy model

Animals were subjected to the LiCl-pilocarpine model of TLE, according to Cavalheiro [9]. Briefly, the rats were treated intraperitoneally with lithium (LiCl, 3 mEq/kg, i.p.) 12–18 h prior to the administration of pilocarpine (45 mg/kg, i.p.) (Sigma, St. Louis, MO, USA). Sham animals also received LiCl at 12–18 h prior to saline (0.9% NaCl, i.p.) administration. Animals were monitored and classified into five stages of an epileptic seizure, according to Racine's scale: (1) mouth and facial movement, (2) head nodding, (3) forelimb clonus, (4) rearing with forelimb clonus, and (5) rearing and falling with forelimb clonus.

We considered SE when animals reached stage 4 and stayed at this stage for more than 30 min. SE induction was stopped after 90 min by administration of diazepam

(10 mg/kg, i.p.) followed by four administrations of HBSS medium (at 1.5, 7, 12, and 24 h after SE onset) containing (in mM) 137 NaCl, 0.63 $Na_2HPO_4$, 4.17 $NaHCO_3$, 5.36 KCl, 0.044 $KH_2PO_4$, 1.26 $CaCl_2.2H_2O$, 0.041 $MgSO_4.7H_2O$, 0.049 $MgCl_2.6H_2O$, and 5.55 glucose, in order to promote a better animal recovery.

For further experiments, only animals that reached stage 4 and presented recurrent seizures were used. These animals were analyzed at different times—1, 14, and 56 days after pilocarpine injection—which correspond to the acute, latent, and chronic phases of epilepsy induced by the Li-pilocarpine model [49].

### First study—evaluation of S100B secretion in the acute hippocampal slices of SE rats

Sixty male rats were divided into (1) sham and (2) SE animals at different times (1, 14, and 56 days) after pilocarpine injection. These animals were killed by decapitation, and their brains were removed and placed in a cold saline medium of the following composition (in mM): 120 NaCl, 2 KCl, 1 $CaCl_2$, 1 $MgSO_4$, 25 HEPES, 1 $KH_2PO_4$, and 10 glucose, adjusted to pH 7.4. The hippocampi were dissected, and transverse slices of 0.3 mm were obtained using a McIlwain Tissue Chopper. Slices were then transferred immediately into 24-well culture plates, each well containing 0.3 ml of saline medium and only one slice. The medium was replaced every 15 min with fresh saline medium at room temperature. Following a 120-min equilibration period, the medium was removed and replaced with basal or specific treatments (high potassium—30 mM KCl; 0.1 μM dexamethasone; vehicle—0.01% DMSO) for 60 min at 30 °C on a warming plate [50].

### S100B secretion

S100B content in the supernatant was measured by ELISA, as described previously [51]. Briefly, 50 μl of sample plus 50 μl of Tris buffer were incubated for 2 h on a microtiter plate that was previously coated with monoclonal anti-S100B SH-B1 (Sigma-Aldrich, St. Louis, MO, USA). Polyclonal anti-S100 (Dako, Carpinteria, CA, USA) was incubated for 30 min, and peroxidase-conjugated anti-rabbit antibody was then added for a further 30 min. The color reaction with OPD was measured at 492 nm. The standard S100B curve ranged from 0.02 to10 ng/ml and data expressed as nanograms per milligram or nanograms per milliliter. Results are shown as percentages of the control.

### Lactate dehydrogenase assay

Slice integrity was evaluated by lactate dehydrogenase (LDH) kinetic activity using a commercial kit (BioClin, Brazil). The assay was performed according to the manufacturer's instructions.

### Second study—effect of dexamethasone on the SE model

Sixty male rats received an administration of vehicle (DMSO, 0.1%, i.p.) or dexamethasone (10 mg/kg, i.p.) 24 and 36 h after SE induction by LiCl-pilocarpine administration. Groups of animals were divided into (1) sham + vehicle, (2) SE + vehicle, and (3) SE + dexamethasone at 1 and 56 days after pilocarpine injection. Herein, the animals were monitored between 1 and 56 days after SE induction and dexamethasone administration. They were video monitored every other day, 4–5 h for behavioral evaluation of occurrence of recurrent spontaneous seizures. All SE animals developed epileptic behavior, i.e., all animals exhibited, at least, score 2 in the Racine's scale between 7 and 25 days after SE induction. Dexamethasone did not change epileptic behavior (see Additional file 2).

### Brain tissue, serum, and CSF samples

Rats were anesthetized by intraperitoneal injection of ketamine (75 mg/kg) and xylazine (10 mg/kg), and the blood was collected by cardiac puncture; serum was obtained by centrifuging at 1000×g for 10 min (Eppendorf 5402, Hamburg, Germany) before storing at − 80 °C. For ventricular access, the anesthetized rats were placed in a stereotaxic apparatus and cerebrospinal fluid (CSF) was obtained carefully by puncturing the cisterna magna with an insulin syringe. A maximum volume of 30 μl was collected over a 3-min period to minimize the risk of brain stem damage. The hippocampi were dissected, and transverse slices of 0.3 mm were obtained using a McIlwain Tissue Chopper as described above. Samples were stored at − 80 °C until biochemical and immunological assays.

### Cytokines and prostaglandin E2 measurement

The hippocampal slices were homogenized in phosphate buffer saline (PBS) containing (in mM) 50 NaCl, 18 $Na_2HPO_4$, and 83 $NaH_2PO_4.H_2O$, pH 7.4, with 1 mM EGTA and 1 mM phenylmethylsulphonyl fluoride (PMSF), followed by centrifugation at 1000×g for 5 min at 4 °C. Cytokines were measured in supernatants using rat TNF-α, IL-1β, IL-10 (eBioscience, San Diego, USA), and PGE2 (Enzo Life Science, Farmingdale, NY, USA) ELISA kits. Serum TNF-α content was also evaluated. Data are expressed in picograms per milligram protein (tissue samples) or picogram per milliliter (serum).

### S100B measurement

Slices were homogenized in PBS with 1 mM EGTA and 1 mM PMSF. The S100B content in the CSF, serum, and brain tissue was measured by ELISA, as described above. Data are expressed in nanograms per milligram protein (tissue samples) or nanogram per milliliter (CSF and serum).

## GFAP measurement

GFAP content was measured by ELISA, as described previously [52]. The ELISA for GFAP was carried out by coating wells of 96-well plates with 100-µl samples containing 70 µg of protein overnight at 4 °C. Wells were incubated with a polyclonal anti-GFAP antibody (Dako, Carpinteria, CA, USA) from rabbit for 2 h, followed by incubation with a secondary antibody conjugated with peroxidase for 1 h, at room temperature. The color reaction with OPD was measured at 492 nm. The standard GFAP (Calbiochem, San Diego, CA, USA) curve ranged from 0.1 to 10 ng/ml. Data are expressed in nanogram per milligram protein.

## Glutamine synthetase activity

The enzymatic assay for glutamine synthetase (GS) was performed, as described previously [53] with modifications. Briefly, the hippocampal slices were homogenized in 50 mM imidazole buffer. Homogenates were then incubated with (mM) 50 imidazole, 50 hydroxylamine, 100 L-glutamine, 25 sodium arsenate dibasic heptahydrate, 0.2 ADP, and 2 manganese chloride, pH 6.2 for 15 min at 37 °C. The reactions were terminated by the addition of 0.2 ml of 0.37 M FeCl$_3$, 200 mM trichloroacetic acid, and 670 mM HCl. After centrifugation, supernatant absorbance was measured at 530 nm. The standard γ-glutamylhydroxamate acid (Sigma-Aldrich, St. Louis, MO, USA) curve ranged from 0.1 to 10 mmol/ml. GS activity is expressed as µmol/h/mg protein.

## Glutathione content

Reduced glutathione (GSH) content was determined based on [50]. Briefly, slices were homogenized in sodium phosphate buffer (0.1 M, pH 8.0), and protein was precipitated with 1.7% meta-phosphoric acid. O-phthaldialdehyde (1 mg/ml methanol) (Sigma) was added to the supernatant at room temperature for 15 min. Fluorescence was measured using excitation and emission wavelengths of 350 and 420 nm, respectively. The standard calibration glutathione (Sigma-Aldrich, St. Louis, MO, USA) solution curve ranged from 0 to 500 µM. Glutathione results are expressed as nanomoles per milligram protein.

## Western blotting

Nitrocellulose membranes were blocked overnight at 4 °C with 2% bovine serum albumin (BSA) in Tris-buffered saline (TBS; in mM 10 Tris, 150 NaCl, pH 7.5, and 0.05% Tween 20®) and then incubated overnight at 4 °C in blocking solution containing the following antibodies: anti-Kir 4.1, anti-AQP-4, anti-COX1, anti-COX2 (diluted 1:1000), and anti-GS (diluted 1:10,000) (Santa Cruz Biotechnology, Inc., Dallas, TX, USA), and anti-actin (1:2000) (Sigma). Subsequently, the membranes were incubated for 1 h at room temperature in a solution containing horseradish peroxidase (HRP)-conjugated anti-rabbit IgG (diluted 1:10,000), HRP anti-mouse IgG (diluted 1:10,000) (GEHealthcare, Sao Paulo, Brazil), or HRP anti-goat diluted 1:10000 (Sigma). A chemiluminescence signal was detected by luminol substrate reaction (ECL Western Blotting System, GEHealthcare®). Immunoblots were quantified by membrane scanning in an Image4000, GE Healthcare®, and optical densities of proteins studied were determined by ImageJ software (Packard Instrument Company) and the protein/actin ratio calculated.

## Protein measurement

Protein was measured by Lowry's method, modified by Peterson, using bovine serum albumin as a standard [54].

## Statistical analysis

All results were expressed as mean ± standard error mean (SEM) and analyzed by one-way analysis of variance (ANOVA) followed by Tukey's or Dunnett's test. The level of statistical significance was set at $p < 0.05$. All analyses were performed using the Prism 5.0 software (GraphPad).

## Results

### S100B secretion in the acute hippocampal slices of epileptic rats

All animals from the Li-pilocarpine group, used in neurochemical assays, reached at least phase 4 of the convulsive Racine's scale within 13 min after pilocarpine administration (data not shown). At 1, 14, and 56 days after Li-pilocarpine injection, we analyzed basal S100B secretion or S100B secretion in the presence of dexamethasone or in high-potassium medium in the acute hippocampal slices from sham and Li-pilocarpine-treated animals (Fig. 1).

S100B secretion in the hippocampal slices from sham animals is presented in panels a, c, and e, which correspond to 1, 14, and 56 days after saline administration. Li-pilocarpine-treated animals are shown in panels b, d, and f. Basal secretion did not differ between the sham and Li-pilocarpine-treated rats at all times (data not shown) and was assumed as 100%. Dexamethasone downregulated S100B secretion ($p = 0.0073$ in a, $p = 0.0184$ in c, and $p = 0.0171$ in e) in high-potassium medium at all times analyzed. Ex vivo S100B secretion of the hippocampi after SE induction of rats by Li-pilocarpine was not different in the normal- or high-potassium medium for all times analyzed. However, dexamethasone downregulated S100B secretion at 1 (panel b) and 56 days (panel f) following SE induction ($p = 0.0184$ and $p = 0.0171$, respectively). Dexamethasone

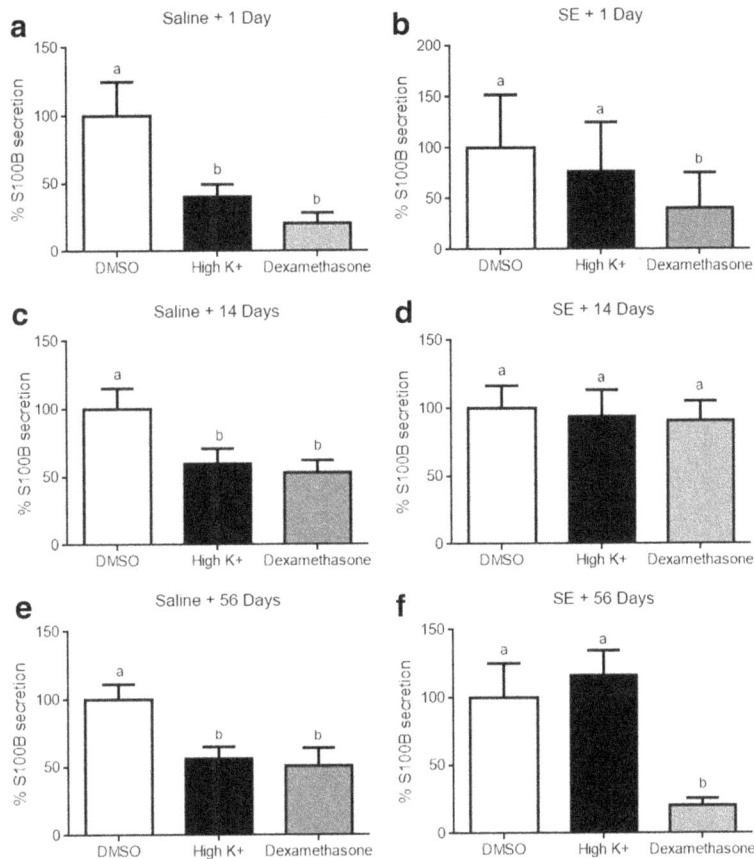

**Fig. 1** Dexamethasone and high potassium levels modulate S100B secretion in the acute hippocampal slices. S100B secretion from the hippocampus was measured by ELISA. Dexamethasone and high potassium levels decreased S100B secretion in sham (saline) animals at 1, 14, and 56 days (**a**, **c**, **e**). Dexamethasone reduced S100B secretion at 1 and 56 days after pilocarpine injection. SE animals were not affected by high potassium at 1, 14, and 56 days (**b**, **d**, **f**). Data are expressed as percentages compared to the basal condition and values represent mean ± standard error, of six to eight animals per group. Data were analyzed by ANOVA, followed by the Dunnet test. Bars without a common letter differ significantly, assuming $p < 0.05$

did not affect S100B secretion at 14 days (panel c) after SE induction ($p = 0.9242$).

### In vivo dexamethasone prevents the increment in inflammatory cytokines, prostaglandin E2 and, cyclooxygenases

Dexamethasone, administered at 24 and 36 h after SE induction, was able to prevent inflammatory signals of hippocampal inflammation caused by SE induction (Fig. 2). Dexamethasone prevented the augmentation in IL-1β (panel a) and PGE2 (panel c) levels in the hippocampus of SE animals at 1 day after pilocarpine injection ($p = 0.0001$ and $p = 0.0002$, respectively). The treatment with dexamethasone reduced TNF-α levels (panel b) when compared with SE and sham animals ($p = 0.0286$). No change was observed in IL-10 at 1 day after SE, and dexamethasone did not affect the levels of this anti-inflammatory cytokine at this time ($p = 0.9221$; panel d). However, interestingly, we observed an increase in hippocampal IL-10 in dexamethasone-treated animals at day 56 after SE ($p = 0.0165$, panel e). At 56 days after SE,

the increment in PGE2 was not significant ($p = 0.572$; panel f) and dexamethasone did not affect this parameter.

The cyclooxygenase (COX1 and 2) content was measured by Western blotting (Fig. 3). The immunocontent of COX1 was the same in all groups at 1 (panel c) and 56 (panel d) days ($p = 0.8938$ and $p = 0.4244$, respectively). However, dexamethasone prevented the increase in COX2 at 1 (panel e) and 56 (panel f) days ($p = 0.0109$ and $p = 0.00913$, respectively).

### Dexamethasone prevents astrogliosis markers, GFAP, and S100B in the epileptic model

The increment in GFAP, induced in the Li-pilocarpine model of epilepsy, was prevented by dexamethasone in animals at 1 (Fig. 4a) and 56 (Fig. 4b) days after pilocarpine injection ($p = 0.0035$ and $p = 0.0245$, respectively). Hippocampal S100B content also increased following SE induction (Fig. 5a, b), and this was prevented by dexamethasone (panel c, $p = 0.0062$). However, the elevation in hippocampal S100B at 56 days in SE animals was

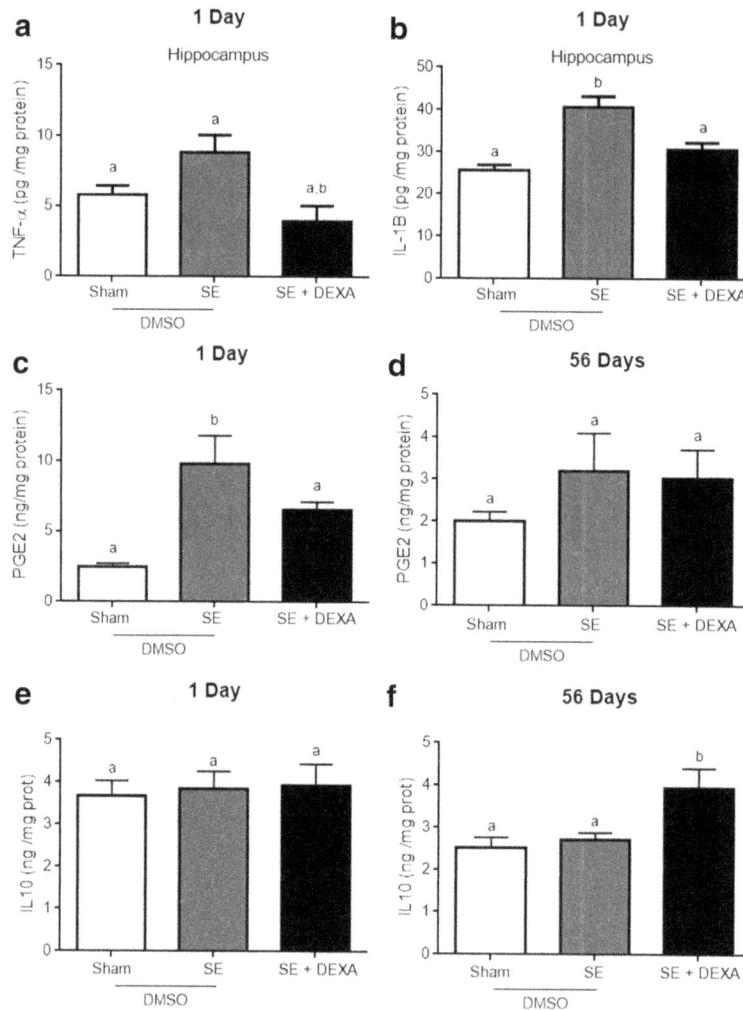

**Fig. 2** Dexamethasone prevents neuroinflammation in the hippocampus. Pro-inflammatory and anti-inflammatory cytokines were measured by ELISA. Dexamethasone decreased TNFα (**a**), reversed IL-1β (**b**), and PGE-2 (**c**) levels at 1 day after treatment. Dexamethasone did not affect PGE2 (**d**) content at 56 days nor IL-10 levels at 1 day after treatment. At 56 days, dexamethasone increased IL-10 content. Values were expressed by mean ± standard error, of four to six animals per group. Data were analyzed by ANOVA, followed by the Tukey test. Bars without a common letter differ significantly, assuming $p < 0.05$

partially prevented by dexamethasone administration (panel b, $p = 0.0445$).

### Dexamethasone prevented the increment in cerebrospinal fluid S100B during the chronic phase of the epileptic model

CSF S100B content was increased after SE induction at 1 (panel c) and 56 (panel d) days ($p = 0.0125$ and $p = 0.0096$, respectively). Dexamethasone was unable to prevent this increase at 1 day after pilocarpine administration (panel c). However, it completely prevented the elevation in CSF S100B at 56 days (panel c). Serum S100B content diminished in SE animals at 1 day ($p = 0.0005$; panel e), and dexamethasone did not affect this change. At 56 days, serum S100B was not different in SE animals or affected by dexamethasone ($p = 0.3719$; panel e).

### Dexamethasone prevents the decrease in glutathione in the Li-pilocarpine model of epilepsy

Based on the astrogliosis signals found in this model, we investigated other astroglial parameters related to astrocyte functionality, namely, glutamine synthetase (GS) activity, GSH content, potassium channel Kir 4.1, and aquaporin-4 (AQP-4). GS activity decreased in epileptic animals (Fig. 6) at 1 (panel a) and 56 (panel b) days ($p = 0.0003$ and $p = 0.0030$, respectively), and dexamethasone did not prevent this change at 1 or 56 days. However, we found a decrease in the hippocampal GSH content at 1 (panel c) and 56 (panel d) days ($p = 0.0174$ and $p = 0.0500$, respectively), possibly reflecting astroglial dysfunction, and dexamethasone administration completely prevented this alteration. In fact, GSH content is not an appropriate marker for astrocytes, but in the brain

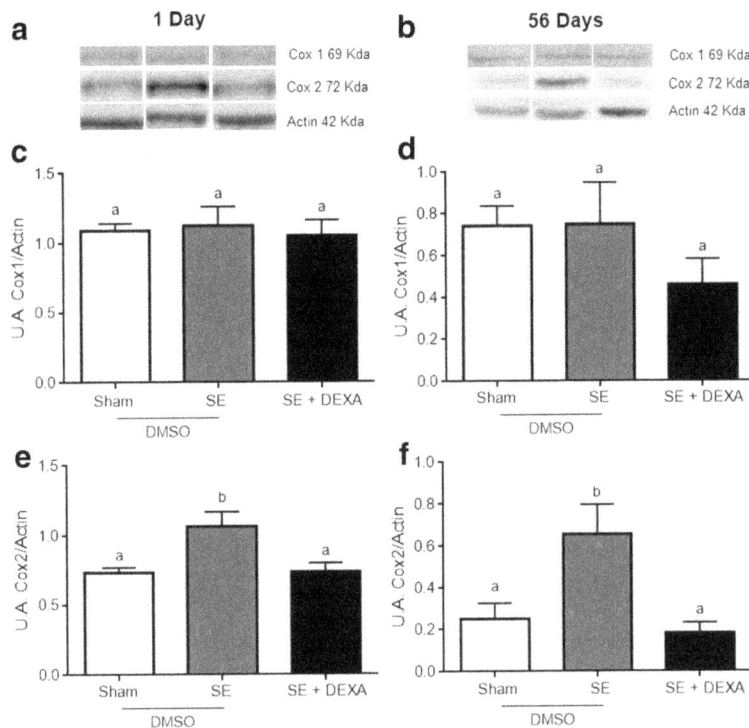

**Fig. 3** Dexamethasone prevents COX2 content in the hippocampus. COX1 and COX2 content were measured by Western blot. Representative images of COX1 and COX2 in the hippocampus at 1 and 56 days after treatment (**a**, **b**). Chemiluminescent quantification of protein/actin of COX 1 (**c**, **d**) and COX 2 (**e**, **f**). Dexamethasone prevented the increase in COX2 content in the hippocampus of SE animals at 1 and 56 days after treatment (**e** and **f**, respectively). Values represent mean ± standard error, of four to six animals per group. Data were analyzed by ANOVA, followed by the Tukey test. Bars without a common letter differ significantly, assuming $p < 0.05$

tissue, its synthesis and recycling are totally dependent on astrocyte activity.

### Dexamethasone prevents the impairment in potassium uptake by astrocytes in epileptic rats

Levels of the Kir 4.1 protein, the main potassium channel in astrocytes, was lower in epileptic rats at 1(Fig. 7c) and 56 (Fig. 7d) days ($p = 0.0024$ and $p = 0.0418$, respectively), and dexamethasone was able to prevent this effect at

56 days after SE induction, but not at 1 day after. There were no differences in AQP-4 levels in epileptic animals at 1 (Fig. 7e) and 56 (Fig. 7f) days ($p = 0.6905$ and $p = 0.1419$, respectively), and dexamethasone did not affect AQP-4 content at 1 and 56 days after SE induction.

### Discussion

Most AED target neuronal activity modulated by ionic channels, particularly GABA$_A$. The steroid sensitivity of

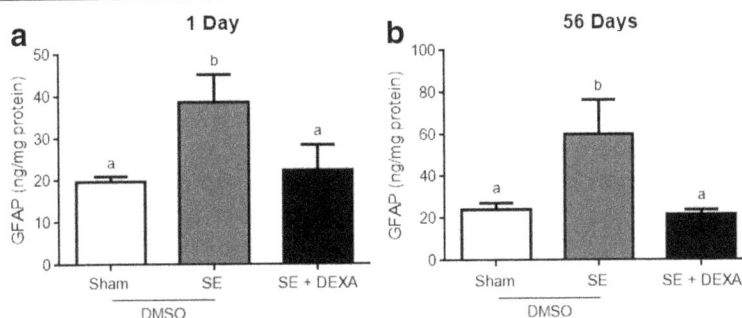

**Fig. 4** Dexamethasone prevents astrogliosis in the hippocampus. GFAP was measured by ELISA. Dexamethasone prevented the increase in GFAP content in the hippocampus of SE animals at 1 and 56 days after treatment (**a** and **b**, respectively). Values represent mean ± standard error, of four to six animals per group. Data were analyzed by ANOVA, followed by the Tukey test. Bars without a common letter differ significantly, assuming $p < 0.05$

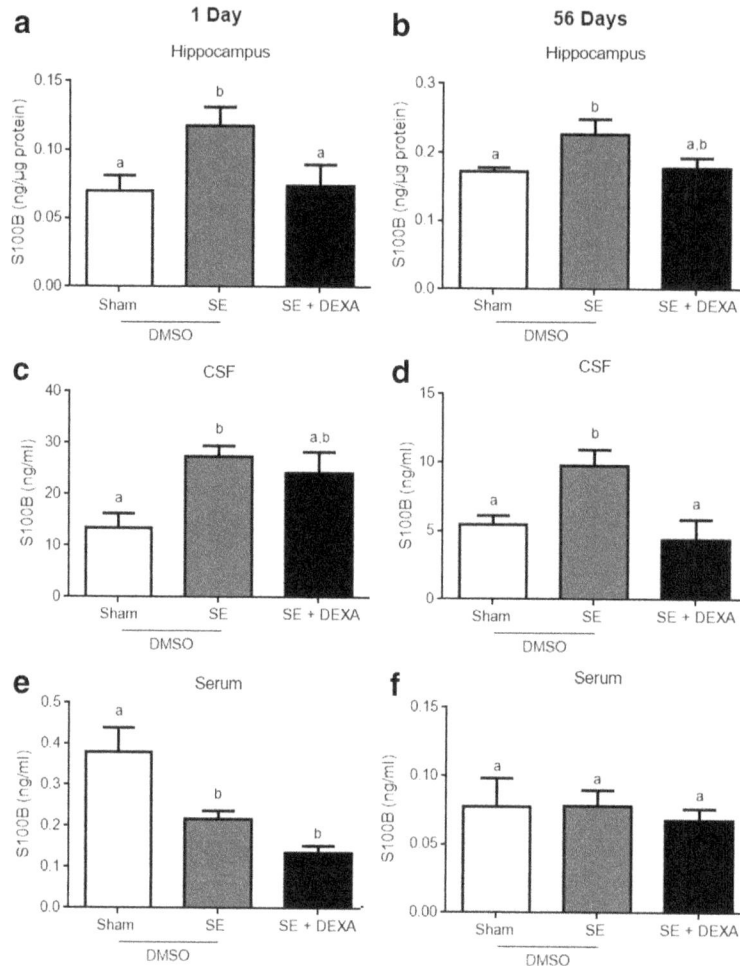

**Fig. 5** Dexamethasone modulates S100B levels in the hippocampus and in the cerebrospinal fluid. S100B content was measured by ELISA. Dexamethasone prevented the augmentation in S100B content in the hippocampus of SE animals at 1 day after treatment (**a**) and did not affect S100B content at 56 days after SE induction (**b**). The augmentation in S100B levels in the CSF was prevented by dexamethasone at 56 days after SE induction (**d**). Serum S100B levels were not altered by dexamethasone at any of the time points (**e**, **f**). Values represent mean ± standard error, of four to six animals per group. Data were analyzed by ANOVA, followed by the Tukey test. Bars without a common letter differ significantly, assuming $p < 0.05$

these channels has led to the use of steroids as adjunctive drugs for epilepsy [55–57]. Moreover, 30% of TLE patients develop resistance to AED [58], and additional strategies for therapeutic approaches are welcome. Mounting evidence suggests that astrocytes and neuroinflammation (which is modulated by astrocytes and microglia in brain tissue) contribute to epileptogenesis and are potential targets for therapies being developed against epileptic disorders [59].

## Dexamethasone affects S100B secretion

As previously mentioned, S100B is widely used as a marker for epileptic disorders [31, 32], and its secretion is modulated by anti-inflammatory drugs [35, 36]. Our studies have suggested that the hippocampal and CSF S100B are altered after SE induction in the Li-pilocarpine model

[14]. We, herein, confirm that the hippocampal slices incubated in high-potassium medium secrete less S100B [60, 61]; this effect was observed in slices from young (14 days old) and adult (70 days old) sham rats. The mechanism underlying this decrease in S100B secretion remains unclear and could be mediated by an undetermined neuronal factor released during high-potassium depolarization, such as glutamate [60]. On the other hand, a direct effect of high-potassium on potassium channels and transporters in astrocytes modulating S100B secretion cannot be ruled out [61].

However, in the hippocampal slices from rats submitted to the Li-pilocarpine model of epilepsy, S100B secretion did not change in high-potassium medium, although the reason for this lack of change in S100B secretion is unclear at the moment [60], as is the mechanism by which

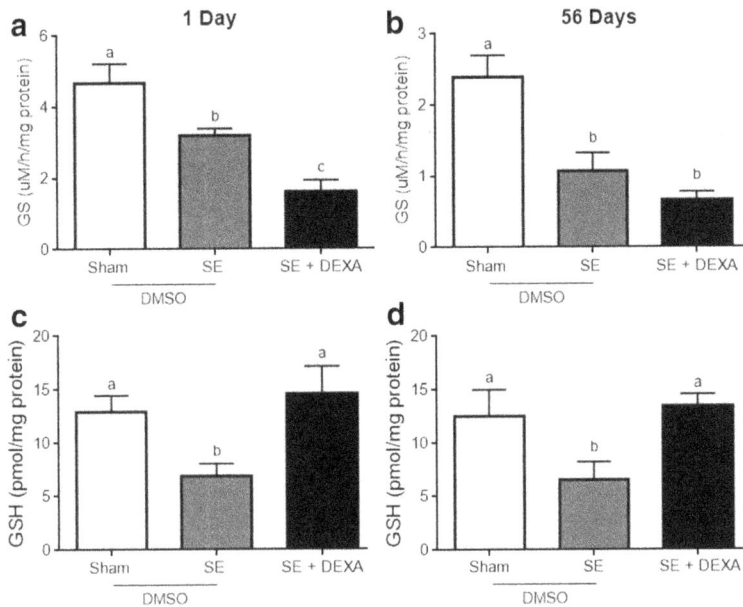

**Fig. 6** Dexamethasone does not modulate decreased GS activity but reverses GSH content in the hippocampus. The decrease in GS activity was not modulated by dexamethasone in the SE animals (**a**, **b**). Dexamethasone prevented the reduction in GSH reduced at 1 and 56 days after treatment (**c**, **d**). Values represent mean ± standard error, of four to six animals per group. Data were analyzed by ANOVA, followed by Tukey test. Bars without a common letter differ significantly, assuming $p < 0.05$

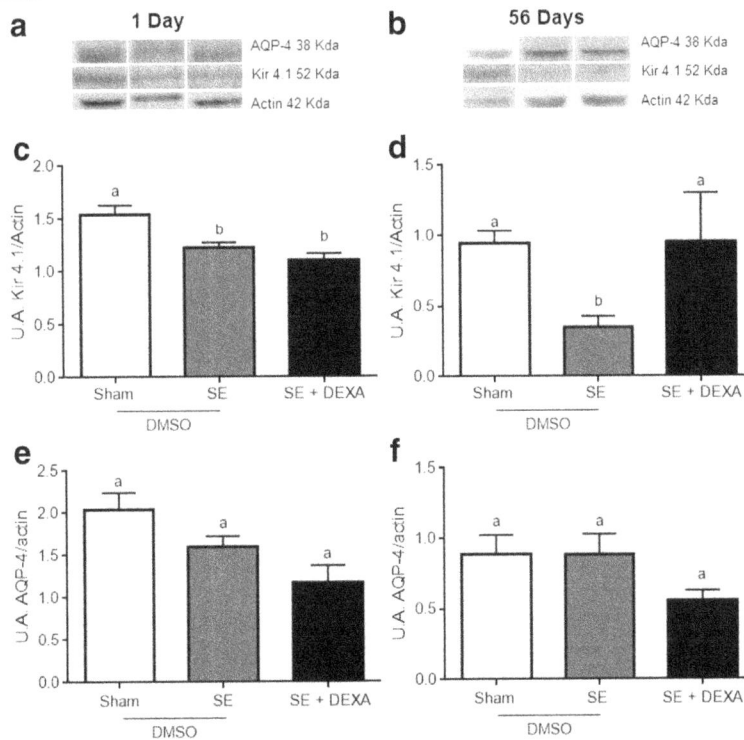

**Fig. 7** Dexamethasone does not alter Kir 4.1 and AQP-4 astrocyte channel content in the hippocampus. Kir 4.1 and AQP-4 contents were determined by Western blot. Representative images of Kir 4.1 and AQP-4 in the hippocampus at 1 and 56 days after treatment (**a**, **b**). Chemiluminescent quantification of Kir 4.1 (**c**, **d**) and AQP-4 (**e**, **f**) protein/actin. Dexamethasone did not reverse the reduction in Kir 4.1 content in the hippocampus of SE animals at 1 day after treatment (**c**); however, dexamethasone prevented Kir4.1 content in SE animals at 56 days after treatment (**d**). No differences in AQP-4 channel expression were observed between groups (**e**, **f**). Values represent mean ± standard error, of four to six animals per group. Data were analyzed by ANOVA, followed by Tukey test. Bars without a common letter differ significantly, assuming $p < 0.05$

S100B secretion occurs [37]. However, it is possible that the decrease in potassium channels in SE animals may contribute to the lower potassium influx in the astrocytes of these animals [49, 62, 63].

A number modulators of S100B secretions have been described [38]. Dexamethasone per se decreased S100B secretion in the acute hippocampal slices from sham animals (at all analyzed times) and in SE animals (at 1 and 56 days after pilocarpine administration). No in vitro effect of dexamethasone occurred at 14 days after SE, which corresponds to the "silent period" of this model [44]. Interestingly, these time-dependent changes in S100B secretion of the hippocampal slices of SE animals coincide with changes of this protein observed in CSF in the Li-pilocarpine model of epilepsy [14]. The acute effect of dexamethasone on the epileptiform activity of the hippocampal slices has been previously reported [64], but the mechanism underlying this activity remains unclear. Based on the effect of dexamethasone on S100B secretion at 1 day after SE induction, we decided to investigate whether dexamethasone administration at 24 and 36 h after pilocarpine injection prevents changes in inflammatory and astroglial markers at 1 and 56 days after dexamethasone injection.

### In vivo dexamethasone prevents neuroinflammation

The long-term effect of dexamethasone observed in astroglial and inflammatory parameters involves changes in gene expression, whereby dexamethasone prevents the increase in IL-1β, TNF-α, and COX2 (and consequently PGE2 levels) in the hippocampus of SE animals at 1 day after dexamethasone administration. Of note, in SE animals treated with dexamethasone, TNF-α was decreased to levels that were lower than those of sham animals, but unfortunately, we did not carry out cytokine measurements in the sham group without dexamethasone. Furthermore, dexamethasone increased IL-10, an anti-inflammatory cytokine, in SE animals at 56 days. Taken together, these data suggest the induction of a non-inflammatory microenvironment by dexamethasone in the hippocampus of Li-pilocarpine-treated animals over the short and long term.

### Dexamethasone prevents astrogliosis

Based on two classical glial markers, GFAP and S100B, we found that dexamethasone administration at 24 and 36 h after pilocarpine-induced SE administration was able to prevent astrogliosis. It is well known that GFAP and S100B expressions are downregulated in glial cultures by dexamethasone [36, 65] and that the in vivo administration of this corticoid has been used to reduce the inflammatory response and gliosis [66, 67]. Moreover, although dexamethasone was not able to reduce CSF S100B during a short time (2 days after SE), it was

effective later on (at 56 days after SE). This effect may be of relevance as chronically elevated levels of this protein contribute to neurodegenerative diseases [37, 38]. Notably, we found a decrease in serum S100B after SE. This could be due to brain "retention" of this protein, as proposed in some cases of acute brain injury [68] or could be due to its peripheral alteration (independent of brain source) [69]. It is also important to mention that, in another model of SE induction using scopolamine/pilocarpine, an increase in serum S100B was reported and that the previous administration of dexamethasone prevented this increment [70].

### Dexamethasone protects against astrocyte dysfunction

Glutamine synthetase (GS) is a specific astrocyte enzyme that is critical to glutamate metabolism in the brain and closely related to glutamatergic and gabaergic neurotransmission and reduced in the human hippocampus in TLE [71]. A reduced expression of GS was reported at 2 weeks after SE in the Li-pilocarpine model [72]. In this study, we detected an earlier decrease in GS that persisted until the chronic phase. It is well known that dexamethasone induces the expression of this enzyme [73]; however, inflammatory cytokines are able to block this induction in astrocyte cultures [74]. We assumed that the hippocampal GS decrease in the Li-pilocarpine model is due to inflammation, but it is unclear at the moment why dexamethasone did not prevent this effect. It is possible that this effect may depend on the dose and time of corticoid administration. On the other hand, the hippocampal oxidative stress observed in this model [75, 76], characterized here by the decrease in GSH, was completely reversed by dexamethasone administration. Rosiglitazone, an agonist of the peroxisome proliferator-activated receptor gamma that has anti-inflammatory activity, also prevented the GSH imbalance in the hippocampus after pilocarpine-induced SE [77].

Neuronal excitability is highly dependent on extracellular levels of $K^+$, which are regulated mainly by the astrocytic Kir 4.1 potassium channels that are in turn functionally coupled to the AQP-4 water channels [30]. In a previous study reporting on the induction of SE in rats with pilocarpine (without lithium), an increase in Kir 4.1 in the cortical regions, but not in the hippocampus, was observed at 8 weeks after SE induction [78]. We found an early (2 days after SE) and persistent (56 days after SE) decrease in Kir 4.1 content in the hippocampus. This apparently contradictory result is possibly due to methodological differences. Dexamethasone prevented the decrease in Kir 4.1 at 56 days after SE induction, but not at 1 day afterward. Accordingly, in the eye retina, dexamethasone (used to treat macular edema) selectively upregulated Kir 4.1 (but not AQP-4) channels [79]. Regardless of the changes in Kir 4.1

observed in SE animals, no changes in AQP-4 were observed in this model.

The use of corticosteroid therapy for epilepsy disorders is a matter of debate, due to the pro- and anticonvulsive effects observed. Experimental studies have administered dexamethasone before SE induction and observed behavioral alterations, changes in the latency period of SE, and mortality, biochemical, neurological, and inflammatory modifications [42, 80, 81]. However, if dexamethasone administration occurred during SE, there were no changes in latency period, increased mortality ratio, and exacerbated cerebral edema [43]. Data relating to COX2 expression in the experimental models suggests that the corticoid effect depends on the dose, the time point of administration, the type of inhibitor (selective or non-selective), and differences among models of SE induction [82].

Although dexamethasone clearly prevented astroglial and inflammatory changes, commonly associated to epileptogenesis, it did not alter the epileptic behavior, such as the beginning of recurrent spontaneous seizures and the scores on Racine's scale (Additional file 2). We are assuming that dexamethasone effect involves a mechanism (direct or indirect) that alters the expression of these glial proteins, as it does with inflammatory proteins (cytokines and COX2). In fact, GFAP, GS, and S100B gene expression are sensitive to dexamethasone and cytokines [36, 83]. GS and GFAP exhibit differing sensitivities to dexamethasone in the hippocampus [36]. Herein, we observed that these proteins are differentially affected in the epilepsy model and that dexamethasone administration did not prevent the change in GS. Kir 4.1 and AQP-4 work together in the brain tissue to provide $K^+$ and water clearance [30]. However, these channels were not affected in the same manner in this model of epilepsy—indicating impairment in the ability to remove $K^+$. Moreover, to our knowledge, there are no data in the literature regarding the effect of dexamethasone on the gene expression of Kir 4.1; the administration of this corticosteroid prevented the decrease of these channels in the Li-pilocarpine model of epilepsy. Figure 8 summarizes the possible changes that occur in astroglial proteins in the model of epilepsy at 56 days after pilocarpine administration, as well as the prevention of such changes by dexamethasone administration. Notice that elevated extracellular levels of $K^+$ decrease S100B secretion under basal conditions [60]. The mechanism involved in this effect is unclear at moment, but such an effect is not observed in the hippocampal slices from animals treated with pilocarpine. However, dexamethasone was able to reduce S100B secretion in the hippocampal slices from and epileptic rats in vitro. Moreover, our data allow us to speculate (but not affirm) that the protection provided by dexamethasone in this model could be useful against other epileptogenic agents such as traumatic

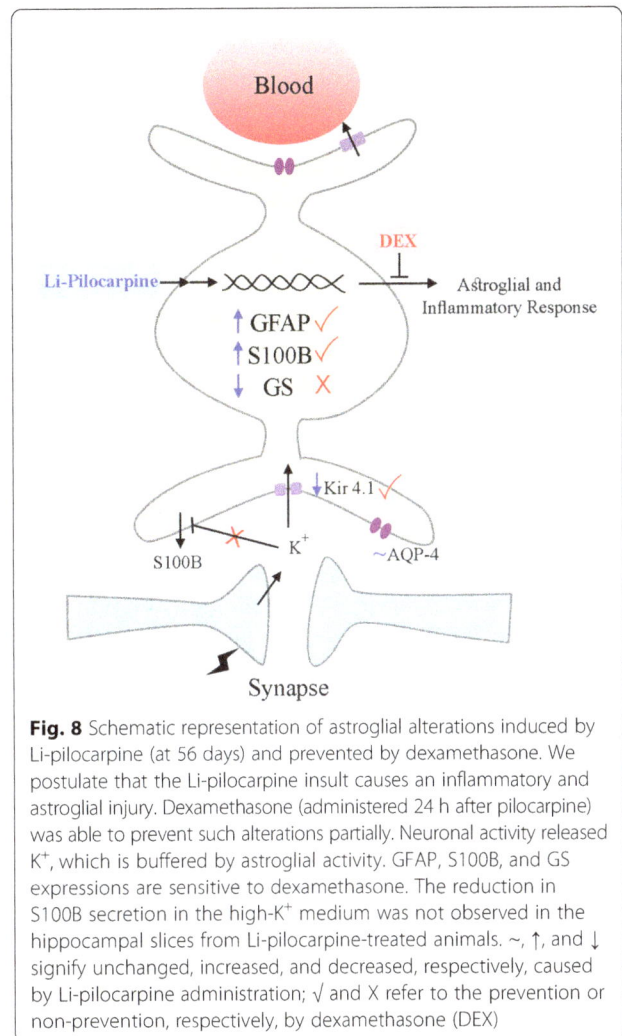

**Fig. 8** Schematic representation of astroglial alterations induced by Li-pilocarpine (at 56 days) and prevented by dexamethasone. We postulate that the Li-pilocarpine insult causes an inflammatory and astroglial injury. Dexamethasone (administered 24 h after pilocarpine) was able to prevent such alterations partially. Neuronal activity released $K^+$, which is buffered by astroglial activity. GFAP, S100B, and GS expressions are sensitive to dexamethasone. The reduction in S100B secretion in the high-$K^+$ medium was not observed in the hippocampal slices from Li-pilocarpine-treated animals. ~, ↑, and ↓ signify unchanged, increased, and decreased, respectively, caused by Li-pilocarpine administration; √ and X refer to the prevention or non-prevention, respectively, by dexamethasone (DEX)

brain injury or ischemia, in which neuroinflammation is present.

Some limitations of this study should be highlighted. Firstly, EEG records at different times would be useful to characterize SE and seizure activities later on. The absence of this data occurred in an effort to avoid surgery and the activation of neuroinflammation and astrogliosis by the lesion incurred by the introduction of electrodes. However, epileptic behavior analysis could provide valid evidence to suggest a protective role of dexamethasone in this model of epilepsy [84, 85]. Secondly, the different time points of 1, 14, and 56 days correspond to acute, latent (silent), and chronic epileptic phases, as determined in a previous study [49]. We did not perform a 14-day group in the second set of experiments to reduce the number of animals used in this study. Thirdly, this study demonstrates that dexamethasone administration (10 mg/kg, 24 and 36 h after SE) has clear neurochemical effects on the acute and chronic phases of Li-pilocarpine model of epilepsy. However, other protocols would be useful to delimit the best "window" and dose for steroid protection in this epilepsy model. Finally, dexamethasone prevented astroglial and inflammatory changes but did not alter the analyzed epileptic behavior, at least, between 7 and 25 days after SE induction, and therefore we cannot rule out the possibility that observed glial alterations constitute an epiphenomenon.

## Conclusions

Our results indicate a decrease in neuroinflammation, astrogliosis, and astroglial dysfunction in the hippocampi of young rats submitted to the Li-pilocarpine model of epilepsy, at 1 and 56 days after intraperitoneal dexamethasone administration. In the acute hippocampal slices prepared at 1, 14, and 56 days after SE induction, basal S100B secretion and S100B secretion in high-K$^+$ medium were not different at 1 and 56 days, in contrast to sham animals in which high-K$^+$ medium induced a decrease in S100B secretion. The addition of dexamethasone to the incubation medium per se induced a decrease in S100B secretion in sham and epileptic rats (1 and 56 days after SE induction). In the second set of experiments, we evaluated the in vivo effect of dexamethasone on hippocampal astroglial parameters (1 day after pilocarpine) in the epileptic model, at 2 and 56 days after SE. In addition to the improvement in inflammatory status (based on cytokine and PGE2 levels), dexamethasone prevented astrogliosis (based on GFAP and S100B content) and partially diminished astroglial dysfunction (based on Kir 4.1 protein and GSH content). The decrease in GS was not abrogated by dexamethasone, and AQP-4 was not altered in this epileptic model. All these parameters, with the exception of AQP-4, were altered, emphasizing the importance of this model for understanding alterations and mechanisms of epileptic disorders. In vivo dexamethasone administration, 24 h after SE induction, prevented most of the parameters analyzed, reinforcing the importance of anti-inflammatory steroid therapy in the Li-pilocarpine model and possibly in other epileptic conditions where neuroinflammation is present. Our data demonstrate specific alterations in astrocytes in this model and clearly contribute to the understanding of the importance of these cells in the pathogenesis of epilepsy, as well as suggest potential therapeutic targets for AED.

## Additional files

**Additional file 1:** Figure studies. Schematic experimental design. Schematic experimental design of the two studies. The first set of experiments analyze S100B secretion in an ex vivo model of hippocampal slices of rats, from sham and SE animals at 1, 14, and 56 days after pilocarpine injection. Hippocampal slices were incubated in high-K$^+$ medium and dexamethasone. The second set of experiments

evaluates dexamethasone treatment at 24 and 36 h after SE induction, in vivo at 1 and 56 days after dexamethasone injection.

**Additional file 2: Table S1.** Behavior resumed. Epilepsy behavioral evaluation of SE animals. Evaluation of the occurrence of spontaneous epileptic seizures in animals submitted to the epilepsy model by Li-pilocarpine administration. Dexamethasone did not prevent behavioral changes. *All animals developed a spontaneous epileptic seizure and jumping and running behavior.

## Abbreviations
AQP-4: Aquaporin channel 4; COX1: Cyclooxygenase 1; COX2: Cyclooxygenase 2; CSF: Cerebrospinal fluid; GFAP: Glial fibrillary acid protein; GS: Glutamine synthetase; GSH: Reduced glutathione; IL-10: Interleukin-10; IL-1β: Interleukin-1β; Kir 4.1: Inwardly rectifying potassium channel 4.1; LDH: Lactate dehydrogenase; PGE2: Prostaglandin E2; SE: Status epilepticus; TNF-α: Tumor necrosis factor-α

## Acknowledgements
The authors would like to thank the undergraduate student, Juliana Furtado, for the help with laboratory analyses.

## Funding
This study was supported by the National Council for Scientific and Technological Development (CNPq, Brazil), Ministry of Education (MEC/CAPES, Brazil), State Foundation for Scientific Research of Rio Grande do Sul (FAPERGS), National Institute of Science and Technology for Excitotoxicity and Neuroprotection (MCT/INCTEN), and project CNPq 27/2014 - Neurodegenerative diseases.

## Authors' contributions
AFKV organized and conducted all studies. FH, EN, and MCL helped with the animal experimentation. DLO and CAG aided in the discussion of data and writing the manuscript. All authors have read and approved of the final manuscript.

## Consent for publication
Not applicable.

## Competing interests
The authors declare that they have no competing interests.

## References
1. Banerjee PN, Filippi D, Allen Hauser W. The descriptive epidemiology of epilepsy—a review. Epilepsy Res. 2009;85:31–45.
2. Dichter MA. Emerging insights into mechanisms of epilepsy: implications for new antiepileptic drug development. Epilepsia. 1994;35(Suppl 4):S51-7.
3. Dalby NO, Mody I. The process of epileptogenesis: a pathophysiological approach. Curr Opin Neurol. 2001;14:187–92.
4. Sander JW. The epidemiology of epilepsy revisited. Curr Opin Neurobiol. 2003;16:165–70.
5. Engel Jr J. Introduction to temporal lobe epilepsy. Epilepsy Res. 1996;26:141–50.
6. Téllez-Zenteno J, Hernánde-Ronquillo L. A review of the epidemiology of temporal lobe epilepsy. Epilepsy Res Treat. 2012;2012:630853. https://doi.org/10.1155/2012/630853.
7. Leite JP, Garcia-cairasco N, Ca EA. New insights from the use of pilocarpine and kainate models. Epilepsy Res. 2002;50:93–103.
8. Wahab A, Albus K, Gabriel S, Heinemann U. In search of models of pharmacoresistant epilepsy. Epilepsia. 2010;51:154–9.
9. Cavalheiro EA, Leite JP, Bortolotto ZA, Turski WA, Ikonomidou C, Turski L. Long-term effects of pilocarpine in rats: structural damage of the brain triggers kindling and spontaneous recurrent seizures. Epilepsia. 1991;32:778–82.
10. Goffin K, Nissinen J, Van Laere K, Pitkänen A. Cyclicity of spontaneous

recurrent seizures in pilocarpine model of temporal lobe epilepsy in rat. Exp Neurol. 2007;205:501–5.

11. Chakir A, Fabene PF, Ouazzani R, Bentivoglio M. Drug resistance and hippocampal damage after delayed treatment of pilocarpine-induced epilepsy in the rat. Brain Res Bull. 2006;71:127–38.

12. Arisi GM, Ruch M, Foresti ML, Mukherjee S, Ribak CE. Astrocyte alterations in the hippocampus following pilocarpine-induced seizures in aged rats. Aging Dis. 2011;2(4):294–300.

13. Borges K. Neuronal and glial pathological changes during epileptogenesis in the mouse pilocarpine model. Exp Neurol. 2003;182:21–34.

14. de Oliveira DL, Fischer A, Jorge RS, da Silva MC, Leite M, Gonçalves CA, et al. Effects of early-life LiCl-pilocarpine-induced status epilepticus on memory and anxiety in adult rats are associated with mossy fiber sprouting and elevated CSF S100B protein. Epilepsia. 2008;49:842–52.

15. Shapiro LA, Wang L, Ribak CE. Rapid astrocyte and microglial activation following pilocarpine-induced seizures in rats. Epilepsia. 2008;49:33–41.

16. Yang F, Liu Z, Chen J, Zhang S. Roles of astrocytes and microglia in seizure-induced aberrant neurogenesis in the hippocampus of adult rats. J Neurosci Res. 2010;88(3):519–29.

17. De Lanerolle NC, Lee T, Spencer DD. Astrocytes and epilepsy. Neurotherapeutics. 2010;7:424–38.

18. Foresti ML, Arisi GM, Shapiro LA. Role of glia in epilepsy-associated neuropathology, neuroinflammation and neurogenesis. Brain Res Rev Elsevier BV. 2010;66:115–22.

19. Perea G, Navarrete M, Araque A. Tripartite synapses: astrocytes process and control synaptic information. Trends Neurosci. 2009;32:421–31.

20. Coulter DA, Steinhauser C. Role of astrocytes in epilepsy. Cold Spring Harb Perspect Med. 2015;5:1–12.

21. Seifert G, Steinhäuser C. Neuron–astrocyte signaling and epilepsy. Exp Neurol Elsevier BV. 2011;244:4–10.

22. Tian G, Azmi H, Takano T, Xu Q, Peng W, Lin J, et al. An astrocytic basis of epilepsy. Nat Med. 2005;11(9):973–81.

23. Bedner P. Astrocyte uncoupling as a cause of human temporal lobe epilepsy. Brain. 2015;138:1208–22.

24. Robel S, Buckingham SC, Boni JL, Campbell SL, Danbolt NC, Riedemann T, et al. Reactive astrogliosis causes the development of spontaneous seizures. J Neurosci. 2015;3:3330–45.

25. Marchi N, Granata T, Janigro D. Inflammatory pathways of seizure disorders. Trends Neurosci. 2014;37:55–65.

26. De Simoni MG, Perego C, Ravizza T, Moneta D, Conti M, Marchesi F, et al. Inflammatory cytokines and related genes are induced in the rat hippocampus by limbic status epilepticus. Eur J Neurosci. 2000;12:2623–33.

27. Ravizza T, Rizzi M, Perego C, Richichi C, Vel J, Mosh SL, et al. Inflammatory response and glia activation in developing rat hippocampus after status epilepticus. Epilepsia. 2005;46:113–7.

28. Rizzi M, Perego C, Aliprandi M, Richichi C, Ravizza T, Colella D, et al. Glia activation and cytokine increase in rat hippocampus by kainic acid-induced status epilepticus during postnatal development. Neurobiol Dis. 2003;14:494–503.

29. Somera-Molina KC, Robin B, Somera CA, Anderson C, Stine C, Koh S, et al. Glial activation links early-life seizures and long-term neurologic dysfunction: evidence using a small molecule inhibitor of proinflammatory cytokine upregulation. Epilepsia. 2007;48:1785–800.

30. Devinsky O, Vezzani A, Najjar S, De Lanerolle NC, Rogawski MA. Glia and epilepsy: excitability and inflammation. Trends Neurosci. 2013;36:174–84.

31. Portela L, Tort A, Walz R, Bianchin M, Trevisol-Bittencourt P, Wille P, et al. Interictal serum S100B levels in chronic neurocysticercosis and idiopathic epilepsy. Acta Neurol Scand. 2003;108:424–7.

32. Chen W, Tan Y, Ge Y. The effects of Levetiracetam on cerebrospinal fluid and plasma NPY and GAL, and on the components of stress response system, hs-CRP, and S100B protein in serum of patients with refractory epilepsy. Cell Biochem Biophys. 2015;73:489–94.

33. Sorci G, Giovannini G, Riuzzi F, Bonifazi P, Zelante T, Bistoni F, et al. The danger signal S100B integrates pathogen–and danger-sensing pathways to restrain inflammation. PLoS Pathog. 2011;7:e1001315.

34. Guerra MC, Tortorelli LS, Galland F, Da Ré C, Negri E, Engelke DS, et al. Lipopolysaccharide modulates astrocytic S100B secretion: a study in cerebrospinal fluid and astrocyte cultures from rats. J Neuroinflammation. 2011;8:128.

35. Leite MC, Galland F, De Souza DF, Guerra MC, Bobermin L, Biasibetti R, et al. Gap junction inhibitors modulate S100B secretion in astrocyte cultures and

acute hippocampal slices gap junction inhibitors modulate S100B secretion in astrocyte cultures and acute hippocampal slices. J Neurosci Res. 2009;87:2439–46.

36. Niu H, Hinkle DA, Wise PM. Dexamethasone regulates basic fibroblast growth factor, nerve growth factor and S100 beta expression in cultured hippocampal astrocytes. Brain Res Mol Brain Res. 1997;51:97–105.

37. Gonçalves CA, Concli Leite M, Nardin P. Biological and methodological features of the measurement of S100B, a putative marker of brain injury. Clin Biochem. 2008;41:755–63.

38. Donato R, Sorci G, Riuzzi F, Arcuri C, Bianchi R, Brozzi F, et al. S100B's double life: intracellular regulator and extracellular signal. Biochim Biophys Acta. 2009;1793(6):1008–22.

39. Yoshikawa M, Suzumura A, Tamaru T, Takayanagi T, Sawada M. Effects of phosphodiesterase inhibitors on cytokine productio n by microglia. Mult Scler. 1999;5:126–33.

40. Chen J, Cai F, Jiang L, Hu Y, Feng C. A prospective study of dexamethasone therapy in refractory epileptic encephalopathy with continuous spike-and-wave during sleep. Epilepsy Behav. 2016;55:1–5.

41. Haberlandt E, Weger C, Sigl SB, Rosta K, Rauchenzauner M, Scholl-bu S, et al. Adrenocorticotropic hormone versus pulsatile dexamethasone in the treatment of infantile epilepsy syndromes. Pediatr Neurol. 2010;42(1):21–7.

42. Al-Shorbagy MY, El Sayeh BM, Abdallah DM. Diverse effects of variant doses of dexamethasone in lithium–pilocarpine induced seizures in rats. Can J Physiol Pharmacol. 2012;90:13–21.

43. Duffy BA, Chun KP, Ma D, Lythgoe MF, Scott RC. Dexamethasone exacerbates cerebral edema and brain injury following lithium-pilocarpine induced status epilepticus. Neurobiol Dis. 2014;63:229–36.

44. Curia G, Longo D, Biagini G, Jones RSG, Avoli M. The pilocarpine model of temporal lobe epilepsy. J Neurosci Methods. 2008;172:143–57.

45. Andersen SL. Changes in the second messenger cyclic AMP during development may underlie motoric symptoms in attention deficit/hyperactivity disorder (ADHD). Behav Brain Res. 2002;130:197–201.

46. Engelhardt B. Development of the blood-brain barrier. Cell Tissue Res. 2003;314:119–29.

47. Nehlig A, De Vasconcelos AP, Boyet S. Postnatal changes in local cerebral blood flow measured by the quantitative autoradiographic [14C] iodoantipyrine technique in freely moving rats. J Cereb Blood Flow Metab. 1989;9:579–88.

48. Ben-Ari Y. Excitatory actions of GABA during development: the nature of the nurture. Nat Rev Neurosci. 2002;3:728–39.

49. Vizuete AFK, Mittmann MH, Gonçalves CA, De Oliveira DL. Phase-dependent Astroglial alterations in Li–pilocarpine- induced status epilepticus in young rats. Neurochem Res. 2017;42:2730–42.

50. Allen S, Shea JM, Felmet T, Gadra J, Dehn PF. A kinetic microassay for glutathione in cells plated on 96-well microtiter plates. Methods Cell Sci. 2000;22:305–12.

51. Leite MC, Galland F, Brolese G, Guerra MC, Bortolotto JW, Freitas R, et al. A simple, sensitive and widely applicable ELISA for S100B: methodological features of the measurement of this glial protein. J Neurosci Methods. 2008;169:93–9.

52. Tramontina F, Leite MC, Cereser K, de Souza DF, Tramontina AC, Nardin P, et al. Immunoassay for glial fibrillary acidic protein: antigen recognition is affected by its phosphorylation state. J Neurosci Methods. 2007;162:282–6.

53. Minet R, Villie F, Marcollet M, Meynial-Denis D, Cynober L. Measurement of glutamine synthetase activity in rat muscle by a colorimetric assay. Clin Chim Acta. 1997;268:121–32.

54. Peterson GL. A simplification of the protein assay method of Lowry et al. which is more generally applicable. Anal Biochem. 1977;83:346–56.

55. Rogawski MA. Diverse mechanisms of antiepileptic drugs in the development pipeline. Epilepsy Res. 2006;69:273–94.

56. Sun C, Mtchedlishvili Z, Erisir A, Kapur J. Diminished neurosteroid sensitivity of synaptic inhibition and altered location of the α4 subunit of GABA a receptors in an animal model of epilepsy. J Neurosci. 2007;27:12641–50.

57. Joshi S, Rajasekaran K, Kapur J. GABAergic transmission in temporal lobe epilepsy: the role of neurosteroids. Exp Neurol. 2013;244:36–42.

58. Ramey WL, Martirosyan NL, Lieu CM, Hasham HA, Lemole GM, Weinand ME. Current management and surgical outcomes of medically intractable epilepsy. Clin Neurol Neurosurg. 2013;115:2411–8.

59. Vezzani A, Lang B, Aronica E. Immunity and inflammation in epilepsy. Cold Spring Harb Perspect Med. 2015;6:a022699.

60. Nardin P, Tortorelli L, Quincozes-Santos A, De Almeida LMV, Leite MC, Thomazi AP, et al. S100B secretion in acute brain slices: modulation by extracellular levels of Ca2+ and K+. Neurochem Res. 2009;34:1603–11.
61. Zanotto C, Abib RT, Batassini C, Tortorelli LS, Biasibetti R, Rodrigues L, et al. Non-specific inhibitors of aquaporin-4 stimulate S100B secretion in acute hippocampal slices of rats. Brain Res. 2013;1491:14–22.
62. Butt AM, Kalsi A. Inwardly rectifying potassium channels (Kir) in central nervous system glia: a special role for Kir4.1 in glial functions. J Cell Mol Med. 2006;10:33–44.
63. Strohschein S, Uttmann KH, Gabriel S, Binder DK. Impact of Aquaporin-4 channels on K 1 buffering and gap junction coupling in the hippocampus. Glia. 2011;980:973–80.
64. Duport S, Stoppini L, Corrèges P. Electophysiological approach of theantiepileptic effect of dexamethasone on hippocampal slice culture using a multirecord system: the physiocard. Life Sci. 1997;60:251–6.
65. Avola R, Di Tullio MA, Fisichella A, Tayebati SK, Tomassoni D. Glial fibrillary acidic protein and vimentin expression is regulated by glucocorticoids and neurotrophic factors in primary rat astroglial cultures. Clin Exp Hypertens. 2004;26:323–33.
66. Bruccoleri A, Pennypacker KR, Harry GJ. Effect of dexamethasone on elevated cytokine mRNA levels in chemical-induced hippocampal injury. J Neurosci Res. 1999;57:916–26.
67. Jaquins-Gerstl A, Shu Z, Zhang J, Liu Y, Weber SG, Michael AC. The effect of dexamethasone on gliosis, ischemia, and dopamine extraction during microdialysis sampling in brain tissue. Anal Chem. 2011;83:7662–7.
68. Kleindienst A, Meissner S, Eyupoglu IY, Parsch H, Schmidt CBM. Dynamics of S100B release into serum and cerebrospinal fluid following acute brain injury. Acta Neurochir Suppl. 2010;106:247–50.
69. Gonçalves CA, Leite MC, Guerra MC. Adipocytes as an important source of serum S100B and possible roles of this protein in adipose tissue. Cardiovasc Psychiatry Neurol. 2010;2010:790431. https://doi.org/10.1155/2010/790431.
70. Marchi N, Granata T, Freri E, Ciusani E, Ragona F, Puvenna V, et al. Efficacy of anti-inflammatory therapy in a model of acute seizures and in a population of pediatric drug resistant epileptics. PLoS One. 2011;6:e18200.
71. Eid T, Behar K, Dhaher R, Bumanglag AV, T-SW L. Roles of glutamine synthetase inhibition in epilepsy. Neurochem Res. 2012;37:2339–50.
72. Van Der W, Hessel E, Bos I, Mulder S, Verlinde S, Van Eijsden P, et al. Persistent reduction of hippocampal glutamine synthetase expression after status epilepticus in immature rats. Eur J Neurosci. 2014;40:3711–9.
73. Patel AJ, Hunt A, Tahourdin CSM. Regulation of in vivo glutamine synthetase activity by glucocorticoids in the developing rat brain. Dev Brain Res. 1983;10:83–91.
74. Huang TL, Banion KO. Interleukin-1B and tumor necrosis factor-a suppress dexamethasone induction of glutamine synthetase in primary mouse astrocytes. J Neurochem. 1998;71:1436–42.
75. Freitas RM, Fonteles MMF. Oxidative stress in the hippocampus after pilocarpine- induced status epilepticus in Wistar rats. FEBS J. 2005;272:1307–12.
76. Waldbaum S, Patel M. Mitochondria, oxidative stress, and temporal lobe epilepsy. Epilepsy Res. 2010;88:23–45.
77. Hong S, Xin Y, Haiqin W, Guilian Z. The PPAR$_\gamma$ agonist rosiglitazone prevents cognitive impairment by inhibiting astrocyte activation and oxidative stress following pilocarpine-induced status epilepticus. Neurol Sci. 2012;33:559–66.
78. Nagao Y, Harada Y, Mukai T, Shimizu S, Okuda A, Fujimoto M, et al. Expressional analysis of the astrocytic Kir 4.1 channel in a pilocarpine-induced temporal lobe epilepsy model. Front Cell Neurosci. 2013;7:1–10.
79. Zhao M, Bousquet E, Valamanesh F, Farman N. Differential regulations of AQP4 and Kir 4.1 by triamcinolone acetonide and dexamethasone in the healthy and inflamed retina. Invest Ophthalmol Vis Sci. 2011;52:6340–7.
80. Fazekas I, Szakács R, Mihály A, Zádor Z, Krisztin-Péva B, Juhász A, et al. Alterations of seizure-induced c- fos immunolabelling and gene expression in the rat cerebral cortex following dexamethasone treatment. Acta Histochem. 2006;108:463–73.
81. Pieretti S, Di Giannuario A, Loizzo A, Sagratella S, Scotti de Carolis A, Capasso A, et al. Dexamethasone prevents epileptiform activity induced by morphine in in vivo and in vitro experiments. J Pharmacol Exp Ther. 1992;263:830–9.
82. Rojas A, Jiang J, Ganesh T, Yang M, Lelutiu N, Dingledine R. Cyclooxygenase-2 in epilepsy. Epilepsia. 2014;55:17–25.
83. Laping NJ, Teter B, Nichols NR, Rozovsky I, Finch CE. Glial fibrillary acidic protein: regulation by hormones, cytokines, and growth factors. Brain Pathol. 1994;1:259–75.
84. Kim J-E, Ryu HJ, Choi SY, Kang T-C. Tumor necrosis factor-α-mediated threonine 435 phosphorylation of p65 nuclear factor-κB subunit in endothelial cells induces vasogenic edema and neutrophil infiltration in the rat piriform cortex following status epilepticus. J Neuroinflammation. 2012;9:1–13.
85. Hung Y-W, Lai M-T, Tseng Y-J, Chou C-C, Lin Y-Y. Monocyte chemoattractant protein-1 affects migration of hippocampal neural progenitors following status epilepticus in rats. J Neuroinflammation. 2013;10:1–11.

# 8

# Brain inflammation is accompanied by peripheral inflammation in Cstb<sup>−/−</sup> mice, a model for progressive myoclonus epilepsy

Brain inflammation is accompanied by peripheral inflammation in $Cstb^{-/-}$ mice, a model for progressive myoclonus epilepsy

Olesya Okuneva[1,2,3†], Zhilin Li[3†], Inken Körber[1,2,3*], Saara Tegelberg[1,2,3], Tarja Joensuu[1,2,3], Li Tian[3,4] and Anna-Elina Lehesjoki[1,2,3]

## Abstract

Progressive myoclonus epilepsy of Unverricht-Lundborg type (EPM1) is an autosomal recessively inherited childhood-onset neurodegenerative disorder, characterized by myoclonus, seizures, and ataxia. Mutations in the cystatin B gene ($CSTB$) underlie EPM1. The CSTB-deficient ($Cstb^{-/-}$) mouse model recapitulates key features of EPM1, including myoclonic seizures. The mice show early microglial activation that precedes seizure onset and neuronal loss and leads to neuroinflammation. We here characterized the inflammatory phenotype of $Cstb^{-/-}$ mice in more detail. We found higher concentrations of chemokines and pro-inflammatory cytokines in the serum of $Cstb^{-/-}$ mice and higher CXCL13 expression in activated microglia in $Cstb^{-/-}$ compared to control mouse brains. The elevated chemokine levels were not accompanied by blood-brain barrier disruption, despite increased brain vascularization. Macrophages in the spleen and brain of $Cstb^{-/-}$ mice were predominantly pro-inflammatory. Taken together, these data show that CXCL13 expression is a hallmark of microglial activation in $Cstb^{-/-}$ mice and that the brain inflammation is linked to peripheral inflammatory changes, which might contribute to the disease pathology of EPM1.

Keywords: Cystatin B, Chemokine, CXCL13, Macrophage, M1/M2, Vascularization

## Introduction

Progressive myoclonus epilepsy of Unverricht-Lundborg type (EPM1, OMIM 254800) is an autosomal recessively inherited neurodegenerative disorder with onset from 6 to 16 years of age and characterized by action-activated and highly incapacitating myoclonus, tonic-clonic epileptic seizures, and ataxia [1]. EPM1 is caused by loss-of-function mutations in the cystatin B ($CSTB$) gene [2, 3], which encodes an inhibitor of lysosomal cysteine cathepsins [4]. CSTB is highly expressed in immune cells, e.g., in blood leukocytes, hepatic lymphocytes, placental macrophages, and microglia [5–9], and it is upregulated in vitro by pro-inflammatory stimulation [8, 10, 11]. In immune cells, the function of CSTB has been linked to chemotaxis [8], expression and secretion of cytokines, and release of

nitric oxide [10, 12, 13], implying a role in the immune response. CSTB function has also been associated with diverse cellular processes, such as regulation of apoptosis [14, 15], bone resorption [16, 17], protection of neurons from oxidative stress [18], and cell cycle progression [19].

A CSTB-deficient mouse model ($Cstb^{-/-}$) mimics key features of EPM1, including myoclonic seizures, ataxia [20], and progressive gray and white matter loss [21]. The brain pathology of $Cstb^{-/-}$ mice is characterized by microglial activation in asymptomatic mice of 2 weeks of age, followed by widespread activation of astrocytes as well as progressive neuronal death and brain volume loss from 1 month of age onwards [22]. Moreover, activated cultured $Cstb^{-/-}$ microglia secrete higher levels of chemokines, such as chemokine (C-C motif) ligand (CCL)2, CCL3, and chemokine (C-X-C motif) ligand (CXCL)1, than control microglia [8]. Gene expression profiling of cultured $Cstb^{-/-}$ microglia revealed impaired interferon signaling and also showed altered chemokine expression [23]. Finally, a striking upregulation of $Cxcl13$ in gene

* Correspondence: anna-elina.lehesjoki@helsinki.fi
†Equal contributors
[1]Folkhälsan Institute of Genetics, Haartmaninkatu 8, 00014 Helsinki, Finland
[2]Research Program's Unit, Molecular Neurology, University of Helsinki, Haartmaninkatu 8, 00014 Helsinki, Finland
Full list of author information is available at the end of the article

expression profiling of postnatal day 30 (P30) $Cstb^{-/-}$ mouse cerebellum was detected [24].

We here confirm the increased CXCL13 expression also on protein level and show that the inflammatory processes in the $Cstb^{-/-}$ brain are linked to peripheral inflammation, which is characterized by increased levels of chemokines and pro-inflammatory cytokines in the serum combined with relatively more pro-inflammatory macrophages, and increased amounts of B lymphocytes in the spleen.

## Materials and methods
### Mice
CSTB-deficient mice ($Cstb^{-/-}$) were obtained from The Jackson Laboratory (129-$Cstb^{tm1Rm}$/SvJ; stock no. #003486). Wild-type mice of the same age and background were used as controls. The research protocols were approved by the Animal Ethics Committee of the State Provincial Office of Southern Finland (decision no. ESAVI/7039/04.10.03/2012, ESAVI/5995/04.10.07/2013, and ESAVI/6288/04.10.07/ 2015).

### Measurement of chemokines and cytokines in mouse serum
Blood samples were obtained by intracardiac puncture of anesthetized P14 and P30 $Cstb^{-/-}$ and control mice. The blood was allowed to clot at room temperature (RT) for 15 min and centrifuged at 2000$g$ for 13 min. The serum was collected and kept at −80 °C until use. The chemokine and cytokine concentrations were assessed using a combination of mouse CXCL10, interleukin (IL)-1α, CXCL1, IL-6, IL-10, IL-18, IL-1β, IL-12, interferon (IFN)-γ, IFN-α, CCL2, CCL3, CCL4, tumor necrosis factor α (TNFα), colony stimulating factor 2 (GM-CSF), and TGF-β1 FlowCytomix Simplex kits for flow cytometry (eBioscience). The CXCL13 concentration was determined using the Quantikine® mouse CXCL13/BLC/BCA-1 Immunoassay ELISA kit (R&D Systems).

### Tissue processing for histochemical analysis
Anesthetized mice (150 mg/kg pentobarbital) were perfused with phosphate-buffered saline (PBS) (pH 7.4) and 4 % paraformaldehyde (PFA)/PBS for 10 min each. The brains were dissected, immersion fixed in 4 % PFA/PBS for 48 h, and cryoprotected in 30 % sucrose/0.05 % $NaN_3$/Tris-buffered saline (TBS) for 3 days. Coronal or sagittal 40-μm sections were cut using a cryostat Leica CM3050 S (Leica Microsystems) and stored in 15 % sucrose/0.05 % $NaN_3$/30 % ethylene glycol/TBS.

### Immunohistochemistry
Adjacent 1-in-12 series of coronal free-floating sections ($n$ = 5 per genotype and age) were incubated with 50 mM $NH_4Cl$ for 30 min to reduce non-specific background

staining and blocked with 15 % fetal calf serum (FCS) diluted in TBS/0.3 %Triton X-100 (TTX) for 1 h. The sections were incubated with the primary antibodies rabbit anti-ionized calcium-binding adaptor molecule 1 (IBA1; Wako) combined with goat anti-CXCL13, goat anti-CXCL10 (both R&D Systems), or rabbit anti-CXCL1 (Novus Biologicals) in 10 % FCS/TTX for 72 h at 4 °C. The secondary antibodies anti-rabbit Alexa Fluor 488 and anti-goat Alexa Fluor 594 (Invitrogen) were applied for 2 h at RT, and mounted sections were examined using a fluorescence microscope.

### Evaluation of brain vascularity
Histochemical detection of blood vessels was performed as described previously [25]. Adjacent 1-in-12 series of sagittal free-floating sections of non-perfused $Cstb^{-/-}$ and control brains (P14 and P30) were incubated in 3,3′-diaminobenzidine (DAB) to detect endogenous peroxidase expression of erythrocytes. From each brain ($n$ = 4 per genotype and age), eight sections were analyzed. Per each brain section, the vascularization was quantified from eight black and white bright-field images (×40, five from cortex and three from cerebellum) as relative DAB-positive section area using ImageJ software.

### Measurement of BBB permeability
Blood-brain barrier (BBB) integrity was analyzed based on its permeability for fluorescein [26, 27] and serum albumin [28]. To measure the fluorescein uptake into the brain, $Cstb^{-/-}$ and control P30 mice were injected i.p. with 100 μl (5 ml per kg) of 100 mg/ml fluorescein sodium salt (NaF, Sigma-Aldrich) in sterile PBS. After 1 h, the mice were perfused with PBS until the liquid leaving the right atrium was colorless. The excised brains were freed from the meninges and the fourth ventricular choroid plexus and weighed. After homogenization in 500 μl PBS and mixing with a vortex for 2 min, 500 μl of 60 % trichloroacetic acid (Sigma-Aldrich) was added to precipitate protein. Homogenized samples were kept at 4 °C for 30 min and centrifuged at 18,000$g$ at 4 °C for 10 min. Fluorescence intensity of the supernatants was measured at excitation 440 nm and emission 525 nm using a microplate reader (WALLAC Victor 2). Fluorescein concentrations were calculated based on a sodium fluorescein standard curve (10 to 200 ng/ml) and expressed as nanogram per milligram brain tissue [29]. For albumin staining, adjacent 1-in-12 series of coronal free-floating sections were incubated with 50 mM $NH_4Cl$ for 30 min, blocked with 15 % FCS/TTX for 1 h, and incubated for 24 h at 4 °C protected from light with goat anti-mouse FITC-conjugated serum albumin IgG (Alpha Diagnostic International) diluted in 10 % FCS/TTX. Mounted sections were examined using a fluorescence microscope.

## Isolation of brain mononuclear cells and nucleated splenocytes

P14 and P30 mice were euthanized with $CO_2$, perfused with ice-cold PBS, and the brain and spleen were dissected. Brain mononuclear cells were isolated as described previously [8]. Splenocytes were collected from spleens by gently grinding through a 40-µm cell strainer, erythrolyzed using VersaLyse lysing solution (Beckman Coulter), and washed with ice-cold PBS.

## Flow cytometry

The above isolated cells were blocked with 10 % normal rat serum/PBS on ice for 30 min. The brain mononuclear cells were stained with a combination of anti-mouse antibodies CD206-FITC + MHCII-PE + F4/80-PE/Cy7 + CD45-APC and the splenocytes with a combination of CD11b-FITC + CD45-PE + F4/80-PE/Cy7 + Gr-1-APC or CD206-FITC + MHCII-PE + F4/80-PE/Cy7 + CD45-APC (all from BioLegend) on ice, protected from light, for 30 min. Cells were washed and resuspended in 500 µl PBS/1 % FCS/0.02 % $NaN_3$. The flow cytometric data were acquired with a two-laser, six-color Gallios flow cytometer and analyzed by Kaluza analysis 1.3 software (Beckman Coulter). Brain mononuclear cells were defined as follows: microglia $CD45^+F4/80^+$, macrophages $CD45^{hi}F4/80^+$, M1-type macrophages $CD45^{hi}F4/80^+MHCII^+CD206^-$, and M2-type macrophages $CD45^{hi}F4/80^+MHCII^{-/+}CD206^+$. Splenocytes were defined as follows: granulocytes $CD45^+F4/80^{-/+}Gr-1^{++}$, monocytes $CD45^+F4/80^-Gr-1^+$, monocyte-derived macrophages $CD45^+CD11b^+F4/80^+Gr-1^-$, tissue-resident macrophages $CD45^+F4/80^{++}Gr-1^{-/+}$, M1-type macrophages $CD45^+F4/80^+MHCII^+CD206^-$, and M2-type macrophages $CD45^+F4/80^+MHCII^{-/+}CD206^+$. Cell populations were calculated as percentages among total leukocytes or macrophages.

## Statistical analyses

Statistical analyses were performed using unpaired, two-sided $t$ test or two-way analysis of variance (ANOVA) test with Sidak's multiple comparison test for comparison between genotypes. All data are presented as mean ± SEM and a value of $p < 0.05$ is considered statistically significant.

Further methods are available in the Supporting Information (Additional file 1).

## Results

### Pro-inflammatory cytokine levels are high in the serum of young Cstb−/− mice

To characterize peripheral inflammatory changes in pre-symptomatic and early symptomatic Cstb−/− mice, we determined the concentrations of 17 cytokines and chemokines in the serum of Cstb−/− and control mice at P14 and P30. At P14, the concentrations of pro-inflammatory chemokines CXCL1 and CXCL10, as well as pro-inflammatory cytokines IL-1α and IL-18, were significantly higher in Cstb−/− than in control mice (Fig. 1a). In contrast, the concentration of anti-inflammatory cytokine TGF-β1 was reduced. The levels of CXCL1, CXCL10, and TNF-α were higher in the serum of P30 Cstb−/− than in control mice, whereas the level of TGF-β1 did not differ between genotypes (Fig. 1b). The level of CXCL13 did not differ at P14, but was increased at P30. In conclusion, these data imply the presence of systemic inflammation, characterized by increased level of chemokines and pro-inflammatory cytokines already in pre-symptomatic Cstb−/− mice at P14.

### Expression of the pro-inflammatory chemokine CXCL13 is highly increased in Cstb−/− microglia

As the expression and secretion of chemokines have previously been shown to be altered in cerebellar tissue and primary microglia of Cstb−/− mice [8, 23, 24], we focused our further analyses on brain expression of chemokines CXCL1, CXCL10, and CXCL13, which were increased in the sera of mice at P30. Using immunohistochemistry in Cstb−/− and control mice, we did not detect expression of CXCL1 and only low level of CXCL10 at P14 and P30 (data not shown). Expression of CXCL13 was higher in Cstb−/− than control brain at both time points (Figs. 2 and 3). In P14 Cstb−/− brain tissue, CXCL13 immunopositivity was restricted to the piriform cortex, the CA3 area of the hippocampus, and the dorsal and ventral part of the anterior pretectal nucleus (Fig. 2), whereas the other cortical areas or the cerebellum did not express CXCL13 (data not shown). At P30, CXCL13 was highly expressed also in other regions of the cortex and in the cerebellum (Fig. 3). CXCL13 immunopositivity co-localized with IBA1 immunopositivity, marking Cstb−/− microglia that have an activated morphology.

### Brain vascularization is enhanced and the BBB is intact in young Cstb−/− mice

Chemokines are involved in the regulation of angiogenesis [30]. Therefore, we analyzed the vascularization in Cstb−/− and control mice at P14 and P30 in non-perfused brains by determining the relative area positive for histochemical DAB staining, which detects endogenous erythrocyte peroxidase (Fig. 4a). At P14, the extent of brain vascularization did not differ significantly between genotypes, but it was more intense in Cstb−/− than in control mice at P30 (Fig. 4b). To determine whether this increased vascularization is associated with higher BBB permeability, we measured the BBB integrity based on the presence of peripherally injected sodium fluorescein or endogenous serum albumin in the brain tissue at P30. Neither method revealed differences in BBB permeability between Cstb−/− and control mice (Additional file 2: Figure S1).

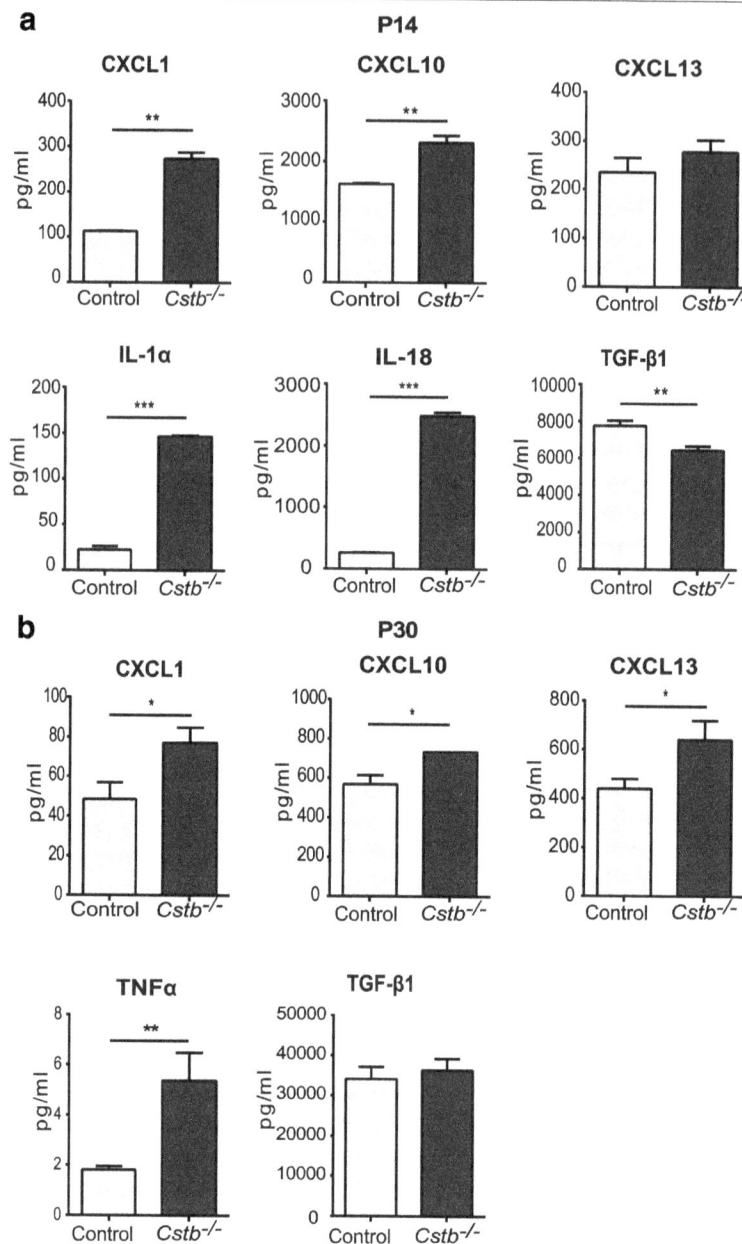

**Fig. 1** Cytokine levels in the serum of control and $Cstb^{-/-}$ mice. **a** Concentrations of CXCL1, CXCL10, CXCL13, IL-1α, IL-18, and TGF-β1 at P14 and **b** CXCL1, CXCL10, CXCL13, TNF-α, and TGF-β1 at P30. Data are presented as mean ± SEM ($n = 3$–6 per genotype; *$p < 0.05$, **$p < 0.01$, ***$p < 0.001$)

**Macrophages are pro-inflammatory in $Cstb^{-/-}$ mice**

To determine whether the high levels of pro-inflammatory cytokines in the serum are associated with changes in immune cell populations, we performed flow cytometric analyses to characterize the composition and activation of different immune cell types in $Cstb^{-/-}$ mouse bone marrow, spleen, and brain at P14 and P30. First, we determined the myeloid cell composition in the spleen and bone marrow (Additional file 3: Figure S2), as well as granulocyte-macrophage and macrophage-dendritic cell progenitors in the bone marrow (Additional file 4: Figure S3). We did not

detect any differences between genotypes at either time point. In addition, because CXCL13 is a chemoattractant for B lymphocytes [31, 32], and it is highly expressed at P30, we determined the relative amount of B lymphocytes among brain, spleen, and bone marrow leukocytes at P30 (Additional file 5: Figure S4A). It was significantly higher in the spleen (Additional file 5: Figure S4B), but did not differ in the brain and bone marrow between genotypes (Additional file 5: Figure S4C, D). Finally, we characterized the immune phenotype of spleen and brain macrophages by specifying the relative amount of pro-inflammatory M1

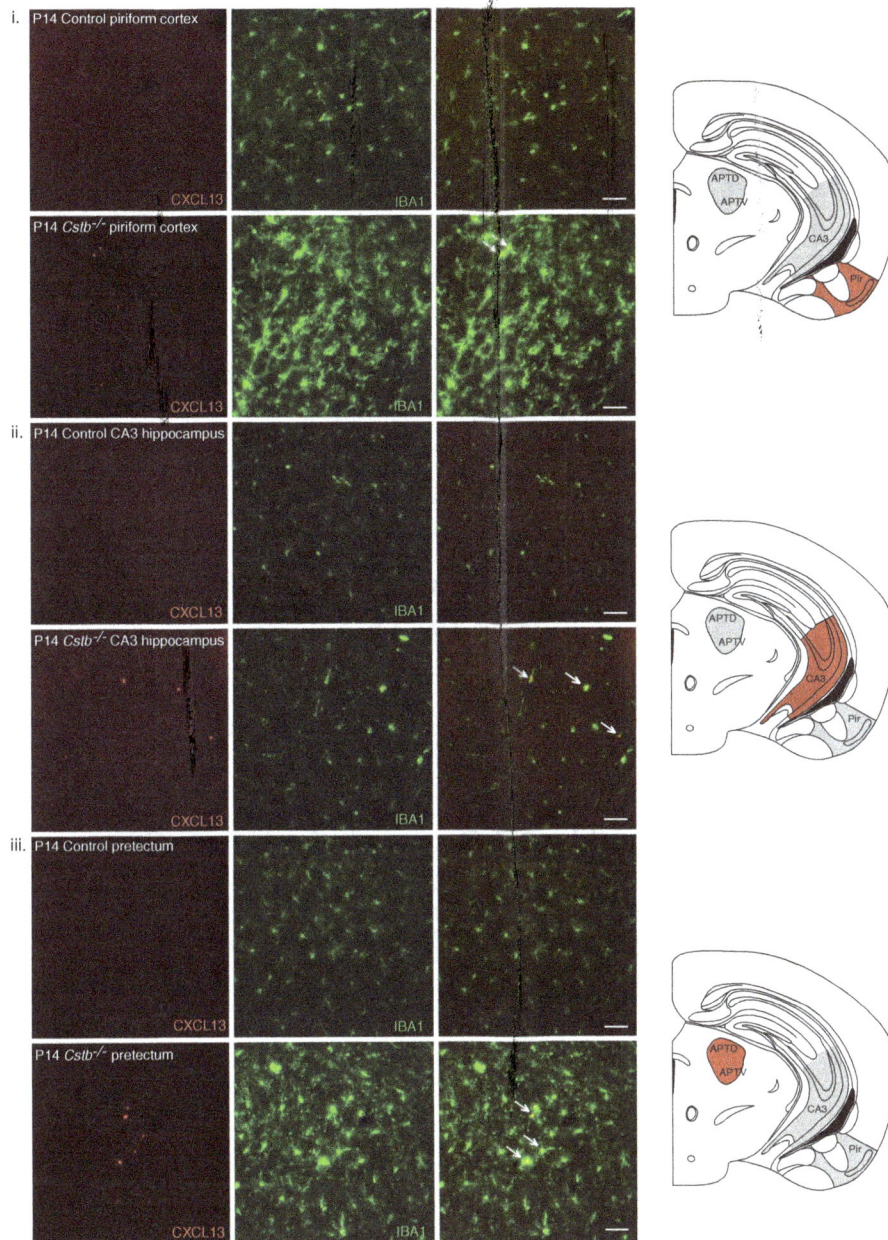

**Fig. 2** Immunohistochemical detection of CXCL13 in control and $Cstb^{-/-}$ mouse brain at P14. CXCL13-positive microglia are shown by double immunofluorescence staining of CXCL13 (*red*) with the microglial marker IBA1 (*green*) in the following brain areas: **i** piriform cortex, **ii** CA3 area of the hippocampus, and **iii** pretectum of control and $Cstb^{-/-}$ mice. Representative CXCL13- and IBA1-double-positive cells in the merged image are marked with arrows. *Scale bar* = 50 μM

and anti-inflammatory M2 macrophages from the total amount of macrophages in each tissue (Fig. 5a and Additional file 6: Figure S5) and determined the ratio (M1:M2) between both types. The ratio was higher in $Cstb^{-/-}$ mice than in controls at P14 and P30 in the spleen (Fig. 5b). In the brain of P30 $Cstb^{-/-}$ mice, the macrophages were also more polarized towards the pro-inflammatory M1 type than control macrophages (Fig. 5d).

## Discussion

In this study, we show that altered levels of chemokines in the serum and brain of young $Cstb^{-/-}$ mice, which indicate systemic inflammation already in pre-symptomatic mice, is linked to increased brain vascularization in the presence of a seemingly intact BBB. Moreover, we show that high CXCL13 expression is a hallmark of activated $Cstb^{-/-}$ microglia and that macrophages in the $Cstb^{-/-}$ spleen and brain are pro-inflammatory.

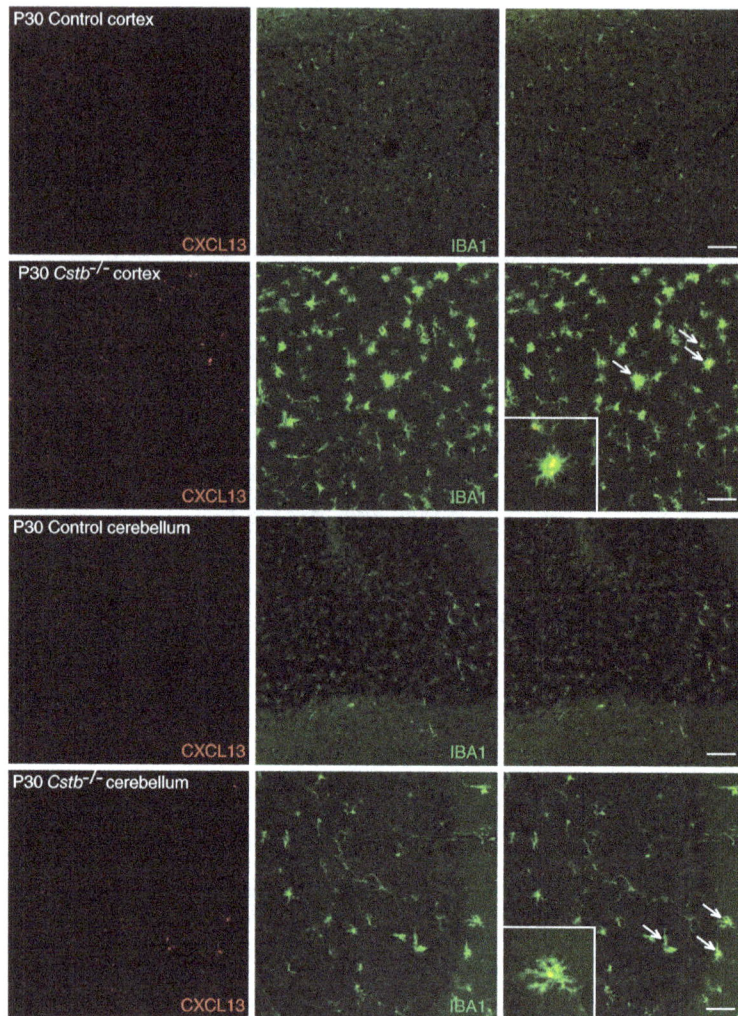

**Fig. 3** Immunohistochemical detection of CXCL13 in control and $Cstb^{-/-}$ mouse brain at P30. CXCL13-positive microglia are shown by double immunofluorescence staining of CXCL13 (*red*) with the microglial marker IBA1 (*green*) in the cortex and cerebellum of control and $Cstb^{-/-}$ mice. Representative CXCL13- and IBA1-double-positive cells in the merged image are marked with *arrows*. The *inserts* show enlargements of one double immuno-positive cell from both brain regions. *Scale bar* = 50 µM

Traumatic brain injury, epileptic seizures, ischemia, multiple sclerosis, and neurodegenerative diseases, which are characterized by a higher prevalence or a reduced threshold for seizures, are all associated with the expression and secretion of cytokines [33, 34]. Cytokines and chemokines are released primarily by cells of the immune system and vascular endothelial cells, and they can actively cross the BBB or stimulate endothelial cells to express mediators that activate brain cells [35, 36]. Previously, it had been shown that the levels of pro-inflammatory cytokines IL-18, IL-1β, and TNFα are increased in the serum of adult $Cstb^{-/-}$ mice after peripheral LPS injection [12]. Interestingly, we identified elevated levels of IL-18 and TNFα already in young $Cstb^{-/-}$ mice without activation of inflammation with LPS, whereas no alterations in the level of IL-1β were seen.

We also identified increased serum levels of chemokine CXCL1, CXCL10, and CXCL13 in $Cstb^{-/-}$ mice. Whether these chemokines are secreted from immune cells or endothelial cells requires further studies. Expression of CXCL13, which binds CXCR4 receptor and regulates B cell migration [32], has been reported to be enhanced in inflammatory CNS diseases, such as multiple sclerosis and encephalitis [37–40]. Our previous gene expression analysis of P30 $Cstb^{-/-}$ cerebellar tissue revealed a striking (29-fold) upregulation of $Cxcl13$ [24]. On the contrary, in transcriptomics profiling of in vitro-cultured $Cstb^{-/-}$ microglia, a slight downregulation of $Cxcl13$ was observed [23], suggesting that the CXCL13 upregulation in $Cstb^{-/-}$ microglia might be specific to the brain in vivo. In line with other studies, which have shown CXCL13 expression in activated mouse microglia and in blood-

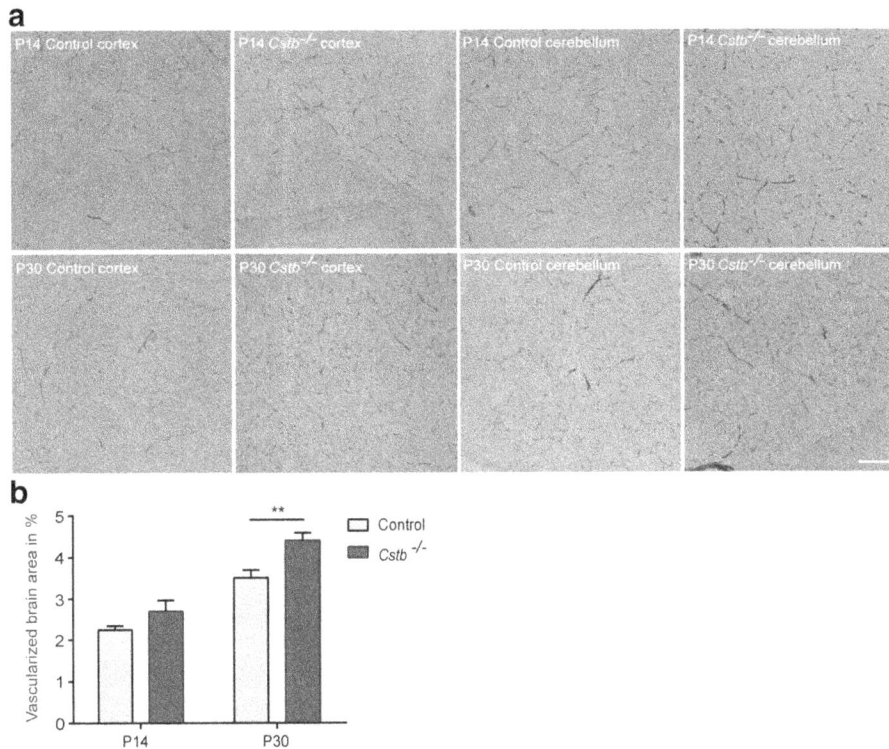

**Fig. 4** Brain vascularization of control and $Cstb^{-/-}$ mice. **a** Histochemical detection of brain vessels in the cortex of control and $Cstb^{-/-}$ mice at P14 and P30 was performed using DAB, which detects erythrocytes based on their endogenous peroxidase expression. **b** Vascularization is quantified at P14 and at P30 as relative DAB-positive area in 64 images from each of four control and four $Cstb^{-/-}$ brains. Data are presented as mean ± SEM (**$p < 0.01$, *scale bar* = 50 μM)

derived human monocytes and macrophages [41–44], we detected increased expression of CXCL13 in IBA1-positive microglia. Therefore, CXCL13 serves as a marker for activated microglia in $Cstb^{-/-}$ mice. Interestingly, the expression of CXCL13 at P14 in $Cstb^{-/-}$ microglia was restricted to the piriform cortex, CA3 area of the hippocampus, and pretectum, but was more widespread at P30.

Chemokines can regulate the integrity of the BBB [45, 46]. In particular, they affect angiogenesis and BBB permeability [30, 45, 46]. The chemokines CXCL10 and CXCL13 have been reported to be angiostatic, i.e., inhibiting the generation of vessels, whereas CXCL1 is angiogenic inducing vessel formation [30, 47]. Our results imply more intense brain vascularization in P30 $Cstb^{-/-}$ mice, which might be mediated by the higher CXCL1 concentration in serum. In addition, CXCL10 and CXCL13 could be upregulated in the serum and in the brain, respectively, to counteract the angiogenic effect of CXCL1. Despite the elevated levels of cytokines in the serum of $Cstb^{-/-}$ mice and the previously shown higher presence of macrophages, T cells, and granulocytes in the brain [8], we did not detect a compromised BBB yet at P30. However, it is likely that the BBB integrity will be impaired in older $Cstb^{-/-}$ mice as a consequence of a prolonged inflammation in the brain.

Although CXCL13 has been reported to function as a B cell chemoattractant [31, 32], we did not detect a greater proportion of B cells in the $Cstb^{-/-}$ brain. In line with our finding, the B cell infiltration after experimental autoimmune encephalomyelitis has been shown to be normal in the brain of CXCL13-deficient mice [48]. We did find an increased B cell population in the spleen of $Cstb^{-/-}$ mice, but the mechanism and significance of this finding warrant further studies.

In response to inflammatory stimuli or pathogens, microglia and macrophages can be broadly classified into pro- (M1) or anti-inflammatory (M2) activated [49–51]. Pro-inflammatory activation is linked to the release of pro-inflammatory cytokines and mediators, whereas anti-inflammatory cells promote tissue repair and survival. However, microglia and macrophages adopt various intermediate phenotypes in vivo depending on the nature of the activating stimuli. Therefore, the M1-M2 classification does not reflect the full spectrum of the intermediate and mutually non-exclusive "activation" states in vivo. A recent report by Murray et al. [52] revised the nomenclature for macrophages in vitro based on the activating stimuli. In relation to this framework, the M1 population in our study, which we identified based on their low mannose receptor (CD206) and high MHCII expression level, can be

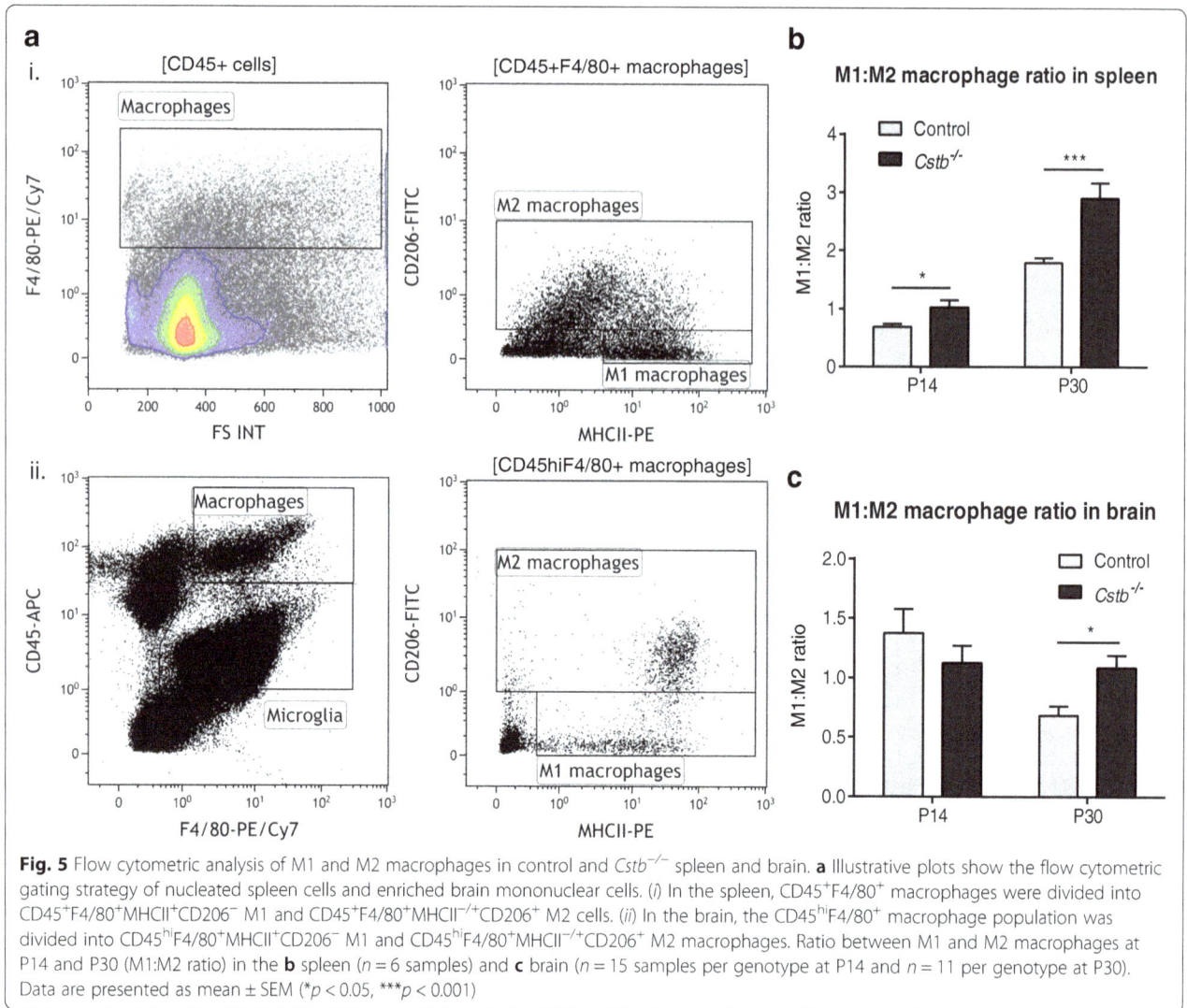

**Fig. 5** Flow cytometric analysis of M1 and M2 macrophages in control and $Cstb^{-/-}$ spleen and brain. **a** Illustrative plots show the flow cytometric gating strategy of nucleated spleen cells and enriched brain mononuclear cells. (*i*) In the spleen, CD45$^+$F4/80$^+$ macrophages were divided into CD45$^{hi}$F4/80$^+$MHCII$^+$CD206$^-$ M1 and CD45$^+$F4/80$^+$MHCII$^{-/+}$CD206$^+$ M2 cells. (*ii*) In the brain, the CD45$^{hi}$F4/80$^+$ macrophage population was divided into CD45$^{hi}$F4/80$^+$MHCII$^+$CD206$^-$ M1 and CD45$^{hi}$F4/80$^+$MHCII$^{-/+}$CD206$^+$ M2 macrophages. Ratio between M1 and M2 macrophages at P14 and P30 (M1:M2 ratio) in the **b** spleen (*n* = 6 samples) and **c** brain (*n* = 15 samples per genotype at P14 and *n* = 11 per genotype at P30). Data are presented as mean ± SEM (*$p < 0.05$, ***$p < 0.001$)

related to the M(IFN-γ) population because MHCII expression is induced by IFN-γ [53, 54]. Moreover, the M2 population, which we defined based on their high CD206 expression level, can be related to M(IL-4) cells because IL-4 stimulation induces CD206 upregulation [52, 55]. Using flow cytometric analysis, we previously showed that microglia directly extracted from the brain are skewed towards the anti-inflammatory phenotype in P14 and towards the pro-inflammatory phenotype in P30 $Cstb^{-/-}$ mice [8]. In line with these findings, also, splenic and brain macrophages show a prevailing pro-inflammatory, M1-type polarization at P30. These data imply that not only microglia but also macrophage cell populations contribute to the emergence of brain and peripheral inflammation.

In conclusion, our results support the previously described association of CSTB deficiency with early inflammatory processes in the brain of $Cstb^{-/-}$ mice. Here, we report altered chemokine and cytokine level in the serum of $Cstb^{-/-}$ mice. Future studies will show whether these findings recapitulate in EPM1 patients and whether altered expression of chemokines and/or cytokines could be useful biomarkers for diagnosis, prognosis, and treatment efficacy. Increased understanding of the inflammatory mechanisms in EPM1 is a prerequisite for the development of novel therapeutic strategies to treat this devastating disease.

## Additional files

**Additional file 1:** Flow cytometric analysis of lymphocytes, bone marrow cells, and bone marrow progenitors.

**Additional file 2: Figure S1.** BBB permeability of control and $Cstb^{-/-}$ mice. (A) Levels of sodium fluorescein (NaF) in the brain of control and $Cstb^{-/-}$ mice at P30 (*n* = 5 per genotype). (B) Immunohistochemical detection of albumin-FITC (green) in the brain of control and $Cstb^{-/-}$ mice at P30 (red: microglial marker IBA1, *n* = 4 per genotype). Data are presented as mean ± SEM (n.s.—statistically not different, scale bar = 50 μM).

**Additional file 3: Figure S2.** Flow cytometric analysis of myeloid cells from control and $Cstb^{-/-}$ mouse spleen and bone marrow. (A) Illustrative plots show the flow cytometric gating strategy of enriched nucleated cells from spleen and bone marrow. In spleen, the CD45$^+$ leukocytes were divided into (i) CD45$^+$F4/80$^{-/+}$Gr-1$^{++}$ granulocytes, CD45$^+$F4/80$^-$Gr-1$^+$ monocytes, CD45$^+$F4/80$^{++}$Gr-1$^{-/+}$ tissue-resident macrophages and (ii) CD45$^+$CD11b$^+$F4/80$^+$Gr-1$^-$ monocyte-derived macrophages. In the bone marrow, the CD45$^+$ leukocytes were divided into (iii) CD45$^+$F4/80$^{-/+}$Gr-1$^{++}$ granulocytes, CD45$^+$F4/80$^-$Gr-1$^+$ monocytes, and CD45$^+$F4/80$^+$Gr-1$^{-/+}$ macrophages. (B) Percentages of granulocytes, monocytes, and tissue-resident and monocyte-derived macrophages in the total CD45$^+$ leukocyte population in spleen of control and $Cstb^{-/-}$ mice at P14 and P30. (C) Percentages of granulocytes, monocytes, and macrophages in the total CD45$^+$ leukocyte population in the bone marrow of control and $Cstb^{-/-}$ mice at P14 and P30. Data are presented as mean ± SEM ($n = 15$ samples per genotype at P14, and $n = 11$ samples per genotype at P30).

**Additional file 4: Figure S3.** Analysis of granulocyte-macrophage progenitors (GMP) and macrophage-dendritic cell progenitors (MDP) in control and $Cstb^{-/-}$ mice. (A) Illustrative plots show the flow cytometric gating strategy of progenitor cells from bone marrow. GMP cells are represented as Lin$^-$c-Kit$^+$Sca-1$^-$CD16/32$^+$CD115$^-$ and MDP cells as Lin$^-$c-Kit$^+$Sca-1$^-$CD16/32$^+$CD115$^+$. Percentages of (B) GMP and (C) MDP cells in the total bone marrow leucocytes of control and $Cstb^{-/-}$ mice at P14 and P30. Data are presented as mean ± SEM ($n = 6$ samples per genotype; each sample containing cells from one mouse).

**Additional file 5: Figure S4.** Analysis of B lymphocytes from the spleen, brain, and bone marrow of control and $Cstb^{-/-}$ mice. (A) Illustrative plots show the flow cytometric gating strategy of lymphocytes from the (i) spleen, (ii) brain, and (iii) bone marrow. Percentage of B lymphocytes in the total CD45$^+$ cell population in the (B) spleen, (C) brain, and (D) bone marrow of control and $Cstb^{-/-}$ mice at P30. Data are presented as mean ± SEM ($n = 5$ samples per genotype; each sample containing cells from one mouse; ***$p < 0.001$).

**Additional file 6: Figure S5.** Flow cytometric analysis of M1 and M2 macrophages in control and $Cstb^{-/-}$ mouse spleen and brain. Percentages of M1 and M2 macrophages in the total macrophage population in the (A and B) spleen and (C and D) brain of control and $Cstb^{-/-}$ mice at P14 and P30. (*$p < 0.05$, **$p < 0.01$, ***$p < 0.001$).

## Abbreviations

BBB: Blood-brain barrier; CSTB: Cystatin B; EPM1: Progressive myoclonus epilepsy of Unverricht-Lundborg type

## Acknowledgements
The authors thank Ms. Paula Hakala for coordinating the mouse breeding. We acknowledge Dmitry Molotkov and the Biomedicum Imaging Unit staff for microscopy service and assistance.

## Funding
This work was supported by Folkhälsan Research Foundation, Academy of Finland (project 1256107 and 1283085 (L.T)), Sigrid Jusélius Foundation, Medicinska Understödsföreningen Liv och Hälsa r.f (Life and Health Medical Fund), and the Doctoral Program in Biomedicine (I.K and Z.L).

## Authors' contributions
OO performed the serum cytokine and the vascularization assays, OO, IK, and ST conducted the IHC and BBB assays, and ZL performed the flow cytometric experiments. LT, TJ, and AEL were responsible for the study design and supervision. OO, IK, and AEL wrote the manuscript. All authors critically revised the manuscript and approved the final version.

## Competing interests
The authors declare that they have no competing interests.

## Consent for publication
Not applicable.

## Author details
[1]Folkhälsan Institute of Genetics, Haartmaninkatu 8, 00014 Helsinki, Finland. [2]Research Program's Unit, Molecular Neurology, University of Helsinki, Haartmaninkatu 8, 00014 Helsinki, Finland. [3]Neuroscience Center, University of Helsinki, Viikinkaari 4, 00014 Helsinki, Finland. [4]Beijing Huilongguan Hospital, Peking University teaching hospital, Beijing, China.

## References
1. Kälviäinen R, Khyuppenen J, Koskenkorva P, Eriksson K, Vanninen R, Mervaala E. Clinical picture of EPM1-Unverricht-Lundborg disease. Epilepsia. 2008;49:549–56.
2. Lalioti MD, Scott HS, Antonarakis SE. What is expanded in progressive myoclonus epilepsy? Nat Genet. 1997;17:17.
3. Pennacchio LA, Myers RM. Isolation and characterization of the mouse cystatin B gene. Genome Res. 1996;6:1103–9.
4. Turk V, Bode W. The cystatins: protein inhibitors of cysteine proteinases. FEBS Lett. 1991;285:213–9.
5. Haves-Zburof D, Paperna T, Gour-Lavie A, Mandel I, Glass-Marmor L, Miller A. Cathepsins and their endogenous inhibitors cystatins: expression and modulation in multiple sclerosis. J Cell Mol Med. 2011;15:2421–9.
6. Lenarcic B, Krizaj I, Zunec P, Turk V. Differences in specificity for the interactions of stefins A, B and D with cysteine proteinases. FEBS Lett. 1996;395:113–8.
7. Luciano-Montalvo C, Ciborowski P, Duan F, Gendelman HE, Melendez LM. Proteomic analyses associate cystatin B with restricted HIV-1 replication in placental macrophages. Placenta. 2008;29:1016–23.
8. Okuneva O, Körber I, Li Z, Tian L, Joensuu T, Kopra O, Lehesjoki AE. Abnormal microglial activation in the Cstb(–/–) mouse, a model for progressive myoclonus epilepsy, EPM1. Glia. 2015;63:400–11.
9. Rinne A, Jarvinen M, Dorn A, Alavaikko M, Jokinen K, Hopsu-Havu VK. Low-molecular cysteine protease inhibitors in the human palatal tonsil. Anat Anz. 1986;161:215–30.
10. Maher K, Zavrsnik J, Jeric-Kokelj B, Vasiljeva O, Turk B, Kopitar-Jerala N. Decreased IL-10 expression in stefin B-deficient macrophages is regulated by the MAP kinase and STAT-3 signaling pathways. FEBS Lett. 2014;588:720–6.
11. Suzuki T, Hashimoto S, Toyoda N, Nagai S, Yamazaki N, Dong HY, Sakai J, Yamashita T, Nukiwa T, Matsushima K. Comprehensive gene expression profile of LPS-stimulated human monocytes by SAGE. Blood. 2000;96:2584–91.
12. Maher K, Jeric Kokelj B, Butinar M, Mikhaylov G, Mancek-Keber M, Stoka V, Vasiljeva O, Turk B, Grigoryev SA, Kopitar-Jerala N. A role for stefin B (cystatin B) in inflammation and endotoxemia. J Biol Chem. 2014;289:31736–50.
13. Verdot L, Lalmanach G, Vercruysse V, Hartmann S, Lucius R, Hoebeke J, Gauthier F, Vray B. Cystatins up-regulate nitric oxide release from interferon-gamma-activated mouse peritoneal macrophages. J Biol Chem. 1996;271:28077–81.
14. Kopitar-Jerala N, Schweiger A, Myers RM, Turk V, Turk B. Sensitization of stefin B-deficient thymocytes towards staurosporin-induced apoptosis is independent of cysteine cathepsins. FEBS Lett. 2005;579:2149–55.
15. Sun L, Wu Z, Hayashi Y, Peters C, Tsuda M, Inoue K, Nakanishi H. Microglial cathepsin B contributes to the initiation of peripheral inflammation-induced chronic pain. J Neurosci. 2012;32:11330–42.
16. Laitala-Leinonen T, Rinne R, Saukko P, Väänänen HK, Rinne A. Cystatin B as an intracellular modulator of bone resorption. Matrix Biol. 2006;25:149–57.
17. Manninen O, Puolakkainen T, Lehto J, Harittu E, Kallonen A, Peura M, Laitala-Leinonen T, Kopra O, Kiviranta R, Lehesjoki AE. Impaired osteoclast homeostasis in the cystatin B-deficient mouse model of progressive myoclonus epilepsy. Bone Reports. 2015;3:76–82.
18. Lehtinen MK, Tegelberg S, Schipper H, Su H, Zukor H, Manninen O, Kopra O, Joensuu T, Hakala P, Bonni A, Lehesjoki AE. Cystatin B deficiency sensitizes neurons to oxidative stress in progressive myoclonus epilepsy, EPM1. J Neurosci. 2009;29:5910–5.
19. Ceru S, Konjar S, Maher K, Repnik U, Krizaj I, Bencina M, Renko M, Nepveu A, Zerovnik E, Turk B, Kopitar-Jerala N. Stefin B interacts with histones and cathepsin L in the nucleus. J Biol Chem. 2010;285:10078–86.
20. Pennacchio LA, Bouley DM, Higgins KM, Scott MP, Noebels JL, Myers RM. Progressive ataxia, myoclonic epilepsy and cerebellar apoptosis in cystatin B-deficient mice. Nat Genet. 1998;20:251–8.

21. Manninen O, Koskenkorva P, Lehtimäki KK, Hyppönen J, Könönen M, Laitinen T, Kalimo H, Kopra O, Kälviäinen R, Gröhn O, et al. White matter degeneration with Unverricht-Lundborg progressive myoclonus epilepsy: a translational diffusion-tensor imaging study in patients and cystatin B-deficient mice. Radiology. 2013;269:232–9.

22. Tegelberg S, Kopra O, Joensuu T, Cooper JD, Lehesjoki AE. Early microglial activation precedes neuronal loss in the brain of the Cstb$^{-/-}$ mouse model of progressive myoclonus epilepsy, EPM1. J Neuropathol Exp Neurol. 2012;71:40–53.

23. Körber I, Katayama S, Einarsdottir E, Krjutškov K, Hakala P, Kere J, Lehesjoki AE, Joensuu T. Gene-expression profiling suggests impaired signaling via the interferon pathway in Cstb$^{-/-}$ microglia. PLoS One. 2016;11:e0158195.

24. Joensuu T, Tegelberg S, Reinmaa E, Segerstråle M, Hakala P, Pehkonen H, Korpi ER, Tyynelä J, Taira T, Hovatta I, et al. Gene expression alterations in the cerebellum and granule neurons of Cstb$^{(-/-)}$ mouse are associated with early synaptic changes and inflammation. PLoS One. 2014;9:e89321.

25. Rigau V, Morin M, Rousset MC, de Bock F, Lebrun A, Coubes P, Picot MC, Baldy-Moulinier M, Bockaert J, Crespel A, Lerner-Natoli M. Angiogenesis is associated with blood–brain barrier permeability in temporal lobe epilepsy. Brain. 2007;130:1942–56.

26. Kaya M, Ahishali B. Assessment of permeability in barrier type of endothelium in brain using tracers: Evans blue, sodium fluorescein, and horseradish peroxidase. Methods Mol Biol. 2011;763:369–82.

27. Morrey JD, Olsen AL, Siddharthan V, Motter NE, Wang H, Taro BS, Chen D, Ruffner D, Hall JO. Increased blood-brain barrier permeability is not a primary determinant for lethality of West Nile virus infection in rodents. J Gen Virol. 2008;89:467–73.

28. Garbuzova-Davis S, Louis MK, Haller EM, Derasari HM, Rawls AE, Sanberg PR. Blood-brain barrier impairment in an animal model of MPS III B. PLoS One. 2011;6:e16601.

29. Aggarwal A, Khera A, Singh I, Sandhir R. S-nitrosoglutathione prevents blood-brain barrier disruption associated with increased matrix metalloproteinase-9 activity in experimental diabetes. J Neurochem. 2015;132:595–608.

30. Romagnani P, Lasagni L, Annunziato F, Serio M, Romagnani S. CXC chemokines: the regulatory link between inflammation and angiogenesis. Trends Immunol. 2004;25:201–9.

31. Gunn MD, Ngo VN, Ansel KM, Ekland EH, Cyster JG, Williams LT. A B-cell-homing chemokine made in lymphoid follicles activates Burkitt's lymphoma receptor-1. Nature. 1998;391:799–803.

32. Legler DF, Loetscher M, Roos RS, Clark-Lewis I, Baggiolini M, Moser B. B cell-attracting chemokine 1, a human CXC chemokine expressed in lymphoid tissues, selectively attracts B lymphocytes via BLR1/CXCR5. J Exp Med. 1998;187:655–60.

33. Galic MA, Riazi K, Pittman QJ. Cytokines and brain excitability. Front Neuroendocrinol. 2012;33:116–25.

34. Murta V, Ferrari CC. Influence of peripheral inflammation on the progression of multiple sclerosis: evidence from the clinic and experimental animal models. Mol Cell Neurosci. 2013;53:6–13.

35. Banks WA. The blood-brain barrier in neuroimmunology: tales of separation and assimilation. Brain Behav Immun. 2015;44:1–8.

36. Rochfort KD, Cummins PM. The blood-brain barrier endothelium: a target for pro-inflammatory cytokines. Biochem Soc Trans. 2015;43:702–6.

37. Festa ED, Hankiewicz K, Kim S, Skurnick J, Wolansky LJ, Cook SD, Cadavid D. Serum levels of CXCL13 are elevated in active multiple sclerosis. Mult Scler. 2009;15:1271–9.

38. Kothur K, Wienholt L, Mohammad SS, Tantsis EM, Pillai S, Britton PN, Jones CA, Angiti RR, Barnes EH, Schlub T, et al. Utility of CSF cytokine/chemokines as markers of active intrathecal inflammation: comparison of demyelinating. Anti-NMDAR and Enteroviral Encephalitis. PLoS One. 2016;11:e0161656.

39. Kuenz B, Lutterotti A, Ehling R, Gneiss C, Haemmerle M, Rainer C, Deisenhammer F, Schocke M, Berger T, Reindl M. Cerebrospinal fluid B cells correlate with early brain inflammation in multiple sclerosis. PLoS One. 2008;3:e2559.

40. Liba Z, Kayserova J, Elisak M, Marusic P, Nohejlova H, Hanzalova J, Komarek V, Sediva A. Anti-N-methyl-D-aspartate receptor encephalitis: the clinical course in light of the chemokine and cytokine levels in cerebrospinal fluid. J Neuroinflammation. 2016;13:55.

41. Chapman KZ, Ge R, Monni E, Tatarishvili J, Ahlenius H, Arvidsson A, Ekdahl CT, Lindvall O, Kokaia Z. Inflammation without neuronal death triggers striatal neurogenesis comparable to stroke. Neurobiol Dis. 2015;83:1–15.

42. Esen N, Rainey-Barger EK, Huber AK, Blakely PK, Irani DN. Type-I interferons suppress microglial production of the lymphoid chemokine, CXCL13. Glia. 2014;62:1452–62.

43. Huang C, Sakry D, Menzel L, Dangel L, Sebastiani A, Krämer T, Karram K, Engelhard K, Trotter J, Schäfer MK. Lack of NG2 exacerbates neurological outcome and modulates glial responses after traumatic brain injury. Glia. 2016;64:507–23.

44. Krumbholz M, Theil D, Cepok S, Hemmer B, Kivisäkk P, Ransohoff RM, Hofbauer M, Farina C, Derfuss T, Hartle C, et al. Chemokines in multiple sclerosis: CXCL12 and CXCL13 up-regulation is differentially linked to CNS immune cell recruitment. Brain. 2006;129:200–11.

45. Chai Q, She R, Huang Y, Fu ZF. Expression of neuronal CXCL10 induced by rabies virus infection initiates infiltration of inflammatory cells, production of chemokines and cytokines, and enhancement of blood–brain barrier permeability. J Virol. 2015;89:870–6.

46. Roberts TK, Eugenin EA, Lopez L, Romero IA, Weksler BB, Couraud PO, Berman JW. CCL2 disrupts the adherens junction: implications for neuroinflammation. Lab Invest. 2012;92:1213–33.

47. Scapini P, Morini M, Tecchio C, Minghelli S, Di Carlo E, Tanghetti E, Albini A, Lowell C, Berton G, Noonan DM, Cassatella MA. CXCL1/macrophage inflammatory protein-2-induced angiogenesis in vivo is mediated by neutrophil-derived vascular endothelial growth factor-A. J Immunol. 2004;172:5034–40.

48. Rainey-Barger EK, Rumble JM, Lalor SJ, Esen N, Segal BM, Irani DN. The lymphoid chemokine, CXCL13, is dispensable for the initial recruitment of B cells to the acutely inflamed central nervous system. Brain Behav Immun. 2011;25:922–31.

49. Butovsky O, Talpalar AE, Ben-Yaakov K, Schwartz M. Activation of microglia by aggregated beta-amyloid or lipopolysaccharide impairs MHC-II expression and renders them cytotoxic whereas IFN-gamma and IL-4 render them protective. Mol Cell Neurosci. 2005;29:381–93.

50. Mills CD, Kincaid K, Alt JM, Heilman MJ, Hill AM. M-1/M-2 macrophages and the Th1/Th2 paradigm. J Immunol. 2000;164:6166–73.

51. Mulder R, Banete A, Basta S. Spleen-derived macrophages are readily polarized into classically activated (M1) or alternatively activated (M2) states. Immunobiology. 2014;219:737–45.

52. Murray PJ, Allen JE, Biswas SK, Fisher EA, Gilroy DW, Goerdt S, Gordon S, Hamilton JA, Ivashkiv LB, Lawrence T, et al. Macrophage activation and polarization: nomenclature and experimental guidelines. Immunity. 2014;41:14–20.

53. Goñalons E, Barrachina M, García-Sanz JA, Celada A. Translational control of MHC class II I-A molecules by IFN-gamma. J Immunol. 1998;161:1837–43.

54. King DP, Jones PP. Induction of Ia and H-2 antigens on a macrophage cell line by immune interferon. J Immunol. 1983;131:315–8.

55. Stein M, Keshav S, Harris N, Gordon S. Interleukin 4 potently enhances murine macrophage mannose receptor activity: a marker of alternative immunologic macrophage activation. J Exp Med. 1992;176:287–92.

# 9

# Sinomenine exerts anticonvulsant profile and neuroprotective activity in pentylenetetrazole kindled rats: involvement of inhibition of NLRP1 inflammasome

Bo Gao[1†], Yu Wu[1†], Yuan-Jian Yang[2†], Wei-Zu Li[1], Kun Dong[1], Jun Zhou[3], Yan-Yan Yin[1], Da-Ke Huang[4] and Wen-Ning Wu[1*]

## Abstract

**Background:** Epilepsy is a common neurological disorder and is not well controlled by available antiepileptic drugs (AEDs). Inflammation is considered to be a critical factor in the pathophysiology of epilepsy. Sinomenine (SN), a bioactive alkaloid with anti-inflammatory effect, exerts neuroprotective activity in many nervous system diseases. However, little is known about the effect of SN on epilepsy.

**Methods:** The chronic epilepsy model was established by pentylenetetrazole (PTZ) kindling. Morris water maze (MWM) was used to test spatial learning and memory ability. H.E. staining and Hoechst 33258 staining were used to evaluate hippocampal neuronal damage. The expression of nucleotide oligomerization domain (NOD)-like receptor protein 1 (NLRP1) inflammasome complexes and the level of inflammatory cytokines were determined by western blot, quantitative real-time PCR and enzyme-linked immunosorbent assay (ELISA) kits.

**Results:** SN (20, 40, and 80 mg/kg) dose-dependently disrupts the kindling acquisition process, which decreases the seizure scores and the incidence of fully kindling. SN also increases the latency of seizure and decreases the duration of seizure in fully kindled rats. In addition, different doses of SN block the hippocampal neuronal damage and minimize the impairment of spatial learning and memory in PTZ kindled rats. Finally, PTZ kindling increases the expression of NLRP1 inflammasome complexes and the levels of inflammatory cytokines IL-1β, IL-18, IL-6, and TNF-α, which are all attenuated by SN in a dose- dependent manner.

**Conclusions:** SN exerts anticonvulsant and neuroprotective activity in PTZ kindling model of epilepsy. Disrupting the kindling acquisition, which inhibits NLRP1 inflammasome-mediated inflammatory process, might be involved in its effects.

**Keywords:** Epilepsy, Inflammation, Sinomenine, Pentylenetetrazole, NLRP1 inflammasome, Neuroprotection

## Background

Epilepsy is one of the most common neurological disorders characterized by recurrent epileptic seizures and cognitive and behavior impairment [1, 2]. In worldwide, approximately 50 million people are suffering from this disorder [3]. Despite numerously available antiepileptic drugs (AEDs) have been used to treat epilepsy, they are not totally efficacious for all epilepsy patients [4]. These compounds are mainly symptomatic and have little effect on the underlying pathology of this disorder [5, 6]. Besides, substantial side effects of currently available AEDs greatly reduce the quality of life of patients [7, 8]. Thus, understanding the molecular mechanisms of epileptogenesis and developing novel antiepileptic agents that modify the epileptic process are still urgently needed.

* Correspondence: wuwn28@hotmail.com
†Bo Gao, Yu Wu, and Yuan-Jian Yang contributed equally to this work.
[1]Department of Pharmacology, School of Basic Medical Sciences, Key Laboratory of Anti-inflammatory and Immunopharmacology, Anhui Medical University, Hefei 230032, People's Republic of China

Accumulating evidences from clinical and experimental studies indicate that brain inflammation might be a cause or a consequence of epilepsy [3]. On the one hand, the expression of pro-inflammatory cytokines, such as IL-1β, IL-6, and TNF-α, is increased in brains of epileptic animals [9, 10]. Similarly, the level of these proinflammatory cytokines is also increased in serum or cerebrospinal fluid of patients with epilepsy [11, 12]. On the other hand, anti-inflammatory treatment also displays antiepileptic and neuroprotective effects [13]. As a critical platform regulating inflammatory responses, inflammasomes have attracted more and more attentions in various CNS disorders [14]. Inflammasomes are multi-protein complexes that consist of a cytosolic pattern-recognition receptor (a member of nucleotide oligomerization domain (NOD)-like receptor (NLR) family or HIN domain-containing (PYHIN) family), an adaptor known as apoptosis-associated speck-like protein containing a caspase-activating recruitment domain (ASC) and pro-caspase-1 [15]. Various stimuli can trigger inflammasome assembly, and then cleave pro-caspase-1 into active capsase-1 resulting in the maturation of proinflammatory cytokines IL-1β and IL-18 [16–18]. Active IL-1β could stimulate the secretion of other cytokines including TNF-α and IL-6 [19, 20]. To date, many inflammasomes have been well characterized, such as NLRP1 (NLR protein 1), NLRP2, NLRP3, NLRC4 (CARD domain-containing protein 4) inflammasome, and AIM2 (absent in melanoma 2) inflammasome [21–25]. The NLRP1 inflammasome is the first to be characterized and expressed in neurons and glial cells [21, 26]. Recent study shows that NLRP1 inflammasome contributes to seizure-induced degenerative process in patients and in the animals with temporal lobe epilepsy (TLE) [27]. These indicate that NLRP1 inflammasome-mediated inflammatory processes might be a critical mediator in the physiopathology of epilepsy.

Sinomenine (SN), a bioactive alkaloid extracted from the Chinese medicinal plant *Sinomenium acutum*, has been used for the clinical treatment of rheumatoid arthritis in China [28]. Previous studies show that SN exhibits a variety of pharmacological effects, including anti-inflammation, immunosuppression, anti-tumor, and neuroprotection [29–31]. Recent studies indicate that SN exerts neuroprotective effect by inhibiting inflammatory processes [32–34]. However, the effect of SN on epilepsy, an inflammation-related neurological disorders, remains little known. In present study, anticonvulsant and neuroprotective effects of SN were investigated in PTZ kindling model of epilepsy. To determine SN's related mechanism of action, we also examined the effects of the drug on NLRP1 inflammasome activation and the associated inflammatory processes.

## Methods
### Animals
Male Sprague-Dawley rats (250–300 g) were obtained from the Experimental Animal Center of Anhui Medical University. They were kept in a controlled environment with a temperature of $22 \pm 2$ °C and humidity of 60% under a 12 h light/dark cycle. Food and water were available ad libitum. All animal procedures were approved by the Committee for Experimental Animal Use and Care of Anhui Medical University.

### Chemicals
SN was purchased from Aladdin Industrial Corporation (Aladdin, Shanghai, China). PTZ and Hoechst 33258 were obtained from Sigma-Aldrich (St. Louis, MO, USA). Primary antibodies of Bax and Bcl-2 were purchased from Cell Signaling Technology Inc. (Danvers, MA, USA). Primary antibodies of NLRP1, caspase-1, IL-1β, IL-6, and TNF-α were purchased from Abcam (San Francisco, CA, USA). Primary antibodies of caspase-3, ASC, and IL-18 were purchased from Santa Cruz Biotechnology (Santa Cruz, CA, USA). Horseradish peroxidase-conjugated secondary antibodies were purchased from Santa Cruz Biotechnology (Santa Cruz, CA, USA). Other general agents were commercially available.

### Kindling procedure
The PTZ kindling epilepsy model was induced as previously described [35]. Briefly, rats were intraperitoneally (i.p.) injected with a sub-convulsive dose of PTZ (35 mg/kg) once every other day for 15 injections (29 days). Rats with three consecutive seizures of stage 4 were considered to be fully kindled [36]. Animals were observed for 30 min after each injection. The seizure intensity was scored as follows [36, 37]: stage 0, no response; stage 1, facial movements, ear, and whisker twitching; stage 2, myoclonic convulsions without rearing; stage 3, myoclonic convulsions with rearing; stage 4, clonic-tonic convulsions; stage 5, generalized clonic-tonic seizures with loss of postural control; stage 6, death. To investigate anticonvulsant and neuroprotective effects of SN, rats were divided into four groups as follow (Table 1): control group that received saline once every day. SN group that received SN (80 mg/kg, i.p.) once every day. PTZ group that received PTZ (35 mg/kg, i.p.) once every other day. PTZ + SN group that received different doses of SN (20, 40, and 80 mg/kg, i.p.) at 30 min prior to PTZ once every day. To further confirm anticonvulsant effect of SN, another experiment was performed to wash out SN. Rats were divided into four groups as follows (Table 2): control group that received saline once every day. PTZ group that received PTZ (35 mg/kg, i.p.) once every other day. PTZ + SN group that received SN (40 mg/kg, i.p.) at 30 min

**Table 1** Experimental group for performing SN's anticonvulsant and neuroprotective effects. PTZ was administered to rats every other day. Saline and SN were administered to rats at 30 min prior to PTZ once every day

| Experimental group | Saline | PTZ | SN |
|---|---|---|---|
| Control | Yes | No | No |
| SN | No | No | 80 mg/kg |
| PTZ | No | 35 mg/kg | No |
| PTZ + SN | No | 35 mg/kg | 20 mg/kg |
| | No | 35 mg/kg | 40 mg/kg |
| | No | 35 mg/kg | 80 mg/kg |

prior to PTZ once every day. SN washout (SNW) group that received SN (40 mg/kg, i.p.) at 30 min prior to PTZ once every day in the beginning. After 14 injections of PTZ, rats in SNW group were not received SN again and were only received PTZ until they were fully kindled.

## Morris water maze test

Morris water maze (MWM) is mainly consisted of a black circular pool (diameter 160 cm, height 60 cm) filled with water (depth 30 cm, temperature $25 \pm 2$ °C) and an circular platform (diameter 10 cm) where animals can escape. The pool was divided into four equal quadrants, and escape platform was placed in a constant quadrant (target quadrant) and was submerged 1.5 cm below the water surface. Several distal extra-maze cues, which used for spatial orientation, were placed around the pool and remained in the same position throughout experiment. MWM test was performed at the end of kindling procedure. Only 1 day prior to the first training trial, animals were allowed an adaptation period (swim freely for 120 s with no platform present) in the pool. For acquisition trial, rats underwent four trials per day with a 30 min intertrial interval for five consecutive days. In each trial, rats were placed into the water starting from one of four quadrants with its head facing towards the wall of the pool. Each rat was allowed to swim until finding the platform. Maximal duration of each trial is 120 s. After climbing on the platform, the rat was allowed to remain there for 15 s, and then was removed and released from the next starting point. The

escape latency and the swimming track were recorded. If the rat failed to find the hidden platform within 120 s, it was guided to platform manually and was allowed to stay there for 15 s. Its escape latency was recorded as 120 s. For the spatial probe test, the hidden platform was removed on the sixth day. The rat was released from quadrant which was opposite to the target quadrant and was allowed to swim freely for 120 s. The times of crossing the former platform area and the time spent in target quadrant were recorded. After the probe trial, visible platform test was performed to evaluated sensorimotor ability and motivation. For this test, the escape platform was raised 2 cm above the water level. The escape latency and swimming speed were recorded. After each swimming session, animals were allowed to warm up and dry off before they were returned to the home cage.

## Histological assay and Hoechst 33258 staining

24 h after last injection of PTZ, rats were anesthetized and the brains were removed quickly and fixed in 4% paraformaldehyde. Paraffinized brains were cut into 5 μm sections using microtome and were stained with hematoxylin and eosin (H.E.). The morphology of hippocampal CA1 and CA3 areas was examined by light microscope (Olympus IX71, Tokyo, Japan). For Hoechst 33258 staining, paraffin sections described above were deparaffinized with xylene twice and then washed with PBS for five times. After incubated with Hoechst 33258 (25 mM) for 15 min, the sections were washed with PBS for three times and mounted onto slides. The cells showing nuclear condensation under fluorescence microscopy (Olympus IX71, Tokyo, Japan) were counted for evaluating neuronal apoptosis.

## Western blotting

24 h after last injection of PTZ, animals were sacrificed by decapitation and hippocampus was isolated. Dissected hippocampal tissues were homogenized in lysis buffer containing 50 mM Tris-base (pH 7.4), 100 mM NaCl, 1% NP-40, 10 mM EDTA, 20 mM NaF, 1 mM PMSF, and protease inhibitors. After being lysed for 30 min on ice, samples were centrifuged at 12,000 $g$ at 4 °C for

**Table 2** Experimental group for performing SN washout. PTZ was administered to rats every other day. Saline and SN were administered to rats at 30 min prior to PTZ once every day. Rats in SNW (SN washout) group was only received PTZ after 14 PTZ injections

| Experimental group | Number of PTZ injection (1–14) | | | Number of PTZ injection (15–19) | | |
|---|---|---|---|---|---|---|
| | Saline | PTZ | SN | Saline | PTZ | SN |
| Control | Yes | No | No | Yes | No | No |
| PTZ | No | 35 mg/kg | No | No | 35 mg/kg | No |
| PTZ + SN | No | 35 mg/kg | 40 mg/kg | No | 35 mg/kg | 40 mg/kg |
| SNW | No | 35 mg/kg | 40 mg/kg | No | 35 mg/kg | No |

15 min. Supernatant was separated, and protein concentration was determined using the BCA protein assay kit (Pierce Biotechnology, Inc., Rockford, IL, USA). Protein samples (30 μg) were separated by 10% SDS-polyacrylamide gel and then transferred onto a polyvinylidencefluoride membrane (Millipore). After blocking with 5% nonfat milk in Tris-buffered saline containing 0.1% Tween-20 (TBST) for 1 h at room temperature, membranes were incubated overnight at 4 °C with different primary antibodies (anti-NLRP1, anti- caspase-1, anti-IL-1β, anti-IL-6 and anti-TNF-α, 1:800 dilution; anti-Bax and anti-Bcl2, 1:500 dilution; anti-caspase-3, anti-ASC, and anti-IL-18, 1:200 dilution) followed by incubation with horseradish peroxidase-conjugated secondary antibodies (1:10000 dilution) in TBST with 1% nonfat milk for 1 h at room temperature. And then membranes were reacted with enhanced chemiluminescence reagents (Amersham Pharmacia Biotech, Inc., Piscataway, NJ, USA) for 5 min and were visualized using chemiluminescence detection system (Bioshine, Shanghai, China).

### Quantitative real-time PCR analysis

Hippocampal tissues were dissected as described above. Total RNA was extracted from hippocampus using TRIzol reagent (Invitrogen, USA) following the manufacturer's instructions. cDNA synthesis was performed using a PrimeScript first Strand cDNA Synthesis Kit (Takara Biotechnology). PCR amplifications of cDNA were performed by standard methods. The following specific primers were used: NLRP1 (forward: 5-GCCC TGGAGACAAAGAATCC-3, reverse: 5-AGTGGGCAT CGTCATGTGT-3); ASC (forward: 5-ACCCCATAG ACCTCACTG AT-3, reverse: 5-ACAGCTCCAGACTC TTCCAT-3); Caspase-1 (forward: 5-ATGCC GTGGAG AGAAACAAG-3, reverse: 5-CCAGGACACATTATCTG GTG-3); β-actin (forward: 5-TTCCTTCCTGGGTA TGGAAT-3, reverse: 5-GAGGAGCAATGATCTT GAT C-3). The fluorescent signals were collected during extension stage, Ct values of the sample were calculated and relative transcript levels were analyzed by $2^{-\Delta\Delta Ct}$ method.

### Enzyme-linked immunosorbent assay (ELISA)

24 h after last injection of PTZ, rats were sacrificed by decapitation and hippocampal tissues were dissected. The protein samples were extracted and protein concentration was determined as described above. The levels of inflammatory cytokines IL-1β, IL-18, IL-6, and TNF-α in hippocampus were measured by commercial ELISA kits (R&D Systems, Minneapolis, MN, USA) according to the manufacturer's protocol.

### Statistical analysis

All data were analyzed by analysis of variance (ANOVA) with the statistical program SPSS 17.0 (Chicago, IL, USA). Data related to seizure stage and escape latency in MWM test were analyzed using two-away ANOVA with repeated measures followed by Bonferroni or Dunnett's T3 post hoc test. Other data were analyzed by one-away ANOVA. Data are expressed as means ± SEM. $P < 0.05$ was considered statistically significant.

## Results

### SN exerts anticonvulsant profile in PTZ kindling model of epilepsy

Firstly, anticonvulsant effect of SN was investigated. Seizure stage scores and fully kindled incidence were recorded. We also recorded the latency (the duration from PTZ administration to seizure event) and duration of generalized seizures (stage 4 or greater). As shown in Fig. 1a, Seizure stage in PTZ group reached 4.40 ± 0.22 after 15 injections. SN alone did not influence the behavior of rats, but 20, 40, and 80 mg/kg SN treatment reduced seizure stage to 3.25 ± 0.15, 2.50 ± 0.74, and 2.5 ± 0.20, respectively. However, SN washout reversed its effect on seizure stage (Fig. 1b), indicating that SN disrupted the kindling acquisition processes. Moreover, 20, 40, and 80 mg/kg SN treatment decreased the incidence of fully kindling from 71.43 to 50, 33.33, and 31.67% in PTZ kindled rats, respectively (Fig. 1c). In addition, SN also significantly increased the latency to generalized seizures and reduced the duration of generalized seizures in a dose-dependent manner (Fig. 1d, e), indicating that SN exhibits anticonvulsant activity in PTZ kindled rats.

### SN minimizes kindling-induced spatial learning and memory deficits in rats

Then, we performed MWM test to assess the effect of SN on spatial learning and memory of PTZ kindling rats. In acquisition trial, the escape latency of all groups decreased gradually during five training days. The escape latency of rats of PTZ group was significant longer than that of control group. There were no statistical differences between SN alone group and control group. However, SN dose-dependently reduced the escape latency (Fig. 2a). While SN washout reversed its effect on escape latency (Fig. 2b). In the fifth training day, rats in PTZ group swam a longer distance to reach the hidden platform compared with control group. Treatment with different doses of SN significantly decreased the swimming distance to find the hidden platform (Fig. 2c, d). In probe trail, rats in PTZ group showed a decrease in the number of times crossing the target quadrant and the time spent in the target quadrant compared with control group. There were no statistical differences between SN

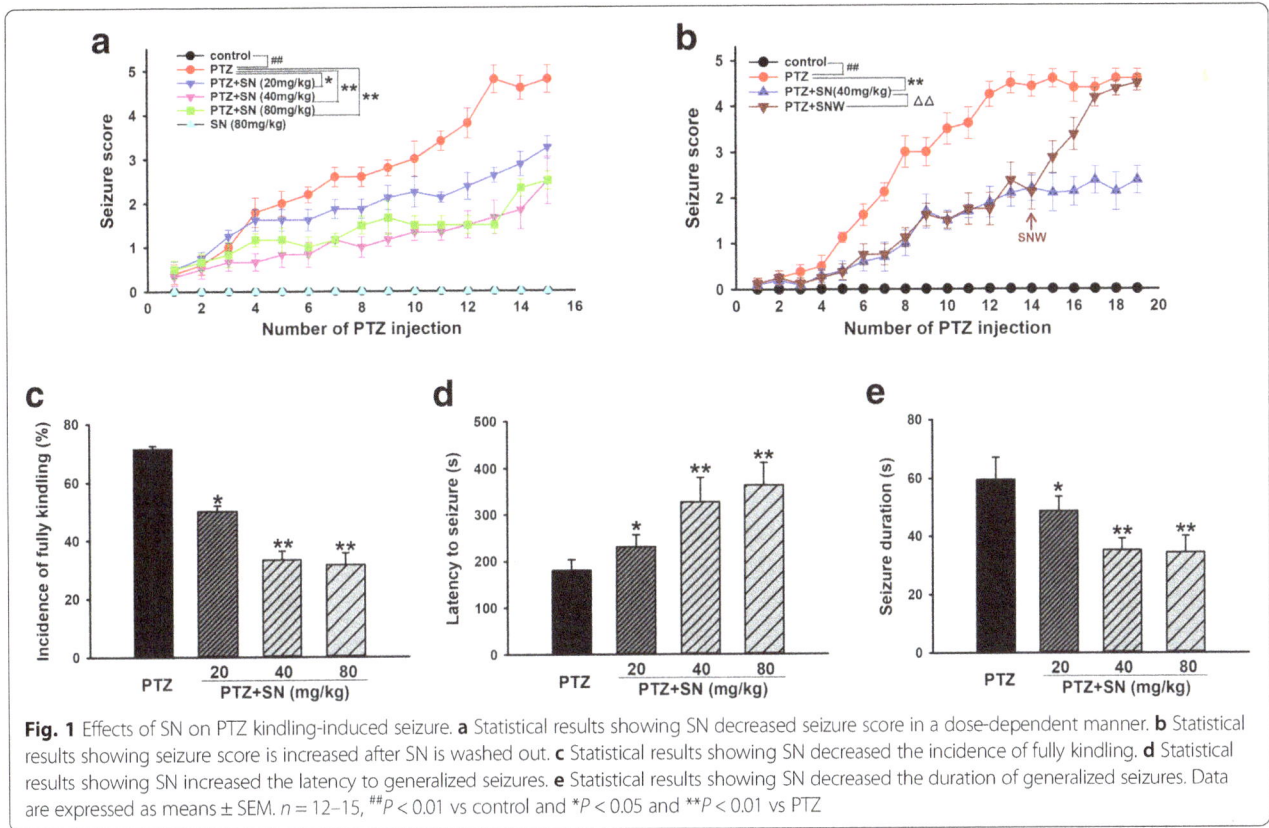

**Fig. 1** Effects of SN on PTZ kindling-induced seizure. **a** Statistical results showing SN decreased seizure score in a dose-dependent manner. **b** Statistical results showing seizure score is increased after SN is washed out. **c** Statistical results showing SN decreased the incidence of fully kindling. **d** Statistical results showing SN increased the latency to generalized seizures. **e** Statistical results showing SN decreased the duration of generalized seizures. Data are expressed as means ± SEM. $n = 12$–15, ##$P < 0.01$ vs control and *$P < 0.05$ and **$P < 0.01$ vs PTZ

alone group and control group. However, SN treatment significantly increased the number of times crossing the target quadrant and the time spent in the target quadrant in a dose-dependent manner (Fig. 2e, f). While SN washout reversed its effect on the number of times crossing the target quadrant and the time spent in the target quadrant (Fig. 2g, h). To rule out the effect of sensorimotor ability and motivation on the results, we performed visible platform test and found there were no statistical differences in the escape latency and

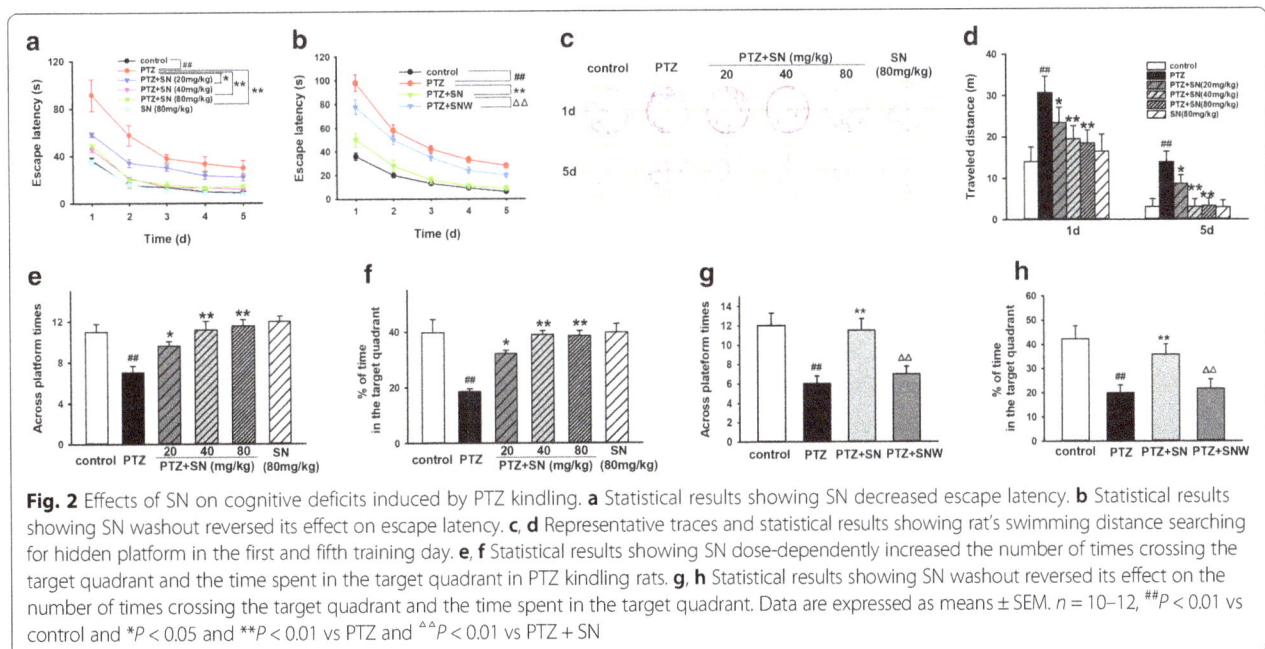

**Fig. 2** Effects of SN on cognitive deficits induced by PTZ kindling. **a** Statistical results showing SN decreased escape latency. **b** Statistical results showing SN washout reversed its effect on escape latency. **c**, **d** Representative traces and statistical results showing rat's swimming distance searching for hidden platform in the first and fifth training day. **e**, **f** Statistical results showing SN dose-dependently increased the number of times crossing the target quadrant and the time spent in the target quadrant in PTZ kindling rats. **g**, **h** Statistical results showing SN washout reversed its effect on the number of times crossing the target quadrant and the time spent in the target quadrant. Data are expressed as means ± SEM. $n = 10$–12, ##$P < 0.01$ vs control and *$P < 0.05$ and **$P < 0.01$ vs PTZ and △△$P < 0.01$ vs PTZ + SN

swimming speed among all groups (Additional file 1), indicating that the alteration of all parameters above did not result from the sensorimotor ability of rats. All these data suggested that SN minimizes the impairment of spatial learning and memory induced by PTZ kindling in rats.

## SN blocks hippocampal neuronal damage in PTZ kindled rats

Hippocampus has long been known as a critical structure for spatial learning and memory [38], so we subsequently investigated the effects of SN on hippocampal neuronal damage induced by PTZ kindling. First, histological examination was performed by H.E. staining. As shown in Fig. 3, hippocampal CA1 and CA3 areas of rats in PTZ group exhibited a serious damage compared with control group. SN dose-dependently blocked hippocampal neuronal damage induced by PTZ kindling. Then, neuronal apoptosis was evaluated by Hoechst 33258 staining. Compared with control group, the number of apoptotic neurons in hippocampal CA1 and CA3 areas was significantly increased in PTZ group. There were no statistical differences between SN alone group and control group. However, SN dose-dependently prevented neuronal apoptosis induced by PTZ kindling (Fig. 4). Finally, apoptosis-related proteins caspase-3, Bax, and Bcl2 in the hippocampus were detected by western blot. Compared with control group, the expression of caspase-3 and Bax was significantly increased, while the expression of Bcl-2 was decreased in PTZ group. The ratio of Bcl-2/Bax was also decreased in PTZ group. There were no statistical differences between SN alone group and control group. However, the effects of PTZ kindling could be inhibited by SN in a dose-dependent manner (Fig. 5). While SN washout reversed its effect on the expression of caspase-3, Bax, and Bcl2 (Additional file 2). All these results suggest that SN blocks hippocampal neuronal damage and apoptosis from PTZ kindling.

## SN inhibits NLRP1 inflammasome activation in PTZ kindled rats

Previous study has demonstrated that NLRP1 inflammasome was activated in TLE patients and electrical kindling model [27]. In order to determine the effect of PTZ kindling on NLRP1 inflammasome activation, NLRP1 inflammasome complexes in hippocampus was detected at protein and mRNA level. As shown in Fig. 6b, the expression of NLRP1 protein of rats in PTZ group is significantly increased compared with control group. Treatment with different doses of SN significant inhibited the effect, while SN alone did not influence NLRP1 expression (Fig. 6a). Similarly, higher doses of SN (40 and 80 mg/kg) also prevented the increase of ASC and caspase-1 expression induced by PTZ kindling (Fig. 6d, e, g, and h) while SN washout reversed its effect on the expression of NLRP1, ASC, and caspase-1 (Additional file 3). Our results also showed that the levels of NLRP1 mRNA, ASC mRNA, and caspase-1 mRNA of rats in PTZ group were significantly higher than those of rats in control group. The effects were significantly inhibited by SN in a dose-dependent manner, while SN alone did not influence the expression of NLRP1, ASC, and caspase-1 at mRNA level (Fig. 6c, f, i). These data suggest that NLRP1 inflammasome activation is associated with acquisition of the fully kindled state in PTZ kindling model and that SN disrupts kindling acquisition which contributes to the inhibition of NLRP1 inflammasome activation.

## SN decreases the levels of inflammatory cytokines in hippocampus of PTZ kindled rats

As a key regulator of innate immune and inflammatory response, inflammasome directly or indirectly promotes

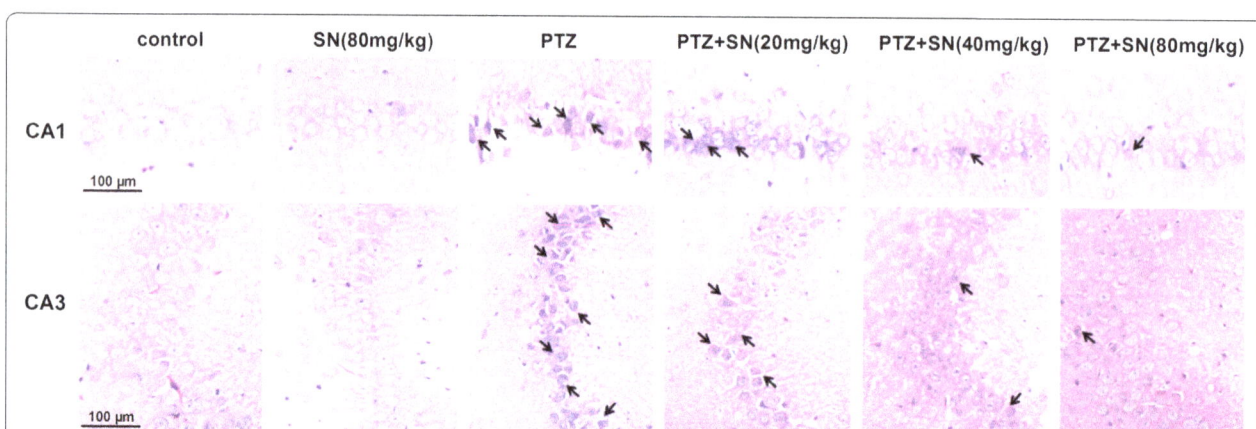

**Fig. 3** Effects of SN on hippocampal neuronal damage induced by PTZ kindling. Representative micrographs (original magnification, × 200) showing SN blocked hippocampal neuronal damage (arrow) induced by PTZ kindling in CA1 and CA3 areas in a dose-dependent manner. Scale bar = 100 μm

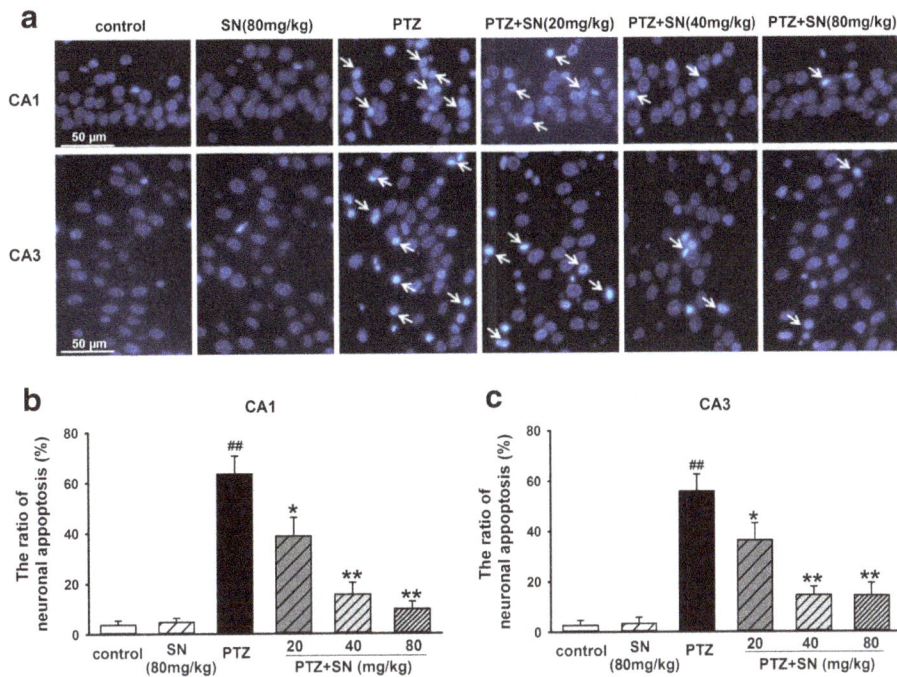

**Fig. 4** Effects of SN on hippocampal neuronal apoptosis induced by PTZ kindling. **a** Representative imagines (original magnification, ×400) showing SN inhibited hippocampal neuronal apoptosis (arrow) induced by PTZ kindling in CA1 and CA3 areas in a dose-dependent manner. Scale bar = 50 μm. Statistical results showing different doses of SN treatment reduced the number of apoptotic neuron in hippocampal CA1 (**b**) and CA3 (**c**) areas. Data are expressed as means ± SEM. $n = 8$–10, $^{##}P < 0.01$ vs control and $^*P < 0.05$ and $^{**}P < 0.01$ vs PTZ

the secretion of inflammatory cytokines, such as IL-1β, IL-18, IL-6, and TNF-α. To further determine the effect of SN on pro-inflammatory cytokines in PTZ kindled rats, we first detected the levels of IL-1β, IL-18, IL-6, and TNF-α in hippocampus by western blot. As shown in Fig. 7b, d, the expression of IL-1β and IL-18 in PTZ group was significant increased compared with control group. The effects were significantly attenuated by SN in a dose-dependent manner, while SN alone did not

influence their expression (Fig. 7a, c). Similarly, higher doses of SN (40 and 80 mg/kg) also prevented the increase of IL-6 and TNF-α expression induced by PTZ kindling (Fig. 7e, f, g, h) while SN washout reversed its effect on the expression of IL-1β, IL-18, IL-6, and TNF-α (Additional file 4). Moreover, we also detected the levels of IL-1β, IL-18, IL-6, and TNF-α in hippocampus by ELISA kits. Compared with control group, the levels of IL-1β, IL-18, IL-6, and TNF-α were significantly

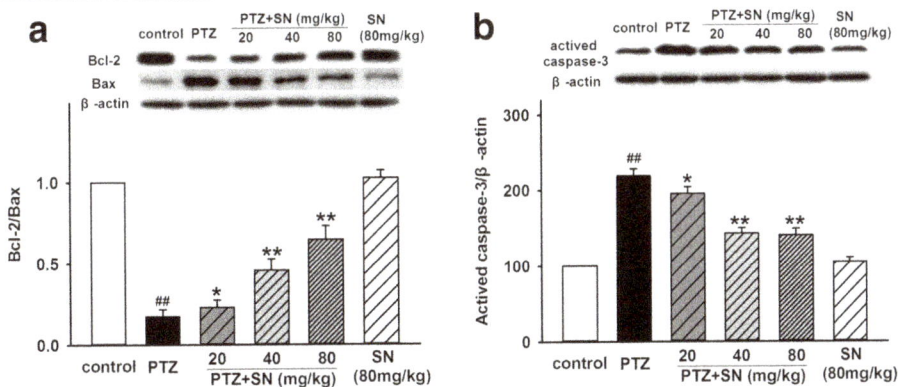

**Fig. 5** Effects of SN on hippocampal apoptosis-related proteins in PTZ kindled rats. **a** Representative immunoreactive bands and statistical results showing SN prevented PTZ-induced decrease in the ratio of Bcl-2/Bax in a dose-dependent manner. **b** Representative immunoreactive bands and statistical results showing SN prevented PTZ-induced increase in the expression of activated caspase-3 in a dose-dependent manner. Data are expressed as means ± SEM. $n = 6$, $^{##}P < 0.01$ vs control and $^*P < 0.05$ and $^{**}P < 0.01$ vs PTZ

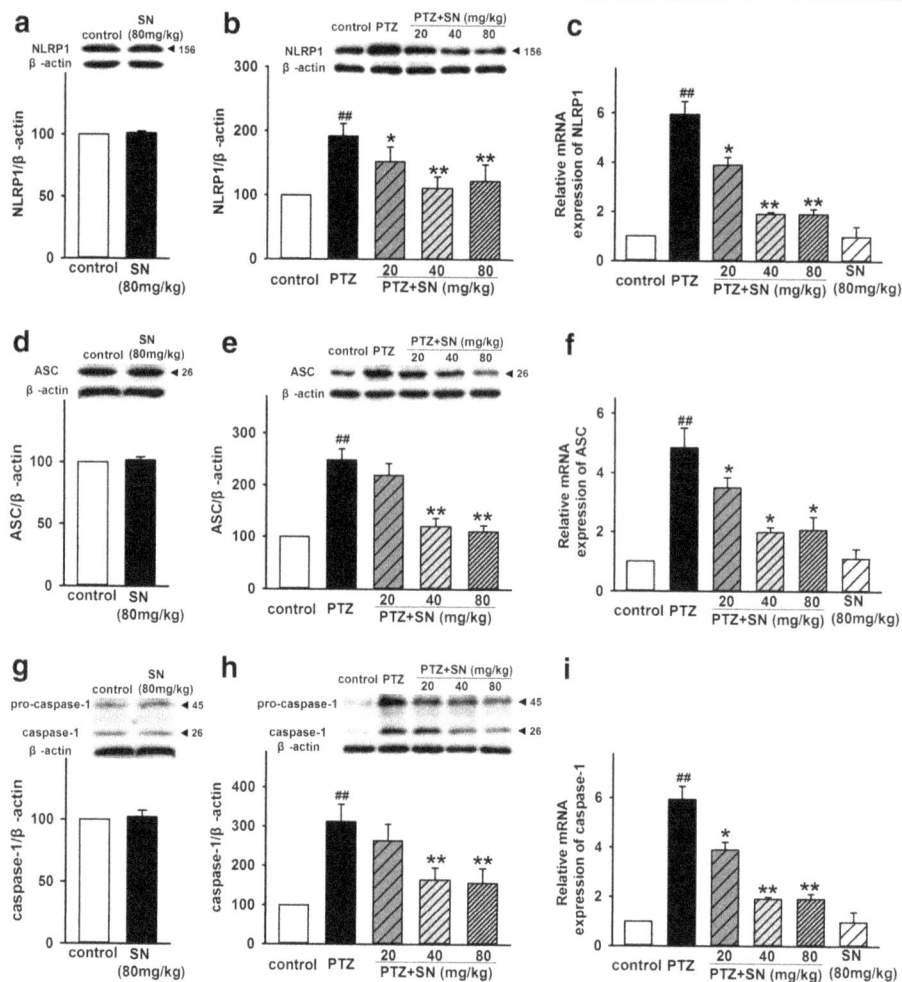

**Fig. 6** Effects of SN on the expression of hippocampal NLRP1 inflammasome complexes in PTZ kindled rats. **a, d,** and **g** Representative immunoreactive bands and statistical results showing SN alone has no influence on the protein expression of NLRP1, ASC, and caspase-1 in protein level. **b, e,** and **h** Representative immunoreactive bands and statistical results showing SN dose-dependently inhibited PTZ-induced increase in the protein expression of NLRP1, ASC, and caspase-1 in protein level. **c, f,** and **i** Statistical results showing SN dose-dependently inhibited PTZ-induced increase in the expression of NLRP1, ASC, and caspase-1 at mRNA level. Data are expressed as means ± SEM. $n = 6$–8, $^{##}P < 0.01$ vs control and $^*P < 0.05$ and $^{**}P < 0.01$ vs PTZ

increased in PTZ group. There were no statistical differences between SN alone group and control group. However, the effects of PTZ were significantly inhibited by SN in a dose-dependent manner (Fig. 8), which is consistent with western blot results. Together, these results indicate that SN inhibits NLRP1 inflammasome-mediated inflammatory processes in PTZ kindled rats.

## Discussion

In the current study, we demonstrated that SN delayed kindling acquisition and decreased the severity of seizure in PTZ kindled rats. Also, we found that SN blocked hippocampal neuronal damage and cognitive deficits. In addition, our results also showed that SN inhibited NLRP1 inflammasome activation and reduced the

secretion of inflammatory cytokines. Interestingly, SN washout blocked these effects, suggesting that disrupting kindling acquisition may be responsible for the anticonvulsant and neuroprotective effects of SN.

Epilepsy is recognized as a complex clinical syndrome. Excessively excitation of CNS resulting from imbalance between excitation and inhibition is considered as the primary cause of epilepsy [39]. However, pathogenesis of epilepsy is still not well understood, and consequently, approximate 30% of patients suffering from seizure episodes under treatment with AEDs [40, 41]. Increasing evidence has shown that inflammatory processes within brain may be a crucial mechanism in the pathophysiology of epilepsy and inflammation is considered as a biomarker of epileptogenesis [42, 43]. Inflammatory mediators can trigger neuronal hyperexcitability by

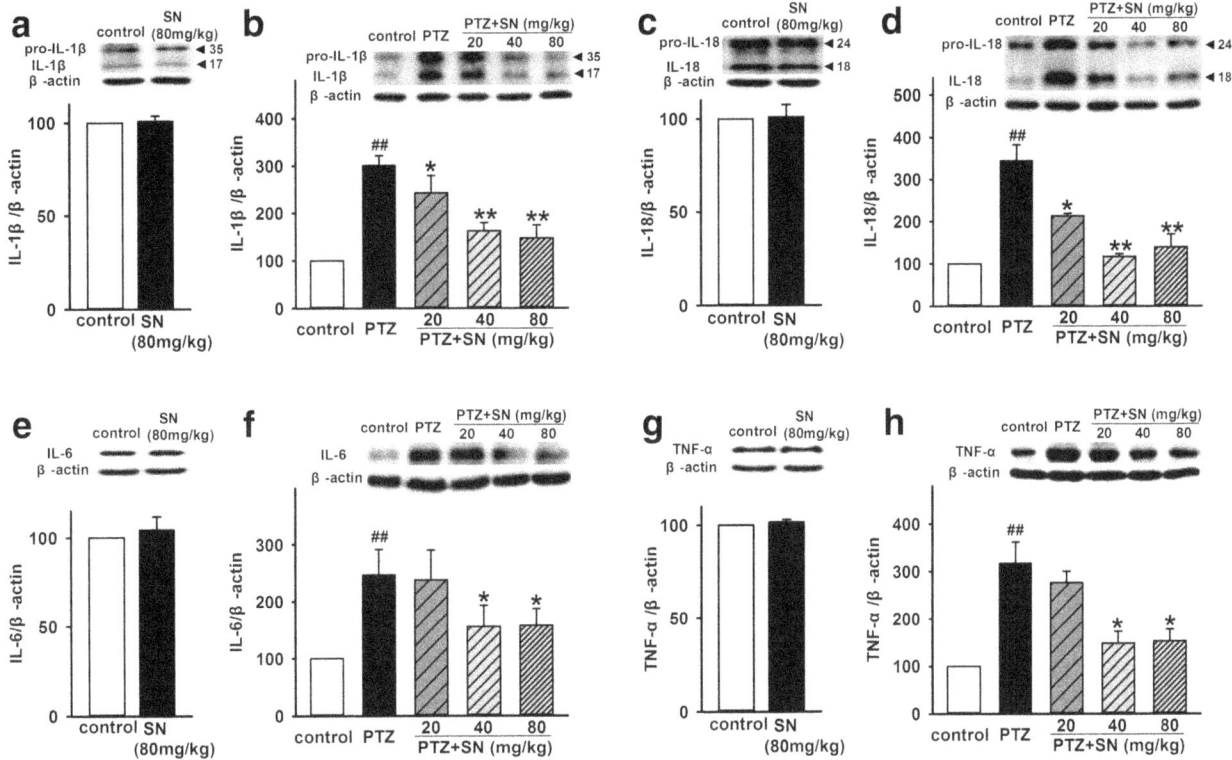

**Fig. 7** Effects of SN on the expression of hippocampal inflammatory cytokines in PTZ kindled rats. Representative immunoreactive bands and statistical results showing SN alone has no influence on the expression of IL-1β (**a**), IL-18 (**c**), IL-6 (**e**), and TNF-α (**g**) in protein level. Representative immunoreactive bands and statistical results showing SN dose-dependently inhibited PTZ-induced increase in the expression of IL-1β (**b**), IL-18 (**d**), IL-6 (**f**), and TNF-α (**h**) in protein level. Data are expressed as means ± SEM. $n = 6$–8, $^{##}P < 0.01$ vs control and $^{*}P < 0.05$ and $^{**}P < 0.01$ vs PTZ

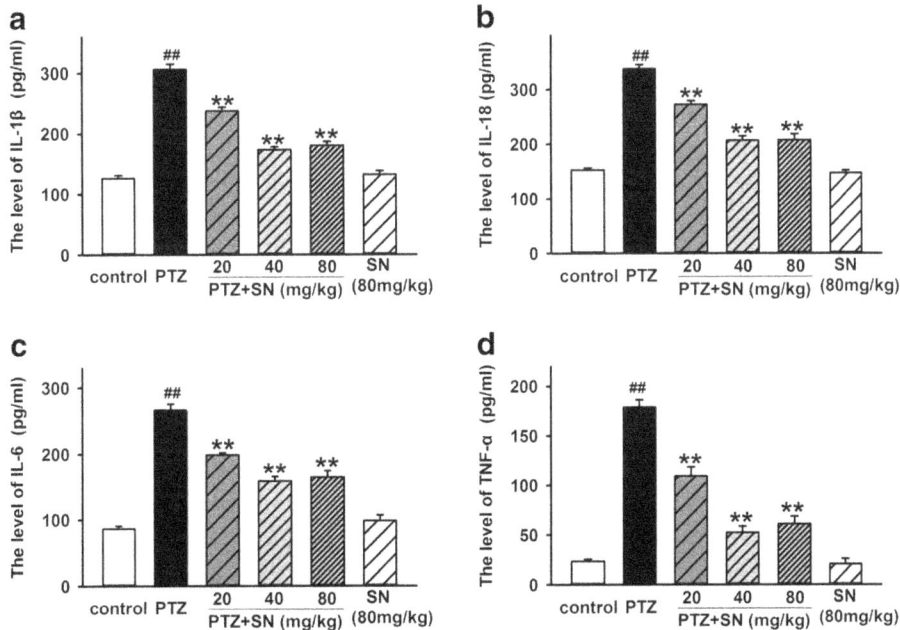

**Fig. 8** Effects of SN on the content of inflammatory cytokines in hippocampus homogenate in PTZ kindled rats. Statistical results showing SN dose-dependently inhibited PTZ-induced increase in the content of IL-1β (**a**), IL-18 (**b**), IL-6 (**c**), and TNF-α (**d**). Data are expressed as means ± SEM. $n = 8$, $^{##}P < 0.01$ vs control and $^{**}P < 0.01$ vs PTZ

activating specific signaling such as NMDA receptor and Toll-like receptor 4, and then result in increased probability of seizure recurrence. Anti-inflammatory treatments can drastically reduce spontaneous seizure frequency and the severity of the disease [13]. In addition, cyclooxy-genase-2 (COX-2) is expressed at low level in hippocampal neurons, but it is markedly increase within an hour after a seizure [44], and diclofenac sodium, a COX-inhibitor, has been reported to reduce the severity of seizure in PTZ kindling model [45].

In view of the above mentioned reasons, we speculated that SN with anti-inflammatory effect, considered as an inhibitor of COX-2 [46], may be able to protect against seizure. To test this hypothesis, a chronic epilepsy model was established by PTZ kindling which could simulate clinical seizure and was widely accepted as an experimental animal model for epileptogenesis. Our results showed that most rats were fully kindled after a subconvulsive dose of PTZ (35 mg/kg, i.p.) was administrated once every other day for 15 injections (29 days). As we expected, SN alone did not influence animal's behavior. However, SN could dose-dependently decrease the severity and incidence of fully kindled seizure, while SN washout increased the severity of seizure (Fig. 1a–c), indicating that SN delayed the kindling acquisition process. Furthermore, SN also significantly increased the latency and reduced the duration of generalized seizures (Fig. 1d, e). These indicate that SN disrupts the kindling acquisition and exerts an anticonvulsant effect in PTZ-induced seizure rats.

As we know, cognitive deficits usually accompany epilepsy. Learning and memory impairments have been found in patients with TLE and electrical kindling model, as well as chemical kindling model induced by PTZ and kainic acid (KA) [47–49]. Although several treatment strategies and AEDs are applied, they exhibit little effectiveness in cognitive deficits even under controlled seizure [50]. Therefore, after determining the anticonvulsant effect of SN, we investigated the effect of SN on cognitive deficits in PTZ kindled rats by MWM test. Our results showed that the escape latency of PTZ kindled rats was still longer compared with control group, indicating PTZ impaired spatial learning ability of rats, which is consistent with previous reports. SN dose-dependently decreased the escape latency and improved spatial learning ability of rats (Fig. 2a), while SN washout increased the escape latency (Fig. 2b). Also, after the hidden platform was removed, the number of times crossing the target quadrant and the time spent in the target quadrant were decreased in PTZ kindled rats. And the effect could be inhibited by SN in a dose-dependent manner, suggesting that SN could alleviate the impairment of spatial memory induced by PTZ kindling (Fig. 2e, f), while SN washout

reversed its effect on spatial learning ability (Fig. 2g, h). In addition, we performed visible platform test to exclude vision and motor interference in behavior test. The results showed that there were no statistical differences in escape latency and swimming speed among all groups (Additional file 1). These data suggest that SN can prevent the impairment of spatial learning and memory from PTZ kindling.

Hippocampus has long been known to be crucial for learning and memory in mammals [51]. Neuronal damage and dysfunction in this area will result in cognitive deficits [52]. Previous studies have shown that PTZ kindled seizure leads to hippocampal neuronal damage followed by spatial learning and memory impairment [35, 53]. Our data showed that SN protected against PTZ-induced seizure and improved the impairment of spatial learning and memory. SN also exhibited neuoprotection in vitro and in vivo [31, 34]. Thus, we proposed that SN might protect against hippocampal neuronal damage induced by PTZ kindling. To test this hypothesis, we first performed a series of experiments to evaluate the effect of SN on hippocampal neuronal damage in PTZ kindled rats. Our results showed SN can dose-dependently block neuronal damage (Fig. 3) and inhibit neuronal apoptosis in the hippocampal CA1 and CA3 areas of PTZ kindled rats (Fig. 4). Moreover, SN inhibited the expression of pro-apoptosis protein Bax and caspase-3 and increased the expression of anti-apoptosis protein Bcl-2 in a dose-dependent manner (Fig. 5), while SN washout reversed its effect on apoptosis-related proteins (Additional file 2). All these suggest that SN can block hippocampal damage induced by PTZ kindling and exhibits a neuroprotective effect, which may contribute to its improvement on behavior and cognitive deficits.

Inflammation is a homeostatic mechanism of defense against noxious stimuli and is designed to limit harm to the host. Neuroinflammation has been found in the pathological processes of many CNS diseases such as autoinmmune, neurodegenerative, epileptic, and psychiatric disorders [54]. Inflammasomes are multi-protein complexes discovered in 2002 [21] and has been known to be responsible for activation of inflammatory processes resulting in the secretion of inflammatory cytokines such as IL-1$\beta$, IL-18, IL-6, and TNF-$\alpha$ [55]. Inflammasomes-mediated inflammatory pathway has involved in various CNS disorders and leads to neuronal damage and changes in behavior [14]. As the first identified inflammasome, NLRP1 inflammasome has been reported to involve in the pathological processes of many nervous system diseases such as spinal cord injury (SCI), traumatic brain injury (TBI), Alzheimer's disease (AD), and nociception [56]. Recent study showed that the level of NLRP1 and caspase-1 is upregulated in TEL patients and electrical kindling model, and NLRP1 or caspase-1 silencing exhibited an antiepileptic and neuroprotective effects [27], indicating NLRP1 inflammasome play a critical role in seizure-induced neuronal damage. Here, we have demonstrated that SN disrupted the kindling acquisition and exerted antiseizure and neuroprotective effects. To further investigate the neuroprotective effects of SN, we investigated the effect of SN on NLRP1 inflammasome activation and associated inflammatory processes in PTZ kindled rats. Similar to previous report, our results showed that PTZ kindling also increased the expression of NLRP1, ASC, and caspase-1 at protein and mRNA levels. And SN can inhibit the effects of PTZ in a dose-dependent manner (Fig. 6). Furthermore, we found that SN also inhibited the upregulation of pro- inflammatory cytokines IL-1β, IL-18, IL-6, and TNF-α in PTZ kindled rats (Figs. 7 and 8), while SN washout reversed its effect on NLRP1 inflammasome activation and inflammatory response (Additional file 3 and 4). These data indicate that disrupting kindling acquisition may contribute to inhibitory effect of SN on NLRP1 inflammasome-mediated inflammatory processes, which may be involved in neuroprotective effects of SN. However, the precise mechanism that SN regulates NLRP1 inflammasome signal is unclear. Further efforts will be made to clarify it in future research.

## Conclusions

The present study showed that SN exerts anticonvulsant profile and neuroprotective effects in PTZ kindling model of epilepsy. These effects may be associated with disrupting kindling acquisition resulting in inhibition of NLRP1 inflammasome-mediated inflammatory processes.

## Additional files

**Additional file 1: Figure S1.** The effect of sensorimotor ability and motivation on the escape latency and swimming speed. (A) and (B) Statistical results showing there were no differences in the escape latency and swimming speed among all groups in visible platform test. Data are expressed as means ± SEM. $n = 10$–12, $P > 0.05$.

**Additional file 2: Figure S2.** SN washout reverses its effect on hippocampal apoptosis-related proteins in PTZ kindled rats. (A) Representative immunoreactive bands and statistical results showing SN washout reversed its effect on the ratio of Bcl-2/Bax. (B) Representative immunoreactive bands and statistical results showing SN washout reversed its effect on the expression of activated caspase-3. Data are expressed as means ± SEM. $n = 6$, $^{##}P < 0.01$ vs control, $^{**}P < 0.01$ vs PTZ and $^{△}P < 0.05$ or $^{△△}P < 0.01$ vs PTZ + SN.

**Additional file 3: Figure S3.** SN washout reverses its effect on the expression of hippocampal NLRP1 inflammasome complexes in PTZ kindled rats. Representative immunoreactive bands and statistical results showing SN washout reversed its effect on the expression of NLRP1 (A), ASC (B), and caspase-1 (C) in protein level. Data are expressed as means ± SEM. $n = 6$, $^{##}P < 0.01$ vs control, $^{**}P < 0.01$ vs PTZ and $^{△}P < 0.05$ or $^{△△}P < 0.01$ vs PTZ + SN.

**Additional file 4: Figure S4.** SN washout reverses its effect on the expression of hippocampal inflammatory cytokines in PTZ kindled rats. Representative immunoreactive bands and statistical results showing SN washout reversed its effect on the expression of IL-1β (A), IL-18 (B), IL-6 (C), and TNF-α (D) in protein level. Data are expressed as means ± SEM. $n = 6$, $^{##}P < 0.01$ vs control, $^{*}P < 0.05$ or $^{**}P < 0.01$ vs PTZ and $^{△}P < 0.05$ or $^{△△}P < 0.01$ vs PTZ + SN.

## Abbreviations

AEDs: Antiepileptic drugs; ASC: Apoptosis-associated speck-like protein containing a caspase-activating recruitment domain; CNS: Central nervous system; ELISA: Enzyme-linked immunosorbent assay; H.E.: Hematoxylin and eosin; MWM: Morris water maze; NLRP1: Nucleotide oligomerization domain (NOD)-like receptor protein 1; TLE: Temporal lobe epilepsy

## Funding

This work was supported by grants from the National Natural Science Foundation of China (NSFC, No. 81671327 and 81201020) to W-NW and the National Natural Science Foundation of China (NSFC, No.81671384) to W-ZL.

## Authors' contributions

W-NW designed the study, analyzed the data, and wrote the manuscript. BG, YW, Y-JY, KD and D-KH performed the experiments and wrote the manuscript. W-ZL, JZ and Y-YY analyzed the data and wrote the manuscript. All authors read and approved the final manuscript.

## Competing interests
The authors declare that they have no competing interests.

## Author details
[1]Department of Pharmacology, School of Basic Medical Sciences, Key Laboratory of Anti-inflammatory and Immunopharmacology, Anhui Medical University, Hefei 230032, People's Republic of China. [2]Department of Psychiatry and Medical Experimental Center, Jiangxi Mental Hospital/ Affiliated Mental Hospital of Nanchang University, Nanchang 330029, People's Republic of China. [3]Department of Pharmacy, Xi'an Chest Hospital, Shaanxi University of Chinese Medicine, Xi'an 710061, People's Republic of China. [4]Synthetic Laboratory, School of Basic Medical Sciences, Anhui Medical University, Hefei 230032, People's Republic of China.

## References
1. Duncan JS, Sander JW, Sisodiya SM, Walker MC. Adult epilepsy. Lancet. 2006; 367:1087–100.
2. Fisher RS, van Emde BW, Blume W, Elger C, Genton P, Lee P, Engel J Jr. Epileptic seizures and epilepsy: definitions proposed by the international league against epilepsy (ILAE) and the International Bureau for Epilepsy (IBE). Epilepsia. 2005;46:470–2.
3. Vezzani A, French J, Bartfai T, Baram TZ. The role of inflammation in epilepsy. Nat Rev Neurol. 2011;7:31–40.
4. Mishra A, Goel RK. Comparative behavioral and neurochemical analysis of phenytoin and valproate treatment on epilepsy induced learning and memory deficit: search for add on therapy. Metab Brain Dis. 2015;30:951–8.
5. Rogawski MA, Loscher W. The neurobiology of antiepileptic drugs. Nat Rev Neurosci. 2004;5:553–64.
6. Pitkanen A, Sutula TP. Is epilepsy a progressive disorder? Prospects for new therapeutic approaches in temporal-lobe epilepsy. Lancet Neurol. 2002;1: 173–81.
7. Schmidt D. The clinical impact of new antiepileptic drugs after a decade of use in epilepsy. Epilepsy Res. 2002;50:21–32.
8. Luoni C, Bisulli F, Canevini MP, De Sarro G, Fattore C, Galimberti CA, Gatti G, La Neve A, Muscas G, Specchio LM, et al. Determinants of health-related quality of life in pharmacoresistant epilepsy: results from a large multicenter study of consecutively enrolled patients using validated quantitative assessments. Epilepsia. 2011;52:2181–91.
9. De Simoni MG, Perego C, Ravizza T, Moneta D, Conti M, Marchesi F, De Luigi A, Garattini S, Vezzani A. Inflammatory cytokines and related genes are

induced in the rat hippocampus by limbic status epilepticus. Eur J Neurosci. 2000;12:2623–33.

10. Minami M, Kuraishi Y, Satoh M. Effects of kainic acid on messenger RNA levels of IL-1 beta, IL-6, TNF alpha and LIF in the rat brain. Biochem Biophys Res Commun. 1991;176:593–8.

11. Sinha S, Patil SA, Jayalekshmy V, Satishchandra P. Do cytokines have any role in epilepsy? Epilepsy Res. 2008;82:171–6.

12. Yamamoto A, Schindler CK, Murphy BM, Bellver-Estelles C, So NK, Taki W, Meller R, Simon RP, Henshall DC. Evidence of tumor necrosis factor receptor 1 signaling in human temporal lobe epilepsy. Exp Neurol. 2006;202:410–20.

13. Vezzani A. Anti-inflammatory drugs in epilepsy: does it impact epileptogenesis? Expert Opin Drug Saf. 2015;14:583–92.

14. Singhal G, Jaehne EJ, Corrigan F, Toben C, Baune BT. Inflammasomes in neuroinflammation and changes in brain function: a focused review. Front Neurosci. 2014;8:315.

15. Schroder K, Tschopp J. The inflammasomes. Cell. 2010;140:821–32.

16. Strowig T, Henao-Mejia J, Elinav E, Flavell R. Inflammasomes in health and disease. Nature. 2012;481:278–86.

17. de Zoete MR, Flavell RA. Interactions between nod-like receptors and intestinal bacteria. Front Immunol. 2013;4:462.

18. Latz E, Xiao TS, Stutz A. Activation and regulation of the inflammasomes. Nat Rev Immunol. 2013;13:397–411.

19. Liu L, Chan C. The role of inflammasome in Alzheimer's disease. Ageing Res Rev. 2014;15:6–15.

20. Alomar SY, Gentili A, Zaibi MS, Kepczynska MA, Trayhurn P. IL-1beta (interleukin-1beta) stimulates the production and release of multiple cytokines and chemokines by human preadipocytes. Arch Physiol Biochem. 2016;122:117–22.

21. Martinon F, Burns K, Tschopp J. The inflammasome: a molecular platform triggering activation of inflammatory caspases and processing of proIL-beta. Mol Cell. 2002;10:417–26.

22. Minkiewicz J, de Rivero Vaccari JP, Keane RW. Human astrocytes express a novel NLRP2 inflammasome. Glia. 2013;61:1113–21.

23. Agostini L, Martinon F, Burns K, McDermott MF, Hawkins PN, Tschopp J. NALP3 forms an IL-1beta-processing inflammasome with increased activity in muckle-wells autoinflammatory disorder. Immunity. 2004;20:319–25.

24. Miao EA, Mao DP, Yudkovsky N, Bonneau R, Lorang CG, Warren SE, Leaf IA, Aderem A. Innate immune detection of the type III secretion apparatus through the NLRC4 inflammasome. Proc Natl Acad Sci U S A. 2010;107: 3076–80.

25. Fernandes-Alnemri T, Yu JW, Datta P, Wu J, Alnemri ES. AIM2 activates the inflammasome and cell death in response to cytoplasmic DNA. Nature. 2009;458:509–13.

26. Abulafia DP, de Rivero Vaccari JP, Lozano JD, Lotocki G, Keane RW, Dietrich WD. Inhibition of the inflammasome complex reduces the inflammatory response after thromboembolic stroke in mice. J Cereb Blood Flow Metab. 2009;29:534–44.

27. Tan CC, Zhang JG, Tan MS, Chen H, Meng DW, Jiang T, Meng XF, Li Y, Sun Z, Li MM, et al. NLRP1 inflammasome is activated in patients with medial temporal lobe epilepsy and contributes to neuronal pyroptosis in amygdala kindling-induced rat model. J Neuroinflammation. 2015;12:18.

28. Xu M, Liu L, Qi C, Deng B, Cai X. Sinomenine versus NSAIDs for the treatment of rheumatoid arthritis: a systematic review and meta-analysis. Planta Med. 2008;74:1423–9.

29. Yamasaki H. Pharmacology of sinomenine, an anti-rheumatic alkaloid from Sinomenium acutum. Acta Med Okayama. 1976;30:1–20.

30. Jiang S, Gao Y, Hou W, Liu R, Qi X, Xu X, Li J, Bao Y, Zheng H, Hua B. Sinomenine inhibits A549 human lung cancer cell invasion by mediating the STAT3 signaling pathway. Oncol Lett. 2016;12:1380–6.

31. Wu WN, Wu PF, Chen XL, Zhang Z, Gu J, Yang YJ, Xiong QJ, Ni L, Wang F, Chen JG. Sinomenine protects against ischaemic brain injury: involvement of co-inhibition of acid-sensing ion channel 1a and L-type calcium channels. Br J Pharmacol. 2011;164:1445–59.

32. Qiu J, Wang M, Zhang J, Cai Q, Lu D, Li Y, Dong Y, Zhao T, Chen H. The neuroprotection of Sinomenine against ischemic stroke in mice by suppressing NLRP3 inflammasome via AMPK signaling. Int Immunopharmacol. 2016;40:492–500.

33. Yang Z, Liu Y, Yuan F, Li Z, Huang S, Shen H, Yuan B. Sinomenine inhibits microglia activation and attenuates brain injury in intracerebral hemorrhage. Mol Immunol. 2014;60:109–14.

34. Shukla SM, Sharma SK. Sinomenine inhibits microglial activation by Abeta and confers neuroprotection. J Neuroinflammation. 2011;8:117.

35. Kaur H, Patro I, Tikoo K, Sandhir R. Curcumin attenuates inflammatory response and cognitive deficits in experimental model of chronic epilepsy. Neurochem Int. 2015;89:40–50.

36. Zhu X, Shen K, Bai Y, Zhang A, Xia Z, Chao J, Yao H. NADPH oxidase activation is required for pentylenetetrazole kindling-induced hippocampal autophagy. Free Radic Biol Med. 2016;94:230–42.

37. Schroder H, Becker A, Lossner B. Glutamate binding to brain membranes is increased in pentylenetetrazole-kindled rats. J Neurochem. 1993;60:1007–11.

38. Hou Y, Aboukhatwa MA, Lei DL, Manaye K, Khan I, Luo Y. Anti-depressant natural flavonols modulate BDNF and beta amyloid in neurons and hippocampus of double TgAD mice. Neuropharmacology. 2010;58:911–20.

39. Scharfman HE. The neurobiology of epilepsy. Curr Neurol Neurosci Rep. 2007;7:348–54.

40. Yu W, Smith AB, Pilitsis JG, Shin DS. Isovaline attenuates generalized epileptiform activity in hippocampal and primary sensory cortices and seizure behavior in pilocarpine treated rats. Neurosci Lett. 2015;599:125–8.

41. Loscher W, Klitgaard H, Twyman RE, Schmidt D. New avenues for anti-epileptic drug discovery and development. Nat Rev Drug Discov. 2013;12: 757–76.

42. Vezzani A, Aronica E, Mazarati A, Pittman QJ. Epilepsy and brain inflammation. Exp Neurol. 2013;244:11–21.

43. Vezzani A, Friedman A. Brain inflammation as a biomarker in epilepsy. Biomark Med. 2011;5:607–14.

44. Vezzani A, Friedman A, Dingledine RJ. The role of inflammation in epileptogenesis. Neuropharmacology. 2013;69:16–24.

45. Vieira V, Glassmann D, Marafon P, Pereira P, Gomez R, Coitinho AS. Effect of diclofenac sodium on seizures and inflammatory profile induced by kindling seizure model. Epilepsy Res. 2016;127:107–13.

46. Hong Y, Yang J, Shen X, Zhu H, Sun X, Wen X, Bian J, Hu H, Yuan L, Tao J, et al. Sinomenine hydrochloride enhancement of the inhibitory effects of anti-transferrin receptor antibody-dependent on the COX-2 pathway in human hepatoma cells. Cancer Immunol Immunother. 2013;62:447–54.

47. Esmaeilpour K, Sheibani V, Shabani M, Mirnajafi-Zadeh J. Effect of low frequency electrical stimulation on seizure-induced short- and long-term impairments in learning and memory in rats. Physiol Behav. 2017;168:112–21.

48. Sayin U, Sutula TP, Stafstrom CE. Seizures in the developing brain cause adverse long-term effects on spatial learning and anxiety. Epilepsia. 2004;45: 1539–48.

49. Liu X, Wu Y, Huang Q, Zou D, Qin W, Chen Z. Grouping pentylenetetrazol-induced epileptic rats according to memory impairment and MicroRNA expression profiles in the hippocampus. PLoS One. 2015;10:e0126123.

50. Eddy CM, Rickards HE, Cavanna AE. The cognitive impact of antiepileptic drugs. Ther Adv Neurol Disord. 2011;4:385–407.

51. Bohbot VD, Corkin S. Posterior parahippocampal place learning in H.M. Hippocampus. 2007;17:863–72.

52. Broadbent NJ, Squire LR, Clark RE. Spatial memory, recognition memory, and the hippocampus. Proc Natl Acad Sci U S A. 2004;101:14515–20.

53. Hassanzadeh P, Arbabi E, Rostami F. The ameliorative effects of sesamol against seizures, cognitive impairment and oxidative stress in the experimental model of epilepsy. Iran J Basic Med Sci. 2014;17:100–7.

54. Vezzani A, Granata T. Brain inflammation in epilepsy: experimental and clinical evidence. Epilepsia. 2005;46:1724–43.

55. Mariathasan S, Newton K, Monack DM, Vucic D, French DM, Lee WP, Roose-Girma M, Erickson S, Dixit VM. Differential activation of the inflammasome by caspase-1 adaptors ASC and Ipaf. Nature. 2004;430:213–8.

56. Wang YC, Li WZ, Wu Y, Yin YY, Dong LY, Chen ZW, Wu WN. Acid-sensing ion channel 1a contributes to the effect of extracellular acidosis on NLRP1 inflammasome activation in cortical neurons. J Neuroinflammation. 2015;12:246.

# 10

# Deep brain stimulation induces antiapoptotic and anti-inflammatory effects in epileptic rats

Beatriz O. Amorim[1], Luciene Covolan[1*], Elenn Ferreira[1], José Geraldo Brito[1], Diego P. Nunes[1], David G. de Morais[1], José N. Nobrega[2], Antonio M. Rodrigues[3], Antonio Carlos G. deAlmeida[3] and Clement Hamani[2,4]

## Abstract

**Background:** Status epilepticus (SE) is a severe condition that may lead to hippocampal cell loss and epileptogenesis. Some of the mechanisms associated with SE-induced cell death are excitotoxicity, neuroinflammation, and apoptosis.

**Objective:** The objective of the present study is to test the hypothesis that DBS has anti-inflammatory and antiapoptotic effects when applied during SE.

**Methods:** Rats undergoing pilocarpine-induced SE were treated with anterior thalamic nucleus (AN) deep brain stimulation (DBS). Inflammatory changes and caspase 3 activity were measured within 1 week of treatment.

**Results:** In pilocarpine-treated rats, DBS countered the significant increase in hippocampal caspase 3 activity and interleukin-6 (IL-6) levels that follows SE but had no effect on tumor necrosis factor α (TNFα).

**Conclusions:** DBS has anti-inflammatory and antiapoptotic effects when given to animals undergoing status.

**Keywords:** Anterior thalamic nucleus, Thalamus, Seizures, Deep brain stimulation, Epilepsy, Apoptosis, Neuroprotection, Caspase

Status epilepticus (SE) is a condition associated with continuous seizure activity that often leads to excitotoxicity and cell death [1]. Deep brain stimulation (DBS) of the anterior thalamic nucleus (AN), an approved treatment for medically refractory partial epilepsy [2], has been shown to reduce seizure rate and increase the latency for the development of SE in different rodent models [3–6]. To date, whether stimulation is protective against SE-induced excitotoxicity is largely unknown.

In Parkinson's disease, subthalamic nucleus DBS has been proposed to induce neuroprotective effects by reducing the glutamatergic drive to the substantia nigra [7]. In a parallel scenario, AN stimulation inhibits the spontaneous activity of local neuronal populations and reduces the firing rate of dentate gyrus cells [8]. Following this line of reasoning, we hypothesize that a decreased drive to the hippocampus following AN DBS could have neuroprotective effects.

In preclinical models [9] and in the clinic [10, 11], neuromodulation treatments that induce antiepileptic effects, such as vagus nerve stimulation (VNS), have been shown to reduce plasmatic levels of cytokines.

In the present study, we test the hypothesis that AN DBS reduces hippocampal apoptosis and neuroinflammation in rats undergoing pilocarpine (Pilo)-induced SE.

## Methods

### Ethics, consent, and permissions

Experiments were approved by the Animal Care committee of the Universidade Federal de São Paulo (1482/11).

### Pilocarpine administration and AN stimulation

Male Wistar rats (~250 g) were anesthetized with ketamine/xylazine (100/7.5 mg/kg i.p.) and had insulated stainless steel electrodes (cathodes; 250-μm diameter; 0.5-mm exposed surface) bilaterally implanted into the AN (anteroposterior −1.5, lateral ± 1.5, depth 5.2) [12]. A

* Correspondence: lucovolan@gmail.com
[1]Disciplina de Neurofisiologia, Universidade Federal de São Paulo, Rua Botucatu, 862 5 andar, 04023-062 São Paulo, Brazil
Full list of author information is available at the end of the article

screw implanted over the right somatosensory cortex was used as the anode. Control animals had holes drilled into the skull but were not implanted with electrodes. Animals undergoing electroencephalography (EEG) recordings were implanted with bipolar cortical electrodes (Plastics One; 3 mm posterior, 4 mm lateral, and 2 mm ventral to the bregma) [12]. One week later, animals received N-methyl-scopolamine (1 mg/kg s.c. Sigma, St Louis, MO) followed, 30 min later, by pilocarpine (320 mg/kg, i.p., Vegeflora, Brazil). SE was characterized by the presence of uninterrupted behavioral seizures [24]. As pilocarpine-induced seizures often last a few seconds, DBS was commenced 1 minute after SE onset. Stimulation settings were in the range of those used in our previous studies: 130 Hz, 90 μs, and 400 μA (St Jude MTS, Plano, TX) [3].

Ninety minutes after SE, the animals received thionembutal (30 mg/kg) to attenuate behavioral status and reduce mortality rate. As animals began to recover 6 h later, DBS was delivered continuously during the first 6 h of status.

EEG was recorded with a BNT-36 system (Lynx, Brazil) using the ENSA software (ENSA, Brazil) for 24 h from the moment Pilo was injected. Signals were amplified, band pass filtered (0.1–30 Hz), and digitized (200 samples/s). Complex Gaussian's wavelet transform analysis was used to investigate the signals in the frequency domain. Placement of DBS electrodes was confirmed in cresyl-violet-stained sections and was similar to that described in our previous reports [13].

## Caspase 3 and cytokine measurements

After removal from the skull, the brains were split in half, and the hippocampus of each hemisphere was dissected. The left hippocampus was used for the study of caspase activity. The right hippocampus was used to measure cytokines.

The hippocampus of each animal was incubated with a homogenization buffer and mechanically homogenized, as previously described [14]. Samples were centrifuged for 40 min, and the total protein content in the supernatant determined using the Bio-Rad Protein Assay, according to the manufacturer's specification (Bio-Rad Labs, Germany). Measurement of caspase 3 activity was obtained using the caspase 3 fluorimetric assay kit (CASP3F, Sigma, USA). Triplicates of each sample (all containing 100 mg of protein) were analyzed. All received the substrate but only one the inhibitor. Activity was measured continuously over 5 h on a FlexStation 3 Spectrofluorimeter (Molecular Probes, USA), using λex = 360 nm and λem = 465 nm. Values obtained from samples containing the inhibitor were subtracted from those recorded from the other samples, and the arithmetic average was calculated. After calibration for AMC, results were expressed as nMol AMC.

For cytokine detection, the right hippocampus was homogenized in 0.01 M Tris hydrochloride (pH 7.6) containing 5.8 % sodium chloride, 10 % glycerol, 1 % Nonidet P40 (NP-40), 0.4 % of ethylenediamine tetraacetic acid (EDTA), and protease inhibitors. Samples were sonicated and stored at –80 °C. Subsequently, samples were centrifuged for 5 min. at $10,000 \times g$ at 4 °C, and concentrations determined with a Millipore multiplex Rat Cytokine Kit (RECYTMAG-65K-03) on the Luminex® xMAP® platform (xPonent/Analyst Software version 4.2). Longitudinal controls were used to assess inter-assay variability. Results are expressed in pg/mg.

## Statistical analysis

Two-way ANOVA (DBS and Pilo as main factors; Tukey post hoc) was used to compare neurochemical data. Electrophysiological results were analyzed with Wilcoxon signed-rank test. Values in the text represent mean ± SEM.

## Results
### Apoptosis and neuroinflammatory changes

Hippocampal caspase 3 activity was studied 7 days following SE, a time frame during which apoptosis reaches maximal levels [15, 16]. At this time point, we found significant Pilo ($F_{(1,16)} = 17.17$; $P = 0.0008$) and DBS effects ($F_{(1,16)} = 10.34$; $P = 0.005$). As can be seen in Fig. 1, caspase 3 activity was increased in pilocarpine-treated rats ($n = 5$) as compared to saline-injected controls ($n = 5$; $P = 0.009$). The administration of DBS significantly reduced such activity ($n = 5$), bringing it to a level that was similar to that of non-epileptic controls ($n = 5$; $P = 0.02$ vs Pilo). In contrast, no significant Pilo ($F_{(1,16)} = 0.01$; $P = 0.95$) or DBS effects ($F_{(1,16)} = 1.97$; $P = 0.18$) were recorded when caspase 3 activity was measured 24 h following status epilepticus (Additional file 1: Figure S1; $n = 5$ animals/group).

Markers of inflammatory activity were studied 1 day following status, when post-SE changes are at high levels [17, 18]. Hippocampal pro-inflammatory IL-6 was influenced by both Pilo ($F_{(1,14)} = 9.85$; $P = 0.007$) and DBS ($F_{(1,14)} = 9.23$; $P = 0.008$) with interaction between both factors ($F_{(1,14)} = 4.53$; $P = 0.05$). Overall, levels of this interleukin were slightly reduced in AN DBS control animals, a response that was further evidenced after status ($P = 0.002$ vs Pilo) (Fig. 1). Although TNFα levels were in the lower limit of the detection of the fluorimetric assay, these were found to be influenced by Pilo ($F_{(1,14)} = 22.60$; $P = 0.0003$) but not DBS.

To investigate whether the protective effects of DBS were due to a decrease in SE severity, EEG recordings were obtained before and during status ($n = 5$ per group). Though tracings looked similar between groups, spectral analysis revealed that animals receiving DBS had a significant decrease in alpha and beta band peaks (Additional

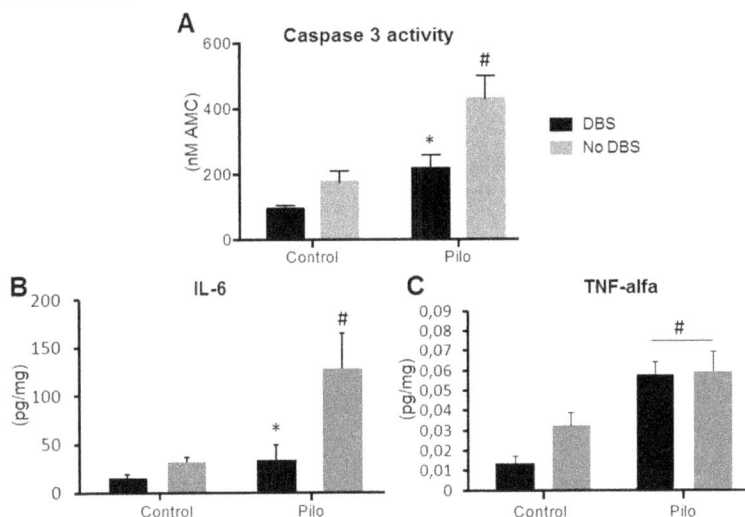

**Fig. 1** DBS, apoptosis, and neuroinflammation. (**a**) Hippocampal caspase 3 activity was increased in pilocarpine-treated rats undergoing SE ($P = 0.009$; vs saline controls), an effect that was significantly reversed in the DBS-treated Pilo group ($P = 0.02$; vs Pilo). Similarly (**b**), hippocampal levels of the pro-inflammatory IL-6 were significantly increased after SE ($P = 0.006$; vs saline-injected controls), an effect that was countered by the administration of AN DBS ($P = 0.02$; vs Pilo). In contrast, SE-induced increases in TNFα ($P = 0.0003$ vs saline-injected controls) were not influenced by DBS (**c**). # indicates differences from *control*, *indicates differences from *Pilo*

file 2: Figure S2). This suggests that DBS may potentially decrease SE severity.

## Discussion

It is well established that seizures and SE can activate intrinsic and extrinsic apoptotic pathways leading to neuronal death. As a common final step, caspase 3 activation invariably leads to an irreversible apoptotic process. In rodents, caspase 3 is active 24–72 h following status but maximally expressed 7 days later [19]. Our results suggest that animals given DBS during status had a significant decrease in hippocampal caspase 3 activity, as measured by a commercial protein assay. While this method was reliable and showed low variability across animals, it did not allow us to determine in which hippocampal subregions apoptosis was occurring. In a preliminary immunohistochemistry experiment (unpublished data), we found that animals undergoing SE with or without DBS had caspase-3-expressing cells in the dentate gyrus, CA1, and CA3 subfields. This technique, however, has only shown sparsely stained cells and a great variability across rats. Whether the effects of DBS are related to a decrease in apoptotic processes or a lower number of hippocampal cells undergoing cell death remains to be elucidated.

Another technical aspect that needs to be discussed is the choice of a control group without electrodes implanted. This was based on our previous studies showing that electrode insertion did not influence the latency for developing SE or the frequency of seizures in pilocarpine-treated rats [3, 20]. Placement of electrodes in the brain often causes a mild local inflammatory response that tends to subside over time. Though it is possible that this might have occurred in the AN, samples in our study were collected at a distance from the target (i.e., in the hippocampus and not in the AN). In addition, an inflammatory response should have theoretically increased pro-inflammatory cytokines. In our study, DBS-treated animals had the opposite effect.

Most cells in the AN are immunocytochemically positive for glutamate and aspartate [21]. Connections between the AN and hippocampus are both direct (e.g., via subiculum and CA1) and indirect (i.e., via anterior cingulum and entorhinal cortex) [22, 23]. In our previous work, AN DBS was shown to induce a strong depolarization block of local neuronal populations and reduce the firing in hippocampal dentate gyrus cells [24]. Bearing this in mind, it is possible that reduced activity within the AN complex and DG following DBS might have decreased glutamate-induced excitotoxicity, reducing hippocampal caspase activity and inflammatory responses. This, however, still needs to be demonstrated.

Another possibility to explain potential neurochemical differences between animals that did or did not receive DBS is that stimulation might have influenced SE severity. Though EEG tracings looked similar between groups, a more detailed spectral analysis revealed that the rats given DBS had a decrease in alpha and beta power. This may represent a milder form of status epilepticus, as the withdrawal of anticonvulsant medications may enhance beta rhythms during continuous seizures [25].

One limitation of the current study is that we cannot infer a direct association between reduced excitotoxicity, anti-inflammatory, and antiapoptotic effects of DBS. Similarly, we are unable to explain why DBS has only influenced certain pro-inflammatory cytokines (i.e., IL-6 but not TNFα).

## Conclusion

As excitotoxicity and inflammatory responses are early occurring events following SE, we postulate that the reduced levels of apoptosis observed after DBS may be due, at least in part, to its anti-inflammatory effects. That said, our results do not allow one to establish a causal relationship between a DBS-induced reduction in cytokines and apoptosis, an aspect that needs to be investigated in the future.

## Additional files

**Additional file 1: Figure S1.** Apoptosis 24 h after pilocarpine-induced status epilepticus. No significant differences were found in hippocampal caspase 3 activity when animals who developed pilocarpine-induced SE with or without DBS were compared to controls.

**Additional file 2: Figure S2.** EEG activity recorded before and during SE in animals that did and did not receive DBS. (A) Traces of a non-stimulated animal before (left) and during (right) SE. Spectral arrays after wavelet transform of corresponding EEG traces show activity in the α and β bands during SE. (B) Traces of a DBS-treated animal before (left) and during (right) SE. Spectral arrays after wavelet transform of the corresponding EEG traces show that activity during SE in the α and β bands are reduced during AN DBS. (C) Box plot showing the mean power spectrum of different frequency bands pre-SE in animals that did not (yellow bars) or did receive AN DBS (blue bars). As stimulation was not turned on at that point, Wilcoxon signed-rank test showed no significant difference between groups ($P > 0.05$, $n = 5$). (D) Box plot showing the mean power spectrum of different frequency bands during SE without (yellow bars) and with AN DBS (blue bars). Wilcoxon signed-rank test showed significant differences between groups in the α and β bands ($P < 0.05$, $n = 5$ animals/group).

## Competing interests

CH is a consultant for St Jude Medical. The other authors have no competing interests.

## Authors' contributions

Surgical procedures to implant electrodes, status induction, caspase 3, and cytokine assays were carried out by BOA, EF, DPN, and DGM. BOA drafted the manuscript. AMR, JGB, and ACGA carried out the quantitative analysis of the EEG. JNN participated in the design of the study and performed the statistical analysis. CH and LC conceived of the study and participated in its design and coordination and helped to draft the manuscript. All authors read and approved the final manuscript.

## Acknowledgements

The authors acknowledge FAPESP (2011/50680-2; 2012/50950-2; 2012/10764-5) for funding this study.

## Author details

¹Disciplina de Neurofisiologia, Universidade Federal de São Paulo, Rua Botucatu, 862 5 andar, 04023-062 São Paulo, Brazil. ²Behavioural Neurobiology Laboratory, Centre for Addiction and Mental Health, Toronto, Canada. ³Departamento de Engenharia de Biossistemas, Universidade Federal de São João del-Rei, São João del-Rei, MG 36301-160, Brazil. ⁴Division of Neurosurgery, Toronto Western Hospital, University of Toronto, Toronto, Canada.

## References

1. Covolan L, Mello LE. Assessment of the progressive nature of cell damage in the pilocarpine model of epilepsy. Braz J Med Biol Res. 2006;39:915–24.
2. Fisher R, Salanova V, Witt T, Worth R, Henry T, Gross R, et al. Electrical stimulation of the anterior nucleus of thalamus for treatment of refractory epilepsy. Epilepsia. 2010;51:899–908.
3. Covolan L, de Almeida AC, Amorim B, Cavarsan C, Miranda MF, Aarao MC, et al. Effects of anterior thalamic nucleus deep brain stimulation in chronic epileptic rats. PLoS One. 2014;9:e97618.
4. Mirski MA, Rossell LA, Terry JB, Fisher RS. Anticonvulsant effect of anterior thalamic high frequency electrical stimulation in the rat. Epilepsy Res. 1997;28:89–100.
5. Takebayashi S, Hashizume K, Tanaka T, Hodozuka A. Anti-convulsant effect of electrical stimulation and lesioning of the anterior thalamic nucleus on kainic acid-induced focal limbic seizure in rats. Epilepsy Res. 2007;74:163–70.
6. Hamani C, Ewerton F, Bonilha S, Ballester G, Mello L, Lozano A. Bilateral anterior thalamic nucleus lesions and high-frequency stimulation are protective against pilocarpine-induced seizures and status epilepticus. Neurosurgery. 2004;54:191–5.
7. Rodriguez M, Obeso J, Olanow C. Subthalamic nucleus-mediated excitotoxicity in Parkinson's disease: a target for neuroprotection. Ann Neurol. 1998;44:S175–88.
8. Hamani C, Dubiela F, Soares J, Shin D, Bittencourt S, Covolan L, et al. Anterior thalamus deep brain stimulation at high current impairs memory in rats. Exp Neurol. 2010;225:154–62.
9. Borovikova LV, Ivanova S, Zhang M, Yang H, Botchkina GI, Watkins LR, et al. Vagus nerve stimulation attenuates the systemic inflammatory response to endotoxin. Nature. 2000;405:458–62.
10. Aalbers MW, Klinkenberg S, Rijkers K, Verschuure P, Kessels A, Aldenkamp A, et al. The effects of vagus nerve stimulation on pro- and anti-inflammatory cytokines in children with refractory epilepsy: an exploratory study. Neuroimmunomodulation. 2012;19:352–8.
11. Majoie HJ, Rijkers K, Berfelo MW, Hulsman JA, Myint A, Schwarz M, et al. Vagus nerve stimulation in refractory epilepsy: effects on pro- and anti-inflammatory cytokines in peripheral blood. Neuroimmunomodulation. 2011;18:52–6.
12. Paxinos G, Watson C. The rat brain stereotaxic coordinates. 2nd ed. London: Academic; 2005.
13. Bittencourt S, Dubiela F, Queiroz C, Covolan L, Andrade D, Lozano A, et al. Microinjection of GABAergic agents into the anterior nucleus of the thalamus modulates pilocarpine-induced seizures and status epilepticus. Seizure. 2010;19:242–6.
14. Malheiros J, Persike D, Castro L, Sanches T, Andrade L, Tannús A, et al. Reduced hippocampal manganese-enhanced MRI (MEMRI) signal during pilocarpine-induced status epilepticus: edema or apoptosis? Epilepsy Res. 2014;108:644–52.
15. Weise J, Engelhorn T, Dorfler A, Aker S, Bahr M, Hufnagel A. Expression time course and spatial distribution of activated caspase-3 after experimental status epilepticus: contribution of delayed neuronal cell death to seizure-induced neuronal injury. Neurobiol Dis. 2005;18:582–90.
16. Narkilahti S, Pirttila TJ, Lukasiuk K, Tuunanen J, Pitkanen A. Expression and activation of caspase 3 following status epilepticus in the rat. Eur J Neurosci. 2003;18:1486–96.
17. Gouveia TL, Scorza FA, Silva MJ, Bandeira Tde A, Perosa SR, Arganaraz GA, et al. Lovastatin decreases the synthesis of inflammatory mediators in the hippocampus and blocks the hyperthermia of rats submitted to long-lasting status epilepticus. Epilepsy Behav. 2011;20:1–5.
18. De Simoni MG, Perego C, Ravizza T, Moneta D, Conti M, Marchesi F, et al. Inflammatory cytokines and related genes are induced in the rat hippocampus by limbic status epilepticus. Eur J Neurosci. 2000;12:2623–33.
19. Lopez-Meraz M-L, Niquet J, Wasterlain C. Distinct caspase pathways mediate necrosis and apoptosis in subpopulations of hippocampal neurons after status epilepticus. Epilepsia. 2010;51:50–60.
20. Hamani C, Hodaie M, Chiang J, del Campo M, Andrade DM, Sherman D, et al. Deep brain stimulation of the anterior nucleus of the thalamus: effects of electrical stimulation on pilocarpine-induced seizures and status epilepticus. Epilepsy Res. 2008;78:117–23.
21. Gonzalo-Ruiz A, Sanz JM, Lieberman AR. Immunohistochemical studies of localization and co-localization of glutamate, aspartate and GABA in the anterior thalamic nuclei, retrosplenial granular cortex, thalamic reticular nucleus and mammillary nuclei of the rat. J Chem Neuroanat. 1996;12:77–84.

22. Shibata H. Topographic organization of subcortical projections to the anterior thalamic nuclei in the rat. J Comp Neurol. 1992;323:117–27.
23. Shibata H. Direct projections from the anterior thalamic nuclei to the retrohippocampal region in the rat. J Comp Neurol. 1993;337:431–45.
24. Malheiros JM, Polli RS, Paiva FF, Longo BM, Mello LE, Silva AC, et al. Manganese-enhanced magnetic resonance imaging detects mossy fiber sprouting in the pilocarpine model of epilepsy. Epilepsia. 2012;53(7):1225–32.
25. Bonati LH, Naegelin Y, Wieser HG, Fuhr P, Ruegg S. Beta activity in status epilepticus. Epilepsia. 2006;47:207–10.

# 11

# P2X7 receptor activation ameliorates CA3 neuronal damage via a tumor necrosis factor-α-mediated pathway in the rat hippocampus following status epilepticus

Ji-Eun Kim[1,2], Hea Jin Ryu[1] and Tae-Cheon Kang[1*]

## Abstract

**Background:** The release of tumor necrosis factor-α (TNF-α) appears depend on the P2X7 receptor, a purinergic receptor. In the present study, we addressed the question of whether P2X7 receptor-mediated TNF-α regulation is involved in pathogenesis and outcome of status epilepticus (SE).

**Methods:** SE was induced by pilocarpine in rats that were intracerebroventricularly infused with saline-, 2′,3′-O-(4-benzoylbenzoyl)-adenosine 5′-triphosphate (BzATP), adenosine 5′-triphosphate-2′,3′-dialdehyde (OxATP), A-438079, or A-740003 prior to SE induction. Thereafter, we performed Fluoro-Jade B staining and immunohistochemical studies for TNF-α and NF-κB subunit phosphorylations.

**Results:** Following SE, P2X7 receptor agonist (BzATP) infusion increased TNF-α immunoreactivity in dentate granule cells as compared with that in saline-infused animals. In addition, TNF-α immunoreactivity was readily apparent in the mossy fibers, while TNF-α immunoreactivity in CA1-3 pyramidal cells was unaltered. However, P2X7 receptor antagonist (OxATP-, A-438079, and A-740003) infusion reduced SE-induced TNF-α expression in dentate granule cells. In the CA3 region, BzATP infusion attenuated SE-induced neuronal damage, accompanied by enhancement of p65-Ser276 and p65-Ser311 NF-κB subunit phosphorylations. In contrast, OxATP-, A-438079, and A-740003 infusions increased SE-induced neuronal death. Soluble TNF p55 receptor (sTNFp55R), and cotreatment with BzATP and sTNFp55R infusion also increased SE-induced neuronal damage in CA3 region. However, OxATP-, sTNFp55R or BzATP+sTNFp55R infusions could not exacerbate SE-induced neuronal damages in the dentate gyrus and the CA1 region, as compared to BzATP infusion.

**Conclusions:** These findings suggest that TNF-α induction by P2X7 receptor activation may ameliorate SE-induced CA3 neuronal damage via enhancing NF-κB p65-Ser276 and p65-Ser311 phosphorylations.

## Background

Status epilepticus (SE) is a medical emergency with significant mortality [1]. SE has been defined as continuous seizure activity, which causes neuronal cell death [2,3], epileptogenesis [3] and learning impairment [4]. Cytokines are critical mediators of specific inflammatory responses and immune reactions in the brain [5]. Tumor necrosis factor-α (TNF-α) is a 17-kDa protein that is mainly produced by activated macrophages and T cells of the immune system. TNF-α is expressed at low levels in the normal brain and is rapidly upregulated in glia, neurons and endothelial cells in various pathophysiological conditions [6]. TNF-α shows various effects on brain function depending on its local tissue concentration, the type of target cells, and especially the specific receptor subtype: TNF receptor I, or p55 receptor (TNFp55R); and TNF receptor II, or p75 receptor (TNFp75R) [7,8]. Basically, TNF-related signal transduction pathways involve NF-κB binding activity for TNFp55R contributing to cell death [9] and downstream

* Correspondence: tckang@hallym.ac.kr
[1]Department of Anatomy & Neurobiology, Institute of Epilepsy Research, College of Medicine, Hallym University, Chunchon, Kangwon-Do 200-702, South Korea
Full list of author information is available at the end of the article

signaling via TNFp75R involves activation of p38 mitogen-activated protein kinase to promote neuronal survival [10]. However, TNFp55R deficiency enhances KA-induced excitotoxic hippocampal injury in mice [11]. Furthermore, Marchetti et al. [12] has reported that TNFp75R-induced persistent NF-κB activity is essential for neuronal survival against excitotoxic stress. Therefore, TNF-α clearly possesses the ability to simultaneously activate both cell death and cell survival pathways, and this balance ultimately determines whether TNF-α promotes neurodegeneration or neuroprotection.

On the other hand, P2X7 receptor, a purinergic receptor, plays a role in intercellular signaling involving ATP and glutamate release. Furthermore, the release of TNF-α appears to be dependent on the P2X7 receptor. Indeed, treatment of microglia in neuron-microglia co-cultures with the P2X7 agonist 2'-3'-O-(benzoyl-benzoyl) ATP (BzATP) leads to significant reductions in glutamate-induced neuronal cell death, and either TNF-α converting enzyme inhibitor or anti-TNF-α IgG readily suppresses this protective effect [13]. In contrast, Choi et al. [14] have reported that the P2X7 receptor antagonist, oxidized ATP (OxATP), is effective in attenuating LPS-induced neuronal damage. These findings encouraged us to speculate that P2X7 receptor-mediated TNF-α regulation is involved in outcomes of SE. In the present study, therefore, we address the question of whether the effects of P2X7 receptor on the TNF-α system represent general features of SE-induced neuronal death in the hippocampus following SE.

## Methods
### Experimental animals and chemicals
This study utilized the progeny of Sprague-Dawley (SD) rats (male, 9-11 weeks old) obtained from Experimental Animal Center, Hallym University, Chunchon, South Korea. The animals were provided with a commercial diet and water *ad libitum* under controlled temperature, humidity and lighting conditions (22 ± 2°C 55 ± 5% and a 12:12 light/dark cycle with lights). Procedures involving animals and their care were conducted in accord with our institutional guidelines that comply with NIH Guide for the Care and Use of Laboratory Animals (NIH Publications No. 80-23, 1996). In addition, we have made all efforts to minimize the number of animals used and their suffering. All reagents were obtained from Sigma-Aldrich (St. Louis, MO), except as noted.

### Intracerebroventricular drug infusion
Rats were divided into eight groups, treated with either (1) saline, (2) vehicle (0.1% DMSO/saline, v/v), (3) BzATP (5 mM in saline), (4) OxATP (5 mM in saline), (5) A-438079 (10 μM in saline; Tocris Bioscience, Ellis-ville, MO), (6) A-740003 (10 μM in 0.001% DMSO/saline, v/v; Tocris

Bioscience, Ellis-ville, MO), (7) soluble TNFp55R (sTNFp55R 50 μg/ml), or (8) BzATP (5 mM) + sTNFp55R (50 μg/ml). The dosage of each compound was determined as the highest dose that did not affect seizure threshold in a preliminary study. Animals were anesthetized (Zolretil, 50 mg/kg, i.m.; Virbac Laboratories) and placed in a stereotaxic frame. For osmotic pump implantation, holes were drilled through the skull to introduce a brain infusion kit 1 (Alzet, Cupertino, CA) into the right lateral ventricle (1 mm posterior; 1.5 mm lateral;−3.5 mm depth; flat skull position with bregma as reference), according to the atlas of Paxinos and Watson [15]. The infusion kit was sealed with dental cement and connected to an osmotic pump (1002, Alzet, Cupertino, CA). The pump was placed in a subcutaneous pocket in the dorsal region. Animals received 0.5 μl/hr of vehicle or compound for 2 weeks [16-18].

### Seizure induction
Three days after the start of vehicle or compound infusion, rats were treated with pilocarpine (380 mg/kg, i.p.) 20 min after methylscopolamine (5 mg/kg, i.p.). Approximately 80% of pilocarpine-treated rats showed acute behavioral features of status epilepticus (SE), including akinesia, facial automatisms, limbic seizures consisting of forelimb clonus with rearing, salivation, masticatory jaw movements, and falling. Diazepam (Valium, 10 mg/kg, i.p.; Hoffman Ia Roche, Neuilly sur-Seine) was administered 2 hours after onset of SE and repeated, as needed. The rats were then observed 3-4 hours a day in a vivarium for general behavior and occurrence of spontaneous seizures. Non-experienced SE rats (which showed only acute seizure behaviors during 10-30 min, n = 21) and age-matched normal rat were used as controls (n = 8).

### Pilocarpine-induced seizure threshold
Three days after the start of vehicle or compound infusion, some animals (n = 3) in each group were anesthetized (urethane, 1.5 g/kg, i.p.) and placed in a stereotaxic frame. Holes were drilled through the skull to introduce electrodes. The coordinates (in mm) were as follows. For the recording electrode (to the dentate gyrus):-3.8 anterior-posterior, 2.5 lateral to bregma, 2.9 depth, at a right angle to the skull surface. For the stimulating electrode (to the angular bundle): 4.2 lateral to lambda, 3.0 depth. Stainless steel electrodes (Plastics One Inc) were used for recording. Reference electrodes were placed in the posterior cranium over the cerebellum. Signals were recorded with DAM 80 differential amplifier (0.1-3000 Hz bandpass, World Precision Instruments) and data were digitized (20 kHz) and analyzed on MacChart 5 (AD Instruments). After establishing a stable baseline for at least 30 min after surgery,

pilocarpine (380 mg/kg, i.p.) was given 20 min after methylscopolamine (5 mg/kg, i.p.), and latency was observed. Latency was determined as seconds from the pilocarpine injection time point to the time point showing the first seizure activity [19]. To analyze changes in EEG power value, root mean square (RMS) values were also measured.

### Tissue processing

At designated time points (Non-SE, 1 day, 2 days, 3 days and 1 week after SE, n = 5, respectively), animals were perfused transcardially with phosphate-buffered saline (PBS) followed by 4% paraformaldehyde in 0.1 M phosphate buffer (PB, pH 7.4) under urethane anesthesia (1.5 g/kg, i.p.). The brains were removed, and postfixed in the same fixative for 4 hr. The brain tissues were cryoprotected by infiltration with 30% sucrose overnight. Thereafter, the entire hippocampus was frozen and sectioned with a cryostat at 30 μm and consecutive sections were placed in six-well plates containing PBS. For stereological study, every sixth section in the series throughout the entire hippocampus was used in some animals [20].

### Immunohistochemistry

Sections were first incubated with 3% bovine serum albumin in PBS for 30 min at room temperature. Sections were then incubated in primary antibody (Table 1) in PBS containing 0.3% Triton X-100 overnight at room temperature. The sections were washed three times for 10 min with PBS, incubated sequentially, in biotinylated horse anti-mouse IgG (Vector, Burlingame, CA) and ABC complex (Vector, Burlingame, CA), diluted 1:200 in the same solution as the primary antiserum. Between incubations, the tissues were washed with PBS three

### Table 1 Primary Antibodies used

| Antigen | Host | Manufacturer | Dilution used* |
|---|---|---|---|
| Calbindin D-28 K | rabbit | Cell signaling | 1:200 (IF) |
| Glial fibrillary acidic protein | mouse | Millipore | 1:5,000 (IF) |
| NeuN (a neuronal maker) | mouse | Millipore | 1:1000 (IF) |
| NF-κB p52-Ser865 | rabbit | Abcam | 1:200 (IH) |
| NF-κB p52-Ser869 | rabbit | Abcam | 1:200 (IH) |
| NF-κB p65-Ser276 | rabbit | Abcam | 1:200 (IH) |
| NF-κB p65-Ser311 | rabbit | Abcam | 1:200 (IH) |
| NF-κB p65-Ser468 | rabbit | Abcam | 1:200 (IH) |
| NF-κB p65-Ser529 | rabbit | Abcam | 1:200 (IH) |
| TNF-α | goat | R&D system | 1:500 (IH) 1:200 (IF) |
| TNFp55R | rabbit | Abcam | 1:200 (IF) |
| TNFp75R | Rabbit | Abcam | 1:200 (IF) |

* IHC, immunohistochemistry; IF, immunofluorescence.

times for 10 min each. The sections were visualized with 3,3'-diaminobenzidine (DAB) in 0.1 M Tris buffer and mounted on gelatin-coated slides. The immunoreactions were observed under an Axiophot microscope (Carl Zeiss, Munchen-Hallbergmoos). All images were captured using an Axiocam HRc camera and Axio Vision 3.1 software [21-23]. To identify the morphological changes induced by SE in the same hippocampal tissue, double immunofluorescent staining was also performed. Brain tissues were incubated in a mixture of goat anti-TNF-α IgG/mouse anti-calbindin D-28 k IgG (a granule cell marker) or mouse anti-GFAP IgG (an astroglial marker)/rabbit anti-TNFp55R IgG or mouse anti-GFAP IgG/TNFp75R IgG in PBS containing 0.3% triton X-100 overnight at room temperature. After washing three times for 10 minutes with PBS, sections were also incubated in a mixture of FITC-or Cy3-conjugated secondary antisera (Amersham, San Francisco, CA) for 1 hr at room temperature. Sections were mounted in Vectashield mounting media with or without DAPI (Vector, Burlingame, CA). For negative controls, rat hippocampal tissues were incubated with only the secondary antibody without primary antibody. All negative controls for immunohistochemistry resulted in the absence of immunoreactivity in any structure (data not shown).

### Fluoro-Jade B staining

Fluoro-Jade B (FJB) staining was used to identify degenerating neurons. Briefly, sections were rinsed in distilled water, and mounted onto gelatin-coated slides and then dried on a slide warmer. The slides were immersed in 100% ethanol for 3 min, followed by 70% ethanol for 2 min and distilled water for 2 min. The slides were then transferred to 0.06% potassium permanganate for 15 min and gently agitated. After rinsing in distilled water for 2 min, the slides were incubated for 30 min in 0.001% FJB (Histo-Chem Inc. Jefferson, AR), freshly prepared by adding 20 ml of a 0.01% stock FJB solution to 180 ml of 0.1% acetic acid, with gentle shaking in the dark. After rinsing for 1 min in each of three changes of distilled water, the slides were dried, dehydrated in xylene and coverslipped with DPX. For stereological study, every sixth section in the series throughout the entire hippocampus was used (see below).

### Stereology

Hippocampal volumes (V) were estimated according to a formula based on the modified Cavalieri method: $V = \Sigma a \times t_{nom} \times 1/ssf$, where $a$ is area of the region of the delineated subfield measured by AxioVision Rel. 4.8 software,, $t_{nom}$ is the nominal section thickness (of 30 μm in this study), and ssf is the fraction of the sections sampled or section sampling fraction (of 1/6 in this study). The subfield areas were delineated with a 2.5 × objective lens. The volumes are reported as mm$^3$ [24,25]. The optical fractionator was used to estimate cell numbers. The optical fractionator (a combination of performing counting with the optical disector, with fractionator sampling) is a stereological method based on a properly designed systematic random sampling method that by definition yields unbiased estimates of population number. The sampling procedure is accomplished by focusing through the depth of the tissue (the optical disector height, $h$; of 15 μm in all cases for this study). The number of each cell type (C) in each of the subregions is estimated as: $C = \Sigma Q^- \times t/h \times 1/asf \times 1/ssf$, where $Q^-$ is the number of cells actually counted in the disectors that fall within the sectional profiles of the subregion seen on the sampled sections, and Asf is the area sampling fraction calculated as the area of the counting frame of the dissector, a(frame) (50 × 50 μm$^2$ in this study) and the area associated with each x, y movement, grid (x, y step) (250 × 250 μm$^2$ in this study) {asf = [a(frame)/a(x, y step)]}. FJB-positive cells were counted with a 40 × objective lens. All FJB-positive cells were counted regardless the intensity of labeling. Cell counts were performed by two different investigators who were blind to the classification of tissues [20].

## Quantification of data

For quantification of immunohistochemical data, images were captured using an AxioImage M2 microscope and AxioVision Rel. 4.8 software (15 sections per each animal). Figures were mounted with Adobe PhotoShop v 8.0. Images were converted to gray and white images. The range of intensity values was obtained from the selected images using Adobe PhotoShop v. 8.0. Based on the mean range of intensity values, each image was normalized by adjusting the black and white range of the image using Adobe PhotoShop v. 8.0. Manipulation of the images was restricted to threshold and brightness adjustments to the whole image [21-23]. After regions were outlined, 10 areas/rat (500 μm$^2$/area) were selected from the hippocampus and gray values were measured. Intensity measurements were represented as the mean number of a 256 gray scale (NIH Image 1.59 software and AxioVision Rel. 4.8 software). Values for background staining were obtained from the corpus callosum. Optical density values were then corrected by subtracting the average values of background noise obtained from 15 image inputs.

## Statistical analysis

All data obtained from the quantitative measurements and electrophysiological study were analyzed using one-way ANOVA to determine statistical significance. Bonferroni's test was used for post-hoc comparisons.

A p-value below 0.05 was considered statistically significant [21-23].

## Results

### Seizure threshold

The criterion for time of seizure onset is the time point showing a paroxysmal depolarizing shift that is defined as lasting > 3 s and consisting of a rhythmic discharge of > 2 Hz and usually between 4 and 10 Hz. Saline-treated animals showed the beginning of epileptiform discharges 768 s after pilocarpine injection (i.p.). BzATP, OxATP, sTNFp55R and BzATP+sTNFp55R-infused animals showed the beginning of SE up to 946, 743, 763 and 816 s after pilocarpine injection, respectively, and maintenance of SE until 2 hr after SE. These findings indicate that BzATP, OxATP, sTNFp55R or BzATP+sTNFp55R-infusion did not affect pilocarpine-induced SE in rats (Figure 1).

### TNF-α expression

In non-SE-induced animals of saline-infused groups, TNF-α immunoreactivity was weakly detected in CA1-3 pyramidal cells and dentate granule cells. In addition, hilar neurons also showed TNF-α immunoreactivity (Figure 2A). This localization pattern of TNF-α immunoreactivity in the hippocampus was consistent with previous studies [26-29]. BzATP-, OxATP-or sTNFp55R-infusion did not affect the localization pattern of TNF-α immunoreactivity in the hippocampus (data not shown). Two days after SE, TNF-α immunoreactivity was slightly increased (not statistically significant) in the hippocampus of saline-infused animals, as compared to non-SE-induced animals (Figures 2A-B). In BzATP-infused animals, TNF-α immunoreactivity in dentate granule cells was significantly increased 1.7-fold as compared with that in saline-infused animals (p < 0.05; Figures 2A-C). In addition, TNF-α immunoreactivity was readily apparent in the mossy fibers (stratum lucidum), while TNF-α immunoreactivity in CA1-3

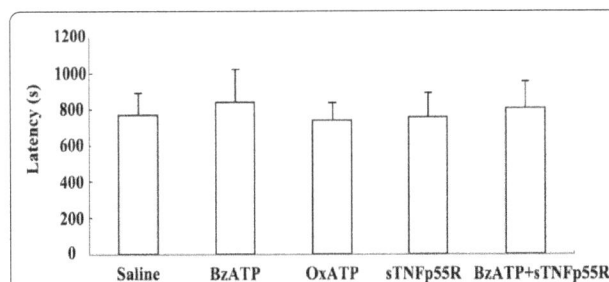

**Figure 1 Effects of BzATP, OxATP, sTNFp55R, and BzATP +sTNFp55R infusions on the timing of pilocarpine (PILO)-induced seizure onset**. There are no differences in seizure latency among the groups.

pyramidal cells was unaltered (p < 0.05; Figures 2A-B and 2D). In OxATP-infused animals, TNF-α immunoreactivity in dentate granule cells was significantly decreased to about 50% that in saline-infused animals (p < 0.05; Figures 2A and 2C). In A-438079-or A-740003-infused animals, alterations in TNF-α immunoreactivity in dentate granule cells were similar to those in OxATP-infused animals (data not shown). In sTNFp55R-and BzATP+sTNFp55R-infused animals, the alterations in TNF-α immunoreactivity were similar those observed in saline-and BzATP-infused animals, respectively (Figures 2A and 2C). One week after SE, TNF-α immunoreactivity in the hippocampus recovered to the level of non-SE-induced animals within every group (Figures 2C-D). TNF-α immunoreactivity was also detected in microglia 1-7 days after SE (data not shown). However, there was no difference in TNF-α immunoreactivity within microglial cells of each group.

## TNFp55R expression

In non-SE-induced animals of saline-infused groups, TNFp55R immunoreactivity was observed mainly in GFAP-positive astrocytes (Figure 3A). Similarly, BzATP-, OxATP-, A-438079, A-740003 or sTNFp55R-infusion did not affect the localization pattern of TNF-α immunoreactivity in the hippocampus of non-SE-induced animals (data not shown). As compared to non-SE-induced animals (Figure 3B), TNFp55R immunoreactivity was gradually reduced in astrocytes 1-7 days after SE (P < 0.05, Figures 3C-D). BzATP, OxATP, A-438079, A-740003, sTNFp55R or BzATP+sTNFp55R infusion did not affect changes in TNFp55R immunoreactivity in the hippocampus following SE (data not shown).

## TNFp75R expression

In non-SE-induced animals of saline-infused groups, TNFp75R immunoreactivity was observed in neurons and GFAP-positive astrocytes (Figures 4A-B). BzATP, OxATP, A-438079, A-740003, sTNFp55R or BzATP+sTNFp55R infusion did not affect changes in TNFp55R immunoreactivity in the hippocampus (data not shown). Two to three days after SE, TNFp75R immunoreactivity was increased, exclusively in CA3 neurons, to 1.3-(2 days after SE) and 1.5-(3 days after SE, data not shown) fold in saline-infused animals, as compared with that in non-SE-induced animals (P < 0.05, Figures 4C-D). In BzATP-infused animals, TNFp75R immunoreactivity was increased, only in CA3 neurons, 1.7-(2 days after SE) and 1.8-(3 days after SE, data not shown) fold as compared with that in saline-infused animals (P < 0.05, Figures 4C-D). OxATP, sTNFp55R or BzATP+sTNFp55R infusions effectively prevented changes in TNFp75R immunoreactivity in the CA3 region following SE (Figures 4C-D). The effect of A-438079-or A-740003 infusion on TNFp75R immunoreactivity was similar to that

of OxATP infusion (data not shown). One week after SE, TNFp75R immunoreactivity in the CA3 region recovered to the levels of non-SE-induced animals within every group (Figure 4D).

## Neuronal damage

In our previous study [30] and in preliminary studies here, neuronal damage was first detectable 3 days after SE. Therefore, we applied FJB stains to 3-day post-SE animals of each group. Few FJB positive neurons were detected in the hippocampus of non-SE-induced animals in any group (data not shown). In saline-infused animals, FJB-positive neurons were detected in CA1-3 pyramidal cells and dentate hilus neurons (Figures 5A-C). The number of FJB-positive neurons in dentate gyrus, CA1 and CA3 regions was 18,215 ± 2,568, 236,145 ± 51,976 and 69,469 ± 4,367, respectively (Figures 5B-C). For BzATP-infused animals, the number of FJB-positive neurons in dentate gyrus, CA1 and CA3 regions was 19,138 ± 2,841, 214,843 ± 42,368 and 12,418 ± 5,714, respectively (Figure 5A). Thus, BzATP infusion attenuated SE-induced neuronal damage in the CA3 region (P < 0.05, Figures 5B-C). In contrast, OxATP-, A-438079, A-740003, sTNFp55R and BzATP+sTNFp55R infusion increased the number of FJB-positive neurons in the CA3 region to 117,428 ± 6,468, 131,456 ± 5,196, 129,345 ± 7,138, 122,987 ± 3,568 and 86,468 ± 9,789, respectively (Figures 5B-C). However, OxATP-, sTNFp55R or BzATP +sTNFp55R infusion could not exacerbate SE-induced neuronal damages in dentate gyrus or the CA1 region, as compared to BzATP-infusion (Figures 5B-C).

## NF-κB phosphorylation

It is well established that TNF-α is a major stimulus to phosphorylation of NF-κB. To confirm TNF-α-mediated signaling following SE, we performed an immunohistochemical study using six phospho-NF-κB antibodies. As compared to control animals, p52-Ser865, p52-Ser869, p65-Ser468, and p65-Ser529 NF-κB phosphorylations were unaltered in nuclei of CA1 and CA3 pyramidal cells, dentate granule cells, and hilar neurons 2 days after SE (data not shown). However, both p65-Ser276 and p65-Ser311 phosphorylations were increased, only in the CA3 region, following SE. In non-SE-induced animals of saline-infused groups, moderate p65-Ser276 immunoreactivity was observed in nuclei of CA3 neurons (Figures 6A-B). p65-Ser311 immunoreactivity was also weakly detected in nuclei of CA3 neurons (Figures 6A-B and 6C). BzATP-, OxATP-, A-438079, A-740003, or sTNFp55R-infusion did not affect the localization patterns of p65-Ser276 or p65-Ser311 immunoreactivity in the hippocampus of non-SE-induced animals (data not shown). Two days after SE, both p65-Ser276 and p65-Ser311 immunoreactivities in CA3 neurons were

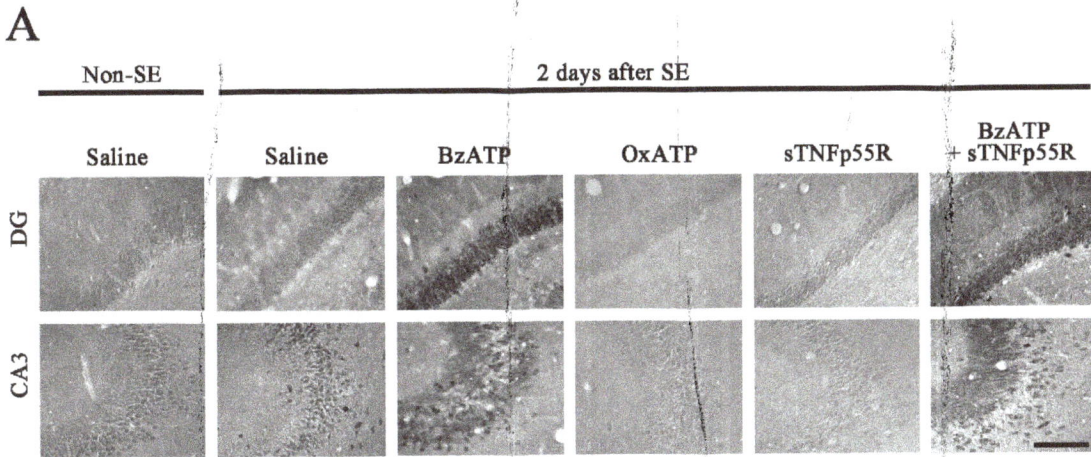

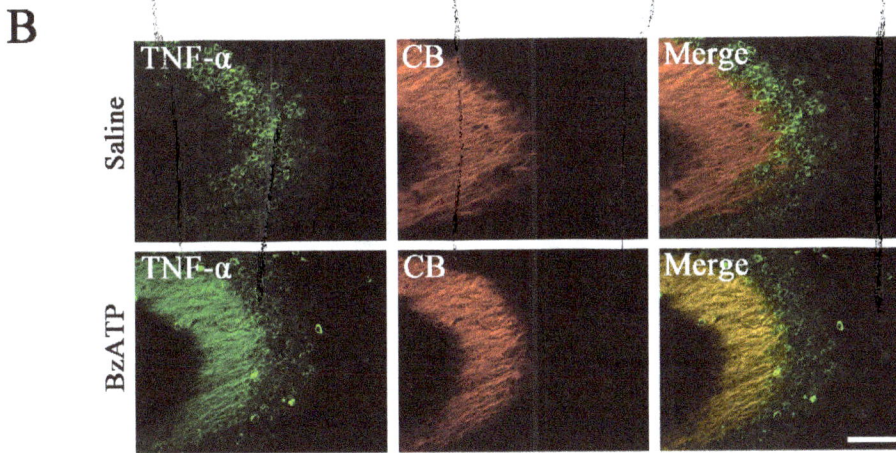

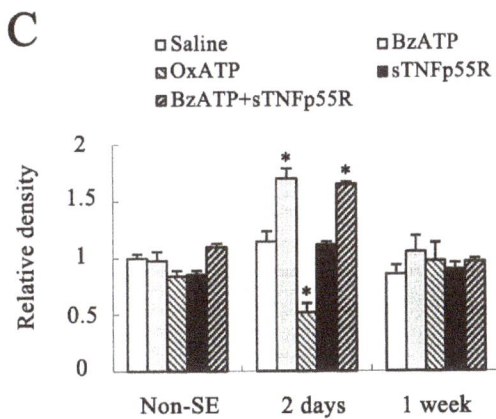

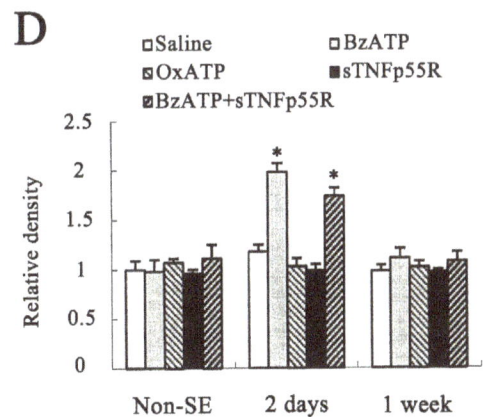

**Figure 2** Effects of BzATP, OxATP, sTNFp55R, and BzATP+sTNFp55R infusion on TNF-α expression following SE. **(A)** TNF-α expression in dentate granule cells and the CA3 region 2 days after SE. Bar = 100 µm (panel 1). **(B)** TNF-α expression in mossy fibers in saline-and BzATP-infused animals 2 days after SE. In BzATP-infused animals, TNF-α immunoreactivity is colocalized with CB, a marker for mossy fibers. Bar = 100 µm (panel 1). **(C)** Quantitative analysis of TNF-α immunoreactivity in dentate granule cells following SE (mean ± S.E.M). *Value is significantly different from saline-infused animals, p < 0.05. **(D)** Quantitative analysis of TNF-α immunoreactivity in the CA3 region following SE (mean ± S.E.M). *Value is significantly different from saline-infused animals, p < 0.05.

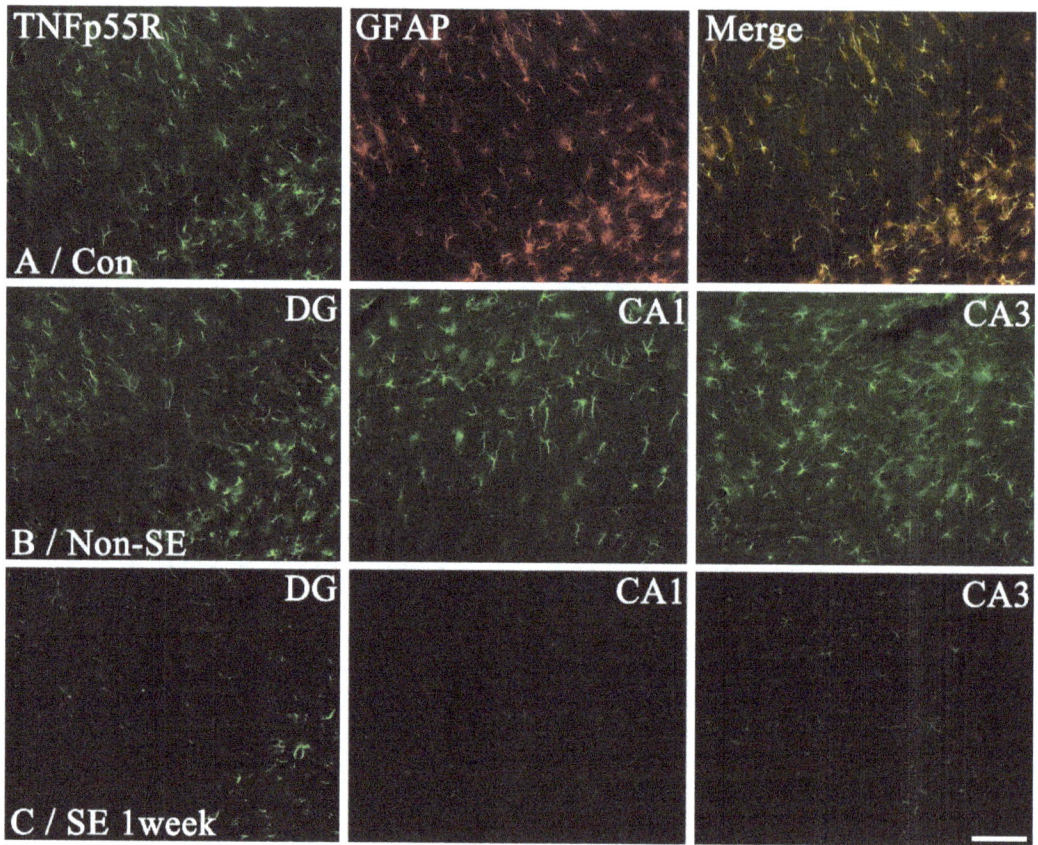

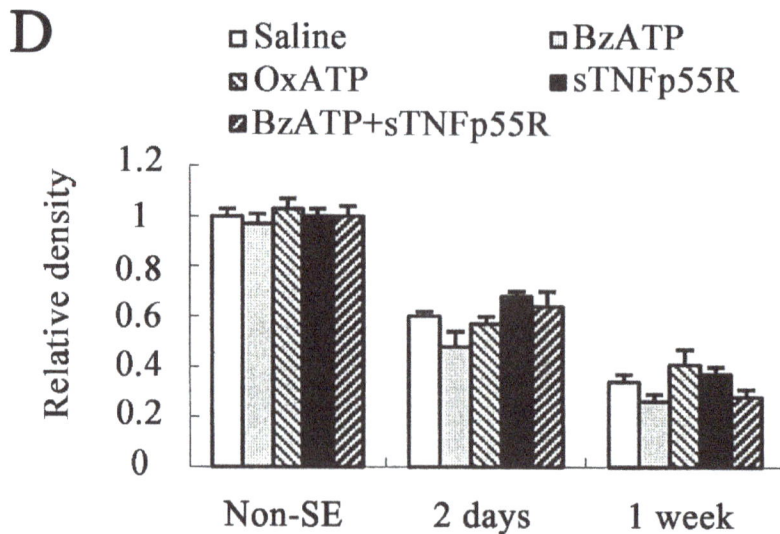

**Figure 3 Effect of SE on TNFp55R expression**. **(A)** Astroglial expression of TNFp55R in control animal. Bar = 100 μm. **(B)** Distribution of TNFp55R immunoreactivity in hippocampus of a non-SE-induced animal in the saline-infused group. Bar = 100 μm. **(C)** Distribution of TNFp55R immunoreactivity in hippocampus of a 1-week post-SE animal in the saline-infused group. Bar = 100 μm. **(D)** Quantitative analysis of TNFp55R immunoreactivity in hippocampus following SE (mean ± S.E.M). There are no differences in TNFp55R immunoreactivity in hippocampus among the groups.

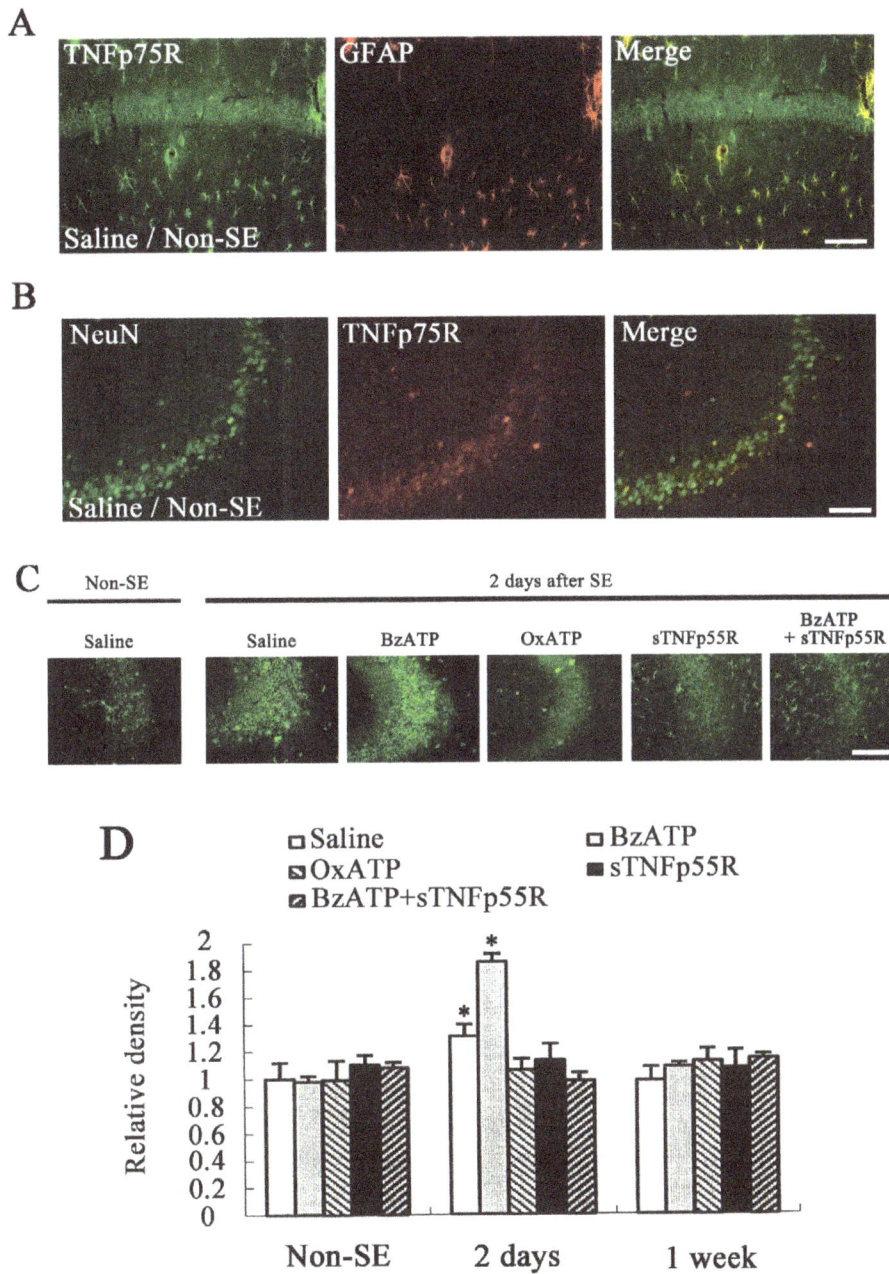

**Figure 4 Effects of BzATP, OxATP, sTNFp55R, and BzATP+sTNFp55R infusions on TNFp75R expression following SE**. (A) Double immunofluorescence for TNFp75R and GFAP in CA1 region of a non-SE-induced animal in the saline-infused group. Bar = 100 μm. (B) Double immunofluorescence for TNFp75R and NeuN in CA3 region of a non-SE-induced animal in the saline-infused group. Bar = 100 μm. (C) TNFp75R expression in the CA3 region 2 days after SE Bar = 100 μm (panel 1). (D) Quantitative analysis of TNFp75R immunoreactivity in the CA3 region following SE (mean ± S.E.M). *Value is significantly different from saline-infused animals, p < 0.05.

enhanced to 1.5-and 1.8-fold in saline-infused animals, respectively (Figures 6A-C). In BzATP-infused animals, both p65-Ser276 and p65-Ser311 immunoreactivities in CA3 neurons were increased 2.1-and 2.9-fold as compared with that in non-SE-induced animals (Figures 6A-C). OxATP-, A-438079, A-740003, sTNFp55R-or BzATP+ sTNFp55R infusions effectively prevented increases in p65-Ser276 and p65-Ser311 immunoreactivities in CA3 neurons following SE (Figures 6A-C). One week after SE, phospho-NF-κB immunoreactivities were decreased to non-SE-induced animal levels (Figures 6B-C). Following SE, however, both p65-Ser276 and p65-Ser311 immunoreactivities were unaltered in CA1 pyramidal cells (Figure 6D) as well as dentate granule cells (Figure 6E). Furthermore, BzATP-,

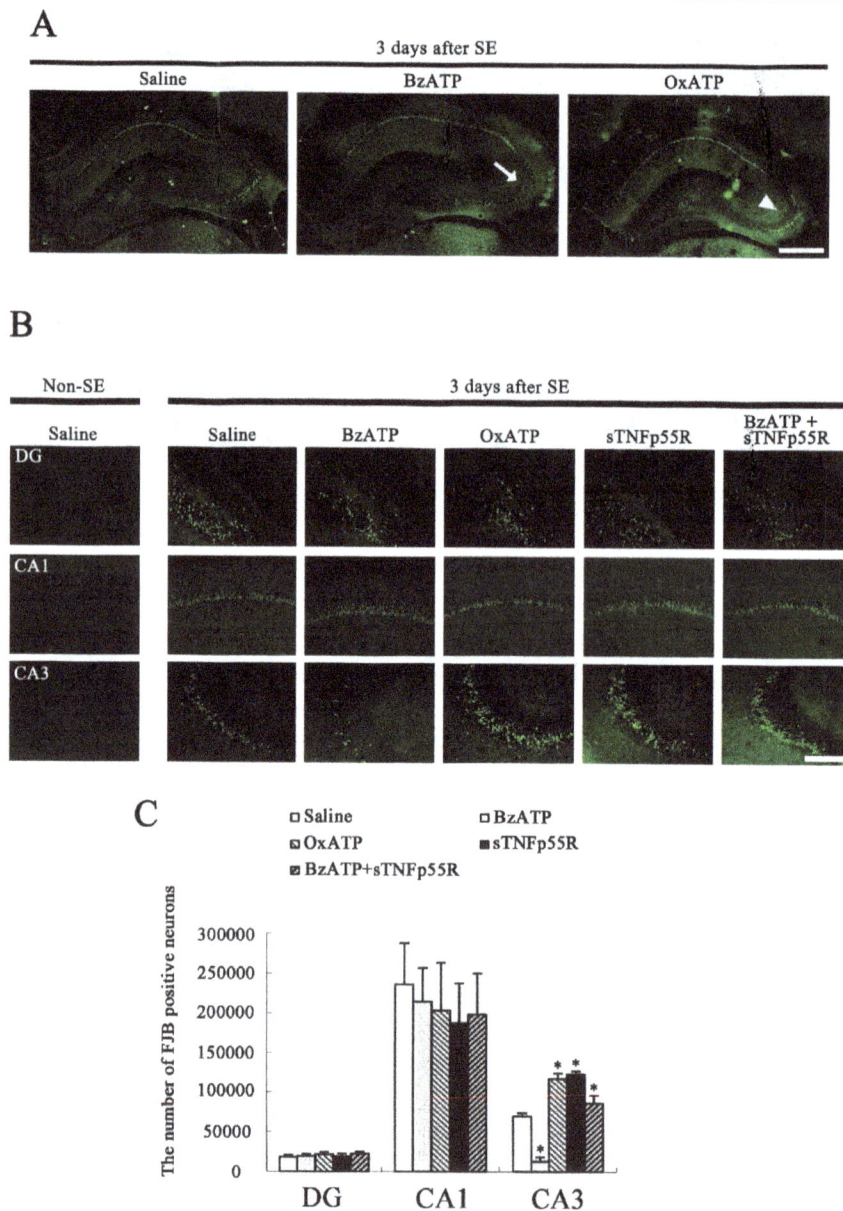

**Figure 5 Effect of BzATP, OxATP, sTNFp55R, and BzATP+sTNFp55R infusions on SE-induced neuronal death**. (A) Representative photographs of FJB staining following SE. As compared to saline-infusion, BzATP infusion attenuates neuronal damage in the CA3 region (arrows), while OxATP infusion worsens it (arrowheads). (B) SE-induced neuronal damages in dentate gyrus, and in the CA1 and CA3 regions 3 days after SE. Bar = 100 μm. (C) Quantitative analysis of neuronal damage in dentate gyrus, and in the CA1 and CA3 regions 3 days after SE (mean ± S.E.M). BzATP infusion alleviates SE-induced neuronal damage only in the CA3 region. However, the other treatments increase SE-induced neuronal damage. *Value is significantly different from saline-infused animals, $p < 0.05$.

OxATP-, A-438079, A-740003, or sTNFp55R infusions did not affect the localization pattern of p65-Ser276 immunoreactivity in these regions following SE (data not shown).

## Discussion

It is well established that normal rat brain constitutive expresses biologically active TNF-$\alpha$ as well as TNF-$\alpha$ mRNA [31-33] and that TNF-$\alpha$ may be produced by neurons themselves [33]. These previous studies reveal that TNF-$\alpha$ may serve as a mediator of neurotransmitter release in the CNS. The P2X7 receptor is identified as a mediator in response to acute brain injury, since the synthesis and membrane localization of P2X7 receptor are rapidly up-regulated in response to various stimuli, including SE [31,34-37]. The P2X7 receptor engages diverse signal cascades, which include initiation of rapid

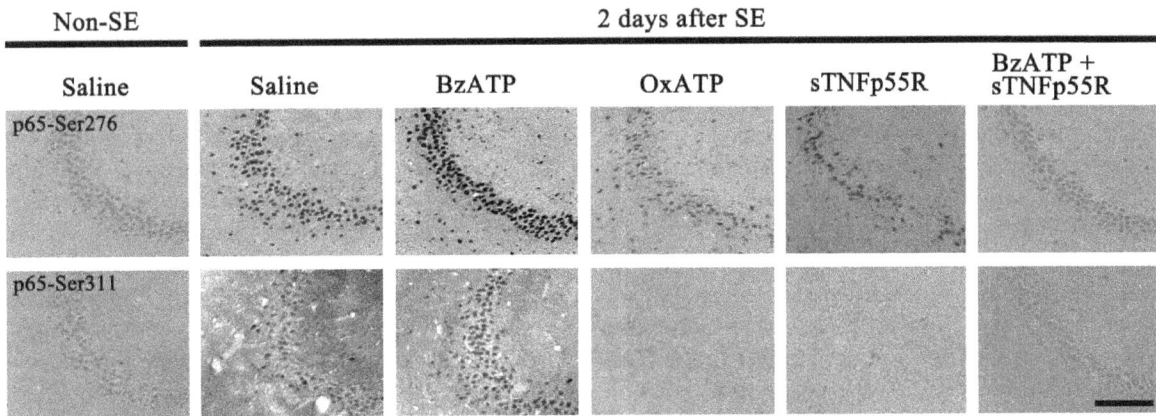

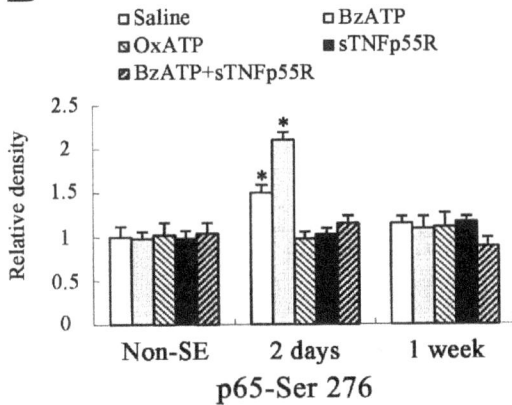

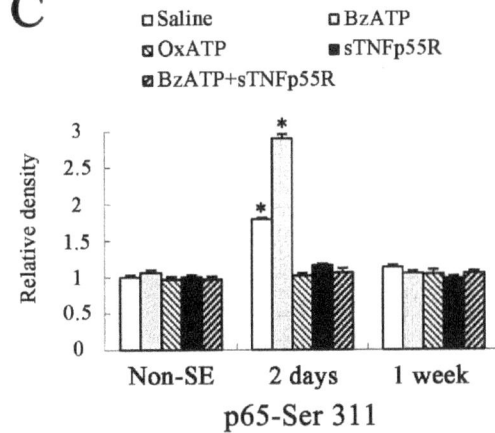

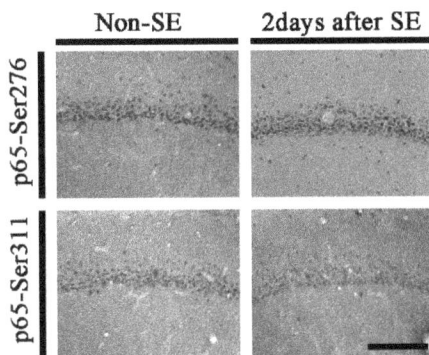

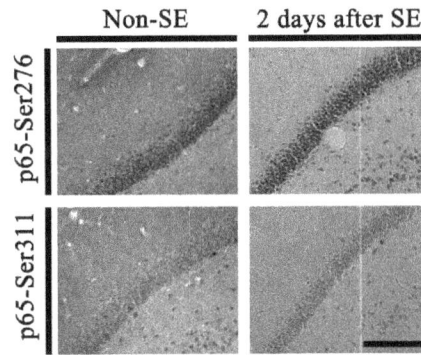

**Figure 6 Effect of BzATP, OxATP, sTNFp55R, and BzATP+sTNFp55R infusions on SE-induced NF-κB phosphorylation**. **(A)** p65-Ser276 and p65-Ser311 phosphorylation in the CA3 region following SE. Bar = 100 μm. **(B)** Quantitative analysis of p65-Ser276 phosphorylation in CA3 region following SE (mean ± S.E.M). *Value is significantly different from saline-infused animals, p < 0.05. **(C)** Quantitative analysis of p65-Ser311 phosphorylation in CA3 region following SE (mean ± S.E.M). *Value is significantly different from saline-infused animals, p < 0.05. **(D-E)** p65-Ser276 and p65-Ser311 phosphorylations in CA1 and in dentate granule cells following SE. As compared to non-SE animals, there is no difference in p65-Ser276 or p65-Ser311 phosphorylations in these regions 2 days after SE. Bar = 100 μm.

release and processing of proinflammatory cytokines including TNF-$\alpha$ [34,36,38]. Similar to previous studies [26-29], the present study shows that TNF-$\alpha$ immunoreactivity is readily apparent in hippocampal neurons as well as dentate granule cells in non-SE-induced animals. Interestingly, BzATP-infusion increased TNF-$\alpha$ immunoreactivity in dentate granule cells following SE, while OxATP-infusion decreased it. These findings indicate that P2X7 receptor-mediated regulation of TNF-$\alpha$ expression may not be a consequence of distinct effects of each drug on seizure activity. This is because BzATP-, OxATP-, A-438079, A-740003, sTNFp55R-and BzATP+sTNFp55R infusions did not affect pilocarpine-induced SE in rats. Furthermore, these infusions could not affect basal level of TNF-$\alpha$ immunoreactivity in the hippocampus. Therefore, the present findings suggest that alterations in SE-induced TNF-$\alpha$ immunoreactivity may be mediated by P2X7 receptor function.

TNF-$\alpha$ clearly possesses the ability to simultaneously activate both cell death and cell survival pathways, and this balance ultimately determines whether TNF-$\alpha$ promotes neurodegeneration or neuroprotection. Basically, TNF-related signal transduction pathways include NF-$\kappa$B binding activity for TNFp55R contributing to cell death [9] and downstream signaling via the TNFp75R involves activation of p38 mitogen-activated protein kinase to promote neuronal survival [10]. In the present study, BzATP-infusion caused a restricted increase in TNF-$\alpha$ immunoreactivity within dentate granule cells and their axons, and mossy fibers, following SE. BzATP-infusion also enhanced TNFp75R expression in response to TNF-$\alpha$ overexpression, only in CA3 neurons, which synapse with mossy fibers. Furthermore, the present study shows that BzATP infusion attenuates SE-induced neuronal damage, only in the CA3 region, while OxATP-, A-438079, A-740003, sTNFp55R and BzATP+sTNFp55R infusions exacerbate neuronal damage as compared to saline-infused animals. Therefore, our findings suggest that TNF-$\alpha$-mediated signaling may play a neuroprotective role against SE.

It has been reported that p65-Ser276 and p65-Ser311 phosphorylations of NF-$\kappa$B induced by TNF-$\alpha$ enhance their transactivation potentials and their interactions with cAMP response element-binding (CREB)-binding protein (CBP), which is also important for the survival of neurons [39-44]. In the present study, BzATP-infusion enhanced TNFp75R expression with intensification of p65-Ser276 and p65-Ser311 immunoreactivities following SE. In addition, sTNFp55R pretreatment could not prevent SE-induced neuronal damages, and BzATP+sTNFp55R infusion did not show protective effect of BzATP. These findings indicate that the activation of TNFp75R may protect CA3 neurons from SE via p65-Ser276 and p65-Ser311 NF-$\kappa$B phosphorylations.

Microglia are a major producer of TNF-$\alpha$ in brain [45,46]. Hide et al. [26] reported that TNF-$\alpha$ release from microglia is induced by BzATP. P2X7 receptor expression is increased in the rat hippocampus following pilocarpine-induced SE [30,47]. With respect to these previous reports, it is likely that TNF-$\alpha$ released from microglia may also play a neuroprotective role in the rat hippocampus following SE. In the present study, however, there was no difference in TNF-$\alpha$ immunoreactivity between microglia of each group. Although the present data could not provide biological mechanism of this phenomenon, it may be considered that the dosages of OxATP, A-438079 and A-740003 applied in the present study are insufficient to inhibit TNF-$\alpha$ expression in microglia due to full P2X7 receptor expression. Further studies are needed to elucidate the effectiveness of P2X7 receptor agonists and antagonists to alter TNF-$\alpha$ expression in activated microglia.

In conclusion, the present study suggests that TNF-$\alpha$ induction by P2X7 receptor activation may ameliorate SE-induced CA3 neuronal damage via enhancement of p65-Ser276 and p65-Ser311 phosphorylations of NF-$\kappa$B.

### Acknowledgements

This work was supported by funds from National Research Foundation of Korea (Grant number: 2009-0064347, 2010K000808 and 2009-0093812).

### Author details

[1]Department of Anatomy & Neurobiology, Institute of Epilepsy Research, College of Medicine, Hallym University, Chunchon, Kangwon-Do 200-702, South Korea. [2]Ji-Eun Kim, Department of Neurology, UCSF, and Veterans Affairs Medical Center, San Francisco, California 94121, USA.

### Authors' contributions

JEK was involved in designing and performing all experiments. HJR, TCK helped in drafting the manuscript. JEK and HJR did the immunohistochemistry, the intracerebroventricular drug infusion, the seizure studies and the acquisition of data and analyses. TCK provided continuous intellectual input, and evaluation and interpretation of data. All authors read and approved the final manuscript.

### Competing interests

The authors declare that they have no competing interests.

### References

1. DeLorenzo RJ, Pellock JM, Towne AR, Boggs JG: Epidemiology of status epilepticus. J Clin Neurophysiol 1995, 12:316-325.
2. Fujikawa DG: Neuroprotective effect of ketamine administered after status epilepticus onset. Epilepsia 1995, 36:186-195.
3. Rice AC, DeLorenzo RJ: NMDA receptor activation during status epilepticus is required for the development of epilepsy. Brain Res 1998, 782:240-247.
4. Stewart LS, Persinger MA: Ketamine prevents learning impairment when administered immediately after status epilepticus onset. Epilepsy Behav 2001, 2:85-591.
5. Allan SM, Rothwell NJ: Cytokines and acute neurodegeneration. Nat Rev Neurosci 2001, 2:734-744.
6. Sriram K, O'Callaghan JP: Divergent roles for tumor necrosis factor-alpha in the brain. J Neuroimmune Pharmacol 2007, 2:140-153.
7. Fotin-Mleczek M, Henkler F, Samel D, Reichwein M, Hausser A, Parmryd I, Scheurich P, Schmid JA, Wajant H: Apoptotic crosstalk of TNF receptors:

TNF-R2-induces depletion of TRAF2 and IAP proteins and accelerates TNF-R1-dependent activation of caspase-8. *J Cell Sci* 2002, 115:2757-2770.

8. Quintana A, Giralt M, Rojas S, Penkowa M, Campbell IL, Hidalgo J, Molinero A: Differential role of tumor necrosis factor receptors in mouse brain inflammatory responses in cryolesion brain injury. *J Neurosci Res* 2005, 82:701-716.

9. Tartaglia LA, Goeddel DV: Tumor necrosis factor receptor signaling. A dominant negative mutation suppresses the activation of the 55-kDa tumor necrosis factor receptor. *J Biol Chem* 1992, 267:4304-4307.

10. Yang L, Lindholm K, Konishi Y, Li R, Shen Y: Target depletion of distinct tumor necrosis factor receptor subtypes reveals hippocampal neuron death and survival through different signal transduction pathways. *J Neurosci* 2002, 22:3025-3032.

11. Lu MO, Zhang XM, Mix E, Quezada HC, Jin T, Zhu J, Adem A: TNF-alpha receptor 1 deficiency enhances kainic acid-induced hippocampal injury in mice. *J Neurosci Res* 2008, 86:1608-1614.

12. Marchetti L, Klein M, Schlett K, Pfizenmaier K, Eisel UL: Tumor necrosis factor (TNF)-mediated neuroprotection against glutamate-induced excitotoxicity is enhanced by N-methyl-D-aspartate receptor activation. Essential role of a TNF receptor 2-mediated phosphatidylinositol 3-kinase-dependent NF-kappa B pathway. *J Biol Chem* 2004, 279:32869-32881.

13. Suzuki T, Hide I, Ido K, Kohsaka S, Inoue K, Nakata Y: Production and release of neuroprotective tumor necrosis factor by P2X7 receptor-activated microglia. *J Neurosci* 2004, 24:1-7.

14. Choi HB, Ryu JK, Kim SU, McLarnon JG: Modulation of the purinergic P2X7 receptor attenuates lipopolysaccharide-mediated microglial activation and neuronal damage in inflamed brain. *J Neurosci* 2007, 27:4957-4968.

15. Paxinos G, Watson C: **The Rat Brain in Stereotaxic Coordinates.** San Diego, Academic Press;, 3 1997.

16. Siuciak JA, Boylan C, Fritsche M, Altar CA, Lindsay RM: BDNF increases monoaminergic activity in rat brain following intracerebroventricular or intraparenchymal administration. *Brain Res* 1996, 710:11-20.

17. Pencea V, Bingaman KD, Wiegand SJ, Luskin MB: Infusion of brain-derived neurotrophic factor into the lateral ventricle of the adult rat leads to new neurons in the parenchyma of the striatum, septum, thalamus, and hypothalamus. *J Neurosci* 2001, 21:6706-6717.

18. Kim JE, Ryu HJ, Yeo SI, Kang TC: P2X7 receptor differentially modulates astroglial apoptosis and clasmatodendrosis in the rat brain following status epilepticus. *Hippocampus* 2010.

19. Kang TC, Kang JH, Kim HT, Lee SJ, Choi UK, Kim JE, Kwak SE, Kim DW, Choi SY, Kwon OS: Anticonvulsant characteristics of pyridoxyl-gamma-aminobutyrate, PL-GABA. *Neuropharmacology* 2008, 54:954-964.

20. Kim DS, Kim JE, Kwak SE, Choi KC, Kim DW, Kwon OS, Choi SY, Kang TC: Spatiotemporal characteristics of astroglial death in the rat hippocampo-entorhinal complex following pilocarpine-induced status epilepticus. *J Comp Neurol* 2008, 511:581-598.

21. Kim JE, Kim DW, Kwak SE, Ryu HJ, Yeo SI, Kwon OS, Choi SY, Kang TC: Pyridoxal-5′-phosphate phosphatase/chronophin inhibits long-term potentiation induction in the rat dentate gyrus. *Hippocampus* 2009, 19:1078-1089.

22. Kim JE, Kwak SE, Kang TC: Upregulated TWIK-related acid-sensitive K+ channel-2 in neurons and perivascular astrocytes in the hippocampus of experimental temporal lobe epilepsy. *Epilepsia* 2009, 50:654-663.

23. Kim JE, Ryu HJ, Yeo SI, Seo CH, Lee BC, Choi IG, Kim DS, Kang TC: Differential expressions of aquaporin subtypes in astroglia in the hippocampus of chronic epileptic rats. *Neuroscience* 2009, 163:781-789.

24. Bedi KS: Early-life undernutrition causes deficits in rat dentate gyrus granule cell number. *Experientia* 1991, 47:1073-1074.

25. Madeira MD, Sousa N, Santer RM, Paula-Barbosa MM, Gundersen HJ: Age and sex do not affect the volume, cell numbers, or cell size of the suprachiasmatic nucleus of the rat: an unbiased stereological study. *J Comp Neurol* 1995, 361:585-601.

26. Nadeau S, Rivest S: Regulation of the gene encoding tumor necrosis factor alpha (TNF-alpha) in the rat brain and pituitary in response in different models of systemic immune challenge. *J Neuropathol Exp Neurol* 1999, 58:61-77.

27. Sairanen TR, Lindsberg PJ, Brenner M, Carpén O, Sirén A: Differential cellular expression of tumor necrosis factor-alpha and Type I tumor necrosis factor receptor after transient global forebrain ischemia. *J Neurol Sci* 2001, 186:87-99.

28. Bette M, Kaut O, Schäfer MK, Weihe E: Constitutive expression of p55TNFR mRNA and mitogen-specific up-regulation of TNF alpha and p75TNFR mRNA in mouse brain. *J Comp Neurol* 2003, 465:417-430.

29. Balosso S, Ravizza T, Perego C, Peschon J, Campbell IL, De Simoni MG, Vezzani A: Tumor necrosis factor-alpha inhibits seizures in mice via p75 receptors. *Ann Neurol* 2005, 57:804-812.

30. Kang TC, Kim DS, Kwak SE, Kim JE, Won MH, Kim DW, Choi SY, Kwon OS: Epileptogenic roles of astroglial death and regeneration in the dentate gyrus of experimental temporal lobe epilepsy. *Glia* 2006, 54:258-271.

31. Ignatowski TA, Noble BK, Wright JR, Gorfien JL, Heffner RR, Spengler RN: Neuronal-associated tumor necrosis factor (TNF alpha): its role in noradrenergic functioning and modification of its expression following antidepressant drug administration. *J Neuroimmunol* 1997, 79:84-90.

32. Ignatowski TA, Spengler RN: Tumor necrosis factor-α: Presynaptic sensitivity is modified after antidepressant drug administration. *Brain Res* 1994, 665:293-299.

33. Ignatowski TA, Chou RC, Spengler RN: Changes in noradrenergic sensitivity to tumor necrosis factor-α in brains of rats administered clonidine. *J Neuroimmunol* 1996, 70:55-63.

34. Guerra AN, Fisette PL, Pfeiffer ZA, Quinchia-Rios BH, Prabhu U, Aga M, Denlinger LC, Guadarrama AG, Abozeid S, Sommer JA, Proctor RA, Bertics PJ: Purinergic receptor regulation of LPS-induced signaling and pathophysiology. *J Endotoxin Res* 2003, 9:256-263.

35. North RA: Molecular physiology of $P_2X$ receptors. *Physiol Rev* 2002, 82:1013-1067.

36. Rothwell N: Interleukin-1 and neuronal injury: Mechanisms, modification, and therapeutic potential. *Brain Behav Immunol* 2003, 17:152-157.

37. Sim JA, Young MT, Sung HY, North RA, Surprenant A: Reanalysis of $P_2X_7$ receptor expression in rodent brain. *J Neurosci* 2004, 24:6307-6314.

38. Verhoef PA, Estacion M, Schilling W, Dubyak GR: $P_2X_7$ receptor-dependent blebbing and activation of rho-effector kinases, caspases and IL-1 release. *J Immmunol* 2003, 170:5728-5738.

39. Bito H, Takemoto-Kimura S: Ca(2+)/CREB/CBP-dependent gene regulation: a shared mechanism critical in long-term synaptic plasticity and neuronal survival. *Cell Calcium* 2003, 34:425-430.

40. Contestabile A: Regulation of transcription factors by nitric oxide in neurons and in neural-derived tumor cells. *Prog Neurobiol* 2008, 84:317-328.

41. Zhong H: Phosphorylation of NF-kB p65 by PKA stimulates transcriptional activity by promoting a novel bivalent interaction with the coactivator CBP/p300. *Mol Cell* 1998, 1:661-671.

42. Zhong H: The phosphorylation status of nuclear NF-kB determines its association with CBP/p300 or HDAC-1. *Mol Cell* 2002, 9:625-636.

43. Vermeulen L: Transcriptional activation of the NF-kBp65 subunit by mitogen-and stress-activated protein kinase-1. *EMBO J* 2003, 22:1313-1324.

44. Duran A: Essential role of RelA Ser311 phosphorylation by zetaPKC in NF-kB transcriptional activation. *EMBO J* 2003, 22:3910-3918.

45. Sawada M, Kondo N, Suzumura A, Marunouchi T: Production of tumor necrosis factor-alpha by microglia and astrocytes in culture. *Brain Res* 1989, 491:394-397.

46. Spanaus KS, Schlapbach R, Fontana A: TNF-alpha and IFN-gamma render microglia sensitive to Fas ligand-induced apoptosis by induction of Fas expression and down-regulation of Bcl-2 and Bcl-xL. *Eur J Immunol* 1998, 28:4398-4408.

47. Vianna EP, Ferreira AT, Naffah-Mazzacoratti MG, Sanabria ER, Funke M, Cavalheiro EA, Fernandes MJ: Evidence that ATP participates in the pathophysiology of pilocarpine-induced temporal lobe epilepsy: Fluorimertric, immunohistochemical, and western blot studies. *Epilepsia* 2002, 43:227-229.

# 12

# Vitexin reduces epilepsy after hypoxic ischemia in the neonatal brain via inhibition of NKCC1

Wen-di Luo[1], Jia-wei Min[1], Wen-Xian Huang[2], Xin Wang[1], Yuan-yuan Peng[1], Song Han[3], Jun Yin[3], Wan-Hong Liu[4], Xiao-Hua He[3] and Bi-Wen Peng[1]* (iD)

## Abstract

**Background:** Neonatal hypoxic-ischemic brain damage, characterized by tissue loss and neurologic dysfunction, is a leading cause of mortality and a devastating disease of the central nervous system. We have previously shown that vitexin has been attributed various medicinal properties and has been demonstrated to have neuroprotective roles in neonatal brain injury models. In the present study, we continued to reinforce and validate the basic understanding of vitexin (45 mg/kg) as a potential treatment for epilepsy and explored its possible underlying mechanisms.

**Methods:** P7 Sprague-Dawley (SD) rats that underwent right common carotid artery ligation and rat brain microvascular endothelial cells (RBMECs) were used for the assessment of $Na^+$-$K^+$-$Cl^-$ co-transporter1 (NKCC1) expression, BBB permeability, cytokine expression, and neutrophil infiltration by western blot, q-PCR, flow cytometry (FCM), and immunofluorescence respectively. Furthermore, brain electrical activity in freely moving rats was recorded by electroencephalography (EEG).

**Results:** Our data showed that NKCC1 expression was attenuated in vitexin-treated rats compared to the expression in the HI group in vivo. Oxygen glucose deprivation/reoxygenation (OGD) was performed on RBMECs to explore the role of NKCC1 and F-actin in cytoskeleton formation with confocal microscopy, N-(ethoxycarbonylmethyl)-6-methoxyquinolinium bromide, and FCM. Concomitantly, treatment with vitexin effectively alleviated OGD-induced NKCC1 expression, which downregulated F-actin expression in RBMECs. In addition, vitexin significantly ameliorated BBB leakage and rescued the expression of tight junction-related protein ZO-1. Furthermore, inflammatory cytokine and neutrophil infiltration were concurrently and progressively downregulated with decreasing BBB permeability in rats. Vitexin also significantly suppressed brain electrical activity in neonatal rats.

**Conclusions:** Taken together, these results confirmed that vitexin effectively alleviates epilepsy susceptibility through inhibition of inflammation along with improved BBB integrity. Our study provides a strong rationale for the further development of vitexin as a promising therapeutic candidate treatment for epilepsy in the immature brain.

**Keywords:** HIBD, Vitexin, NKCC1, F-actin, Blood-brain barrier, Inflammation, Epilepsy

* Correspondence: pengbiwen@whu.edu.cn
[1]Department of Physiology, Hubei Provincial Key Laboratory of Developmentally Originated Disorder, School of Basic Medical Sciences, Wuhan University, Hubei Donghu Rd 185#, Wuhan 430071, Hubei, China
Full list of author information is available at the end of the article

## Background

Perinatal hypoxic-ischemic encephalopathy (HIE) secondary to perinatal asphyxia remains a major cause of neonatal mortality and is associated with long-term neurologic comorbidities both in the late preterm and term neonate [1]. Approximately 15 to 25% of newborns die in the postnatal period, and 25% develop severe and permanent neuropsychological sequelae, including cerebral palsy, visual impairment, mental retardation, learning impairment, and epilepsy [2–5]. It has also been reported that HIE is one of the most common devastating etiologies associated with neonatal seizures, constituting 50–60% of the total number of seizures reported in neonates [6, 7]. However, HIE-associated neonatal seizures are often unresponsive to conventional antiepileptic drugs (AEDs), and the seizures cannot be controlled in 30% of children due to drug resistance [8, 9]. In the past decade, the mainstay of treatment for HIE remains comprehensive treatment, including hyperbaric oxygen therapy and mild hypothermia therapy, and medication. Although this therapy has been shown to improve survival and neurodevelopmental outcome, the neuroprotective response is limited by timing of initiation and severity of encephalopathy [10]. Thus, it is an urgent need to develop effective agents that target vulnerable periods in HIE-induced neonatal epilepsy.

The blood-brain barrier (BBB) plays an important role in brain damage. BBB dysfunction facilitates the infiltration of inflammatory factors and neutrophils, which contribute to morbidity in multiple sclerosis, encephalitis, traumatic brain injury, neurodegenerative diseases, brain tumors, and ischemic and hemorrhagic stroke [11]. BBB leakage occurs after the initial brain insult and is postulated to trigger epileptogenesis by permitting infiltration of inflammatory molecules into the brain [12–15]. Furthermore, inflammation in brain tissue has been fully described in human epilepsy of various etiologies and in experimental rodents with seizures [16–18], indicating that epilepsy could be a cause of the inflammatory response and endothelium impairments [14].

The Na-K-Cl co-transporter (NKCC), which consist of two isoforms (NKCC1 and NKCC2), is a critical transmembrane protein family playing an important role in cellular ion homeostasis and the subsequent accumulation of intracellular water [19, 20]. And NKCC is one of the major pathways to transport $Cl^-$ into cells [21]. NKCC1 is a member of the critical transmembrane protein family, which plays an important role in maintaining CNS functions, such as cell migration, astrocyte swelling [22], and neuroblast migration [23]. NKCC1 expression is developmentally regulated in the human and rodent brain, peaking in neurons, astrocytes, and oligodendrocytes in early perinatal development before declining in adulthood [20, 22, 24–26]. In addition to acting as an ion transporter, NKCC1 also participates in interactions with the actin cytoskeleton, and there is decreased expression of F-actin content upon NKCC1 knockdown [27, 28]. F-actin stress fibers present in injured endothelial cells, which leads to endothelial contraction and dismantlement of ZO-1, which maintains the integrity of the BBB [29]. The proposed ZO-1-regulatory mechanisms that are affected by F-actin may be based on the unique C-terminal half of ZO-1, which co-precipitates with F-actin. In contrast, the construct encoding the N-terminal half of ZO-1 is specifically associated with tight junctions (TJs) [30]. It has also been well documented that inhibition of NKCC1 may protect against traumatic brain injury-induced BBB breakdown [26]. Moreover, an increase in NKCC1 in neurons partially elevates excitability in neonatal seizures [25, 31], and the pharmacomodulation of chloride co-transporters has been investigated in treating refractory neonatal seizures [32–34].

Vitexin, which is a naturally derived flavonoid compound found in many medicinal plants, has recently received increasing attention due to its numerous pharmacological properties. Previous studies have shown that in vivo and in vitro treatment of flavonoid exerts protective effects by reducing pro-inflammatory cytokine secretion and restoring the levels of tight junction proteins of the BBB [35–38]. For instance, vitexin possesses a cardio-protective effect, which may be associated with its anti-oxidative effects, activation of ER stress, and inhibition of inflammatory cytokine release [39–41]. Vitexin also attenuated neuronal death and reduced neonatal brain injury in rats induced by hypoxia-ischemia via rescuing BBB collapse [42]. In addition, vitexin provides short- and long-term neuroprotection in pilocarpine-induced seizures in rats and exerts antiepileptic activity and neuroprotection [43]. Investigations of the underlying mechanism of action have come to the assumption that vitexin seems to be a ligand for benzodiazepine receptor, which could allosterically modulate $GABA_A$ receptors by binding to the benzodiazepine receptor site [44–46].

Nevertheless, although there have been a few studies demonstrating the antiepileptic activity of vitexin using in vivo and in vitro experimental models, none of these investigated its potential mechanism involved in NKCC1. The present study firstly showed that vitexin is beneficial to the treatment of HI insult through disturbing the NKCC1/F-actin pathway, which potentially protects against the severity of BBB collapse. Therefore, this study was designed to investigate the effect of vitexin in alleviating seizures during neonatal brain damage through preserving the integrity of the BBB via inhibition of NKCC1.

## Methods

### Experimental animals and groups

Sprague-Dawley (SD) rats (postnatal day 7) were provided by the Animal Biosafety Level 3 Laboratory (ABSL-3,

Wuhan University, China). All rats were housed at the standard laboratory animal facility ($25 \pm 2$ °C, 12-h light/dark cycle) with access to food and water ad libitum in individual cages.

The rats ($n = 128$) were randomly assigned to four groups ($n = 32$ rats each): hypoxia-ischemia group (abbreviated: HI group), rats underwent the ligation of the right common carotid artery and had hypoxic injury, the details of which are discussed in the following experimental methods; sham-operated group (abbreviated: sham group), rats underwent the same operation, without ligation of the right common carotid artery nor the hypoxia treatment; HI+bumetanide group (abbreviated: HI+Bum group), bumetanide (0.5 mg/kg, intraperitoneal injection, i.p., Cat. sc-200727, Santa Cruz) was diluted with saline and administered 5 min after HI; bumetanide, an inhibitor of NKCC1, served as positive group in our study. HI+vitexin group (abbreviated: HI+Vit group), vitexin (45 mg/kg, intraperitoneal injection, i.p., Cat. E-0310, Tauto Biotech) was diluted with saline and administered 5 min after HI.

### Neonatal hypoxia-ischemia model

All procedures of the neonatal HI model in this study were based on the Rice-Vanucci study [47, 48]. Animal surgical procedures and experimental protocols were reviewed and approved by the Committee on the Ethics of Animal Experiments of Wuhan University (China). Briefly, P7 SD rats (13–19 g, equal males and females have been chosen for each group) were anesthetized by inhalation of isoflurane. The right common carotid artery (CCA) was exposed and ligated with 5-0 surgical silk. After ligation for 2 h, the rat pups were then placed in an airtight, transparent chamber at 37 °C and exposed to 8% $O_2$ in $N_2$ for 3 h to create hypoxic injury after brain ischemia. Thereafter, the littermates were returned to their mothers when they can move freely. Meanwhile, sham-operated rats were subjected to isolation and stringing of vessels without ligation and subsequent ischemia. The rats were sacrificed at 24 h after HI insult, and their ipsilateral hemispheres were collected for follow-up experiments.

### Cell culture and oxygen glucose deprivation (OGD) progression

Lines of rat brain microvascular endothelial cells (RBMECs) were purchased from BeNa Culture Collection (Cat. BNCC337880). RBMEC cultures were expanded and maintained in 89% basal medium, 10% fetal bovine serum (FBS), and 1% penicillin/streptomycin solution (P/S). They were then incubated in a humidified atmosphere containing 5% $CO_2$ at 37 °C.

OGD was conducted as described previously. Briefly, RBMECs were grown in complete growth media as monolayers in cell culture incubator (95% $O_2$ and 5%

$CO_2$ at 37 °C). To initiate OGD in vitro, the cells at 4 DIV (days in vitro) were washed with 1× PBS three times, switched to OGD medium (serum- and glucose-free DMEM), and placed in a hypoxic/anoxic chamber (1% $O_2$, 5% $CO_2$, and 94% $N_2$ at 37 °C) to mimic OGD injury in incubator. Following the OGD carried out for 3.5 h, cells were removed from the anaerobic chamber, and the OGD medium in the cultures was then changed back to DMEM medium for an additional 24-h reperfusion under normal conditions. At the same time, control glucose-containing cultures remained in a regular incubator (5% $CO_2$ and 95% $O_2$). The supernatants and cell extracts were collected after OGD for the following experiments.

### Protein isolation and western blot

Membrane protein was extracted according to the manufacturer's protocol from cultured RBMECs and the ischemic penumbra of the rat cortex with a Membrane and Cytosol Protein Extraction Kit (Cat. P0033, Beyotime, Shanghai, China). The concentrations were determined with a BCA protein assay kit (Cat. P0012, Beyotime, Shanghai, China). Samples were denatured for 10 min at 100 °C and frozen at $-20$ °C before assay. Approximately 20 μl of the samples were separated by 8–12% SDS–PAGE gel and then transferred to polyvinylidene fluoride (PVDF) membranes. Subsequently, the membranes were blocked in 5% BSA for 1 h at room temperature following incubation with primary antibodies overnight at 4 °C. Dilutions for primary and secondary antibodies were listed in Table 1. Membranes were washed three times in TBST and specific binding was visualized by ECL reaction. The density of bands was detected using an imaging densitometer (Bio-Rad, Foster City, CA, USA), and the gray value of the bands was quantified using ImageJ Software (version 1.41).

### Real-time PCR

Total RNA was extracted from the ischemic cerebral cortices ($n = 6$ per group) for the detection of NKCC1, IL-1β, IL-6, and TNF mRNA at 24 h after HI using Trizol Reagent (Invitrogen Life Technologies Corporation, USA) according to the manufacturer's protocol. The quantity of total RNA was measured with a UV spectrophotometer (Biochrom Ltd., UK). Next, reverse transcription was performed using a cDNA synthesis kit (TaKaRa Biotechnology). Briefly, 2 μl of total RNA was combined with 4 μl of 5× Prime Script® Buffer. RNase Free ddH$_2$O was added to 20 μl, after which the mixture was heated at 37 °C for 15 min and then 85 °C for 5 s. Quantitative PCR was performed with SYBR-Green premix (Trans Gen Biotech) at the following conditions (denaturing at 95 °C for 10 s, followed by 40 cycles of 95 °C for 5 s and 60 °C for 30 s) and detected by a real-time

**Table 1** Antibodies applied for western blot

| Antibody | Host | Company | Cat. no. | Dilution | Duration |
|---|---|---|---|---|---|
| NKCC1 | Goat | Santa Cruz Biotechnology | Sc-21545 | 1:500 | Overnight 4 °C |
| ZO-1 | Rabbit | Invitrogen | RA231621 | 1:100 | Overnight 4 °C |
| β-actin | Mouse | Protein tech | HRP-60008 | 1:10000 | Overnight 4 °C |
| Anti-goat IgG-HRP | Rabbit | Protein tech | SA00001-4 | 1:1000 | 1 h RT |
| Anti-rabbit IgG-HRP | Goat | PMK Biotech | PMK-014-090 | 1:100000 | 1 h RT |

PCR system (Step One, Applied Biosystems). The expression of target genes was measured in triplicate and normalized to β-actin as an internal control. The $\Delta\Delta Ct$ values of each group were analyzed, and mRNA expression levels were normalized to $2-\Delta\Delta Ct$. Primers are listed in Table 2 (Sangon Biotech, Shanghai, Co., Ltd.).

### Enzyme-linked immunosorbent assay (ELISA)

The protein concentrations of IL-1β, IL-6, and TNF in each group of animals were quantified using an ELISA kit (purchased from 4A Biotech Co., Ltd) according to the manufacturer's instruction. Absorbance at 450 nm was recorded and the concentration of the target protein was calculated according to the standard curve and normalized against the protein of the samples. Result was expressed as pg/mg protein.

### Immunofluorescence

Immunofluorescence staining was carried out to detect ZO-1 and CD31 expression in peri-ischemic brain tissue or ZO-1, NKCC1, and F-actin expression in RBMECs.

Rats in each group were deeply anesthetized with 10% chloral hydrate and transcardially perfused first with PBS and then fixed in 4% paraformaldehyde solution at room temperature, dehydrated, and embedded in paraffin at 24 h after HI. Post-fixation, the brains were removed and cryoprotected in 20% sucrose and 30% sucrose solutions and dehydrated by 30% sucrose for 72 h at 4 °C. Serial coronal sections (5-µm-thick with injury epicenter located centrally) prepared with cryotome (Leica, Wetzlar, Germany) were used for immunofluorescence labeling. Sections were incubated with a blocking solution (5% FBS) for 30 min at 37 °C. The tissue slices were then incubated overnight with the anti-ZO-1 and anti-CD31 antibodies. On the following day, the

**Table 2** Primer sequences applied for q-PCR

| Primer | Forward prime 5'-3' | Reverse prime 5'-3' |
|---|---|---|
| NKCC1 | AGACTTCAACTCAGCCACTGT | CAAGGTCAAACCTCCATCATCA |
| ZO-1 | TTGCCACACTGTGACCCTAA | GTTCACACTGCTTAGTCCAGC |
| IL-1β | GGAACCCGTGTCTTCCTAAAG | CTGACTTGGCAGAGGACAAAG |
| IL-6 | TAGTCCTTCCTACCCCAATTTCC | TTGGTCCTTAGCCACTACTTC |
| TNF | CCAACAAGGAGGAGAAGTTCC | CTCTGCTTGGTGGTTTGCTAC |
| β-actin | GATCAAGATCATTGCTCCTCCTG | AGGGTGTAAAACGCAGCTCA |

sections protected from light were washed and subsequently incubated with secondary antibodies Cy3-conjugated Goat Anti-Rabbit IgG (H+L) and Alexa Fluor® 488 Conjugates for 2 h at 37 °C. Dilutions for antibodies were listed in Table 3. Images were obtained using a confocal microscope (Leica-LCS-SP8-STED).

For the assessment of ZO-1, NKCC1, and F-actin expression in RBMECs, cells were fixed with methanol, washed with PBS-T, and incubated at 4 °C with anti-NKCC1, anti-F-actin, and anti-ZO-1 antibodies. Subsequently, cells were washed with PBS-T before incubation with mixtures of secondary antibodies: Alexa Fluor® 488 Conjugates, Cy3-conjugated Rabbit Anti-Goat IgG (H+L), and Cy3-conjugated Goat Anti-Rabbit IgG (H+L) diluted in blocking buffer for 2 h in the dark at room temperature. Dilutions for antibodies were also listed in Table 3. The cells were washed three times in PBS-T before they were mounted using DAPI. Finally, cellular co-localization was captured using confocal microscope (Leica-LCS-SP8-STED).

### Immunohistochemistry

To evaluate the expression of NKCC1and the severity of HI-induced inflammation, the slices from paraffin-embedded tissues were subjected to immunohistochemical staining for NKCC1 and myeloperoxidase (MPO), respectively. MPO is a representative marker of neutrophils and is an important index for evaluating the severity of inflammation. It also reflects the extent of inflammation in brain tissue [49]. The sections were washed with PBS and blocked in 5% BSA for 2 h. Thereafter, the primary antibody goat anti-NKCC and rabbit anti-MPO polyclonal antibody were applied. After being rinsed with PBS, the sections were incubated with corresponding secondary antibodies, and nuclei were stained with DAPI. Images were obtained using a confocal laser-scanning microscope (Leica-LCS-SP8-STED).

### Phalloidin staining

For visualization of cytoskeleton F-actin, the cultured RBMECs were processed for direct confocal imaging with FITC-conjugated phalloidin (Cat. P5282, Sigma), which specifically combines with F-actin. Monolayers were rinsed with PBS solution, fixed with 4% paraformaldehyde for 30 min at 4 °C, and permeabilized with

**Table 3** Antibodies applied for flow cytometry, immunohistochemistry, and fluorescence staining

| Antibody | Host | Company | Cat. no. | Dilution | Applied | Stored |
|---|---|---|---|---|---|---|
| NKCC1 | Goat | Santa Cruz | Sc-21545 | 1:50 | ICC,FCM,IHC | Overnight 4 °C |
| NeuN | Mouse | Millipore | #2742283 | 1:100 | ICC | Overnight 4 °C |
| Phalloidin | | Sigma | P5282 | 5 µg/ml | ICC | 1 h RT |
| Alexa Fluor® 488 | Mouse | Cell Signaling Technology | #4408 | 1:250 | ICC | 1 h RT |
| Anti-goat IgG-Cy3 | Rabbit | Protein tech | SA00009-4 | 1:50 | ICC | 1 h RT |
| Anti-rabbit IgG-Cy3 | Goat | Protein tech | SA00009-2 | 1:50 | ICC | 1 h RT |
| ZO-1 | Rabbit/IgG | Invitrogen | RA231621 | 0.25 mg/ml | ICC,IF | Overnight 4 °C |
| MPO | Rabbit | Abcam | ab9535 | 1:100 | IHC | Overnight 4 °C |
| CD31 | Mouse | Thermo Fisher Scientific | MA3100 | 1:50 | IF | Overnight 4 °C |
| Anti-rabbit IgG | Goat | PMK Biotech | PMK-014-090 | 1:100000 | IHC | 1 h RT |
| F-actin | Mouse | Abcam | ab205 | 1:100 | ICC | Overnight 4 °C |
| Anti-goat IgG-FITC | Rabbit | Protein tech | SA00003-4 | 1:50 | ICC | 1 h RT |
| DAPI | | Beyotime | C1002 | 1:2000 | ICC,IF,IHC | 1 min RT |

0.3% Triton X-100 for 30 min. The cells were incubated with FITC-phalloidin (5 µg/ml, Sigma) for 1 h at room temperature in the dark. Cells were then counterstained with DAPI for nuclear labelling. Visualization was performed with a Leica-LCS-SP8-STED confocal microscope (Leica Microsystems).

## Measurement of intracellular Cl⁻ concentration ($[Cl^-]_i$)

$N$-(ethoxycarbonylmethyl)-6-methoxyquinolinium bromide (MQAE), a chloride-sensitive fluorescent indicator inversely related to intracellular chloride ion concentration, was used to detect $[Cl^-]_i$ as previously described [50]. This dye detects the ion via diffusion-limited collisional quenching. The cultured RBMECs were then incubated with 10 mM MQAE (Cat. E3101, Invitrogen) in a Kreb HEPES-buffered isotonic solution [DMEM, 0.1% BSA, 10 mM 4-(2-hydroxyethyl)-1 piperazine-ethanesulfonic acid (HEPES), pH 7.5] for 1 h at 37 °C in the dark. Subsequently, cells were washed with DMEM three times. Fluorescence was excited every 60 s at 340 nm, and emission fluorescence at 460 nm was recorded. Images were collected and analyzed with the Image-Pro Plus 6.0 image-processing software.

## Flow cytometry

The number of NKCC1⁺ RBMECs was analyzed by flow cytometry. Single-cell suspensions were harvested at 24 h after OGD and flushed with PBS. The suspensions were then stained with fluorescently labeled antibodies, anti-NKCC1 antibody, and FITC rabbit anti-goat antibodies. The staining was performed according to the manufacturer's instructions. Flow

cytometric analysis was performed using Flow Jo (version 9.2; Tree Star Inc.).

## Electrode implantation and EEG recording

For the recording of the electrical activity of the brain, electrodes were implanted in rats ($n = 15$ per group) on P28. The rats were anesthetized with 10% chloral hydrate (3 ml/kg) and then fixed into the stereotaxic apparatus. The electrodes were bipolar twisted silver steel and embedded in the skull with dental cement. These electrodes were implanted into the bilateral hippocampal CA3 (3.5 mm posterior to bregma, 3.5 mm lateral, 3.5 mm ventral to the dura mater), according to the coordinates derived from the atlas of Paxinos and Watson. Spontaneous EEG seizures in the dentate gyrus were recorded in freely moving animals after 3 days of recovery, which were then individually placed in a cage and connected to a neurophysiology workstation (AD Instruments Lab Chart 8) through a flexible cable that prevents twisting [51]. The frequency and mean duration of these spontaneous EEG seizures during an EEG recording session were examined for 2 h. The EEG signals were digitized with Lab Chart software (AD Instruments). Seizure severity was classified into five levels by Racine's scale [52]: I, facial movement; II, head nodding; III, unilateral forelimb clonus; IV, bilateral forelimb clonus; V, tonic clonic seizure, rearing, and failing. The rats in which seizure severity reached a level III were identified as grand mal seizure disorder. Seizures were also identified by consistent changes in the power of the fast Fourier transform of EEG, including changes in the frequency of activity during the course of the event. These criteria have been used successfully by experts in the field [53].

## Statistical analysis

Statistical differences between groups were analyzed with either an unpaired $t$ test or one-way analysis of variance (ANOVA) where appropriate. Post hoc analysis was performed with the Newman-Keuls multiple-comparison test. Differences were considered statistically significant at a critical value of $*P < 0.05$. All values are presented as the mean ± standard error of the mean (SEM).

## Results

### NKCC1 mRNA and protein expression in the peri-ischemic brain tissue

To determine the profile of NKCC1, we analyzed the protein and mRNA expression of NKCC1 at 24 h following HI. We induced the HI model in P7 neonatal rats, and samples were extracted from the ipsilateral cerebral cortex at 24 h after HI (Fig. 1a). Our results showed an upregulation of the protein and mRNA expression of NKCC1 in the peri-ischemic brain tissue. The optical density of the immune-reactive bands of NKCC1 protein levels that appeared at approximately 170 kDa were significantly increased at 24 h following HI compared with that in the sham group (Fig. 1c). However, after treatment with vitexin, the structure of which is depicted in Fig. 1b, the optical density was decreased significantly when compared with the optical density in ischemic rats (Fig. 1d, $*P < 0.05$). NKCC1 mRNA expression was significantly increased in the peri-ischemic brain tissue at 24 h following HI rats in comparison with the expression in the sham-operated rats. However, after treatment with bumetanide, which acted as a positive control, or vitexin, the level of NKCC1 mRNA expression in the peri-ischemic brain tissue was significantly decreased when compared with that in the ischemic rats (Fig. 1e, $*P < 0.05$). Moreover, we performed immunohistochemistry of coronal sections from the ipsilateral cortex to detect NKCC1$^+$ cells using anti-NKCC1 antibody (Fig. 1f, gf, $***P < 0.001$). NKCC1$^+$ cells were rarely observed in the sham-operated rats, whereas they were more abundant and more extensively distributed in the HI group, particularly in the ischemic penumbra (Fig. 1f, g). After treatment with bumetanide or vitexin, NKCC1$^+$ cells in the ipsilateral penumbra were dramatically reduced compared with those in the HI group (Fig. 1f, g). In addition, NKCC1 is located predominantly in the luminal membrane of BBB endothelial cells in situ [54, 55].

### Expression of NKCC1 in RBMECs after OGD treatment

Our previous studies have shown that vitexin has a protective effect on the BBB in HI neonatal brain injury [47]. To further investigate the mechanisms underlying HI-induced BBB disruption, we adopted an in vitro BBB model composed of a monolayer of RBMECs and subjected this model to the ischemia-like insult OGD for 3.5 h [47]. Subsequently, the expression of NKCC1 in RBMECs was confirmed by confocal imaging (Fig. 2a).

To further confirm NKCC1 expression in RBMECs under different conditions, flow cytometry was also used. As shown in Fig. 2b, the number of NKCC1-positive cells increased after OGD compared to that in controls. The cell quantities in both the bumetanide (100 mM; 24 h) and vitexin (100 mM; 24 h) groups were decreased compared to those in the OGD group. In addition, we performed MQAE to analyze the concentration of Cl$^-$ in RBMECs (Fig. 2c). This was studied by preloading the cells with the Cl$^-$ fluorescent indicator, MQAE, with subsequent analysis of the changes in fluorescence that occurred with changes in the intracellular Cl$^-$ levels, which were inversely related to the intracellular chloride ion concentration ($[Cl^-]_i$). Compared with the fluorescence intensity in the controls, the fluorescence intensity of RBMECs was significantly decreased in the OGD group, indicating that $[Cl^-]_i$ was enhanced following OGD (Fig. 2d). Fluorescence was dramatically decreased with treatment with bumetanide or vitexin. Taken together, these results suggested that vitexin effectively suppresses intracellular $[Cl^-]_i$, which indirectly represents the expression of NKCC1.

### Vitexin rapidly reduces actin stress fiber expression in RBMECs after OGD

In addition to its conventional function as an ion transporter, NKCC1 also modulates cell migration ability by interacting with the cytoskeleton and acting as an anchor that transduces contractile forces [27, 28]. We therefore examined the NKCC1-positive cells co-stained with the F-actin antibody with confocal microscopy. Our results showed that NKCC1 was localized to F-actin in cultured RBMECs at 24 h following HI (Fig. 3a–c). We also investigated the effects of vitexin on cytoskeletal proteins in RBMECs after OGD (Fig. 3d, e). Representative confocal images of RBMECs showed F-actin cytoskeleton staining with FITC-phalloidin. In the control group, phalloidin staining in RBMECs demonstrated no obvious stress fiber formation, which appeared as large bundles of actin filaments. Instead, the cells showed an apparent increase in stress fiber formation in the OGD group. Treatment of OGD-exposed cells with bumetanide (100 mM; 24 h) or vitexin (100 mM; 24 h) resulted in a decrease in F-actin stress fiber formation (Fig. 3b).

Consistent with the above findings, western blot analysis of lysates from cultured RBMECs also proved that the significant increase in F-actin levels after OGD could be rescued by bumetanide (100 mM; 24 h) or vitexin (100 mM; 24 h) treatment (Fig. 3c). These results further validated our hypothesis that vitexin inhibits OGD-induced stress fiber formation in RBMECs through the NKCC1/F-actin pathway.

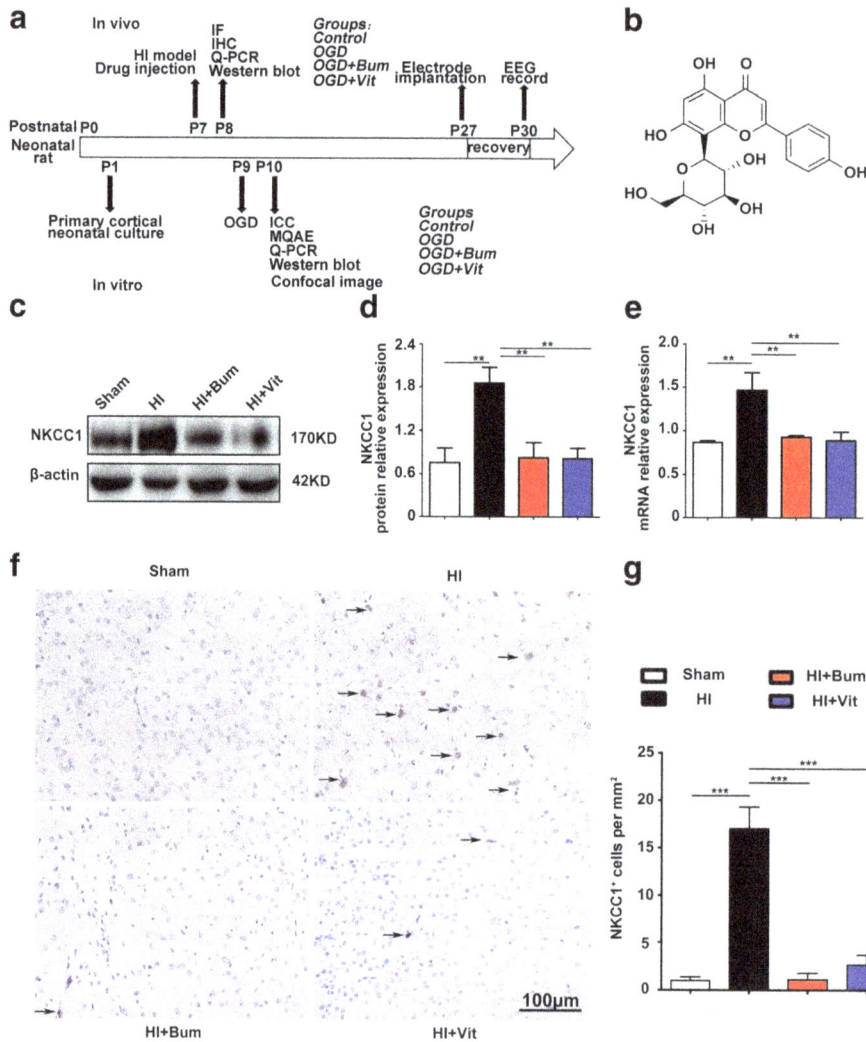

**Fig. 1** Structure and effect of vitexin on HI-induced NKCC1 expression in hypoxia-ischemia brain tissue. **a** Diagram of the experimental design. **b** The structure of vitexin. **c**, **d** Representative protein expression levels of NKCC1 (170 kDa) and β-actin (42 kDa) in the cerebral tissue of the sham, HI, HI+Bum, and HI+Vit groups were evaluated. **e** The graphical representation of the fold changes in NKCC1 mRNA expression in each group as quantified by normalization to β-actin as an internal control. Data are shown as the mean ± SEM; **$P < 0.01$ compared to the HI group, $n = 4$ per group, based on a one-way ANOVA. **f** Cortical penumbral regions of coronal sections from the rats of each group were subjected to immunohistochemistry using an anti-NKCC1 antibody, and stereological counts of NKCC1$^+$ cells (arrows) in each group are shown. Scale bar = 100 μm. **g** The graph shows the mean number of NKCC1$^+$ cells per square millimeter. Data are expressed as the mean ± SEM; one-way ANOVA, ***$P < 0.005$ in comparison with the HI group, $n = 4$ per group

## Vitexin restored the expression of ZO-1 and alleviated BBB breakdown

Robust actin polymerization and stress fiber formation in RBMECs lead to cell contraction and redistribution/disassembly of tight-junction proteins (TJs) [48]. Confocal imaging demonstrated that OGD weakened ZO-1 expression at extracellular cell–cell contact sites (Fig. 4a). In the control group, the subcellular location of ZO-1 was presented continuously at the RBMEC membrane, outlining the points of cell–cell contact and presumably the TJs. When cells were exposed to OGD, ZO-1 showed a discontinuous and diffuse pattern of staining at regions of cell–cell contact (Fig. 4a). Compared with the OGD group, those treated with vitexin exhibited more areas where the membrane-bound location of ZO-1 was maintained (Fig. 4a).

Alteration in TJ-associated proteins such as ZO-1 has been reported to contribute to the loss of BBB function in many CNS diseases and disorders [56]. Next, ZO-1 expression in the brain tissue from animals of each group was detected by immunofluorescence staining. ZO-1 expression was greatly reduced in CD31-positive capillaries in the ischemic penumbra region, which is indicative of a damaged BBB (Fig. 4b). However, after

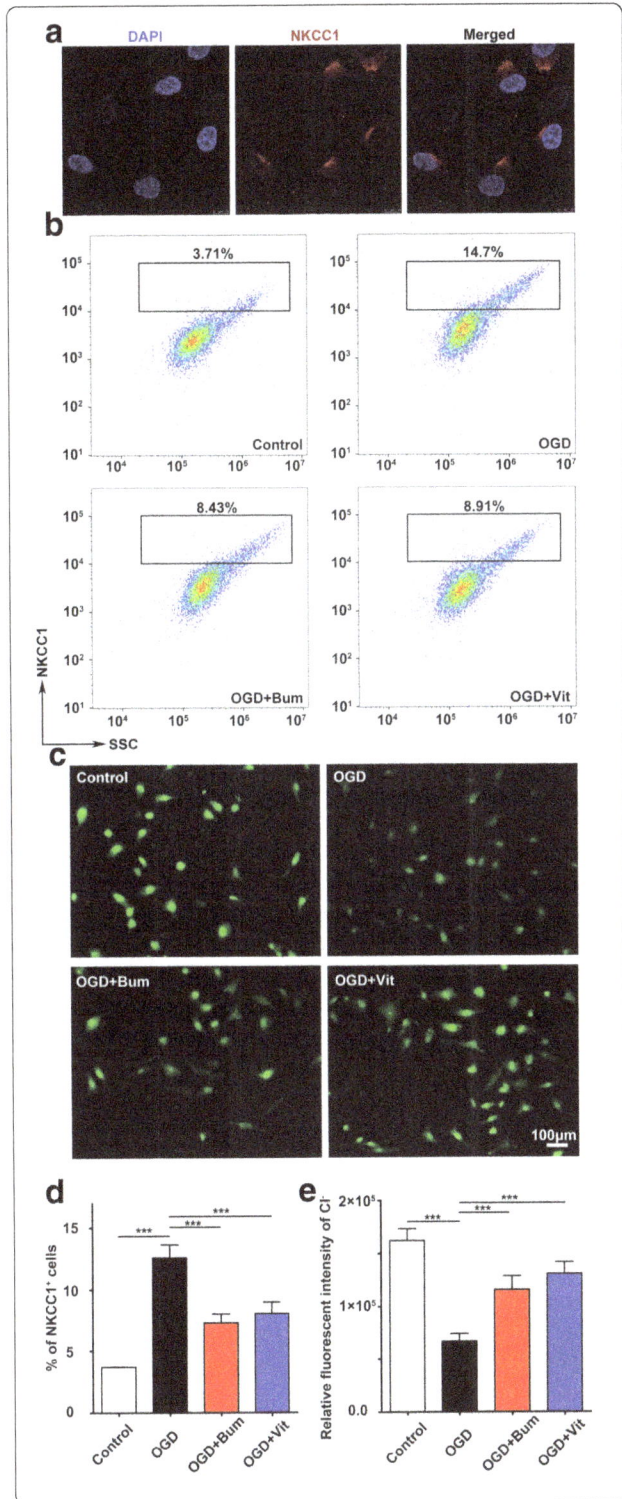

Fig. 2 Expression of NKCC1 in RBMECs after OGD. a Confocal image demonstrated that NKCC1 expression was localized in RBMECs. RBMECs were fixed and stained with anti-NKCC1 (red) and DAPI-stained nuclei (blue) in the control group, OGD conditions, OGD+Bum group, and OGD+Vit group. Images shown are representative of at least three independent experiments. b, d Flow cytometry analysis and the quantification of NKCC1-positive cell numbers in RBMECs. Cells were obtained at 24 h after OGD and were subjected to analysis using a flow cytometer after being immunostained with NKCC1 antibodies. Representative results from three to four tests of NKCC1-positive cells from each group are shown. c, e Fluorescence imaging of Cl⁻ via MQAE stained in RBMECs. The green fluorescence indicated the intracellular level of Cl⁻ in RBMECs and the fluorescence intensity of the controls was high while the RBMECs subjected to OGD were markedly decreased. These changes are readily reversible after treatment of OGD-exposed cells with bumetanide (100 mM; 24 h) or vitexin (100 mM; 24 h). Data are shown as the mean ± SEM; $***P < 0.005$ compared to the OGD condition, $n = 8\sim10$ per group, scale bar = 100 μm, based on a one-way ANOVA

western blotting and q-PCR also proved that the significant reduction in ZO-1 expression after HI could be rescued by vitexin treatment (Fig. 4c, d). Based on these experiments, we concluded that vitexin protected ischemic brain damage through increasing ZO-1 expression, which consequently improved the integrity of the BBB and protected vasogenic edema.

### Vitexin reduces hypoxia-ischemia-induced neutrophil infiltration and IL-1β, IL-6, and TNF expression

Mounting evidence suggests that inflammation is a key contributor to the severity of CNS hypoxia-ischemia injury. In rats subjected to 3.5 h of HI, their ipsilateral hemispheres displayed an inflammatory response as shown by increased expression of hallmark cytokines such as IL-1β, IL-6, and TNF. We further evaluated changes in the mRNA and protein levels of pro-inflammatory cytokine at 24 h after HI insult by q-PCR and ELISA. We demonstrated that HI caused a significant increasement ($***P < 0.001$) in the secretion of IL-1β, IL-6, and TNF when compared to sham treatment. However, treatment with vitexin (45 mg/kg) reduced IL-β, IL-6, and TNF mRNA at 24 h after HI (Fig. 5a–c, $*P < 0.05$, $***P < 0.001$). Correspondingly, a significant decrease of protein levels of IL-β, IL-6, and TNF had also been detected (Fig. 5d–f). In sum, these results illustrate that vitexin is a potent suppressor of HI-induced inflammation. To investigate the effect of vitexin on neutrophil infiltration into ipsilateral hemispheres at 24 h after HI, we performed immunohistochemistry of coronal sections from the ipsilateral cortex to detect MPO⁺ cells

treatment with bumetanide or vitexin, a certain degree of rescue of ZO-1 expression was observed, suggesting that BBB destruction after HI was attenuated. Similarly,

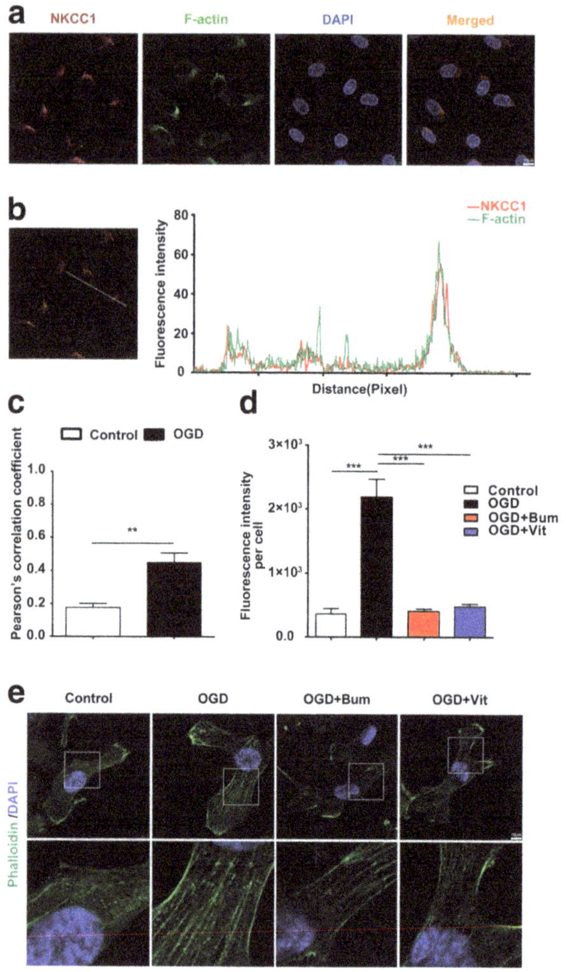

**Fig. 3** Vitexin downregulated F-actin expression in RBMECs after OGD. FITC-conjugated phalloidin staining for F-actin⁺ stress fiber formation demonstrated changes in cytoskeletal assembly following OGD in RBMECs. **a** Confocal images show co-localization of NKCC1 and F-actin in RBMECs. Scale bar = 10 μm. **b** Merged views of indicated NKCC1 show complete co-localization (**b**, left). A side overlap of two peaks was taken as a partial co-localization (**b**, right). **c** Pearson's correlation coefficient is shown in graph (**c**) from five independent experiments analyzed. **d**, **e** The distribution of F-actin⁺ stress fibers was shown by confocal imaging in Control, OGD, OGD +Bum, and OGD+Vit groups. Arrows indicate actin stress fiber formation. The intensity of F-actin fluorescence was determined in 10 fields/well and divided by the number of cells counterstained with DAPI. Each experimental group consisted of three replicates. Scale bar = 10 μm

using anti-MPO antibodies. MPO activity is an indicator of inflammation and is used to evaluate neutrophil accumulation [57]. Neutrophils were rarely observed in the sham-operated rats, whereas they were more abundant and more extensively distributed in the HI group, particularly in the ischemic penumbra (Fig. 5g, h). After treatment with bumetanide or vitexin, the number of MPO⁺ cells in the ipsilateral penumbra was dramatically reduced compared with that in the

HI group (Fig. 5g, h). Collectively, these findings strongly suggest that vitexin can reduce the infiltration of neutrophils to a large extent under HI conditions.

### Effects of vitexin on the spontaneous EEG seizures

Based on a previous study, we provided evidence that hypoxia-ischemia induced neonatal seizure which is thought to contribute to abnormal brain activity [51]. We therefore performed EEG monitoring to examine whether vitexin treatment in the early phase after HI has a long-term effect on HI rats. Rats were sorted into a sham group, HI group, or vitexin treatment group at P30 (Fig. 1a). The P7 rats were treated with HI and were then injected with vitexin (45 mg/kg, 5 min after HI). Electrodes were implanted in rats ($n = 15$ per group) on P28, and after 3 days of recovery, spontaneous EEG seizures were recorded in freely moving animals (Fig. 6a). During the EEG recording session, no spontaneous EEG seizures were observed in rats in the sham group. Rats in the HI+Vit group, which were given an intraperitoneal injection of vitexin, exhibited less intense spontaneous EEG seizures than rats in the HI group. Vitexin-treated animals also exhibited a marked reduction in the mean duration of spontaneous EEG seizures from 38.22 s/seizures (min. 14.0 s/seizures; max. 61.0 s/seizures) in the HI group to 7.75 s/seizures (min. 5.0 s/seizures; max. 21.0 s/seizures) in the HI+Vit group (Fig. 6b). Also, vitexin treatment significantly decreased the frequency of spontaneous EEG seizures in rats in the HI+Vit group (0.62 (min. 0; max. 2)) compared with the frequency in rats in the HI group (1.72 (min. 1; max. 3); Fig. 6b; *$P < 0.05$). Taken together, our results demonstrated that treatment with vitexin during a vulnerable period was able to decrease pentylenetetrazol (PTZ)-induced seizure in rats after HI.

### Discussion

In this research, we revealed that vitexin could be an effective neuroprotective agent to reduce the severity of seizures in hypoxic-ischemic rat model. Such neuroprotective effects were potentially mediated through inhibition of NKCC1/F-actin expression, which subsequently improved the tight junctions and, therefore, the integrity of the BBB and reduced infiltration of neutrophils. In summary, our data showed a previously unexplored mechanism by which vitexin exerts its neuroprotective effect after HI-induced injury through diminished NKCC1 expression.

Flavonoids are polyphenolic structures that are naturally present in most plants and consumed daily with no adverse effects reported. Of interest, flavonoids and their glycosides have been shown to exert mild to potent activity in several seizure and epilepsy

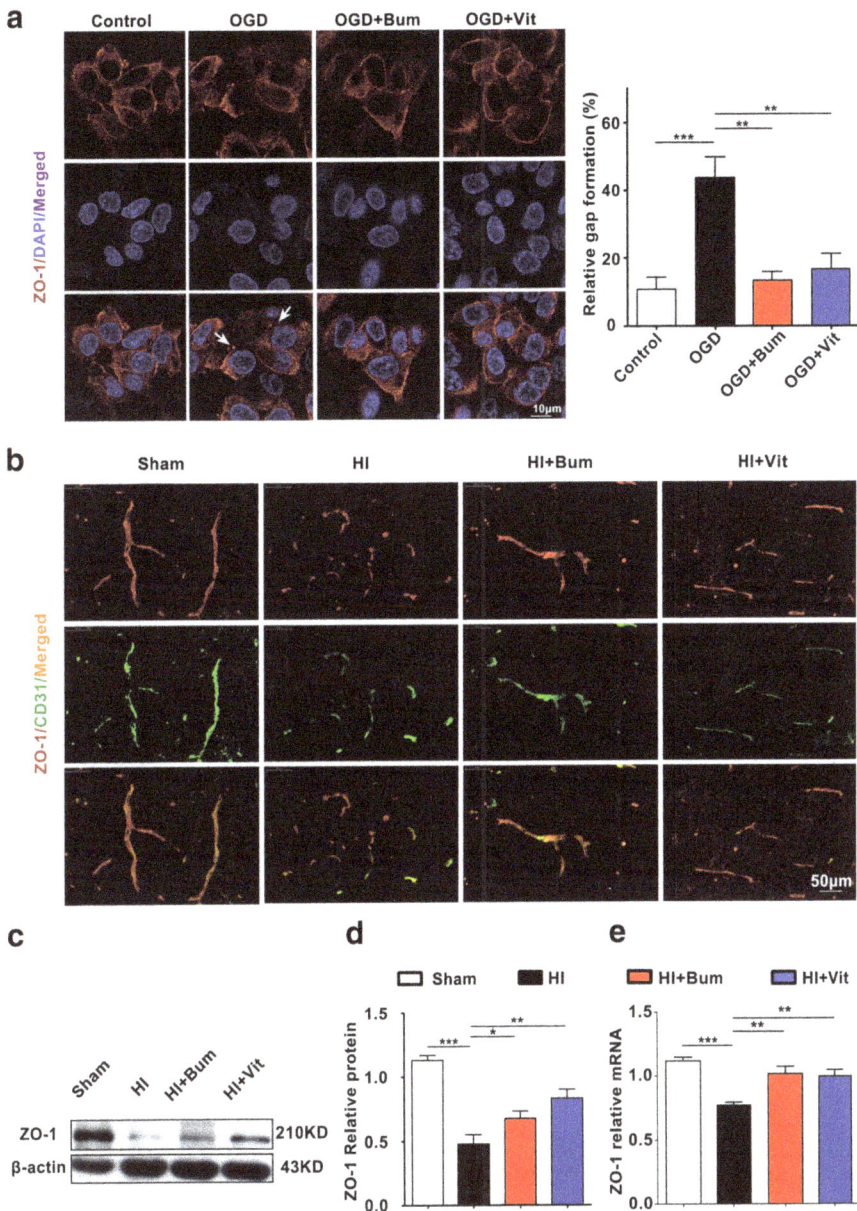

**Fig. 4** Vitexin inhibited HI-induced BBB destruction assayed by tight junction-related ZO-1. **a** TJs are characteristically located at cell–cell contact sites and are intact under physiological conditions. Confocal image of ZO-1 demonstrated disruption of the tight junctions and gap formation following OGD in RBMECs. Arrows indicate tight junction disruption. Scale bar = 50 μm. **b** Immunofluorescence staining for ZO-1 (red) and CD31 (green), a capillary endothelia marker, in the ischemic cortex of the sham, HI, HI+Bum, and HI+Vit groups 24 h after HI. Merged images of ZO-1 and CD31 staining are also shown. Scale bar = 50 μm. **c**, **d** Representative western blot for ZO-1 protein levels in the cerebral cortex from rats of each group. Densitometric value of the protein bands normalized to the respective β-actin is also shown. *$P < 0.05$, **$P < 0.01$, ***$P < 0.001$. **e** The mRNA expression of ZO-1 in the ipsi-ischemic brain tissue of each group was analyzed by real-time quantitative PCR. Data are shown as the mean ± SEM; **$P < 0.01$, ***$P < 0.001$ in comparison with the HI group, $n = 4$~6 per group, based on a one-way ANOVA

animal models [58, 59]. Investigations of the underlying mechanism of action have led to the assumption that these structures allosterically modulate $GABA_A$ receptors by binding to the benzodiazepine receptor site [46]. Thus, vitexin seems to be a ligand for benzodiazepine receptors [44–46]. To the best of our knowledge, there has been no report on the antiepileptic effect of vitexin in an HI-induced epileptic rat model (Fig. 7).

Many of the available anti-seizure drugs block seizures by enhancing inhibitory $GABA_A$ receptor activity in the brain. The inhibitory activity of $GABA_A$ receptor activation depends on low $[Cl^-]_i$, which is modulated by the opposing regulation of NKCC1 and KCC2 in neurons

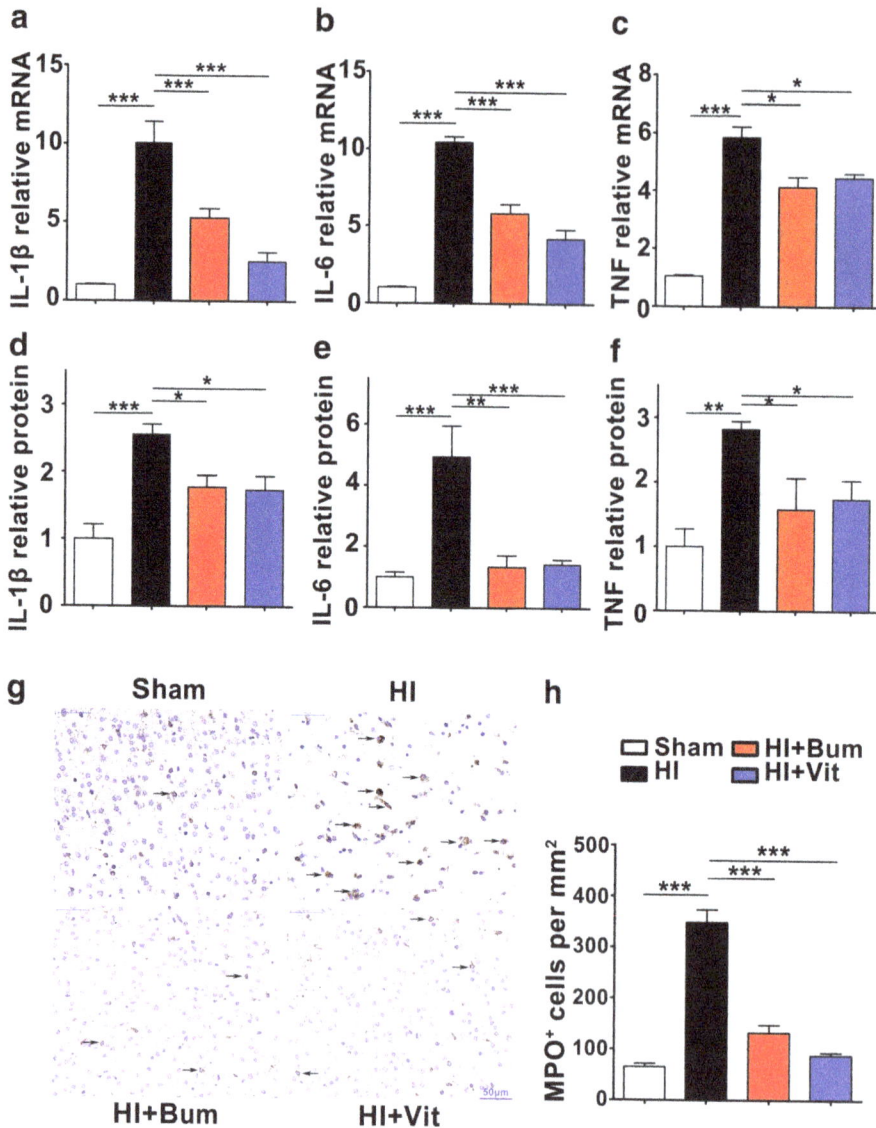

**Fig. 5** Vitexin alleviated HI-induced neutrophil infiltration and inflammatory cytokine expression. Panels **a**, **b**, and **c** show the graphical representation of the fold changes in IL-1β, IL-6, and TNF mRNA, respectively. Relative protein levels of IL-1β (**d**), IL-6 (**e**), and TNF (**f**) in brain tissue samples were measured with ELISA. Data were normalized against the protein level of the sham group, from six separate experiments. **g** Cortical penumbral regions of coronal sections from the rats of each group were subjected to immunohistochemistry using an anti-MPO antibody, and stereological counts of MPO⁺ cells (arrows) in each group are shown. Scale bar = 50 μm. **h** The graph shows the mean number of MPO⁺ cells per square millimeter. Data are expressed as the mean ± SEM; one-way ANOVA, *$P < 0.05$, **$P < 0.01$, ***$P < 0.001$ in comparison with the HI group, $n = 5$ per group

[60, 61]. NKCC1 is frequently expressed in developing CNS regions, and its activity has been associated with the depolarizing actions of GABA [62, 63]. The increase in NKCC1 levels has been shown to be involved in neonatal seizures [64, 65]. Inappropriate activation and increased expression of NKCC1 will contribute to increased $[Cl^-]_i$, which in turn renders GABAergic input less inhibitory and more seizure-prone. Thus, we sought drugs targeting NKCC1 to reduce seizures by lowering $[Cl^-]_i$. Taken together, our results are the first to reveal that vitexin disturbs the expression of NKCC1 in vivo and in vitro, which may subsequently protect the brain against seizures.

With regard to the fact that seizures are a process that includes BBB dysfunction and neuronal death, we aimed to investigate the protective role of vitexin in seizures. A previous study on other flavonoids proved its neuroprotective effect after SAH in rats through upregulating the expression of ZO-1 and occludin following subarachnoid hemorrhage (SAH), which was closely related to the

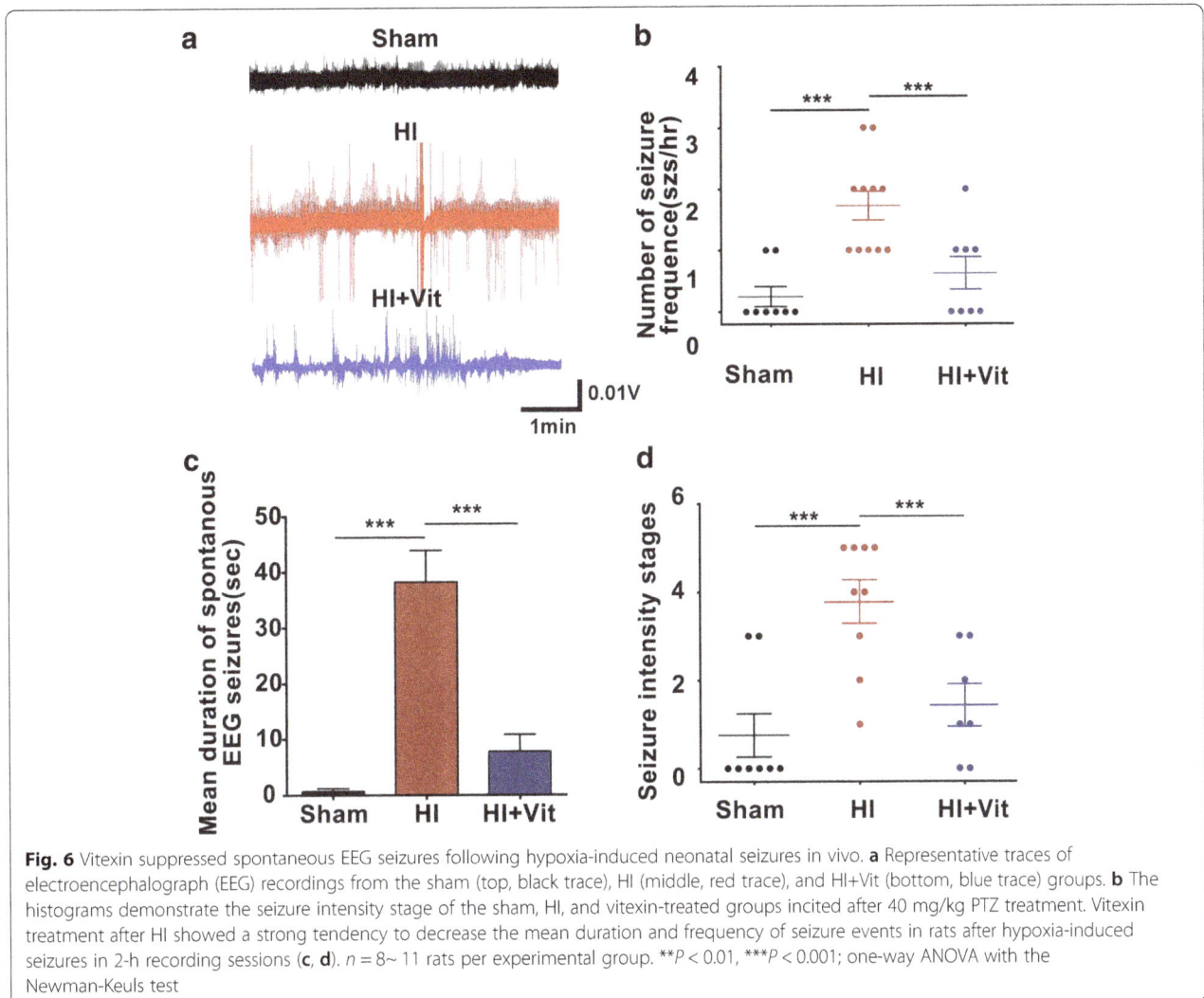

**Fig. 6** Vitexin suppressed spontaneous EEG seizures following hypoxia-induced neonatal seizures in vivo. **a** Representative traces of electroencephalograph (EEG) recordings from the sham (top, black trace), HI (middle, red trace), and HI+Vit (bottom, blue trace) groups. **b** The histograms demonstrate the seizure intensity stage of the sham, HI, and vitexin-treated groups incited after 40 mg/kg PTZ treatment. Vitexin treatment after HI showed a strong tendency to decrease the mean duration and frequency of seizure events in rats after hypoxia-induced seizures in 2-h recording sessions (**c**, **d**). $n = 8 \sim 11$ rats per experimental group. $**P < 0.01$, $***P < 0.001$; one-way ANOVA with the Newman-Keuls test

integrity of the BBB [28]. Injuries such as ischemia and traumatic brain injury lead to a disruption and reconstruction of ZO-1 and occludin and an increase in BBB permeability [57]. Studies have demonstrated that hypoxia mainly influences the distribution of ZO-1, resulting in a disruption of TJ proteins at cell–cell contacts and an increase in endothelial cell permeability [58]. A reduction in BBB permeability alleviates cerebral ischemia injury in both transient and permanent cerebral ischemia [57, 59, 60]. As our previous study has shown, vitexin attenuated neuronal cell death and brain edema and preserved BBB disruption after neonatal HI in a rat pup model [37]. Further research is needed to evaluate the molecular mechanism underlying BBB preservation by vitexin.

Furthermore, flavonoids are also known to exert potent anti-inflammatory effects in the brain [66] and directly modulate key components of the inflammatory cascade [67]. Concomitantly, the heightened expression of the pro-inflammatory cytokines such as IL-1β, IL-6,

TNF, and neutrophils was significantly attenuated by vitexin treatment in the HI-stimulated brain, further demonstrating diminished inflammation by this agent (Fig. 5). Our results are in partial agreement with the results of Borghi et al., which demonstrated an analgesic effect of vitexin through reducing TNF-α and IL-1β expression in mice [68]. In addition to increasing inflammatory cytokines, neutrophil infiltration also induces endothelial injury and increases BBB permeability [69].

A previous study concluded that NKCC1 not only regulates migration but also alters the actin cytoskeleton, the migratory engine of cells [19, 65]. Therefore, the relationship between NKCC1 and actin appears to be important for understanding NKCC1 functions [66]. In an effort to dissect NKCC1's role in actin regulation, we use confocal imaging to study NKCC1 protein-interacting partners. We found that NKCC1 interacts with F-actin, which plays a key role in actin polymerization/depolymerization in RBMECs (Fig. 3a, b). The disruption of the BBB and the increase in permeability were related

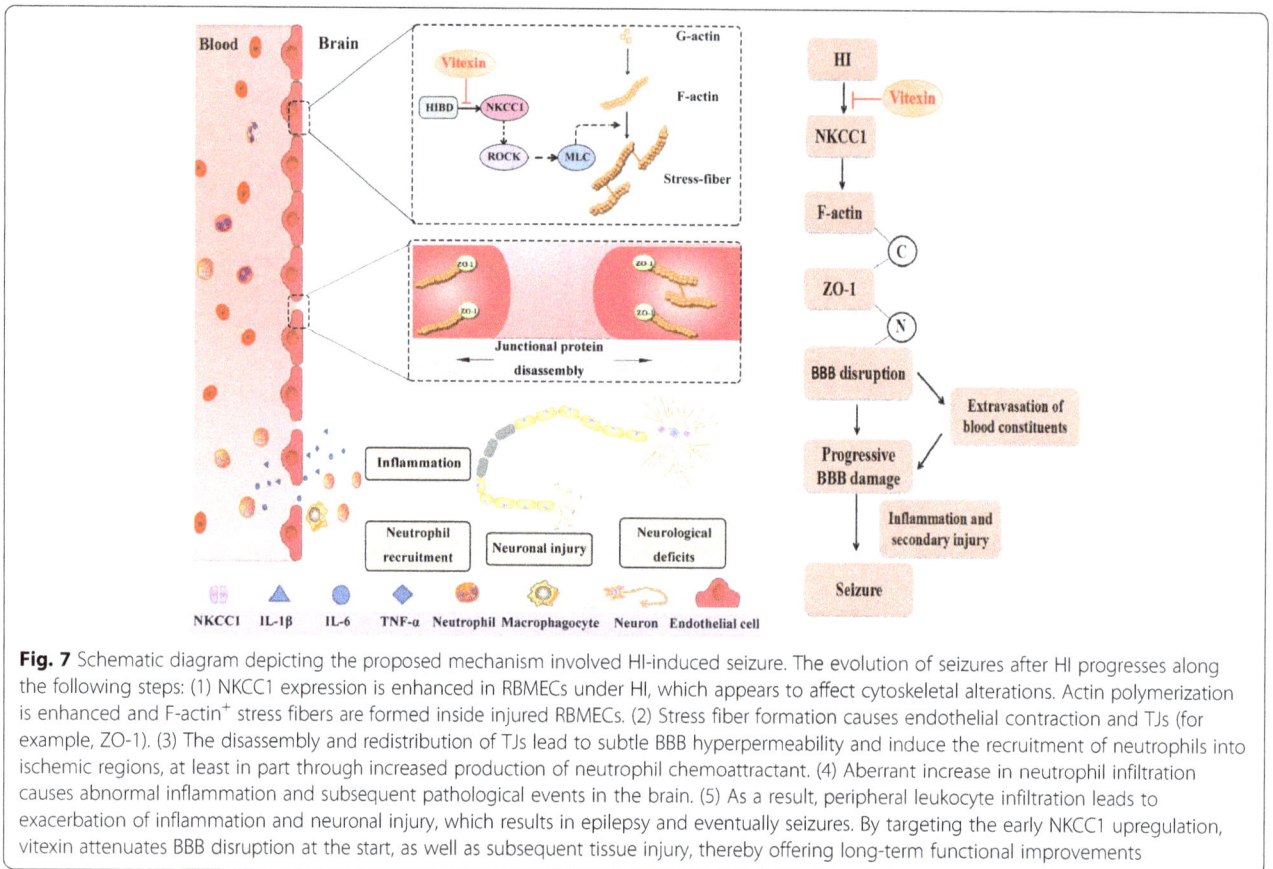

**Fig. 7** Schematic diagram depicting the proposed mechanism involved HI-induced seizure. The evolution of seizures after HI progresses along the following steps: (1) NKCC1 expression is enhanced in RBMECs under HI, which appears to affect cytoskeletal alterations. Actin polymerization is enhanced and F-actin+ stress fibers are formed inside injured RBMECs. (2) Stress fiber formation causes endothelial contraction and TJs (for example, ZO-1). (3) The disassembly and redistribution of TJs lead to subtle BBB hyperpermeability and induce the recruitment of neutrophils into ischemic regions, at least in part through increased production of neutrophil chemoattractant. (4) Aberrant increase in neutrophil infiltration causes abnormal inflammation and subsequent pathological events in the brain. (5) As a result, peripheral leukocyte infiltration leads to exacerbation of inflammation and neuronal injury, which results in epilepsy and eventually seizures. By targeting the early NKCC1 upregulation, vitexin attenuates BBB disruption at the start, as well as subsequent tissue injury, thereby offering long-term functional improvements

to increased F-actin and enhanced stress fiber formation during hypoxia/reoxygenation [29, 70–72]. In summary, we found that inhibition of NKCC1 not only controls the Cl⁻ concentration but also decreases the formation of stress fibers through regulating the actin cytoskeleton, which eventually leads to the destruction of the BBB.

In summary, our data revealed a previously unexplored neuroprotective effect of vitexin through inhibition of the NKCC1/F-actin pathway, subsequently ameliorating the BBB collapse and inflammatory responses in the context of HIBD. In addition, another potential mechanism by which vitexin inhibits the onset of epilepsy may be the direct inhibition of the occurrence of neutrophil infiltration. Therefore, with these specific properties, vitexin plays a vital role in preventing various diseases associated with NKCC1 upregulation, such as cardiovascular, glioblastoma, stroke, and neurodegenerative disease.

## Conclusions

Collectively, our results and results of previous study strongly indicate that NKCC1 is a vital contributor to secondary damage after HI in rats. Vitexin is beneficial in the treatment of ischemic insult, which potentially occurs via disturbances in the NKCC1/F-actin signaling pathways, alleviating the severity of BBB collapse, controlling inflammation, and improving neurological recovery after HI. Vitexin is a widely used drug with few adverse effects, and the utilization of this long-established drug for a new use may be a promising way to develop an effective therapy for HIBD-induced epilepsy.

**Abbreviations**
BBB: Blood-brain-barrier; DAPI: 4:6-diamidino-2-phenylindole; EEG: Electroencephalography; HIBD: Hypoxia-ischemia brain damage; HIE: Hypoxic-ischemic encephalopathy; IL-1β: Interleukin 1β; IL-6: Interleukin 6; NKCC1: Na⁺-K⁺-Cl⁻ co-transporter1; OGD: Oxygen glucose deprivation; PBS: Phosphate-buffered saline; RBMECs: Rat brain microvascular endothelial cells; TJ: Tight-junction protein; TNF: Tumor necrosis factor; ZO-1: Zona occludens-1

**Acknowledgements**
We thank Jiangjian-Hu for critically reading and revising the manuscript. We wish to sincerely thank Xingliang-Yang and Junchen-Liu for their valuable comments and for the technical assistance during the experiments. We are also grateful to Boqun-Pan from the University of Wuhan for sharing their expertise in the confocal operation.

**Funding**
This research is supported by the Natural Science Foundation of China (Grant No. 81370737, No. 81571481, and No. 81601325) and Independent Scientific Research Project Fund of Wuhan University (No. 2042017kt0066).

## Authors' contributions

LWD, PBW, and MJW conceived and designed the experiments. LWD, WX, and PYY performed the experiments. LWD, WX, and MJW analyzed the data. HXH, LWH, HS, YJ, and HWX contributed to the reagents/materials/analysis tools. LWD, PBW, and MJW wrote the paper. All authors reviewed and approved the final manuscript.

## Consent for publication

Not applicable.

## Competing interests

The authors declare that they have no competing interests.

## Author details

[1]Department of Physiology, Hubei Provincial Key Laboratory of Developmentally Originated Disorder, School of Basic Medical Sciences, Wuhan University, Hubei Donghu Rd 185#, Wuhan 430071, Hubei, China. [2]Department of Pathology, Renmin Hospital, Wuhan University, Wuhan, China. [3]Department of Pathophysiology, School of Basic Medical Sciences, Wuhan University, Wuhan, China. [4]Department of Immunology, School of Basic Medical Sciences, Wuhan University, Wuhan, China.

## References

1. Lehtonen L, Gimeno A, Parra-Llorca A, Vento M. Early neonatal death: a challenge worldwide. Semin Fetal Neonatal Med. 2017;22:153–60.
2. Bass JL, Corwin M, Gozal D, Moore C, Nishida H, Parker S, Schonwald A, Wilker RE, Stehle S, Kinane TB. The effect of chronic or intermittent hypoxia on cognition in childhood: a review of the evidence. Pediatrics. 2004;114: 805–16.
3. Graham EM, Ruis KA, Hartman AL, Northington FJ, Fox HE. A systematic review of the role of intrapartum hypoxia-ischemia in the causation of neonatal encephalopathy. Am J Obstet Gynecol. 2008;199:587–95.
4. Williams PA, Dou P, Dudek FE. Epilepsy and synaptic reorganization in a perinatal rat model of hypoxia-ischemia. Epilepsia. 2004;45:1210–8.
5. Jacobs SE, Berg M, Hunt R, Tarnow-Mordi WO, Inder TE, Davis PG. Cooling for newborns with hypoxic ischaemic encephalopathy. Cochrane Database Syst Rev. 2013;1:CD003311.
6. Tekgul H, Gauvreau K, Soul J, Murphy L, Robertson R, Stewart J, Volpe J, Bourgeois B, du Plessis AJ. The current etiologic profile and neurodevelopmental outcome of seizures in term newborn infants. Pediatrics. 2006;117:1270–80.
7. Miller SP, Ramaswamy V, Michelson D, Barkovich AJ, Holshouser B, Wycliffe N, Glidden DV, Deming D, Partridge JC, Wu YW, et al. Patterns of brain injury in term neonatal encephalopathy. J Pediatr. 2005;146:453–60.
8. Dalic L, Cook MJ. Managing drug-resistant epilepsy: challenges and solutions. Neuropsychiatr Dis Treat. 2016;12:2605–16.
9. Moshe SL, Perucca E, Ryvlin P, Tomson T. Epilepsy: new advances. Lancet. 2015;385:884–98.
10. Gluckman PD, Wyatt JS, Azzopardi D, Ballard R, Edwards AD, Ferriero DM, Polin RA, Robertson CM, Thoresen M, Whitelaw A, Gunn AJ. Selective head cooling with mild systemic hypothermia after neonatal encephalopathy: multicentre randomised trial. Lancet. 2005;365:663–70.
11. Neuwelt EA, Bauer B, Fahlke C, Fricker G, Iadecola C, Janigro D, Leybaert L, Molnar Z, O'Donnell ME, Povlishock JT, et al. Engaging neuroscience to advance translational research in brain barrier biology. Nat Rev Neurosci. 2011;12:169–82.
12. Michalak Z, Sano T, Engel T, Miller-Delaney SF, Lerner-Natoli M, Henshall DC. Spatio-temporally restricted blood-brain barrier disruption after intra-amygdala kainic acid-induced status epilepticus in mice. Epilepsy Res. 2013; 103:167–79.
13. Marchi N, Teng Q, Ghosh C, Fan Q, Nguyen MT, Desai NK, Bawa H, Rasmussen P, Masaryk TK, Janigro D. Blood-brain barrier damage, but not parenchymal white blood cells, is a hallmark of seizure activity. Brain Res. 2010;1353:176–86.
14. Kim SY, Buckwalter M, Soreq H, Vezzani A, Kaufer D. Blood-brain barrier dysfunction-induced inflammatory signaling in brain pathology and epileptogenesis. Epilepsia. 2012;53(Suppl 6):37–44.
15. Oby E, Janigro D. The blood-brain barrier and epilepsy. Epilepsia. 2006;47: 1761–74.
16. Vezzani A, Granata T. Brain inflammation in epilepsy: experimental and clinical evidence. Epilepsia. 2005;46:1724–43.
17. Fu L, Liu K, Wake H, Teshigawara K, Yoshino T, Takahashi H, Mori S, Nishibori M. Therapeutic effects of anti-HMGB1 monoclonal antibody on pilocarpine-induced status epilepticus in mice. Sci Rep. 2017;7:1179.
18. Vezzani A, French J, Bartfai T, Baram TZ. The role of inflammation in epilepsy. Nat Rev Neurol. 2011;7:31–40.
19. Hannemann A, Christie JK, Flatman PW. Functional expression of the Na-K-2Cl cotransporter NKCC2 in mammalian cells fails to confirm the dominant-negative effect of the AF splice variant. J Biol Chem. 2009;284:35348–58.
20. Haas M, Forbush B 3rd. The Na-K-Cl cotransporter of secretory epithelia. Annu Rev Physiol. 2000;62:515–34.
21. Alvarez-Leefmans FJ, Gamino SM, Giraldez F, Nogueron I. Intracellular chloride regulation in amphibian dorsal root ganglion neurones studied with ion-selective microelectrodes. J Physiol. 1988;406:225–46.
22. Chen H, Sun D. The role of Na-K-Cl co-transporter in cerebral ischemia. Neurol Res. 2005;27:280–6.
23. Mejia-Gervacio S, Murray K, Lledo PM. NKCC1 controls GABAergic signaling and neuroblast migration in the postnatal forebrain. Neural Dev. 2011;6:4.
24. Lorin-Nebel C, Boulo V, Bodinier C, Charmantier G. The Na+/K+/2Cl-cotransporter in the sea bass Dicentrarchus labrax during ontogeny: involvement in osmoregulation. J Exp Biol. 2006;209:4908–22.
25. Dzhala VI, Talos DM, Sdrulla DA, Brumback AC, Mathews GC, Benke TA, Delpire E, Jensen FE, Staley KJ. NKCC1 transporter facilitates seizures in the developing brain. Nat Med. 2005;11:1205–13.
26. Kaila K, Price TJ, Payne JA, Puskarjov M, Voipio J. Cation-chloride cotransporters in neuronal development, plasticity and disease. Nat Rev Neurosci. 2014;15:637–54.
27. Schiapparelli P, Guerrero-Cazares H, Magana-Maldonado R, Hamilla SM, Ganaha S, Goulin Lippi Fernandes E, Huang CH, Aranda-Espinoza H, Devreotes P, Quinones-Hinojosa A. NKCC1 regulates migration ability of glioblastoma cells by modulation of actin dynamics and interacting with cofilin. EBioMedicine. 2017;21:94–103.
28. Garzon-Muvdi T, Schiapparelli P, ap Rhys C, Guerrero-Cazares H, Smith C, Kim DH, Kone L, Farber H, Lee DY, An SS, et al. Regulation of brain tumor dispersal by NKCC1 through a novel role in focal adhesion regulation. PLoS Biol. 2012;10:e1001320.
29. Shi Y, Zhang L, Pu H, Mao L, Hu X, Jiang X, Xu N, Stetler RA, Zhang F, Liu X, et al. Rapid endothelial cytoskeletal reorganization enables early blood-brain barrier disruption and long-term ischaemic reperfusion brain injury. Nat Commun. 2016;7:10523.
30. Fanning AS, Jameson BJ, Jesaitis LA, Anderson JM. The tight junction protein ZO-1 establishes a link between the transmembrane protein occludin and the actin cytoskeleton. J Biol Chem. 1998;273:29745–53.
31. Cleary RT, Sun H, Huynh T, Manning SM, Li Y, Rotenberg A, Talos DM, Kahle KT, Jackson M, Rakhade SN, et al. Bumetanide enhances phenobarbital efficacy in a rat model of hypoxic neonatal seizures. PLoS One. 2013;8:e57148.
32. Gagnon M, Bergeron MJ, Lavertu G, Castonguay A, Tripathy S, Bonin RP, Perez-Sanchez J, Boudreau D, Wang B, Dumas L, et al. Chloride extrusion enhancers as novel therapeutics for neurological diseases. Nat Med. 2013;19: 1524–8.
33. Puskarjov M, Kahle KT, Ruusuvuori E, Kaila K. Pharmacotherapeutic targeting of cation-chloride cotransporters in neonatal seizures. Epilepsia. 2014;55: 806–18.
34. Marguet SL, Le-Schulte VT, Merseburg A, Neu A, Eichler R, Jakovcevski I, Ivanov A, Hanganu-Opatz IL, Bernard C, Morellini F, Isbrandt D. Treatment during a vulnerable developmental period rescues a genetic epilepsy. Nat Med. 2015;21(12):1436–44.
35. Zhang T, Su J, Guo B, Wang K, Li X, Liang G. Apigenin protects blood-brain barrier and ameliorates early brain injury by inhibiting TLR4-mediated inflammatory pathway in subarachnoid hemorrhage rats. Int Immunopharmacol. 2015;28:79–87.
36. Wang CX, Xie GB, Zhou CH, Zhang XS, Li T, Xu JG, Li N, Ding K, Hang CH, Shi JX, Zhou ML. Baincalein alleviates early brain injury after experimental subarachnoid hemorrhage in rats: possible involvement of TLR4/NF-kappaB-mediated inflammatory pathway. Brain Res. 2015;1594:245–55.
37. Cheng X, Yang YL, Yang H, Wang YH, Du GH. Kaempferol alleviates LPS-induced neuroinflammation and BBB dysfunction in mice via inhibiting HMGB1 release and down-regulating TLR4/MyD88 pathway. Int Immunopharmacol. 2018;56:29–35.

38. Lv H, Yu Z, Zheng Y, Wang L, Qin X, Cheng G, Ci X. Isovitexin exerts anti-inflammatory and anti-oxidant activities on lipopolysaccharide-induced acute lung injury by inhibiting MAPK and NF-kappaB and activating HO-1/Nrf2 pathways. Int J Biol Sci. 2016;12:72–86.

39. Dong LY, Li S, Zhen YL, Wang YN, Shao X, Luo ZG. Cardioprotection of vitexin on myocardial ischemia/reperfusion injury in rat via regulating inflammatory cytokines and MAPK pathway. Am J Chin Med. 2013;41:1251–66.

40. Sun Z, Yan B, Yu WY, Yao XP, Ma XJ, Sheng GL, Ma Q. Vitexin attenuates acute doxorubicin cardiotoxicity in rats via the suppression of oxidative stress, inflammation and apoptosis and the activation of FOXO3a. Exp Ther Med. 2016;12:1879–84.

41. Ashokkumar R, Jamuna S, Sakeena Sadullah MS, Niranjali Devaraj S. Vitexin protects isoproterenol induced post myocardial injury by modulating hipposignaling and ER stress responses. Biochem Biophys Res Commun. 2018;496:731–7.

42. Min JW, Hu JJ, He M, Sanchez RM, Huang WX, Liu YQ, Bsoul NB, Han S, Yin J, Liu WH, et al. Vitexin reduces hypoxia-ischemia neonatal brain injury by the inhibition of HIF-1 alpha in a rat pup model. Neuropharmacology. 2015;99:38–50.

43. Aseervatham GS, Suryakala U, Doulethunisha SS, Bose PC, Sivasudha T. Expression pattern of NMDA receptors reveals antiepileptic potential of apigenin 8-C-glucoside and chlorogenic acid in pilocarpine induced epileptic mice. Biomed Pharmacother. 2016;82:54–64.

44. Hanrahan JR, Chebib M, Johnston GA. Flavonoid modulation of GABA(A) receptors. Br J Pharmacol. 2011;163:234–45.

45. Johnston GA. Flavonoid nutraceuticals and ionotropic receptors for the inhibitory neurotransmitter GABA. Neurochem Int. 2015;89:120–5.

46. Abbasi E, Nassiri-Asl M, Shafeei M, Sheikhi M. Neuroprotective effects of vitexin, a flavonoid, on pentylenetetrazole-induced seizure in rats. Chem Biol Drug Des. 2012;80:274–8.

47. Min JW, Hu JJ, He M, Sanchez RM, Huang WX, Liu YQ, Bsoul NB, Han S, Yin J, Liu WH, et al. Vitexin reduces hypoxia-ischemia neonatal brain injury by the inhibition of HIF-1alpha in a rat pup model. Neuropharmacology. 2015;99:38–50.

48. Rice JE 3rd, Vannucci RC, Brierley JB. The influence of immaturity on hypoxic-ischemic brain damage in the rat. Ann Neurol. 1981;9:131–41.

49. Koh HS, Chang CY, Jeon SB, Yoon HJ, Ahn YH, Kim HS, Kim IH, Jeon SH, Johnson RS, Park EJ. The HIF-1/glial TIM-3 axis controls inflammation-associated brain damage under hypoxia. Nat Commun. 2015;6:6340.

50. Griffon N, Jeanneteau F, Prieur F, Diaz J, Sokoloff P. CLIC6, a member of the intracellular chloride channel family, interacts with dopamine D(2)-like receptors. Brain Res Mol Brain Res. 2003;117:47–57.

51. Hu JJ, Yang XL, Luo WD, Han S, Yin J, Liu WH, He XH, Peng BW. Bumetanide reduce the seizure susceptibility induced by pentylenetetrazol via inhibition of aberrant hippocampal neurogenesis in neonatal rats after hypoxia-ischemia. Brain Res Bull. 2017;130:188–99.

52. Racine RJ, Gartner JG, Burnham WM. Epileptiform activity and neural plasticity in limbic structures. Brain Res. 1972;47:262–8.

53. Sivakumaran S, Maguire J. Bumetanide reduces seizure progression and the development of pharmacoresistant status epilepticus. Epilepsia. 2016;57:222–32.

54. O'Donnell ME, Tran L, Lam TI, Liu XB, Anderson SE. Bumetanide inhibition of the blood-brain barrier Na-K-Cl cotransporter reduces edema formation in the rat middle cerebral artery occlusion model of stroke. J Cereb Blood Flow Metab. 2004;24:1046–56.

55. Yuen N, Lam TI, Wallace BK, Klug NR, Anderson SE, O'Donnell ME. Ischemic factor-induced increases in cerebral microvascular endothelial cell Na/H exchange activity and abundance: evidence for involvement of ERK1/2 MAP kinase. Am J Physiol Cell Physiol. 2014;306:C931–42.

56. Liu T, Zhang T, Yu H, Shen H, Xia W. Adjudin protects against cerebral ischemia reperfusion injury by inhibition of neuroinflammation and blood-brain barrier disruption. J Neuroinflammation. 2014;11:107.

57. Huang J, Li Y, Tang Y, Tang G, Yang GY, Wang Y. CXCR4 antagonist AMD3100 protects blood-brain barrier integrity and reduces inflammatory response after focal ischemia in mice. Stroke. 2013;44:190–7.

58. Sucher NJ, Carles MC. A pharmacological basis of herbal medicines for epilepsy. Epilepsy Behav. 2015;52:308–18.

59. Zhu HL, Wan JB, Wang YT, Li BC, Xiang C, He J, Li P. Medicinal compounds with antiepileptic/anticonvulsant activities. Epilepsia. 2014;55:3–16.

60. Fu P, Tang R, Yu Z, Huang S, Xie M, Luo X, Wang W. Bumetanide-induced NKCC1 inhibition attenuates oxygen-glucose deprivation-induced decrease in proliferative activity and cell cycle progression arrest in cultured OPCs via p-38 MAPKs. Brain Res. 2015;1613:110–9.

61. Modol L, Santos D, Cobianchi S, Gonzalez-Perez F, Lopez-Alvarez V, Navarro X. NKCC1 activation is required for myelinated sensory neurons regeneration through JNK-dependent pathway. J Neurosci. 2015;35:7414–27.

62. Delpy A, Allain AE, Meyrand P, Branchereau P. NKCC1 cotransporter inactivation underlies embryonic development of chloride-mediated inhibition in mouse spinal motoneuron. J Physiol. 2008;586:1059–75.

63. Ge S, Goh EL, Sailor KA, Kitabatake Y, Ming GL, Song H. GABA regulates synaptic integration of newly generated neurons in the adult brain. Nature. 2006;439:589–93.

64. Rangroo Thrane V, Thrane AS, Wang F, Cotrina ML, Smith NA, Chen M, Xu Q, Kang N, Fujita T, Nagelhus EA, Nedergaard M. Ammonia triggers neuronal disinhibition and seizures by impairing astrocyte potassium buffering. Nat Med. 2013;19:1643–8.

65. Wang F, Wang X, Shapiro LA, Cotrina ML, Liu W, Wang EW, Gu S, Wang W, He X, Nedergaard M, Huang JH. NKCC1 up-regulation contributes to early post-traumatic seizures and increased post-traumatic seizure susceptibility. Brain Struct Funct. 2017;222:1543–56.

66. Diniz TC, Silva JC, de Lima-Saraiva SR, Ribeiro FP, Pacheco AG, de Freitas RM, Quintans-Junior LJ, Quintans Jde S, Mendes RL, Almeida JR. The role of flavonoids on oxidative stress in epilepsy. Oxidative Med Cell Longev. 2015;2015:171756.

67. Shamri R, Melo RC, Young KM, Bivas-Benita M, Xenakis JJ, Spencer LA, Weller PF. CCL11 elicits secretion of RNases from mouse eosinophils and their cell-free granules. FASEB J. 2012;26:2084–93.

68. Borghi SM, Carvalho TT, Staurengo-Ferrari L, Hohmann MS, Pinge-Filho P, Casagrande R, Verri WA Jr. Vitexin inhibits inflammatory pain in mice by targeting TRPV1, oxidative stress, and cytokines. J Nat Prod. 2013;76:1141–9.

69. Chopp M, Zhang ZG, Jiang Q. Neurogenesis, angiogenesis, and MRI indices of functional recovery from stroke. Stroke. 2007;38:827–31.

70. Wachtel M, Frei K, Ehler E, Bauer C, Gassmann M, Gloor SM. Extracellular signal-regulated protein kinase activation during reoxygenation is required to restore ischaemia-induced endothelial barrier failure. Biochem J. 2002;367:873–9.

71. Lai CH, Kuo KH, Leo JM. Critical role of actin in modulating BBB permeability. Brain Res Brain Res Rev. 2005;50:7–13.

72. Witt KA, Mark KS, Hom S, Davis TP. Effects of hypoxia-reoxygenation on rat blood-brain barrier permeability and tight junctional protein expression. Am J Physiol Heart Circ Physiol. 2003;285:H2820–31.

# 13

# Altered morphological dynamics of activated microglia after induction of *status epilepticus*

Elena Avignone[1,2]*, Marilyn Lepleux[1,2], Julie Angibaud[1,2] and U. Valentin Nägerl[1,2]*

## Abstract

**Background:** Microglia cells are the resident macrophages of the central nervous system and are considered its first line of defense. In the normal brain, their ramified processes are highly motile, constantly scanning the surrounding brain tissue and rapidly moving towards sites of acute injury or danger signals. These microglial dynamics are thought to be critical for brain homeostasis. Under pathological conditions, microglial cells undergo "activation," which modifies many of their molecular and morphological properties. Investigations of the effects of activation on motility are limited and have given mixed results. In particular, little is known about how microglial motility is altered in epilepsy, which is characterized by a strong inflammatory reaction and microglial activation.

**Methods:** We used a mouse model of *status epilepticus* induced by kainate injections and time-lapse two-photon microscopy to image GFP-labeled microglia in acute hippocampal brain slices. We studied how microglial activation affected the motility of microglial processes, including basal motility, and their responses to local triggering stimuli.

**Results:** Our study reveals that microglial motility was largely preserved in kainate-treated animals, despite clear signs of microglial activation. In addition, whereas the velocities of microglial processes during basal scanning and towards a laser lesion were unaltered 48 h after *status epilepticus*, we observed an increase in the size of the territory scanned by single microglial processes during basal motility and an elevated directional velocity towards a pipette containing a purinergic agonist.

**Conclusions:** Microglial activation differentially impacted the dynamic scanning behavior of microglia in response to specific acute noxious stimuli, which may be an important feature of the adaptive behavior of microglia during pathophysiological conditions.

**Keywords:** Microglia, Microglial dynamics, Epilepsy, Inflammation, Two-photon microscopy, Laser lesion

## Background

Microglia are the resident macrophages of the central nervous system (CNS), acting as its first line of defense to cordon off brain lesions, to phagocytize cellular debris, and to release signaling molecules critical for cell survival [1].

Under physiological conditions, microglia show a uniform distribution and occupy distinct spatial domains with minimal overlap [2]. A hallmark of microglia is their highly dynamic and motile nature, which allows them to react rapidly and intervene locally for effective maintenance and control of brain homeostasis. Indeed, they continuously scan the parenchyma of the brain in an apparently random fashion (called basal motility), rapidly extending and retracting their highly branched processes [3–6] and contacting practically all other cell types and neuronal compartments, including synapses [7, 8].

In response to an acute lesion, microglia rapidly project their processes towards sites of danger signals (called directional motility; [3, 4, 9]), presumably to probe and contain the damage and to protect the surrounding cells [10].

* Correspondence:
elena.avignone@u-bordeaux.fr; valentin.nagerl@u-bordeaux.fr
[1]Interdisciplinary Institute for Neurosciences, CNRS UMR 5297, 33077 Bordeaux, France

Due to their role as immune-competent cells, a variety of signals are expected to attract microglial processes. In particular, they are attracted by adenosine triphosphate (ATP) and its derivatives. Indeed, activation of purinergic receptors plays a major role for microglial dynamics [3, 11]. In particular, extracellular ATP affects basal motility [3, 12], while activation of purinergic P2Y12 receptors (P2Y12R) mediates directional motility induced by laser lesions [13, 14].

Under pathological conditions, microglia change many of their morphological and molecular properties through a series of long-term transformations, called microglial activation [15, 16]. Microglial activation plays a critical role in the inflammatory reaction associated with a variety of diseases, and it is a prominent feature in the brain following *status epilepticus* (SE). SE is a seizure lasting several minutes and that may occur in patients with a history of epilepsy or as a consequence of a variety of insults, such as trauma, febrile seizure, and stroke. The inflammatory reaction induced by SE may contribute to the progression towards recurrent (chronic) epilepsy and to common associated neuropsychiatric comorbidities such as depression, memory impairment, and autism spectrum disorders [17]. Microglial activation, which plays a central role in orchestrating the inflammatory reaction, is accompanied by morphological and functional changes that may influence their motility and could thus compromise their housekeeping capacities. In the context of SE, it is unclear how microglial activation affects the motility of microglia and their ability to respond to noxious signals. A down- or up-regulation of microglial motility is conceivable as microglia are known to retract their processes and to exhibit boosted purinergic responses at the same time after SE [18–20].

To explore this question, we performed time-lapse two-photon imaging of microglia in acute hippocampal brain slices two days after induction of SE in mice. We assessed the impact of microglial activation on basal and directional microglial motility in response to focal laser lesions as well as to local application of an ATP analog.

## Methods

### Animals and SE model

All experiments followed Inserm and European Union and institutional guidelines for the care and use of laboratory animals (Council directive 2010/63/EU) and have been validated by the local ethics committee of Bordeaux (n° A50120200). The heterozygous CX3CR1$^{+/eGFP}$ mice used in this study were obtained by crossing CX3CR1$^{eGFP/eGFP}$ with C57BL/6 (Janvier, Le Genest Saint Isle, France) wild-type mice. To avoid non-specific activation of microglia, animals were kept in an animal facility free of specific pathogenic organisms until the experiments.

To induce SE, 30- to 40-day-old male mice received two intraperitoneal (i.p.) kainate (KA) injections (15 and 5 mg/kg) at an interval of 30 min. Littermate male mice injected with PBS were used as control. The KA injections induced crises scored according to the Racine scale of level 3 (rear into a sitting position with forepaws shaking) to 5 (continuous rearing and falling). Mice, which did not reach level 3 after 1 h received a third injection (5 mg/kg). The multiple injection protocol provided a better control of the crisis and reduced mortality (less than 10 %).

The overall crisis of each animal was evaluated according to a modified Racine scale, which also considered the duration of the crisis. The crisis was classified as mild (level 2 of Racine's scale: rigid posture with straight and rigid tail), intermediate (level 3 of Racine's scale, duration shorter than 2 h), intense (level 3 of Racine's scale with episode 4 or 5, duration shorter than 3 h), or severe (erratic behavior such as jumping or walking backwards or crisis duration longer than 3 h).

### Preparation of acute brain slices

Hippocampal slices were prepared 48 h after i.p. injections. Mice were sacrificed by cervical dislocation. The brain was then quickly removed and placed in ice-cold artificial cerebrospinal fluid (aCSF) saturated with carbogen (95 % $O_2$/5 % $CO_2$) and in which NaCl was replaced by sucrose (in mM: 210 sucrose, 2 KCl, 26 NaHCO$_3$, 1.25 NaH$_2$PO$_4$, 10 glucose, 0.2 CaCl$_2$, 6 MgCl$_2$; pH 7.4, osmolarity 310 mOsm). Transverse 350-μm-thick slices were cut using a vibratome (VT1200, Leica, Mannheim, Germany), transferred to a heated (33 °C) holding chamber containing carbogenated (95 % $O_2$/5 % $CO_2$) standard aCSF (in mM: 124 NaCl, 3 KCl, 26 NaHCO$_3$, 1.25 NaH$_2$PO$_4$, 10 glucose, 2 CaCl$_2$, 1 MgCl$_2$, pH 7.4, osmolarity 305 mOsm/L) for 45 min, and then maintained until the experiment at room temperature for a maximum of 3 h.

### Time-lapse two-photon imaging

Individual slices were transferred to a submerged recording chamber and continuously perfused with carbogenated aCSF (3 ml/min) at 33 °C. Images were acquired with a 40X water immersion objective (NA 1.0), using a commercial upright two-photon laser-scanning fluorescence microscope (Ultima, Prairie Technologies, Middleton, Wisconsin, USA and Axio Examiner, Zeiss, Oberkochen, Germany). For two-photon excitation, a Ti:Sapphire laser (Mai Tai, Spectra-Physics, Darmstadt, Germany) was tuned to 900 nm. Four-dimensional image stacks (x, y, z, t) were acquired in the *strata radiatum/lacunosum-moleculare* in the CA1 area of the hippocampus. The voxel size was $200 \times 200 \times 1000$ nm$^3$ in all experiments measuring basal motility and responses to laser lesion, while it was $300 \times 300 \times 1000$ nm$^3$ in most of the experiments with the ATP analog. The $z$-stacks were 11 to 25 μm thick and acquired at intervals between 25 and 60 s. We did not detect any signs of photo-induced damage during extended time-lapse acquisitions lasting up to 1 h.

To induce a small laser lesion, a region of $1.6 \times 1.6$ μm was repeatedly illuminated for 20–50 times with an elevated intensity of the two-photon laser, which reliably induced a microglial response.

A puff of the P2Y12R agonist 2-Methylthioadenosine diphosphate trisodium salt (2Me-ADP, 100 μM) was applied by manual pressure through a glass pipette gently inserted in the slice to limit mechanical damage. No microglial responses were observed when a pipette containing aCSF was inserted and a similar pressure was applied.

To reduce effects from the slicing procedure, we imaged microglia that were fully embedded in the brain slice, at least 50 μm below the surface of the slice, which is a depth where neurons are usually intact [21]. At this imaging depth, microglial morphology was comparable to what has been observed in perfusion-fixed animals (data not shown) and in vivo [3, 4]. Furthermore, in our experimental conditions, basal motility was similar to what has been reported for cortex and spinal cord in vivo [3, 4, 9].

## Image analysis

Analysis was carried out with ImageJ (National Institute of Health). Analysis of microglial cell body size was performed on maximal intensity projection images, considering only the cells having the cell soma fully contained within the 3D image stack. Image analysis was done blindly with respect to crisis level. In order to avoid subjective interpretation of the crisis level, only scores by the same person were considered for the correlation between crisis level and microglial morphology. Cell bodies were measured using the "magic wand" tool in ImageJ on the maximal intensity projection image. When objects from a different focal plane contaminated the measurement, a subset of images containing only the cell body was used for the projection. The number of primary processes was assessed in 3D stacks. The longest process was verified in the 3D stack, then drawn by hand and measured in the 2D projection. Images of microglia were taken in two to three hippocampal slices per animal. Morphological parameters were measured in all images, and the median was taken as a representative value of each animal. To assess the relationship between cell body size and dynamics, the median of cell body measurements per slice in each experiment was taken as representative value.

To compensate for $x$-$y$ movements, images of the temporal series were aligned using the following ImageJ plug-ins: StackReg, MultistackReg, and PoorMan3Dreg [22]. To analyze the movement of single processes, the plug-in MtrackJ [23] and custom written programs in MATLAB (MathWorks, France) were used. Each movement was classified as elongation, retraction, or stationary, according to its velocity relative to a fixed reference point (lesion site or pipette tip for directional motility). In the case of basal motility, the reference point was defined by where the process emerged from the parent process. The territory explored was calculated as maximum-minimum distance from the point of reference.

To estimate the overall velocity at which the fluorescent processes elongated towards the target (pipette or laser lesion site), a series of concentric circles were drawn as a region of interest and the fluorescence was measured in concentric rings (Additional file 1: Figure S1). The velocity was defined as the distance between two rings divided by the time between their maxima of the fluorescence signal. We considered only the experiments in which we could clearly identify at least three peaks of fluorescence in three coronal sections, thus two velocities, and the mean was taken as the representative velocity of each experiment (Additional file 1: Figure S1).

The territory explored by a single process was calculated as the linear distance between the most distant and closest points reached by a single process with respect to its parent branch, irrespective of elongation or retraction. For each slice, 7–10 processes from several cells were analyzed.

## Statistics

Data values are presented as mean ± SEM or median with quartile. Statistical significance was established with statistical tools in MATLAB or Origin (OriginLab, RITME Informatique, France). First, we tested whether data were sampled from populations that follow Gaussian distributions using the method of Kolmogorov and Smirnov. For sample populations with non-Gaussian and Gaussian distributions, a non-parametric (Mann-Whitney) or parametric tests ($t$ test with Welch's correction) were used to assess differences in the median (or mean). In case of paired data, the non-parametric Wilcoxon signed-rank test was used. The Kolmogorov and Smirnov test was used to compare distributions of pooled values across all experiments between two groups of animals. Statistical significance was established at $p < 0.05$ and $p < 0.01$. $N$ represents the number of animals, while $n$ represents the number of cells, experiments, or processes as indicated in the text.

## Results
### Microglial activation after status epilepticus

We imaged microglia in acute hippocampal brain slices from Cx3Cr1$^{+/\text{eGFP}}$ mice by two-photon microscopy and analyzed their morphological dynamics. As previously described [18, 21, 24], 48 h after injection, we observed an increase in the number of microglia in KA-treated animals, indicative of microglial activation. Furthermore, in KA-treated animals, microglial cell bodies were substantially larger and processes were shorter compared to control animals (Fig. 1a, b). We checked whether the degree of morphological changes after SE induction correlated with the severity of SE, as classified according to a modified Racine scale (see Methods for details). While no significant differences in cell body sizes were observed between control ($n = 163$, $N = 10$) and animals with mild seizures ($n = 21$, $N = 2$, KS test, $p = 0.29$), the cumulative probability plot of the distribution obtained from animals with intermediate ($n = 106$, $N = 5$), intense ($n = 43$, $N = 4$), and severe seizures ($n = 126$, $N = 8$, KS test, $p < 0.01$, compared to previous level; Fig. 1c, d) was progressively shifted to the right. Moreover, in experiments where the animals exhibited intense and protracted seizures, microglia took on an amoeboid shape and migrated to the pyramidal cell body layer (Additional file 2: Figure S2). Microglial cell shape varied widely in KA-treated animals, even within the same slice. The variation was larger for severe crises, where we could observe hyper-ramified cells, as well as amoeboid-like shapes. We analyzed two morphological parameters: the number of primary processes and the longest process identifiable in each cell. The number of primary process was not statistically different between the control (median 6, $n = 85$) and animal with intermediate seizure (median 5.5, $n = 56$; KS test 0.99), while it was different between control animals and animals with severe seizure (median 7, $n = 36$; KS test 0.028). Similar to cell body size, we observed a progressive behavior, with the process length shifting towards smaller values for more intense crises (Fig. 1f, h). The median values were 38.5, 31.8, 26, and 22 µm for control ($n = 96$, $N = 10$), intermediate ($n = 91$, $N = 5$), intense ($n = 49$, $N = 4$), and severe ($n = 115$, $N = 8$) crisis levels, respectively. All distributions were significantly different from the respective previous level (KS < 0.01), except between the severe and intense crisis (KS = 0.08). These results are in general agreement with changes reported in the literature in different animal models [24–27].

Taken together, these results show that there is a strong correlation between seizure severity and morphological changes (Fig. 1e–h), indicating that cell body size can be used as a reliable proxy of seizure intensity and microglial activation.

## Effect of microglial activation on basal motility of microglial processes

To establish whether and how microglial activation induced by SE affects the ability of microglia to patrol brain parenchyma, we tracked the morphological dynamics of

microglial processes by time-lapse two-photon imaging in acute hippocampal slices.

First, we analyzed the motility of microglial processes under baseline conditions in control and KA-treated animals (Fig. 2). To this end, we measured the average velocity of the tips of individual microglial processes based on the maximal intensity projections of 3D image stacks acquired every 45 s for up to 8 min.

The average tip velocity was indistinguishable between KA-treated and control tissue (ctrl: $2.38 \pm 0.08$ µm/min, $N = 7$; KA: $2.46 \pm 0.10$ µm/min $N = 6$; $p = 0.58$, $t$ test). Similarly, no difference was found between the velocity distributions of all processes for the two groups (Fig. 2b; ctrl: $n = 89$; KA: $n = 71$; KS = 0.99), despite the significant difference in their average cell body size (ctrl: $42.2 \pm 2.5$ µm$^2$; KA: $73.5 \pm 9.1$ µm$^2$; $p = 0.004$), confirming that KA injections indeed had induced microglial activation.

Performing extended time-lapse imaging experiments (acquiring 3D image stacks every 30 s for up to 30 min), we also analyzed the speed at which individual microglial processes elongated and retracted, which is a more refined measure of microglial process motility. Comparing elongation and retraction velocity in the same process did not turn up any significant differences, neither in control ($p = 0.46$; Wilcoxon signed-rank test; $n = 51$ processes; obtained in experiments in three animals) nor KA-treated animals ($p = 0.95$; Wilcoxon signed-rank test; $n = 136$ processes; obtained in nine experiments in five animals; data not shown).

Finally, we determined the size of the territory explored by microglial processes as the maximal linear covered distance (see Methods for details). The size of the territory was highly variable (ranging from 1 to 15 µm). Yet, on the whole, microglial processes explored a significantly larger territory in KA-treated than in control animals (median ctrl: $4.18$ µm; $n = 51$ processes; $n = 3$ experiments; three animals; median KA: $5.38$ µm; $n = 152$ processes; $n = 9$ experiments; five animals; $p = 0.019$; Fig. 2c). Moreover, there was a strong positive correlation between microglial cell body size (median value per animal) and the average distance covered by microglial processes in KA-treated animals ($r = 0.8$; Fig. 2d).

Taken together, our analysis indicates that basal motility of microglia was preserved after microglial activation. Microglial processes moved at the same speed but covered a larger distance in KA-treated animals as compared with control animals.

## Directional motility towards a pipette containing P2Y12R agonist

We next assessed the ability of activated microglia to rapidly react to potentially noxious signals. Consistently with previous reports, microglial processes were attracted

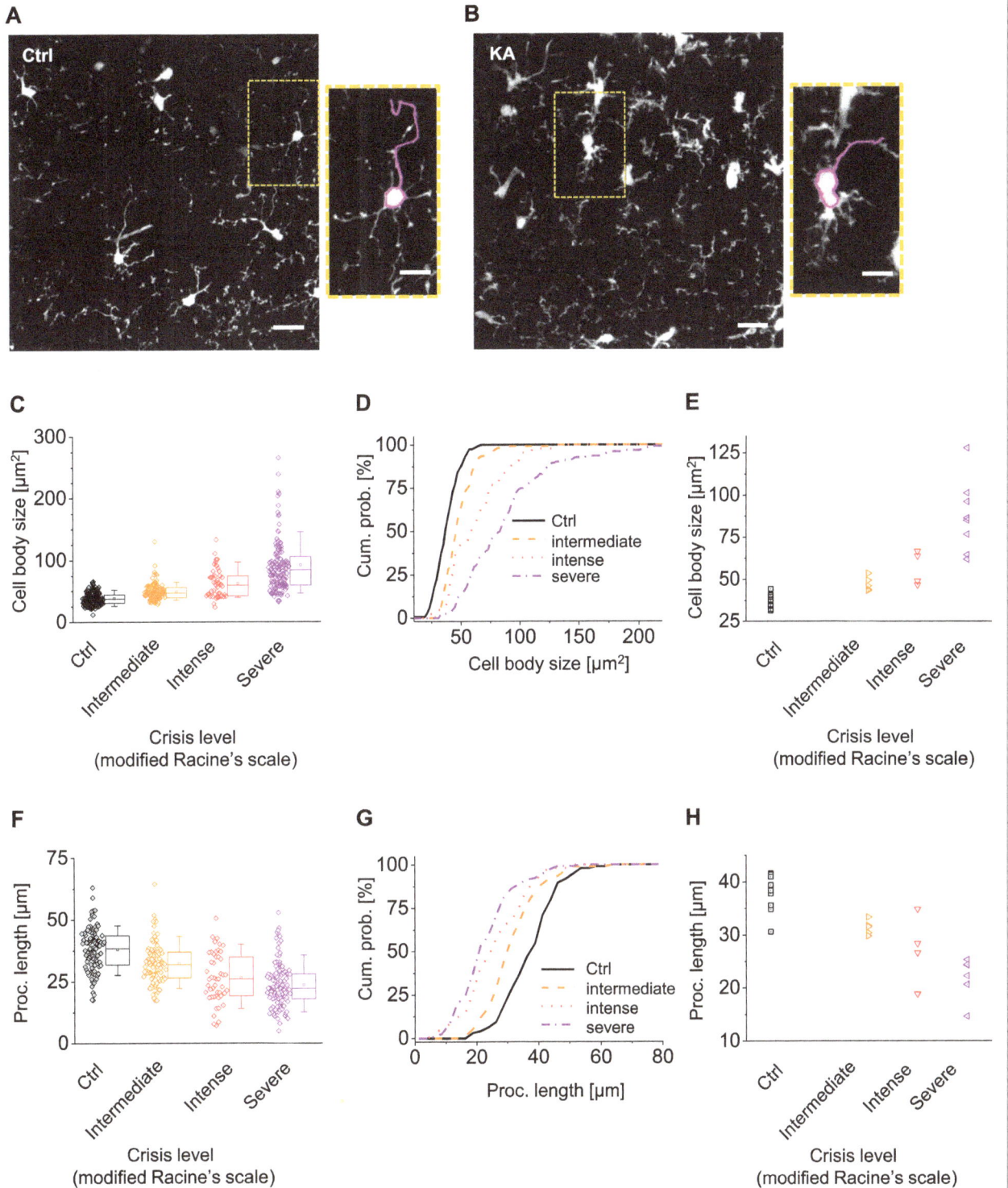

**Fig. 1** (See legend on next page.)

(See figure on previous page.)
**Fig. 1** Cell body size correlates with the severity of *status epilepticus*. **a, b** Maximal intensity projection (MIP, $z = 19$ μm) images of microglial cells obtained in control mice (**a**) and in mice two days after kainate i.p. injection (**b**). The insets show higher magnification images. The *line around cell bodies* was drawn in a semi-automatic way to measure cell body size. The *line on the process* was based on the 3D image stack to avoid projection artifacts. Note the increase in cell body size of microglia and decrease of the longest process after SE. Scale bars 10 and 6 μm in the insets. **c** Soma size measurements obtained in all experiments classified according to the crisis level of animals, their median, and quartile value. **d** Cumulative probability of cell body size grouped according to the crisis level of animals, scored according to modified Racine's scale. Note the progressive shift to the right with the increase of the severity of the induced SE. **e** Relationship between the median of cell body size for each animal and its crisis level or in control (*ctrl, black*). **f** Measurements of longest processes obtained in all experiments classified according to crisis level of animals, their median, and quartile value. **g** Cumulative probability of data represented in (**f**) grouped according to crisis level. Note the progressive shift to the left with increasing crisis severity. **h** Relationship between the median of the longest processes for each animal and its crisis level or in control (*ctrl, black*)

by ATP analog 2Me-ADP (Additional file 3; Additional file 4), an agonist of P2Y12R, while cell bodies did not move during the observation time (up to 1 h) [3, 13, 18, 28]. We tracked individual microglial processes during their movements towards a patch pipette containing the P2Y12R agonist. We observed that it took microglial processes about half the time to reach the pipette tip in KA-treated animals compared to control experiments (ctrl: $58.2 \pm 5.7$ min, $n = 6$, $N = 4$; KA: $29.0 \pm 3.7$ min, $n = 6$, $N = 4$; $p < 0.01$, $t$ test; Fig. 3a), confirming a previous study based on wide-field imaging in acute brain slices [18].

In two KA experiments, microglial processes failed to be attracted by the 2Me-ADP-containing pipette. In both cases, slices were obtained from mice, which had undergone particularly strong crisis and whose microglia showed signs of extreme activation. Indeed, their cell bodies were very large and fragmented and mostly devoid of processes (Additional file 2: Figure S2), suggestive of strong phagocytic activity. This data set was excluded from the statistical analysis of the morphological dynamics.

To analyze the directional motility in greater details, we compared the distributions of all elongation steps made by single microglial processes. The distribution observed in KA-injected animals was substantially shifted to the right compared to the control case, indicating increased velocity (ctrl: median 1.49 μm/s, $n = 1450$ movements; KA: median 2.25 μm/s, $n = 740$ movements; KS test, $p < 0.001$; Fig. 3b). We then calculated the mean velocity of several single processes in each experiment (Fig. 3c), which confirmed the difference between the two experimental groups ($t$ test, $p < 0.01$). Similar results were obtained by measuring the fluorescence of microglial processes passing through concentric rings drawn around the pipette (global velocity, see the "Methods" section for details). The mean velocity was $1.30 \pm 0.17$ μm/min ($n = 6$) for the control group and $2.68 \pm 0.22$ μm/min ($n = 5$) for the KA group ($p < 0.01$, $t$ test; Fig. 3c).

The analysis of single processes revealed that some of them abruptly stopped and retracted and/or started to scan the territory in an apparent random fashion, even though initially they appeared to move towards the pipette tip. Therefore, we compared the retraction velocity

between KA-treated and control animals. In contrast to elongation velocity, the distributions of retracting velocity were not statistically different (ctrl: median 1.38 μm/min, $n = 97$; KA median 1.73 μm/min, $n = 57$; $p = 0.18$, KS test). Consistently, elongation was more rapid than retraction in the KA group ($p < 0.001$, KS test), while in the control group elongation and retraction were not statistically different ($p = 0.19$, KS test; data not shown).

Taken together, our analysis shows that microglial activation affected the motility of microglial processes towards a pipette containing a purinergic agonist by specifically boosting the elongation speed, while the retraction speed was unaltered.

### Directional motility towards a laser lesion

In order to assess how microglial activation affects the ability of microglia to direct their processes towards sites of acute physical injury in brain tissue, we induced a laser lesion in a small region ($1.6 \times 1.6$ μm) and measured the velocity of microglial processes moving towards the lesion site. Laser lesions have been used before in in vivo [3, 4] and acute slice studies [10]. In agreement with previous reports, we observed that many microglial processes rapidly switched from a basal scanning mode to directional motility towards the lesion site (Fig. 4a, Additional file 5; Additional file 6). In many instances, newly formed processes grew out from the cell body and from existing processes and moved towards the lesion site. Similar to the case of the ATP analog, cell bodies did not move during observation time (up to 30 min). The number of processes involved in the response was highly variable between experiments, depending on the distance to the lesion site and presumably also on the type of the affected region (e.g., neuronal dendrites or soma, astrocyte, blood vessel).

Microglial processes typically reached the lesion site within a few minutes (examples in Fig. 4a, Additional file 5; Additional file 6) for both experimental groups (ctrl: median values 4.23 min; $n = 9$, $N = 6$; KA: 4.48 min; $n = 11$, $N = 6$; $p = 0.17$; Mann-Whitney test), even though their median cell body sizes were substantially different (ctrl: $38.6 \pm 2.64$; KA: $64.7 \pm 5.8$; $p = 0.001$).

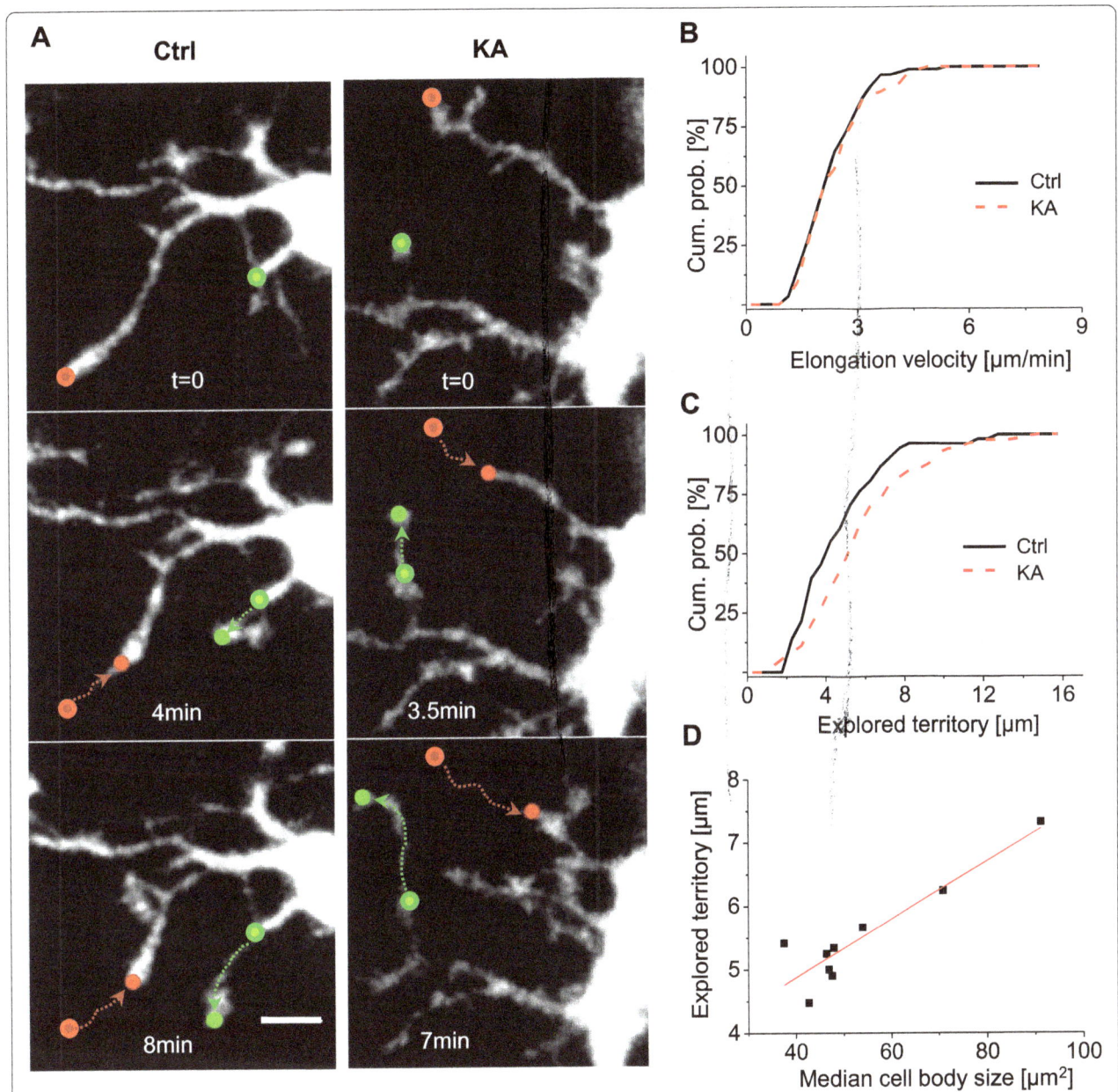

**Fig. 2** Activated microglia scan larger territory, without changing their velocity. **a** Maximal intensity projection of time-lapse two-photon images at different time points during spontaneous movements of microglial processes in control (*left column*) and 48 h after induction of SE (*right column*). The figure shows retracting (*red symbols*) and elongating processes (*green symbols*), with the starting/arriving points marked by *circles*. Scale bar, 5 μm. **b** Cumulative probability of all elongation movements by single process tips measured in control (*black*) and KA-injected (*red*) animals shows no difference between the two groups (*p* = 0.99, KS test). **c** Cumulative probability of territory explored by all single process tips measured in control (*black*) and KA-injected (*red*) animals. *p* = 0.019, KS test. **d** Relationship between the median of explored territory by microglial processes versus the median of the cell body size in each experiment. The *red line* represents the linear fit (*r* = 0.8)

We then analyzed the global and elongation velocity of each process induced by the laser lesion. The elongations made by all analyzed processes did not show any statistically significant differences between the experimental groups (ctrl: median 3.84 μm/s; *n* = 817 movements, *N* = 6; KA: median 3.99; *n* = 1231 movements, *N* = 6; *p* = 0.4; KS test; Fig. 4b). Similarly, no statistically significant difference was found in the elongation velocity measured in each experiment (assessed as a mean of single processes) (ctrl: 4.22 ± 0.23 μm/min, *n* = 9, *N* = 6; KA: 4.53 ± 0.26 μm/min; *n* = 10, *N* = 6, *p* = 0.40, *t* test; Fig. 4c). Likewise, no differences were observed for global velocity between the experimental groups (ctrl: 3.75 ± 0.43 μm/min, *n* = 7; KA: 4.16 ± 0.2 μm/min, *n* = 9; *p* = 0.38, *t* test; Fig. 4c).

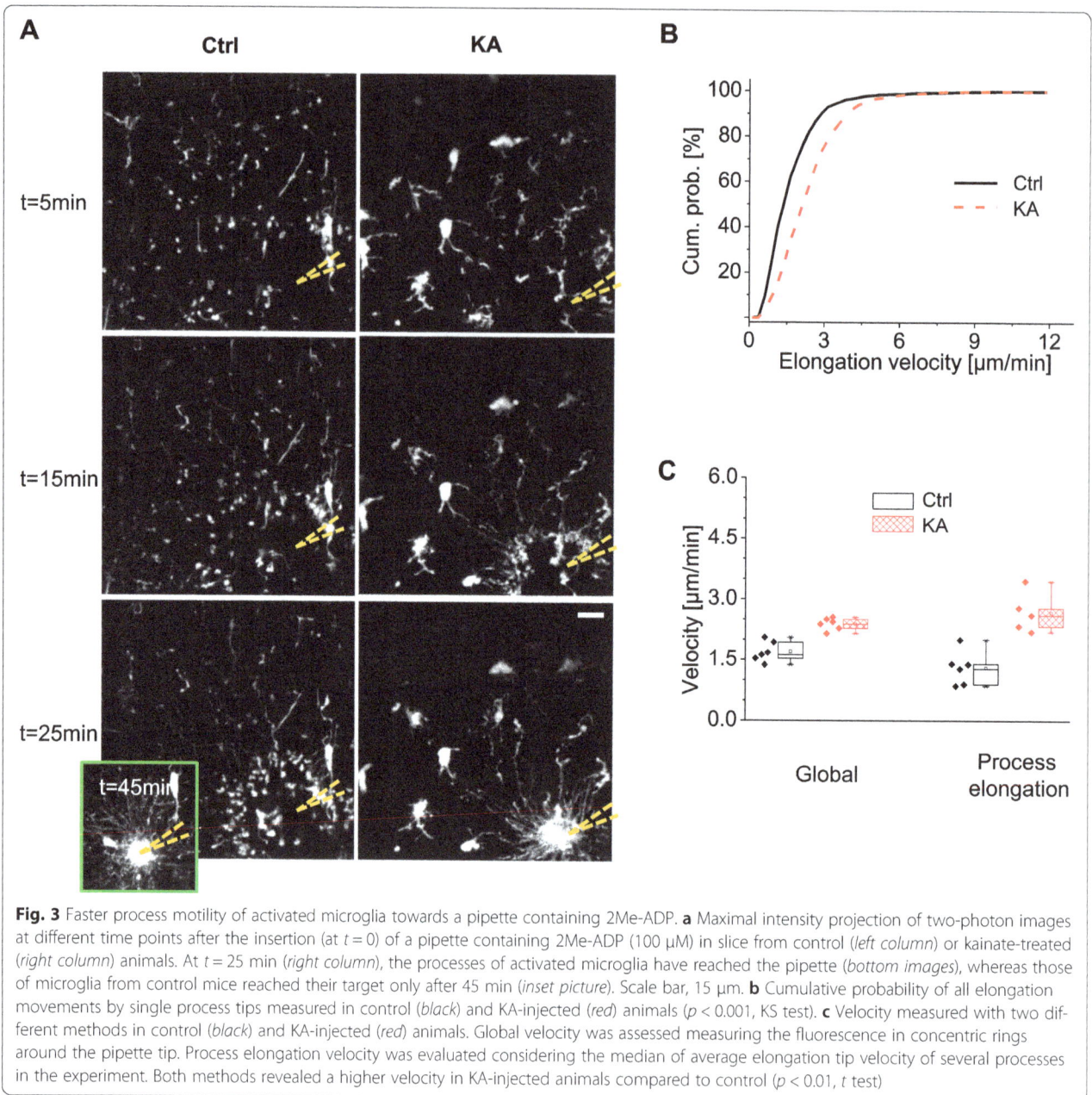

**Fig. 3** Faster process motility of activated microglia towards a pipette containing 2Me-ADP. **a** Maximal intensity projection of two-photon images at different time points after the insertion (at $t = 0$) of a pipette containing 2Me-ADP (100 μM) in slice from control (*left column*) or kainate-treated (*right column*) animals. At $t = 25$ min (*right column*), the processes of activated microglia have reached the pipette (*bottom images*), whereas those of microglia from control mice reached their target only after 45 min (*inset picture*). Scale bar, 15 μm. **b** Cumulative probability of all elongation movements by single process tips measured in control (*black*) and KA-injected (*red*) animals ($p < 0.001$, KS test). **c** Velocity measured with two different methods in control (*black*) and KA-injected (*red*) animals. Global velocity was assessed measuring the fluorescence in concentric rings around the pipette tip. Process elongation velocity was evaluated considering the median of average elongation tip velocity of several processes in the experiment. Both methods revealed a higher velocity in KA-injected animals compared to control ($p < 0.01$, $t$ test)

In summary, unlike the elevated directional motility towards a 2Me-ADP-containing pipette, the velocity towards a laser lesion was not measurably affected by microglial activation.

## Spatial extent of microglial responses to 2Me-ADP and laser lesions

In our experimental conditions, the velocity of the directional motility induced by laser lesions was roughly three times higher than the velocity induced by the P2Y12R agonist. However, the time it took to completely surround the pipette tip was almost 15 times longer than the time to surround the lesion site. To better

understand this apparent discrepancy, we characterized in more detail the effects of 2Me-ADP application and laser lesions on directional motility.

We determined the spatial extent of the microglial reaction, i.e., the area over which microglial processes responded to a locally applied trigger stimulus.

Microglial processes were attracted over large distances in response to 2Me-ADP (ctrl: >100 μm, Additional file 3). By comparison, the distance was much smaller for laser lesions (laser maximal distance, ctrl: $35.8 \pm 1.7$ μm, $n = 9$, Fig. 4d). Interestingly, not all processes that initially responded (responding process) actually reached the target area (arriving process), both for 2Me-ADP application

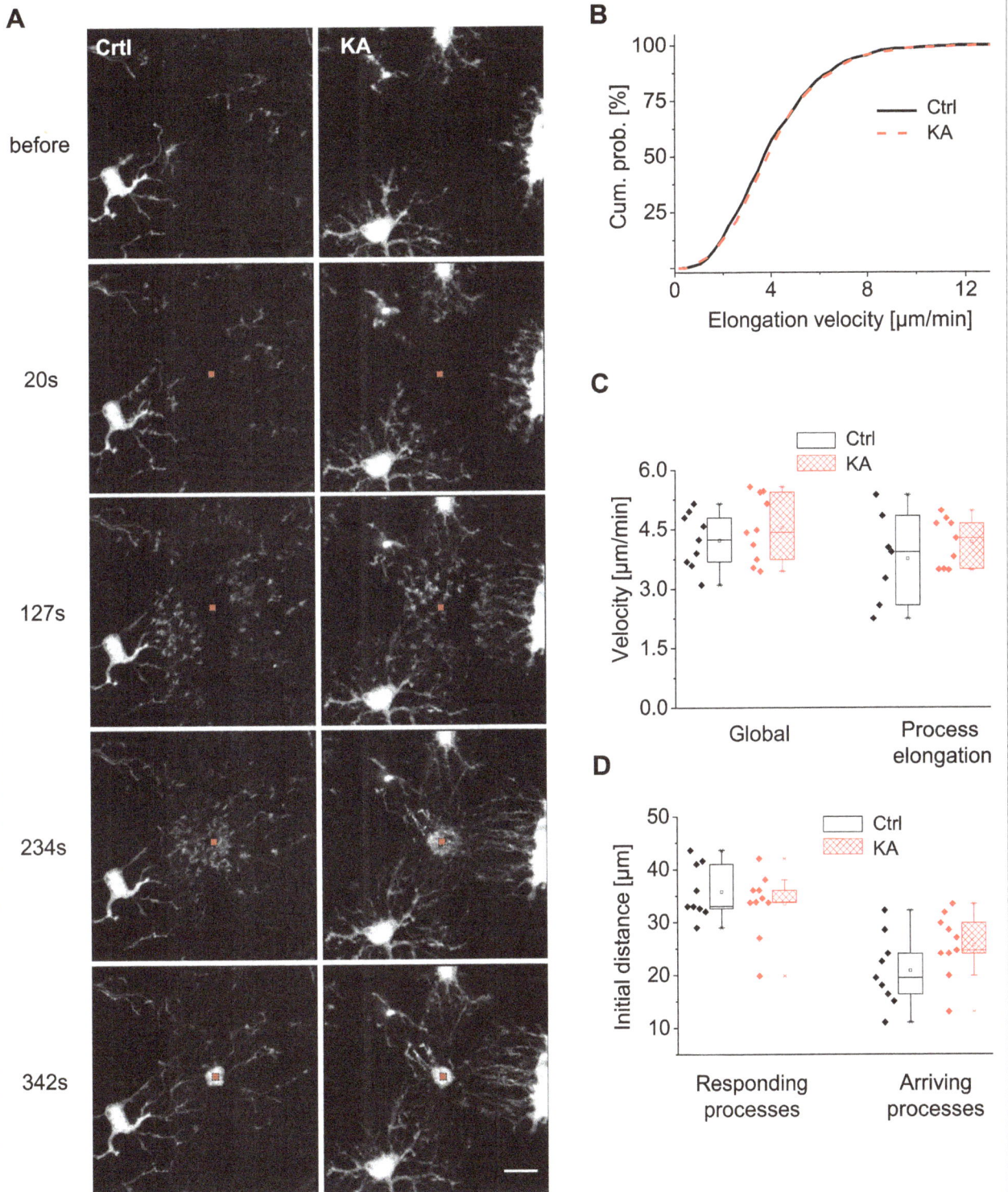

**Fig. 4** Microglial activation does not affect process motility towards a laser-induced lesion. **a** Examples of maximal intensity projection of two-photon images at different time points after the induction of lesion with a laser in a small portion of the slice (*red square*) in control (*left column*) and in KA-injected (*right column*) animal. Scale bar, 10 μm. **b** Cumulative probability of all elongation movements by single process tip measured in control (*black*) and KA-injected (*red*) animals. *p* = 0.17, KS test. **c** Global velocity and process elongation velocity measured in control (*black*) and KA-injected animals (*red*). None of the two methods shows a statistically significant difference between the two groups (*p* = 0.38 and 0.40 for global and process elongation, respectively, *t* test). **d** Evaluation of the area of influence of the laser lesion in control (*black*) and KA-injected (*red*) animals. Each *dot* represents the most distant process that still reacted to the lesion (*responding processes*) or actually arrived at the lesion site (*arriving processes*). None of the two groups showed a statistically significant difference (*p* = 0.39 and *p* = 0.16 for responding and arriving, respectively, *t* test)

and laser lesion (maximal distance arriving process, ctrl: $20.8 \pm 2.4$ μm, $n = 9$, Fig. 4d). The maximal distance of arriving or responding processes was not significantly different in KA-treated animals ($p = 0.38$ for responding, $p = 0.16$ for arriving), suggesting that despite the dramatic changes in morphology, the response zone of microglia to a laser lesion was not affected.

Interestingly, the responses to 2Me-ADP application frequently seemed to be coordinated among processes from different microglia. We observed that processes, which were closer to the pipette, started to move only after the more distal ones had caught up with them (Additional file 3; Additional file 4; Additional file 7: Figure S3), both in the control and KA groups. By comparison, this striking effect of coordination across many microglia cells in response to the ATP analog was much less obvious in the response to laser lesions, where microglial processes rushed to the lesion site more precipitously (Additional file 8: Figure S4, Additional file 5; Additional file 6).

Thus, 2Me-ADP application and laser lesions both effectively triggered microglial directional motility. However, the responses to these two triggers differed with respect to their sensitivity to/modulation by SE, their velocity, and the spatial extent of their responses as well as the level of coordination in their collective behavior, which resulted in large differences in the time to reach the target.

## Discussion

Microglia play a critical role in the health and homeostasis of the CNS. One of their main responsibilities is to avert impending threats by continuously scanning brain parenchyma and removing noxious substances and cellular debris that would otherwise accumulate and disrupt brain physiology. This ability is particularly important during neurodegenerative diseases when neural cell death and damage are rampant. Thus, it is important to understand how microglial motility is affected by pathological states. Using time-lapse two-photon imaging in acute brain slices, we examined in detail the ability of microglia to scan brain tissue and to respond to acute danger signals in the context of an animal model of SE. We observed that the basal velocity of microglial processes and their directional motility towards a laser lesion were unaffected, while the size of the territory scanned by individual microglial processes and their velocity towards a source of ATP analogs were markedly increased after the induction of SE. Our experiments indicate that microglial motility was not compromised by the activation of microglia caused by the induction of SE. Instead, microglial activation resulted in an enhanced scanning behavior, which may represent a state of heightened vigilance.

The mechanisms underlying microglial motility are not well understood yet. However, purinergic signaling

seems to play a major role [6, 11]. The ATPase apyrase and the purinergic antagonist suramin both slow down baseline motility, while ATP increases it [3, 12]. Directional motility towards laser lesion strongly depends on P2Y12R, since it is almost abolished in P2Y12R knockout animals [13, 14]. Forty-eight hours after SE, P2Y12R are up-regulated [18], which would be expected to lead to an increase in directional motility. Here, we confirmed that the velocity towards a pipette containing the P2Y12R agonist is indeed increased. Surprisingly, we did not find any difference in directional motility between KA-injected and control animals in response to laser lesions. However, the two types of directional motility could be mediated by different mechanisms. While the P2Y12R agonist activates a specific signaling pathway, laser lesions are a blunter trigger, which is likely to engage multiple signaling pathways that define the microglial response. Microglial dynamics depend on actin polymerization [10]. In other cell types, motility and actin polymerization are largely controlled by small GTPases [29–31], which can be differently modulated by the activation of several receptors, including purinergic receptors [32, 33]. Thus, stimulation of different microglial membrane receptors may induce distinct forms of directional motility. Consistently, the spatial extent and collective behavior of microglial processes were quite distinct for the two types of induced directional motility. Furthermore, the velocity of the processes was higher for laser lesions than in response to the ATP analog, and it might have been already at the maximal speed the cell could sustain. Indeed, as far as we know, no increase in the velocity of laser-induced directional motility has been reported following any type of treatment.

The relationship between activation and motility has been investigated before in several mouse models of neurological disorders, showing highly heterogeneous results. In amyotrophic lateral sclerosis (ALS) at the preclinical stage, basal motility was reported to be similar to control, while the response to laser lesion involved more microglial processes, which moved with unaltered velocity [34]. However, at the clinical stage, amoeboid and activated microglia reportedly showed reduced injury-directed response as well as reduced basal motility [34]. In contrast, in an Alzheimer's model, microglial processes moved faster towards an ATP-containing pipette [35], while responses to a laser lesion and phagocytosis were impaired [36], and basal motility remained unaffected [37]. A low dose of intraperitoneal injection of lipopolysaccharide (LPS), which activates microglia, showed no effects after two days on basal motility in vivo [38], although a decrease was observed 2 h after injection in acute slices [39]. However, higher LPS doses increased basal motility without affecting the time to reach the site of the laser lesion [40]. Interestingly, the relationship between activation and actin dynamics may be bi-directional, since impairment of actin dynamics shapes microglial functions [41].

Thus, the effects of microglia activation on motility cannot be easily generalized, because they unfold dynamically over time and depend strongly on the disease model. Furthermore, the type of motility must be taken into account when comparing different models, because they may be differently affected by microglial activation as our experiments demonstrate. We speculate that differential expression of P2Y12R may partially account for the variety in observations, as it seems to vary with activation status and mode of activation. On the one hand, enhanced P2Y12R expression is observed in the spinal cord three days after partial sciatic nerve ligation [42], as well as in human microglia under pathological conditions that promote alternative activation (M2; IL4- and IL-13, [43]). On the other hand, in post-mortem samples from the cerebral cortex of patients with multiple sclerosis (MS), P2Y12R expression is absent in microglia within the lesion zone [44]. Consistently, it gradually decreases in ALS and MS animal models [45]. Similar effects are observed when microglia activation is induced by LPS [13]. Thus, high activation characterized by an amoeboid shape may diminish P2Y12R expression. The lack of response in this study to a P2Y12R agonist in slices obtained from two animals, which had undergone a particularly long and severe crisis, is consistent with this hypothesis.

In addition to the velocity of microglial processes, it is important to consider the territory they explore, because it may influence their ability to interact with each other. Under physiological conditions, microglial processes hardly ever come into physical contact with each other. The avoidance behavior is abandoned when they detect danger signals and act together to isolate the source of the putative problem, implying that their mutual repulsion is dynamically regulated.

After SE, the spatial distribution of microglia was altered. Besides the twofold increase in the number of microglia [18], several cell bodies and cellular processes were found in the immediate proximity of each other (Additional file 9: Figure S5), which may reflect an alteration of the rules governing their physical interactions. Furthermore, the territory spanned by single processes was larger in KA-treated than control animals, which might reflect a compensation for shorter processes, allowing an efficient scanning of the territory. These phenomena could be due to the reduction of the signaling molecule(s) used for mediating the repulsive interactions.

## Conclusions

This study shows that, in contrast to other models of microglial activation, the state of activation induced 48 h

after induction of SE does not hamper the sentinel role of microglia. Indeed, they can still patrol the environment, and they can react to stimuli, possibly even in a more efficient way. Furthermore, our study reveals that microglia exhibit a variety of motility behaviors, which are differentially affected by microglial activation, indicating that the dynamic behavior of microglia depends on their state of activation as well as the nature of the stimulus, which triggers the motility.

## Additional files

**Additional file 1: Figure S1.** Method to assess global velocity of microglial processes. **A** Concentric rings are drawn around the area of interest (laser lesion spot or 2Me-ADP-containing pipette) in the maximal intensity projection (MIP) image. **B** Global velocity is calculated by observing the fluorescent wave passing through the rings in the MIP video. Each curve represents the evolution of the normalized fluorescence in time in the corresponding ring (matched color in A).

**Additional file 2: Figure S2.** Example of hyper-activated microglial cells in a slice obtained from a mouse with a long and severe crisis. Maximal intensity projection of two-photon images of the CA1 region in a hippocampal slice obtained from a KA-injected animal, which showed a particularly severe crisis. Microglia almost completely retracted their processes and accumulated around the *stratum pyramidale*, indicated by the dotted line. Scale bar, 30 μm.

**Additional file 3: Microglial response to P2Y12R agonist in control animal.** This movie shows the microglia response to a pipette containing 2Me-ADP in control animal. Processes distant as far as 100 μm responded to the stimulus. The processes coordinate their response to form a circle and arrive at the ATP analog source at the same time. New processes of microglia closer to stimulus start to be formed but started to move only after the more distal ones had caught up with them. Time expressed in minutes. Images are maximal intensity projection over a stack of 20 μm. Scale bar, 10 μm. Pixel sizes, 500, 300, and 200 nm.

**Additional file 4: Microglial response to P2Y12R agonist in KA-injected animal.** This movie shows the microglia response to a pipette containing 2Me-ADP in animal injected with KA. Comparing to control, processes reach the target in about half time. Time expressed in minutes. Images are maximal intensity projection over a stack of 20 μm. Scale bar, 10 μm. Pixel size, 250 nm.

**Additional file 5: Microglial response to laser ablation in control animal.** This movie shows the microglia movement before and after a small (1.6 × 1.6 μm) laser lesion (red spot) in control animal. Newly formed processes grew out from the cell body and from existing processes and moved towards the lesion site. Images are maximal intensity projection over a stack of 10 μm. Time expressed in minutes and seconds. Scale bar, 10 μm. Pixel size, 200 nm.

**Additional file 6: Microglial response to laser ablation in KA-injected animal.** This movie shows the microglia response to a small (1.6 × 1.6 μm) laser lesion (red spot) in KA-injected animal. In this movie, we can see that the response is not completely synchronized and processes do not approach the lesion site as a circle. Images are maximal intensity projection over a stack of 10 μm. Time expressed in minutes and seconds. Scale bar, 10 μm. Pixel size, 200 nm.

**Additional file 7: Figure S3.** Microglial processes converge towards a 2Me-ADP-containing pipette in a synchronized way. **A–B** Examples of maximal intensity projection in the *z* direction and in time for 6 min of two-photon images in slices where 2Me-ADP (100 μM)-containing pipette have been introduced (at *t* = 0) in control (A) and 48 h after the induction of a *SE* (B). Scale bar, 20 μm.

**Additional file 8: Figure S4.** The synchronization of microglial processes is less evident in the movement induced by laser lesion. Maximal intensity projections in the *z* direction and in time for 135 s (five time frames) of two-photon images in control. Processes arriving from the cell on the left reached the lesion before other processes, and there is no organization in circle as observed when a 2Me-ADP-containing pipette is inserted (see Additional file 7: Figure S3).

**Additional file 9: Figure 5.** Activated microglia lose their spatial segregated distribution. Three-dimensional reconstruction of 2-P image stacks obtained in control (top row) and KA-injected (bottom row) animals. Imaris software was used to reconstruct the morphology of single microglial cells, and to each cell, a different color was associated. Scale grid, 10 μm.

## Abbreviations
2Me-ADP: 2-Methylthioadenosine diphosphate trisodium salt; aCSF: artificial cerebrospinal fluid; KA: kainate; SE: status epilepticus.

## Competing interests
Authors declare no competing interests.

## Authors' contributions
EA and UVN conceived the study; EA, ML and UVN designed the experiments; EA and ML performed the experiments; EA, ML, and JA performed the analysis; UVN provided funding and supervised the study; EA and UVN wrote the manuscript.

## Acknowledgements
This study was supported by grants from the Agence Nationale de la Recherche (ANR-09-CEXC-012-01; ANR-2010-BLAN-1419, ANR-12-NEUR-0007-03). We are grateful to E. Audinat for fruitful discussions and comments on the manuscript and thank T. Pfeiffer, T. Amedé, and A. Panatier for comments on the manuscript and M. Jany for technical assistance. 3D image reconstructions were done in the Bordeaux Imaging Center, which is a service unit of CNRS, INSERM and the University of Bordeaux and a member of the national infrastructure 'France BioImaging'.

## Author details
[1]Interdisciplinary Institute for Neurosciences, CNRS UMR 5297, 33077 Bordeaux, France. [2]Université de Bordeaux, CNRS UMR 5297, 33077 Bordeaux, France.

## References
1. Kettenmann H, Hanisch U-K, Noda M, Verkhratsky A. Physiology of microglia. Physiol Rev. 2011;91:461–553.
2. Kettenmann H, Kirchhoff F, Verkhratsky A. Microglia: new roles for the synaptic stripper. Neuron. 2013;77:10–8.
3. Davalos D, Grutzendler J, Yang G, Kim JV, Zuo Y, Jung S, et al. ATP mediates rapid microglial response to local brain injury in vivo. Nat Neurosci. 2005;8:752–8.
4. Nimmerjahn A, Kirchhoff F, Helmchen F. Resting microglial cells are highly dynamic surveillants of brain parenchyma in vivo. Science. 2005;308:1314–8.
5. Parkhurst CN, Gan W-B. Microglia dynamics and function in the CNS. Curr Opin Neurobiol. 2010;20:595–600.
6. Madry C, Attwell D. Receptors, ion channels, and signaling mechanisms underlying microglial dynamics. J Biol Chem. 2015;290:12443–50.
7. Wake H, Moorhouse AJ, Jinno S, Kohsaka S, Nabekura J. Resting microglia directly monitor the functional state of synapses in vivo and determine the fate of ischemic terminals. J Neurosci Off J Soc Neurosci. 2009;29:3974–80.
8. Tremblay M-È, Lowery RL, Majewska AK. Microglial interactions with synapses are modulated by visual experience. PLoS Biol. 2010;8, e1000527.
9. Dibaj P, Nadrigny F, Steffens H, Scheller A, Hirrlinger J, Schomburg ED, et al. NO mediates microglial response to acute spinal cord injury under ATP control in vivo. Glia. 2010;58:1133–44.
10. Hines DJ, Hines RM, Mulligan SJ, Macvicar BA. Microglia processes block the spread of damage in the brain and require functional chloride channels. Glia. 2009;57:1610–8.
11. Domercq M, Vázquez-Villoldo N, Matute C. Neurotransmitter signaling in the pathophysiology of microglia. Front Cell Neurosci. 2013;7:49.
12. Fontainhas AM, Wang M, Liang KJ, Chen S, Mettu P, Damani M, et al. Microglial morphology and dynamic behavior is regulated by ionotropic glutamatergic and GABAergic neurotransmission. PLoS One. 2011;6, e15973.
13. Haynes SE, Hollopeter G, Yang G, Kurpius D, Dailey ME, Gan W-B, et al. The P2Y12 receptor regulates microglial activation by extracellular nucleotides. Nat Neurosci. 2006;9:1512–9.
14. Sieger D, Moritz C, Ziegenhals T, Prykhozhij S, Peri F. Long-range Ca2+ waves transmit brain-damage signals to microglia. Dev Cell. 2012;22:1138–48.
15. Hanisch U-K, Kettenmann H. Microglia: active sensor and versatile effector cells in the normal and pathologic brain. Nat Neurosci. 2007;10:1387–94.
16. Ransohoff RM, Perry VH. Microglial physiology: unique stimuli, specialized responses. Annu Rev Immunol. 2009;27:119–45.
17. Vezzani A, Aronica E, Mazarati A, Pittman QJ. Epilepsy and brain inflammation. Exp Neurol. 2013;244:11–21.
18. Avignone E, Ulmann L, Levavasseur F, Rassendren F, Audinat E. Status epilepticus induces a particular microglial activation state characterized by enhanced purinergic signaling. J Neurosci Off J Soc Neurosci. 2008;28:9133–44.
19. Ulmann L, Levavasseur F, Avignone E, Peyroutou R, Hirbec H, Audinat E, et al. Involvement of P2X4 receptors in hippocampal microglial activation after status epilepticus. Glia. 2013;61:1306–19.
20. Jimenez-Pacheco A, Mesuret G, Sanz-Rodriguez A, Tanaka K, Mooney C, Conroy R, et al. Increased neocortical expression of the P2X7 receptor after status epilepticus and anticonvulsant effect of P2X7 receptor antagonist A-438079. Epilepsia. 2013;54:1551–61.
21. Eyo UB, Peng J, Swiatkowski P, Mukherjee A, Bispo A, Wu L-J. Neuronal hyperactivity recruits microglial processes via neuronal NMDA receptors and microglial P2Y12 receptors after status epilepticus. J Neurosci Off J Soc Neurosci. 2014;34:10528–40.
22. Thévenaz P, Ruttimann UE, Unser M. A pyramid approach to subpixel registration based on intensity. IEEE Trans Image Process Publ IEEE Signal Process Soc. 1998;7:27–41.
23. Meijering E, Dzyubachyk O, Smal I. Methods for cell and particle tracking. Methods Enzymol. 2012;504:183–200.
24. Kozlowski C, Weimer RM. An automated method to quantify microglia morphology and application to monitor activation state longitudinally in vivo. PLoS One. 2012;7, e31814.
25. Papageorgiou IE, Fetani AF, Lewen A, Heinemann U, Kann O. Widespread activation of microglial cells in the hippocampus of chronic epileptic rats correlates only partially with neurodegeneration. Brain Struct Funct. 2015;220:2423–39.
26. Shapiro LA, Wang L, Ribak CE. Rapid astrocyte and microglial activation following pilocarpine-induced seizures in rats. Epilepsia. 2008;49 Suppl 2:33–41.
27. Morrison HW, Filosa JA. A quantitative spatiotemporal analysis of microglia morphology during ischemic stroke and reperfusion. J Neuroinflammation. 2013;10:4.
28. Wu LJ, Vadakkan KI, Zhuo M. ATP-induced chemotaxis of microglial processes requires P2Y receptor-activated initiation of outward potassium currents. Glia. 2007;55:810–21.
29. Ridley AJ. Life at the leading edge. Cell. 2011;145:1012–22.
30. Sadok A, Marshall CJ. Rho GTPases: masters of cell migration. Small GTPases. 2014;5, e29710.
31. Murali A, Rajalingam K. Small Rho GTPases in the control of cell shape and mobility. Cell Mol Life Sci CMLS. 2014;71:1703–21.
32. Soulet C, Hechler B, Gratacap M-P, Plantavid M, Offermanns S, Gachet C, et al. A differential role of the platelet ADP receptors P2Y1 and P2Y12 in Rac activation. J Thromb Haemost JTH. 2005;3:2296–306.
33. Erb L, Weisman GA. Coupling of P2Y receptors to G proteins and other signaling pathways. Wiley Interdiscip Rev Membr Transp Signal. 2012;1:789–803.
34. Dibaj P, Steffens H, Zschüntzsch J, Nadrigny F, Schomburg ED, Kirchhoff F, et al. In vivo imaging reveals distinct inflammatory activity of CNS microglia versus PNS macrophages in a mouse model for ALS. PLoS One. 2011;6, e17910.
35. Brawek B, Schwendele B, Riester K, Kohsaka S, Lerdkrai C, Liang Y, et al. Impairment of in vivo calcium signaling in amyloid plaque-associated microglia. Acta Neuropathol (Berl). 2014;127:495–505.
36. Krabbe G, Halle A, Matyash V, Rinnenthal JL, Eom GD, Bernhardt U, et al. Functional impairment of microglia coincides with beta-amyloid deposition in mice with Alzheimer-like pathology. PLoS One. 2013;8, e60921.
37. Bolmont T, Haiss F, Eicke D, Radde R, Mathis CA, Klunk WE, et al. Dynamics of the microglial/amyloid interaction indicate a role in plaque maintenance. J Neurosci Off J Soc Neurosci. 2008;28:4283–92.

38. Kondo S, Kohsaka S, Okabe S. Long-term changes of spine dynamics and microglia after transient peripheral immune response triggered by LPS in vivo. Mol Brain. 2011;4:27.

39. Madore C, Joffre C, Delpech JC, De Smedt-Peyrusse V, Aubert A, Coste L, et al. Early morphofunctional plasticity of microglia in response to acute lipopolysaccharide. Brain Behav Immun. 2013;34:151–8.

40. Gyoneva S, Davalos D, Biswas D, Swanger SA, Garnier-Amblard E, Loth F, et al. Systemic inflammation regulates microglial responses to tissue damage in vivo. Glia. 2014;62:1345–60.

41. Uhlemann R, Gertz K, Boehmerle W, Schwarz T, Nolte C, Freyer D, et al. Actin dynamics shape microglia effector functions. Brain Struct Funct. 2015.

42. Kobayashi K, Yamanaka H, Fukuoka T, Dai Y, Obata K, Noguchi K. P2Y12 receptor upregulation in activated microglia is a gateway of p38 signaling and neuropathic pain. J Neurosci Off J Soc Neurosci. 2008;28:2892–902.

43. Moore CS, Ase AR, Kinsara A, Rao VTS, Michell-Robinson M, Leong SY, et al. P2Y12 expression and function in alternatively activated human microglia. Neurol Neuroimmunol Neuroinflammation. 2015;2, e80.

44. Amadio S, Montilli C, Magliozzi R, Bernardi G, Reynolds R, Volonté C. P2Y12 receptor protein in cortical gray matter lesions in multiple sclerosis. Cereb Cortex. 2010;20:1263–73.

45. Amadio S, Parisi C, Montilli C, Carrubba AS, Apolloni S, Volonté C. P2Y(12) receptor on the verge of a neuroinflammatory breakdown. Mediators Inflamm. 2014;2014:975849.

# Protein expression profiling of inflammatory mediators in human temporal lobe epilepsy reveals co-activation of multiple chemokines and cytokines

Anne A Kan[1], Wilco de Jager[2], Marina de Wit[1], Cobi Heijnen[5], Mirjam van Zuiden[5], Cyrill Ferrier[3], Peter van Rijen[3], Peter Gosselaar[3], Ellen Hessel[1], Onno van Nieuwenhuizen[4] and Pierre N E de Graan[1*]

## Abstract

Mesial temporal lobe epilepsy (mTLE) is a chronic and often treatment-refractory brain disorder characterized by recurrent seizures originating from the hippocampus. The pathogenic mechanisms underlying mTLE remain largely unknown. Recent clinical and experimental evidence supports a role of various inflammatory mediators in mTLE. Here, we performed protein expression profiling of 40 inflammatory mediators in surgical resection material from mTLE patients with and without hippocampal sclerosis, and autopsy controls using a multiplex bead-based immunoassay. In mTLE patients we identified 21 upregulated inflammatory mediators, including 10 cytokines and 7 chemokines. Many of these upregulated mediators have not previously been implicated in mTLE (for example, CCL22, IL-7 and IL-25). Comparing the three patient groups, two main hippocampal expression patterns could be distinguished, pattern I (for example, IL-10 and IL-25) showing increased expression in mTLE + HS patients compared to mTLE-HS and controls, and pattern II (for example, CCL4 and IL-7) showing increased expression in both mTLE groups compared to controls. Upregulation of a subset of inflammatory mediators (for example, IL-25 and IL-7) could not only be detected in the hippocampus of mTLE patients, but also in the neocortex. Principle component analysis was used to cluster the inflammatory mediators into several components. Follow-up analyses of the identified components revealed that the three patient groups could be discriminated based on their unique expression profiles. Immunocytochemistry showed that IL-25 IR (pattern I) and CCL4 IR (pattern II) were localized in astrocytes and microglia, whereas IL-25 IR was also detected in neurons. Our data shows co-activation of multiple inflammatory mediators in hippocampus and neocortex of mTLE patients, indicating activation of multiple pro- and anti-epileptogenic immune pathways in this disease.

**Keywords:** Temporal lobe epilepsy, Immune system, Network analysis

## Background

Epilepsy is a common brain disorder that affects approximately 50 million people worldwide [1]. Mesial temporal lobe epilepsy (mTLE) is a type of epilepsy where seizure activity originates from the hippocampal structures, and is the most common type of partial epilepsy [2]. Approximately 30% of mTLE patients experience seizures that do not respond to treatment with current anti-epileptic medication [3,4]. A common hallmark of mTLE is hippocampal sclerosis; it is characterized by hippocampal neuronal loss combined with gliosis and aberrant axonal sprouting [5,6]. To develop new treatment strategies for drug-refractory patients, there is an urgent need to unravel the molecular mechanisms of epileptogenesis, the complex cascade of molecular, cellular and network changes leading to mTLE [7]. A rapidly growing body of clinical and experimental evidence supports the involvement of the immune system in seizure generation and epileptogenesis [8,9]. For instance, genome-wide mRNA expression

* Correspondence: p.n.e.degraan@umcutrecht.nl
[1]Department of Neuroscience and Pharmacology, Rudolf Magnus Institute of Neuroscience, Universiteitsweg 100, 3584 CG, Utrecht, The Netherlands
Full list of author information is available at the end of the article

profiling in tissue resected from mTLE patients revealed upregulation of multiple genes coding for inflammatory mediators [10,11]. The inflammatory mediators which have been most extensively studied in mTLE are members of the cytokine and chemotactic cytokine (chemokine) families.

Cytokines are soluble polypeptides that play a crucial role in mediating the immune response in both the periphery and the central nervous system (CNS). Prototypical proinflammatory cytokines, such as IL-6, TNFα and the IL-1 family, have been extensively studied in the CNS and are implicated in human mTLE [10,12-14]. Rodent studies have provided evidence for a pro-epileptogenic role of these proinflammatory cytokines (reviewed in [9,15,16]). Tissue resected from mTLE patients also contains increased levels of chemokine transcripts, a specific class of cytokines that provides chemoattractant cues for immune-competent cells such as microglia and leukocytes [17]. Upregulated chemokine transcripts include CCL2, CCL3 and CCL4 (Chemokine (C-C motif) ligand 2 to 4) [10,11], which are considered to be proinflammatory markers in the brain [9,18].

As the inflammatory mediators mentioned above are considered to be pro-epileptogenic, it is expected that interference with inflammatory pathways would ameliorate epileptogenesis and mTLE. However, treatment strategies employing general or specific anti-inflammatory agents in animal models for mTLE have not been fully effective thus far [19-25]. The limited success of anti-inflammatory treatment could be due to the fact that the key targets in epileptogenesis have not yet been identified. Alternatively, the treatment may not only affect proinflammatory pathways, but may concomitantly inhibit beneficial anti-inflammatory pathways. A third possibility is that specific targeting of only one component in the complex pathways of the innate immune response is not sufficient to affect epileptogenesis [26-28].

To address these issues it is essential to map changes in expression of multiple immune mediators in human mTLE tissue. mRNA expression profiling studies have provided the first insight into the regulation of immunological networks in mTLE [10,11]. However, these studies need verification at the protein level, because it is not known whether changes in mRNA expression translate into protein differences. Moreover, recent evidence indicates that large scale post-transcriptional regulation plays a role in mTLE [29,30].

In the present study, we performed protein expression profiling of multiple immune mediators in tissue resected from mTLE patients. We analyzed 40 proteins in each tissue sample using a bead-based multiplex immunoassay (MIA) and compared protein expression levels in homogenates of mTLE patients with hippocampal sclerosis (HS, mTLE + HS), (mTLE-HS) and of non-epileptic autopsy controls. We identified 21 differentially expressed inflammatory mediators, predominantly cytokines and chemokines. Principal component analysis clustered the inflammatory mediators into several components, and follow-up analysis revealed that patient groups could be discriminated based on their unique expression profiles. Our data indicates the upregulation of multiple immune pathways in mTLE and provides new targets for the development of immunological intervention strategies.

## Materials and methods
### Patient selection and tissue collection
Neocortical (medial temporal gyrus) (CX) and hippocampal (HC) tissue samples of pharmaco-resistant mTLE patients were obtained after surgery at the University Medical Centre Utrecht. Patients were selected for surgery according to the criteria of the Dutch Epilepsy Surgery Program [31]. The excision was based on clinical evaluations, interictal and ictal electroencephalography (EEG) studies, magnetic resonance imaging (MRI) and intraoperative electrocorticography (iEcOG). Informed consent was obtained from all patients and all procedures were approved by the Institutional Review Board. Immediately after resection, the tissue was cooled in physiological saline (4°C) and cut on a precooled plate. The neocortex sample was cut in half perpendicular to the surface of the gyrus, the hippocampus into three slices perpendicular to its longitudinal axis. One half of the neocortex sample and the two outer parts of the hippocampus were used for clinical pathological analysis. The remaining neocortical and hippocampal tissue samples were once more divided into a part that was immediately frozen on powdered dry ice and a part that was immersion-fixed in 4% paraformaldehyde in 0.1 M phosphate buffer for 24 h at 4°C. Following fixation, tissue was embedded in paraffin and stored at 4°C. Frozen samples were stored at −80°C. Frozen and paraffin-embedded control brain tissue samples were obtained from non-epileptic post mortem cases without hippocampal aberrations from the Netherlands Brain Bank (NBB no. 618, www.brainbank.nl). All control material was collected from donors with written informed consent for brain autopsy and the use of the material and clinical information for research purposes. Only patient samples obtained after a relatively short post mortem delay (range 4 to 20.5 h; mean 6.8 h) and with a pH value close to 6.5 (range 6.36 to 6.88; mean 6.68) were used. Detailed histological examination of the brain material from all patients used in this study showed that all samples were devoid of tumor tissue. Neocortical samples that displayed cortical dysplasia or any other abnormalities that might trigger an immunological response were excluded from the study [32,33]. The quality of all

tissue samples was further analyzed in a parallel study [30], showing that after RNA isolation all samples had RNA integrity values (RIN) >6 (range 6.4 to 8.4; mean 7.2) and RIN values did not significantly differ between autopsy control and mTLE patient samples. Table 1 provides a summary of the clinical data of all patients included in the study. Cortical and hippocampal specimens were divided into three groups: a non-epileptic autopsy control group (control, n = 10), a group of mTLE patients without signs of hippocampal sclerosis (mTLE-HS, n = 10) and an mTLE group with hippocampal sclerosis (mTLE + HS, n = 10). The severity of HS was determined by a neuropathologist using the Wyler classification method [34] defining W0 as hippocampal tissue without HS and W4 as tissue with the most severe type of HS. Wyler classification was independently verified on sections of paraffin-embedded tissue.

## Multiplex bead-based immunoassay analysis

Nissl-stained cryosections were generated to ensure that neocortical samples contained 50% gray and 50% white matter, and that in hippocampal samples all anatomical subregions were equally represented. Subsequently 25 μm cryosections were cut until approximately 20 mg of tissue was collected. This material was stored at –80°C until all samples were collected. The frozen slices were homogenized at 4°C in 400 μl lysis buffer (Lysis M, Roche, Basel, Switzerland), sonicated, centrifuged and passed through a filtering column (0.22 μm, Spin-X, Costar, Sigma-Aldrich, St Louis, MO, USA), frozen and stored (final concentration 0.5ug/ul) at –80°C [36].

Concentrations of 39 immune modulators (listed in Table 2) were measured using a multiplex bead-based immunoassay (MIA) as previously described. [37]. Capture and detection antibody pairs and recombinant proteins used for the standard curves were purchased from commercial sources as described previously [38] (and Table 3). Carboxylated polystyrene microspheres were purchased from Bio-Rad Laboratories (Hercules, CA, USA). Covalent coupling of the capture antibodies to the microspheres was performed as previously described [37,38]. Optimal working conditions and sample dilutions were determined for each antibody and calibration curves from recombinant protein standards were prepared using two-fold dilution steps in Lysis M buffer used for homogenization [38]. All assays were carried out directly in a 96 well 1.2 μm filter plate (Millipore, Billerica, MA, USA) at room temperature and protected from light. A mixture containing 1000 microspheres per antigen (total volume 10 μl/well) was incubated together with a standard, homogenate or lysis buffer for 1 h at room temperature. Next, 10 μl of a cocktail of biotinylated antibodies (16.5 μg/ml each) was added to each well and incubated for an additional 60 min Beads were

then washed with phosphate buffered saline (PBS) supplemented with 1% bovine serum albumin (BSA) and 0.5% Tween 20 at pH of 7.4. After incubation for 10 min with 50 ng/well streptavidin R-phycoerythrin (BD Biosciences, San Diego CA, USA) and washing twice with PBS-1% BSA-0.5%-Tween 20 pH 7.4. Fluorescence intensity of the beads was measured in a final volume of 100 μl HPE buffer (Sanquin Reagents, Amsterdam, The Netherlands) and buffer values were subtracted from all readings. Measurements and data analysis were performed using the Bio-Plex system in combination with the Bio-Plex Manager software version 4.1 (Bio-Rad Laboratories). CCL4 levels were measured separately using a fluorokine kit (R&D Systems, Abingdon, UK) according to the manufacturer's instructions.

MIA was performed on selected chemokines, cytokines, growth factors and adhesion molecules. HC and CX protein levels were determined in controls and two mTLE patient groups (– and + HS). Inflammatory proteins are listed in order of overall significance (ANOVA/Kruskal-Wallis). Proteins in bold show significant changes between groups (ANOVA/Kruskal-Wallis, $P < 0.0015$). Levels are presented as medians and range (between brackets). Abbreviations: b. d., below detection; HGF, hepatocyte growth factor; ICAM1, intercellular cell adhesion molecule 1; IFNα, interferon type 1α; IP10, interferon gamma-induced protein 10; MCP1. monocyte chemotactic protein-1; MDC, macrophage-derived chemokine; MIF, macrophage migration inhibitory factor; MIG, monokine induced by interferon γ; MIP1α, macrophage inflammatory protein-1α; MIP1β, macrophage inflammatory protein-1β; MIP3β, macrophage inflammatory protein-3β; PARC, pulmonary and activation-regulated chemokine; RANTES, regulated upon activation normal T cell express sequence; TARC, thymus- and activation-regulated chemokine; TIMP-1, tissue inhibitor of metalloproteinases; TNFα. tumor necrosis factor; VCAM1, vascular cell adhesion molecule 1; VEGF, vascular endothelial growth factor.

## Immunohistochemistry and immunofluorescence

Hippocampal immunohistochemistry (IHC) was performed on 7 μm paraffin sections of the same patients (n = 6 per group) as used in the MIA (CCL4 polyclonal goat, 1:200, Santa Cruz Biotechnology, Santa Cruz, CA, USA; IL-25 monoclonal mouse, 1:800, R&D systems, Abingdon, UK). We tested several antibodies against immune modulators with pattern 1 and 2 (Figure 1). Based on their superior quality for immunocytochemistry on paraffin section we choose IL-25 and CCL4. Serial antibody dilution curves were prepared in phosphate buffered saline (PBS) containing 0.2%Triton-X100 to determine optimal working concentrations. After rehydration, all sections were subjected to antigen retrieval using microwave treatment (in 0.01 M, Na$^+$ Citrate pH

**Table 1 Clinical data of mTLE and Control patients**

| Patient group | Age | Sex | Pathology/COD | Tissue used | Seizure frequency | iEcOG spikes | Anti-epileptic drugs | Engel score (1 yr) |
|---|---|---|---|---|---|---|---|---|
| 1) Control | 73 | F | subdural hematoma | HC | NA | NA | NA | NA |
| 2) Control | 58 | M | unknown. ALS patient | HC & CX | NA | NA | NA | NA |
| 3) Control | 62 | M | unknown, non-demented control | HC & CX | NA | NA | NA | NA |
| 4) Control | 94 | F | CVA | HC & CX | NA | NA | NA | NA |
| 5) Control | 71 | M | pancreas carcinoma | HC & CX | NA | NA | NA | NA |
| 6) Control | 64 | F | respiratory failure | HC & CX | NA | NA | NA | NA |
| 7) Control | 70 | M | sepsis with broncopneumonia | HC | NA | NA | NA | NA |
| 8) Control | 50 | F | metastasized broncocarcinoma | HC & CX | NA | NA | NA | NA |
| 9) Control | 48 | M | DMT I induced organ failure | HC | NA | NA | NA | NA |
| 10) Control | 74 | M | pulmonary carcinoma | HC & CX | NA | NA | NA | NA |
| 11) Control | 62 | F | renal carcinoma (euthanasia) | CX | NA | NA | NA | NA |
| 12) Control | 93 | F | heart failure | CX | NA | NA | NA | NA |
| 13) Control | 92 | F | cachexia/dehydration | CX | NA | NA | NA | NA |
| 14) non-HS | 45 | M | W0, FCD type1 to 2A in cortex | HC | 6 | CX | LTG, PHT | 1A |
| 15) non-HS | 46 | F | W0, MCD type 1 in cortex | HC | 12 | CX | CBZ, VPA | 1A |
| 16) non-HS | 46 | M | W0, epilepsy after head trauma | HC | 90 | HC & CX | CBZ, VPA, TPR | 1B |
| 17) non-HS | 42 | F | W0, DNT WHO grade I | HC & CX | 1 | CX | CBZ, LTG, LEV | 1A |
| 18) non-HS | 34 | F | W0, cortical cavernoma | HC | 1.5 | HC & CX | CBZ | 1A |
| 19) non-HS | 40 | F | W0, MCD type 1 in cortex | HC | 8 ( C ) | HC & CX | LEV, LTG, CBZ | 1A |
| 20) non-HS | 43 | F | W0, therapy resistant epilepsy | HC & CX | 40 ( C ) | HC & CX | PHT, LTG | 1A |
| 21) non-HS | 47 | M | W0, therapy resistant epilepsy | HC | 30 | HC | CBZ, VPA, LTG, LEV | 3A |
| 22) non-HS | 28 | M | W0, MCD type 1 in cortex | HC | 60 | HC & CX | CBZ, TPR. | 1A |
| 23) non-HS | 54 | M | W0, ganglioglioma WHO grade I | HC & CX | 1.5 | HC & CX | OXC, LTG, CLO | 1A |
| 24) non-HS | 30 | M | W0, therapy resistant epilepsy | CX | 8 | HC & CX | OXC, LEV, CLO | 1A |
| 25) non-HS | 37 | F | W0, therapy resistant epilepsy | CX | 1 | not measured | LTG, CLO | 1A |
| 26) non-HS | 61 | M | W0, therapy resistant epilepsy | CX | 5.5 | HC & CX | PHT, CBZ | 2A |
| 27) non-HS | 19 | M | W0, ganglioglioma WHO grade II | CX | 1 | None | VPA, LEV | 1A |
| 28) non-HS | 27 | F | W0, therapy resistant epilepsy | CX | 16 | HC & CX | LEV | 1A |
| 29) non-HS | 46 | M | W0, cavernoma in uncus | CX | 60 | HC | CBZ, VPA, OXC, LEV, LTG | 1A |
| 30) non-HS | 44 | M | W0, therapy resistant epilepsy | CX | 18 | HC & CX | TPR, OXC | 1A |
| 31) HS | 41 | M | MTS W4 | HC & CX | 12 | not measured | PHT, CLO, CBZ, LTG | 1A |
| 32) HS | 44 | F | MTS W2 | HC | 8 ( C ) | not measured | CBZ, OXC, CLO | 1A |
| 33) HS | 41 | M | MTS W4 | HC | 3 | not measured | CBZ | 1A |
| 34) HS | 52 | F | MTS W4 | HC & CX | 10 | not measured | CBZ, CLO, DZP | 2D |
| 35) HS | 50 | M | MTS W4 | HC | 18 | not measured | CBZ, GBP | 2A |
| 36) HS | 36 | F | MTS W4 | HC & CX | 2 | not measured | OXC, LZP | no info |
| 37) HS | 42 | M | MTS W4 | HC & CX | 2 | not measured | LEV, LTG | 2A |
| 38) HS | 36 | M | MTS W4 | HC & CX | 10 | HC & CX | OXC, PGB | 1B |
| 39) HS | 49 | F | MTS W4 | HC | 8 ( C ) | not measured | OXC, CLO | 1A |
| 40) HS | 42 | F | MTS W4 | HC | 4.5 | not measured | LEV, LTG, PBT | 1A |
| 41) HS | 36 | M | MTS W4 | CX | 5 | not measured | PGB, LTG | 1A |
| 42) HS | 34 | F | MTS W4 | CX | 10 ( C ) | HC & CX | LTG, CBZ, VPA,CLO | 2A |
| 43) HS | 49 | M | MTS W3 | CX | 1 | None | LTG, CBZ, CLO | 1A |

**Table 1 Clinical data of mTLE and Control patients** *(Continued)*

| | | | | | | | | | |
|---|---|---|---|---|---|---|---|---|---|
| **44) HS** | 45 | M | MTS W4 | | CX | 0.5 | not measured | GBP, LTG | 1A |
| **45) HS** | 48 | M | MTS W4 | | CX | 3.5 | not measured | CBZ, LTG, VPA | 1A |

Hippocampal (HC) and neocortical (CX) homogenates were prepared from tissue of the listed patients as indicated in column 5. All epilepsy patients suffered therapy resistant epilepsy, any additional pathologies are listed in column 4. Seizure frequencies are listed as an average of monthly activity, patients who suffered clustered attacks are marked (C). iEcOG spikes indicate epileptic spike activity detected by iEcOG at surgery. Engel scores were recorded 1 year after surgery [35]. Abbreviations: *ALS* amyotrophic lateral sclerosis, *CBZ* Carbamazepine, *COD* cause of death, *CLO* Clobazam, *CVA* cerebrovascular accident, *CX* temporal neocortex, *DMT I* diabetes mellitus type I, *DNT* Dysembryonic neuroepithelial tumor, *DZP* diazepam, *FCD* focal cortical dysplasia, *GBP* Gabapentin, *HC* hippocampus, *HS* hippocampal sclerosis, *iEcOG* intraoperative electrocorticography, *LEV* Levetiracetam, *LTG* Lamotrigine, *LZP* Lorazepam, *MCD* malformation of cortical development, *MTS* mesial temporal sclerosis, *NA* not applicable, *OXC* Oxcarbazepine, *PBT* Phenobarbital, *PGB* Pregabaline, *PHT* Phenytoin, *PMD* post mortem delay, *RIN* RNA integrity number, *TPR* Topiramate; *VPA* Valproinic acid, *W0 till 4* Wyler score, *WHO grade* world health organization grading scale of malignancy.

6.0), non-specific binding was blocked by incubating sections with 0.3% $H_2O_2$ for 30 min at room temperature and with fetal calf serum (IL-25) or normal rabbit serum (CCL4) for 30 min at 37°C. Sections were incubated with primary antibodies overnight at 4°C. The secondary antibodies used were biotinylated rabbit anti-goat and biotinylated horse anti-mouse (Dako Cytomation, Glostrup, Denmark). Signals were visualized using the avidin-biotin method (Vectastain ABC Elite kit; Vector Laboratories, Burlingame, CA, USA) with 3,3′-diaminobenzidinetetrachloride (DAB) as the chromogen (Sigma Chemical Co., St. Louis, MO, USA). By visual inspection, sections were ranked according to overall IR levels by two independent observers blinded to the experimental design. No immunostaining was observed when the protocol was completed with primary antibodies preabsorbed with their respective antigens, or without the primary antibodies.

Double immunofluorescence labeling was performed as described for IHC, but without the 0.3% $H_2O_2$ blocking step. Anti-GFAP (polyclonal rabbit, 1:6000 Dako Cytomation, Glostrup, Denmark), Iba1 (polyclonal rabbit, 1:200, WAKO Pure Chemical Industries, Neuss, Germany), Vimentin (monoclonal mouse,1:2400, Dako Cytomation, Glostrup, Denmark) and NeuN (polyclonal rabbit, 1:800, Millipore, Billerica, MA, USA) were used as CNS cell-type markers. Secondary antibodies used were donkey anti-goat Alexa 488 and goat anti-mouse Alexa 488 (Invitrogen, Molecular Probes, Eugene, OR, USA) for CCL4 and IL-25, donkey anti-mouse Alexa 555 and donkey anti-rabbit Alexa 555 (Invitrogen, Molecular Probes, Eugene, OR, USA) for the cell-type markers. Finally, Sudan Black dye was used to reduce autofluorescence [39]. Controls without primary antibody were devoid of fluorescent staining.

## Statistical analyses

To determine overall statistical significance of differences in protein expression between patient groups, data from all detectable inflammatory mediators were analyzed using a one-way ANOVA (if normally distributed) or Kruskal-Wallis test (if not normally distributed). When significant group differences were present

(Bonferroni corrected for multiple testing: $P = <0.0015$), additional post hoc tests (Table 4) were performed (Students *t*-test or Mann–Whitney U with Bonferroni correction: $P = <0.008$).

A univariate general linear model analysis was used to assess possible confounding effects of age and gender. Using age or gender as covariate did not result in loss of significance for any of the previously significant group differences ($P = <0.0015$), nor did age and gender significantly predict the outcome.

In the autopsy control data set Pearson's correlation tests did not reveal significant correlations between protein expression and brain pH or post mortem delay (PMD), thus ruling out pH and PMD as confounders ($CC < 0.7$ $P = > 0.0015$). Also, using RNA integrity numbers (RIN) measured for a different study of these control samples, no correlation was found between inflammatory mediator levels and RIN values [30]. To assess correlations between expression levels of inflammatory mediators (all proteins with $P = <0.05$) and known clinical parameters (Engel score, seizure frequency, iEcOG spikes), we performed correlation analyses using a Pearson's correlation (if normally distributed) or a Spearman's rank test (if not normally distributed). The cut-off for a correlation was set at 0.8 with a Bonferroni corrected $P$ value $P = <0.0017$. All positive correlations between inflammatory mediators were plotted to form networks using Cytoscape.

Finally, all data from the detectable inflammatory mediators were clustered into components (factors) using an unbiased principle component analysis (PCA) (see Marengo *et al.* 2010 [40]) (in SPSS also known as factor analysis). As bivariate analyses showed that expression data for multiple proteins were correlated, which is in line with functional relations between cytokines, we chose the oblimin rotation, which allows correlation between factors, rather than the often used varimax rotation, which does not allow correlation between factors. The number of extracted components was based on examination of the scree plot and eigenvalues (>1.0). Interpretation of the components was based on mediators with factor loadings above 0.4 (16% explained variance). When there were missing values (in one patient, for two cytokines) they were replaced

**Table 2 Protein levels inflammatory mediators**

| Protein | Hippocampal expression (pg/ml) | | | Cortical expression (pg/ml) | | | P-value |
|---|---|---|---|---|---|---|---|
| | Cntrl | mTLE-HS | mTLE + HS | Cntrl | mTLE-HS | mTLE + HS | |
| **Chemokines** | | | | | | | |
| CCL22/MDC | 0.3 (0–0.7) | 0.8 (0.4-1.6) | 0.9 (0.3-1.4) | 0.2 (0–0.6) | 0.6 (0.3-1.2) | 0.9 (0.7-1.3) | 1.74E-08 |
| CCL5/RANTES | 8.1 (4–15.8) | 77.4 (40.9-238.1) | 49.4 (18.5-167.7) | 10.9 (1.6-18.5) | 26.0 (18.5-122.3) | 31.5 (17.4-38.5) | 1.60E-08 |
| CCL4/MIP1β | 0 (0–0) | 19.4 (4-122.3) | 18.9 (6.2-95.3) | 0 (0–0) | 0 (0–7.6) | 0.0 (0-33.6) | 2.11E-08 |
| CXCL9/MIG | 3.2 (1.1-11) | 9.0 (6.7-16.7) | 11.0 (4.4-17.1) | 5.7 (2.4-7.7) | 8.3 (5.7-12) | 10.7 (7.0-12.3) | 5.99E-07 |
| CCL2/MCP1 | 1.1 (0–4.3) | 11.4 (2.1-52.8) | 9.3 (2.1-29.0) | 0.0 (0–2.9) | 0.7 (0-4.6) | 0.3 (0-18.2) | 4.13E-06 |
| CCL3/MIP1α | 44.4 (11.2-106.2) | 94.5 (62-177.4) | 94.6 (62-317.1) | 35.6 (20.1-57.4) | 62.0 (35.6-104.9) | 85.1 (59.0-97.2) | 9.13E-05 |
| CCL19/MIP3β | 0 (0–0) | 0.5 (0-1.6) | 0 (0-1) | 0 (0–0) | 0 (0-1.7) | 0.4 (0-1.3) | 9.90E-05 |
| CCL18/PARC | 16.6 (0.2-151.6) | 24.2 (1.8-177.4) | 14.0 (0-29.5) | 13.7 (0-132.7) | 3.3 (0-31.9) | 0.7 (0-37.6) | 0.001966 |
| CXCL8/IL-8 | 0.8 (0-13.8) | 2.7 (0-26) | 1.0 (0.3-20.1) | 0.6 (0-1.6) | 0.5 (0-10.3) | 0.9 (0-3.6) | 0.02352 |
| CCL11/Eotaxin | 0 | 0 | 0 | 0 | 0 | 0 | b.d. |
| CCL17/Tarc | 0 | 0 | 0 | 0 | 0 | 0 | b.d. |
| CXCL10/IP-10 | 0 | 0 | 0 | 0 | 0 | 0 | b.d. |
| **Cytokines** | | | | | | | |
| IL-7 | 0 (0-5.6) | 8.3 (3.8-9.6) | 7.3 (0.6-12.2) | 0.9 (0.0-4.6) | 8.7 (4.6-14.5) | 11.0 (8-12.7) | 5.07E-15 |
| IL-13 | 2.6 (0.9-6.8) | 13.4 (7.9-20.5) | 11.2 (8.1-17.4) | 6.4 (2.6-12.5) | 12.7 (10.3-17.4) | 15.4 (10.7-16.5) | 7.60E-13 |
| IL-22 | 92.5 (58.3-212.2) | 351.2 (236.6-540.6) | 304.1 (244.8-449.9) | 212.2 (122.8-359.4) | 380.0 (293.8-548.8) | 425.2 (261.1-499.3) | 1.65E-12 |
| IL-5 | 0 (0-1.2) | 2.8 (1.5-7.4) | 2.8 (0.3-5.5) | 0 (0-1) | 2.3 (1-6.7) | 5.0 (2-6.1) | 2.06E-07 |
| IL-25/IL-17E | 726.9 (273.4-1780) | 868.3 (348.3-1616) | 1976.4 (258.5-2499) | 303.3 (109.9-757.4) | 673.5 (483.8-1234.5) | 922.1 (468.7-1327.5) | 1.93E-05 |
| IL-1RA | 13.5 (6.7-26.8) | 19.0 (13.5-33.4) | 20.7 (12.3-29) | 15.7 (13.5-31.2) | 29.0 (13.5-165.2) | 53.1 (26.8-92.2) | 2.96E-05 |
| IL-1a | 0 (0-0.2) | 0.3 (0-3) | 0.3 (0-1.3) | 0 (0-0) | 0 (0-0.9) | 0.3 (0-1.6) | 5.06E-05 |
| IL-27 | 40.9 (0-153.8) | 33.7 (0-133.4) | 132.1 (0-370.5) | 0 (0-42.3) | 28.6 (0-89.7) | 49.4 (29.4-78.7) | 8.93E-05 |
| IL-10 | 2.2 (0-5.9) | 1.4 (0-3.4) | 7.8 (0-12.4) | 0 (0-2.2) | 0.5 (0-1.9) | 0.9 (0-3.4) | 1.02E-04 |
| IFNα | 22.5 (12.8-41.5) | 31.5 (22.7-58.5) | 66.3 (10.1-114.3) | 27.0 (4.1-73.1) | 41.3 (26.9-51.5) | 38.5 (30.7-59) | 3.40E-04 |
| MIF | 11135.4 (7054-13156) | 8200.7 (6406-19843) | 6907.3 (4910-9650) | 11062.2 (4645-17980) | 7112.0 (4645-9872) | 7180.8 (5547-9470) | 0.0024 |
| IL-1β | 0.2 (0-0.9) | 0.8 (0.2-1.7) | 0.9 (0.2-1.7) | 0.2 (0-0.9) | 0.5 (0-1.5) | 0.9 (0-1.7) | 0.0063 |
| IL-23 | 298.9 (190.4-568.7) | 575.1 (473.2-675) | 556.2 (311.2-691) | 308.1 (238.2-717) | 500.2 (286.7-633) | 543.2 (372.9-710) | 0.0063 |
| IL-4 | 0 (0-0.1) | 0.1 (0-0.2) | 0 (0-0.2) | 0 (0-0) | 0 (0-0.2) | 0.1 (0-0.2) | 0.0234 |
| IL-6 | 0 (0-11.7) | 0 (0-3.9) | 0 (0-1.1) | 0 (0-2.1) | 0 (0-0) | 0.0 (0-0) | 0.0428 |
| IL-21 | 336.5 (117.7-944.2) | 510.6 (0-944.2) | 831.0 (55.8-1270.4) | 431.2 (0-1009.1) | 415.4 (0-847.1) | 654.1 (179.9-1534) | 0.0848 |
| TNFα | 10.4 (8.6-12.7) | 11.5 (7.0-13.2) | 11.2 (8.2-13.2) | 9.3 (6.3-12.9) | 10.6 (6.9-12.3) | 10.5 (9.2-13.2) | 0.1341 |
| IL-18 | 3.7 (1.7-14.2) | 3.2 (1.5-5.2) | 2.1 (1.1-23.8) | 5.0 (1.6-163.1) | 2.9 (1.7-12.4) | 2.9 (2.2-4.8) | 0.1481 |
| IL-6R | 1.4 (0-10) | 1.4 (0-5.6) | 4.5 (1.4-8.9) | 3.4 (0-17) | 3.4 (0-10) | 4.5 (0-7.8) | 0.4944 |
| IL-2 | 0 | 0 | 0 | 0 | 0 | 0.0 | b.d. |

**Table 2 Protein levels inflammatory mediators** *(Continued)*

| | | | | | | | | | | | | | b.d. |
|---|---|---|---|---|---|---|---|---|---|---|---|---|---|
| IL-12p70 | 0 | | 0 | | 0 | | 0 | | 0 | | 0.0 | | |
| **Other** | | | | | | | | | | | | | |
| **VCAM1** | 219.7 | (33.9–828.3) | 985.5 | (548–1722.6) | 1181.3 | (364.5–1649) | 210.3 | (67.3–527.2) | 817.5 | (444.9–1287) | 1239.9 | (740.4–1551) | **2.71E-11** |
| **VEGF** | 10.0 | (0.4–28.8) | 30.3 | (18.6–47) | 31.1 | (7.2–59.3) | 4.5 | (0–12.8) | 22.9 | (12.8–39.3) | 32.6 | (17.1–36.3) | **3.70E-10** |
| **HGF** | 33.0 | (26.7–54.5) | 105.2 | (65.8–157.4) | 90.3 | (34.6–156.4) | 24.0 | (19–50.3) | 71.3 | (37–207.7) | 52.4 | (32.2–83.6) | **1.38E-07** |
| **ICAM1** | 9099.6 | (3364–17901) | 5400.2 | (3174–9985) | 16011.1 | (5781–26620) | 5039.5 | (1532–16739) | 3440.4 | (1532–10754) | 4698.9 | (1861–8725) | **9.13E-05** |
| Cathepsin S | 463.3 | (284.2–1010) | 311.9 | (129.1–525.7) | 218.0 | (160.4–425.5) | 350.6 | (198.2–993.6) | 303.8 | (198.2–478.7) | 327.2 | (190.4–413) | 0.0025 |
| TIMP-1 | 101.0 | (36.2–2243.7) | 124.3 | (81.6–382.5) | 103.2 | (50.7–204) | 81.6 | (53.7–137.7) | 97.7 | (64.5–324.4) | 112.5 | (83.5–305.6) | 0.2672 |
| Adiponectin | 415.0 | (14–1412.5) | 727.8 | (193.3–1643) | 480.3 | (221–1787.4) | 722.4 | (22.4–1979.9) | 490.0 | (22.4–940.7) | 349.3 | (0–1751) | 0.4253 |

MIA was performed on selected chemokines, cytokines, growth factors and adhesion molecules. HC and CX protein levels were determined in controls and 2 mTLE patient groups (– and +HS).Inflammatory proteins are listed in order of **overall** significance (**ANOVA/Kruskal-Wallis**). Proteins in bold show significant changes between groups (ANOVA/Kruskal-Wallis, p < 0.0015). Levels are presented as medians and range (between brackets). Abbreviations: *b.d.* below detection, *HGF* hepatocyte growth factor, *ICAM1* intercellular cell adhesion molecule 1, *IFNα* interferon type 1α, *IP10* Interferon gamma-induced protein 10, *MCP1* macrophage derived chemokine, *MDC* macrophage derived chemokine, *MIF* Macrophage migration inhibitory factor, *MIG* monokine induced by interferon γ, *MIP1α* Macrophage inflammatory protein-1α, *MIP1β* Macrophage inflammatory protein-1β, *MIP3β* Macrophage inflammatory protein-3β, *PARC* pulmonary and activation-regulated chemokine, *RANTES* Regulated upon activation normal T cell express sequence, *TARC* thymus and activation regulated chemokine, *TIMP-1* tissue inhibitor of metalloproteinases, *TNFα* tumor necrosis factor, *VCAM1* vascular cell adhesion molecule 1, *VEGF* vascular endothelial growth factor.

**Table 3 Recombinant proteins and antibody sets used in MIA**

| Antigen | Protein source | Antibody set |
|---|---|---|
| CCL4 | R&D | R&D |
| CCL19 | R&D | R&D |
| IL-1RA | R&D | Bioledgend |
| IL-6R | R&D | Sanquin |
| IL-7 | BD | BD |
| IL-21 | Abnova | eBioscience |
| IL-22 | Peprotech | Peprotech |
| IL-23 | R&D | eBioscience |
| IL-25 | R&D | R&D |
| IL-27 | R&D | R&D |
| IFNa | eBioscience | eBioscience |
| VEGF | R&D | R&D |
| HGF | R&D | R&D |
| Cathepsin S | R&D | R&D |
| TIMP1 | R&D | R&D |
| Adiponectin | R&D | R&D |

R&D systems, UK; Bioledgend, USA; Sanquin, The Netherlands; Abnova, Taiwan; Peprotech, USA; eBioscience, USA.

with the group mean. Rotations for all data converged within 50 iterations. All inflammatory mediators were used to calculate individual components scores for each participant (using regression to determine the component or factor scores). These were saved and subsequently used to analyze group differences and construct PCA plots.

Programs used for the statistical analyses and graphical representations were SPSS (SPSS 15 for Windows), Graphpad Prism 4 and Cytoscape 2.8.

## Results

### Protein expression profiling of the immune system in human mTLE

To generate protein expression profiles of inflammatory mediators in individual mTLE patients, we analyzed 40 proteins in each brain sample using a multiplex bead-based immunoassay. To assess mTLE-associated differences in expression profiles in hippocampus (HC) and neocortex (CX), we compared three patient groups, mTLE patients without HS (mTLE-HS), mTLE patients with HS (mTLE + HS), and autopsy controls (for patient details see Table 1). This experimental setup has been previously used by us and others [41-44]. In samples of mTLE patients, we could reliably detect 35 proteins, whereas due to the lower expression levels in autopsy control tissue we could reliably detect 32 proteins. Table 2 summarizes the data set (median and concentration range) of all inflammatory mediators measured in all HC

and CX samples in the three patient groups. Statistical analysis revealed that 21 inflammatory mediators showed differential expression across patient groups (Bonferroni-corrected $P$ value <0.0015); mediators are ranked according to level of significance. A univariate general linear approach and Pearson's correlation tests revealed no significant covariate influence or correlations for gender, age, post mortem delay, anti-epileptic drugs (AED) or pH. Post hoc testing showed that all 21 differentially expressed mediators were upregulated in mTLE + HS and/or mTLE-HS tissue compared to autopsy controls. Two inflammatory mediators (MIF, $P = 0.0024$ and Cathepsin S, $P = 0.0025$) showed a tendency to upregulation in autopsy controls compared to both mTLE groups (Table 2 and Figure 2D), but this upregulation did not pass the strict Bonferroni correction.

### Inflammatory mediators show distinct patterns of upregulation across patient groups and tissues

To further analyze the upregulation of individual inflammatory mediators between patient groups, we generated scatter plots per mediator showing the protein concentration in the HC and CX of each individual patient (Figure 1 and Figure 2). These plots clearly showed that upregulation of mediators in HC and CX tissue can be divided into two patterns (classified as pattern I and II). For instance, IL-10 and IL-25 showed upregulation in mTLE + HS tissue compared to mTLE-HS and autopsy controls (pattern I, Figure 1A and 1B), whereas CCL4 and IL-7 showed upregulation in both mTLE groups compared to autopsy controls (pattern II, Figure 1C and 1D). Interestingly, IL-1RA was only upregulated in the CX of mTLE + HS patients (Figure 1E).

Upregulation of some mediators, which we classified type A, was only found in the hippocampus (Figure 1A and 1C), whereas others (classified as type B) showed upregulation in both hippocampal and neocortical tissue (Figure 1B and 1D). A summary of the response types of all significantly upregulated mediators is provided in Figure 1G.

These results show that in both mTLE-HS and mTLE + HS patients multiple components of the immune response are upregulated. Upregulation can be found in the HC and the CX, and inflammatory mediators show distinct patterns of upregulation.

### Cellular localization of IL25 and CCL4

Our next step was to independently verify upregulation and to analyze the distribution and cell types expressing one inflammatory mediator in each of the two major expression patterns. We performed immunohistochemistry (IHC) for IL-25 (pattern I) and CCL4 (pattern II) on hippocampal sections of a subset (n = 6) of patients from each of the three groups also used in the MIA. Visual inspection of overall immunoreactivity (IR) for IL-25 revealed

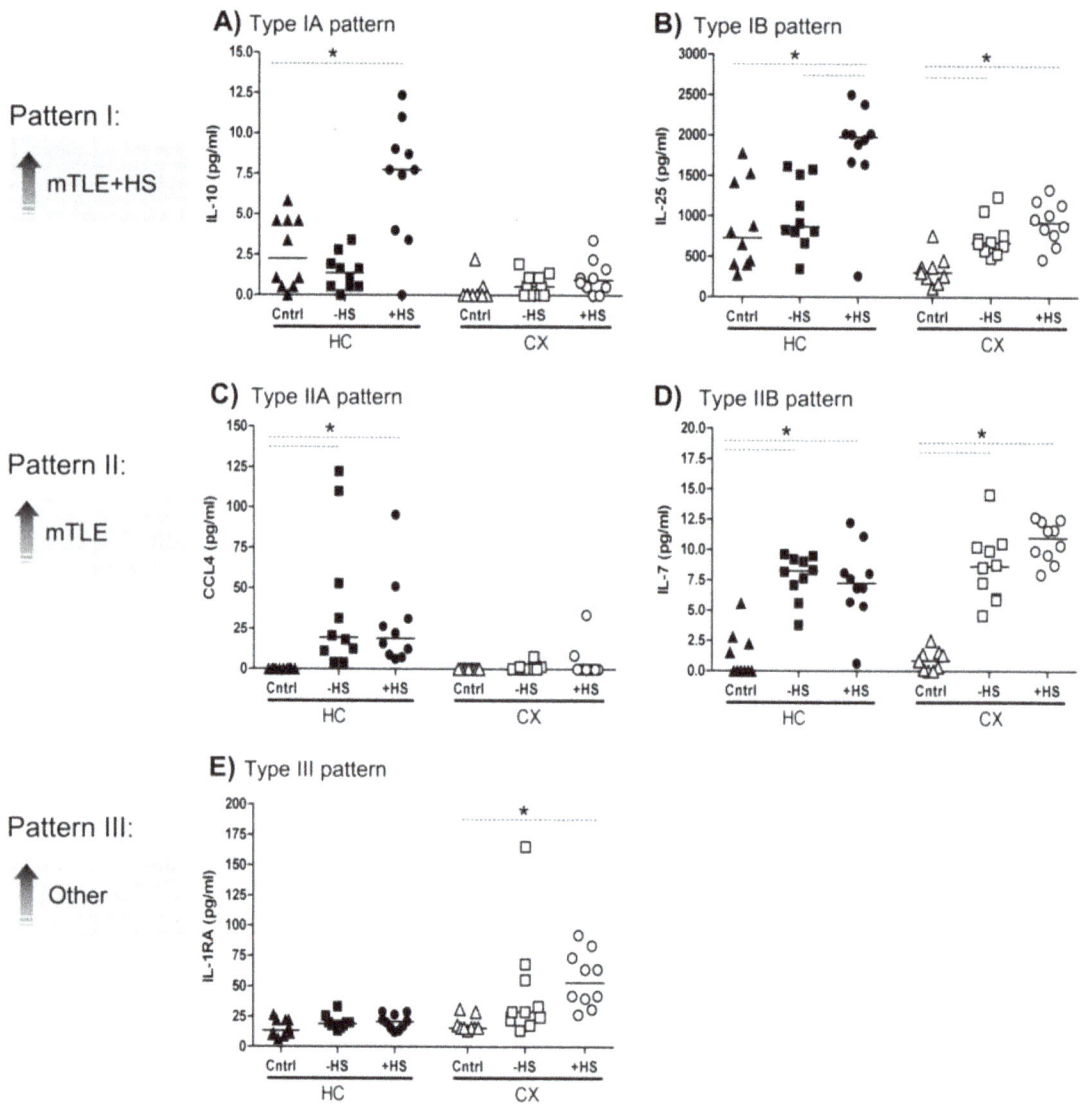

**A)** Type IA pattern

Pattern I:

↑ mTLE+HS

**B)** Type IB pattern

**C)** Type IIA pattern

Pattern II:

↑ mTLE

**D)** Type IIB pattern

**E)** Type III pattern

Pattern III:

↑ Other

**G)** Expression patterns of inflammatory mediators

| Pattern of up-regulation | Chemokines | Cytokines | Other |
|---|---|---|---|
| IA | - | IL-10, IFNα | ICAM1 |
| IB | - | IL-25, IL-27 | - |
| IIA | CCL2, CCL4 | - | - |
| IIB | CCL5, CCL22, CXCL9, CCL3 , CCL19 | IL-5, IL-7, IL-13, IL-22, IL-1α | HGF,VCAM1, VEGF |
| III | | IL-1ra | |

**Figure 1 HC and CX expression patterns of inflammatory proteins in mTLE.** Scatter plots of protein levels per individual patient, per group. Horizontal lines represent the median expression level of the group. Post-hoc analysis of the data revealed three expression patterns among the patient groups. We classified them as Type I to III (I: **A** and **B**, II: **C** and **D**, III: **E**). Additionally, different patterns were detected depending on the type of tissue, hence we classified an up-regulation in HC only as **A** (**A** and **C**) and an up-regulation in both HC and CX as **B** (**B** and **D**). * indicates significant difference. All significantly changed proteins showed one of these three expression patterns (**G**) (see Figure 2).

**Table 4 Summary of all p-values for the post hoc tests**

| Parameter | HC +HS vs – HS | HC +HS vs Cntrl | HC-CX +HS vs + HS | HC -HS vs Cntrl | HC-CX -HS vs –HS | CX +HS vs Cntrl | CX -HS vs Cntrl |
|---|---|---|---|---|---|---|---|
| IL1 RA | 0.64497528 | 0.116 | **0.0008** | 0.137 | 0.108 | **0.0005** | 0.027 |
| IL1a | 0.24252404 | **0.0007** | 0.687 | **0.003** | 0.0722 | **0.0021** | 0.171 |
| IL-5 | 0.706 | **0.0002** | 0.0261 | **0.001** | 0.705 | **1.32E-06** | **0.001** |
| IL-7 | 0.853 | **6.65E-05** | 0.007 | **3.28E-07** | 0.469 | **1.78E-10** | **7.37E-06** |
| IL-10 | **4.1619E-06** | **0.004** | **2E-06** | 0.138 | 0.079 | 0.068 | 0.305 |
| IL-13 | 0.25819279 | **2.78E-06** | 0.0449 | **7.35E-07** | 0.518 | **1.16E-06** | **4.90E-05** |
| IL-22 | 0.491 | **4.86E-07** | 0.0149 | **9.13E-07** | 0.478 | **1.23E-05** | **0.00023** |
| IL-25 | **1.8845E-05** | **0.001** | **1E-07** | 0.470 | 0.0865 | **3.81E-05** | **0.001** |
| CCL2 | 0.376 | **0.0009** | 0.0185 | **0.0006** | **0.0001** | 0.372 | 0.227 |
| CCL3 | 0.521 | *0.015* | 0.106 | **0.002** | 0.0132 | **1.34E-06** | **0.002** |
| CCL5 | 0.250 | **0.006** | 0.0661 | **0.001** | 0.0166 | **5.78E-07** | **0.0002** |
| CCL19 | 0.258 | 0.045 | 0.203 | **0.0015** | 0.2107 | **0.002** | 0.126 |
| CCL22 | 0.99 | **0.00029** | 0.5204 | **0.0002178** | 0.1207 | **2.00E-07** | **0.001** |
| CXCL9 | 0.168 | **0.00020** | 0.0958 | **0.001** | 0.249 | **1.70E-05** | **0.003** |
| HGF | 0.327 | **0.001** | **0.0021** | **9.61E-08** | 0.142 | **0.001** | **0.006** |
| sICAM1 | **5.9897E-05** | **0.004** | **2E-05** | 0.052 | 0.281 | 0.136 | 0.147 |
| sVCAM1 | 0.326 | **3.01E-05** | 0.9371 | **7.48E-05** | 0.1186 | **6.88E-09** | **0.00011** |
| VEGF | 0.714 | **0.001** | 0.5836 | **8.71E-05** | 0.0925 | **3.09E-10** | **3.07E-05** |
| IFNa | **0.00177** | **0.002** | *0.014* | 0.036 | 0.1402 | 0.327 | 0.318 |
| IL-27 | **0.0012** | *0.008* | **0.0051** | 0.933 | 0.4785 | **3.62E-06** | 0.022 |
| CCL4 | 0.795 | **0.0000108** | 0.022 | **0.00001** | **0.00004** | 0.49 | 0.27 |

All significantly different inflammatory mediators (ANOVA/Kruskal-Wallis) were subjected to post-hoc testing (Students-*T* test/Mann–Whitney U). Significant p-values are depicted in bold.

increased expression in all sections from mTLE + HS patients compared to mTLE-HS and autopsy control patients, thus confirming our MIA data (Figure 1B).

IL-25 IR was found in all three patient groups in the principle neuronal layers of the hippocampus, the pyramidal layer of the cornu ammonis (CA) (subfields 1 to 4) and the granule cell layer in the dentate gyrus (DG). In mTLE patients the increased IL-25 IR was most apparent in the CA1 (Figure 3A) and the DG-CA4 region (Figure 3B) of the hippocampus. This increase in IL-25 IR was due to labeling of cells with a glial morphology (see also Figure 4A and 4B). As expected, the number of IL-25 IR neurons was decreased in mTLE patients compared to mTLE-HS and controls as a result of neuron loss in the sclerotic hippocampus [5].

Hippocampal CCL4 IR was higher in all sections of both mTLE groups compared to autopsy controls (Figure 3), thus confirming our MIA data (Figure 1C). CCL4 expression in both mTLE groups was most pronounced in the CA1 and the hilar region of the hippocampus (Figure 3).

To identify the cell types expressing IL-25 and CCL4 IR, we performed double-label immunofluorescence on mTLE + HS patients (Figure 4 and Figure 5). IL-25 IR co-localized with Iba1-positive microglial cells, GFAP-positive astrocytes and NeuN-positive neuronal cells (Figure 4). CCL4 was predominantly detected in Vimentin-positive reactive (Figure 5A) and GFAP-positive astrocytes (Figure 5B). Interestingly, both IL-25 and CCL4 IR were also detected in GFAP-positive astrocytic endfeet surrounding blood vessels (Figure 4B and 5A, small insets). To exclude T cells as prominent source of cytokines we performed IHC for these cells (data not shown). In line with results published by others [12,45], we only detected a small number of T cells in the hippocampus of mTLE patients. Together, our immunocytochemistry data show distinct hippocampal staining patterns for IL-25 and CCL4, particularly in the dentate gyrus, where IL-25 but not CCL4 expression is prominent in the principle neurons in the granule cell layer. In mTLE + HS patients the increased IL-25 and CCL4 expression (compared to controls) appears to involve glia cells, whereas increased IL-25 expression is also found in principle neurons.

### Principle component analyses revealed pathology-associated immunological profiles in mTLE

To investigate relationships between various upregulated mediators, we conducted unbiased correlation network

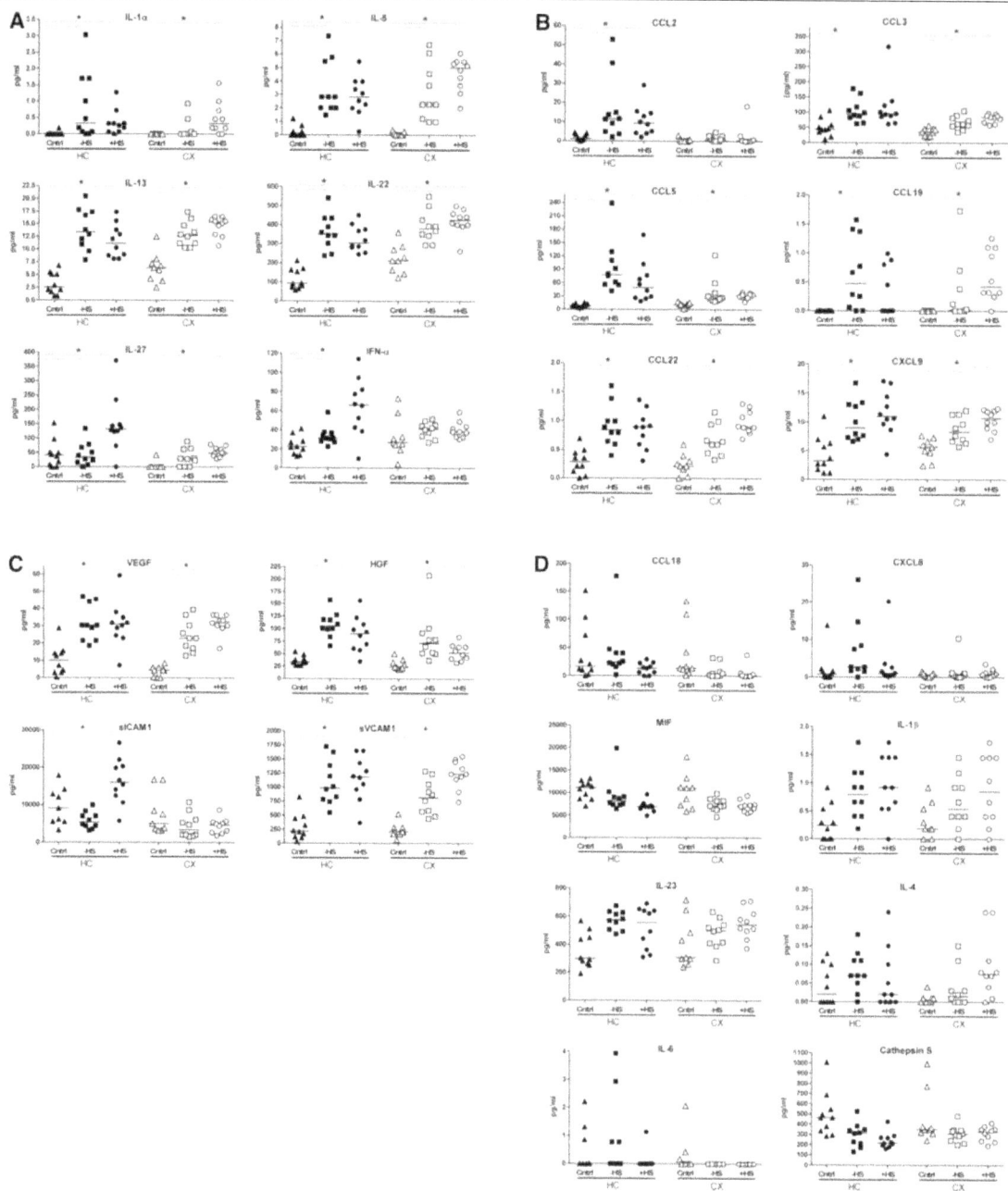

**Figure 2 HC and CX expression patterns of other inflammatory proteins.** Interleukins (**A**), chemokines (**B**), miscellaneous inflammatory proteins (**C**), and inflammatory proteins with p-values 0.0017-0.05 which were not tested post-hoc (**D**). Scatterplots of individual protein levels per patient group. Horizontal lines represent the median expression level of the group.

and principle component analyses on data from all patients, irrespective of their pathology. First, correlation analyses using Pearson's correlation showed that many cytokines were co-regulated in patterns that were remarkably similar in the three patient groups and segregated in two main networks (Figure 6). In most cases, patients with high expression of proteins in the first network had lower levels of proteins in the second network, and vice versa (data not shown).

Principle component analyses (PCA) on all inflammatory mediators above the detection limit (see Table 2), confirmed the correlation analyses and revealed clustering of the proteins in eight principle components. These eight components explained 88.5% (HC) and 84% (CX) of the variance detected in all samples (Table 5A and B). The major components, which explained 63% (HC) and 50.1% (CX) of the variance, are depicted in Figure 7 with their corresponding plots. The first and the third HC

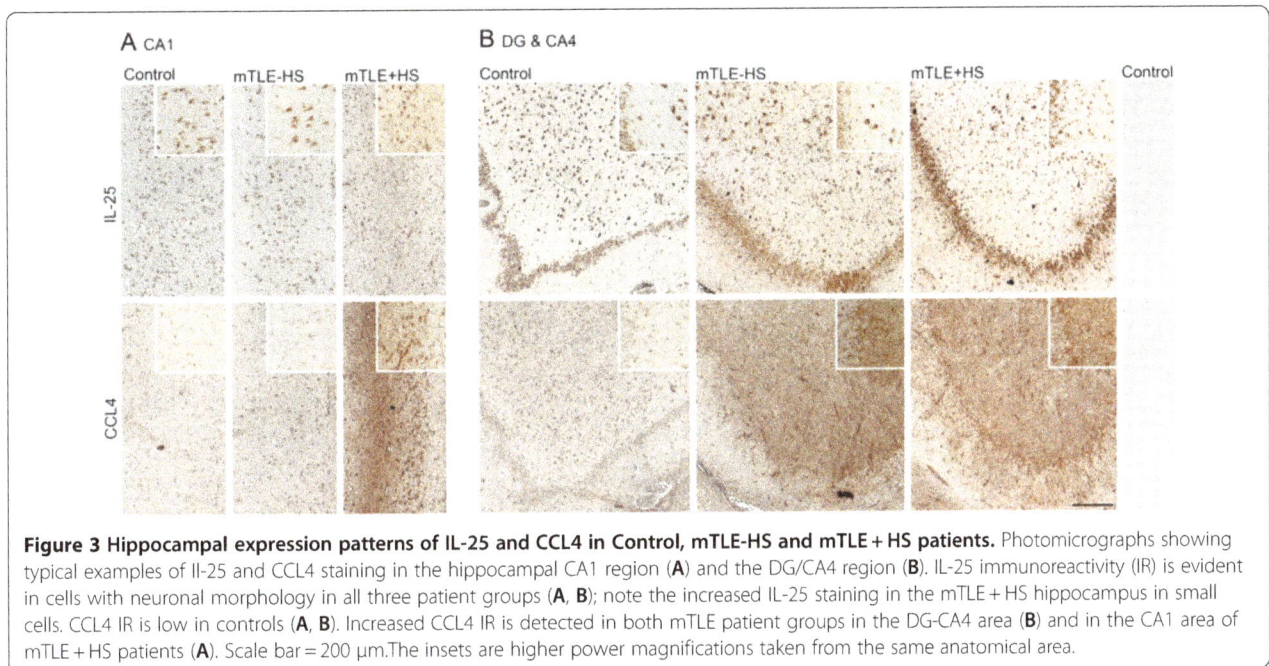

**Figure 3 Hippocampal expression patterns of IL-25 and CCL4 in Control, mTLE-HS and mTLE + HS patients.** Photomicrographs showing typical examples of Il-25 and CCL4 staining in the hippocampal CA1 region (**A**) and the DG/CA4 region (**B**). IL-25 immunoreactivity (IR) is evident in cells with neuronal morphology in all three patient groups (**A**, **B**); note the increased IL-25 staining in the mTLE + HS hippocampus in small cells. CCL4 IR is low in controls (**A**, **B**). Increased CCL4 IR is detected in both mTLE patient groups in the DG-CA4 area (**B**) and in the CA1 area of mTLE + HS patients (**A**). Scale bar = 200 μm.The insets are higher power magnifications taken from the same anatomical area.

components contained all three types of inflammatory mediators we investigated (chemokines, interleukins, growth factors and adhesion molecules), while the second HC component predominantly consisted of chemokines (Figure 7A). Follow-up analysis on the individual factor scores obtained from the PCA, revealed that HC components 1 and 2 differed as whole clusters between both mTLE groups and controls, whereas the HC component 3 differed between mTLE + HS versus mTLE-HS and controls (Table 5A). The PCA plots (Figure 7A, bottom panel) clearly showed that patient groups can be discriminated based on the expression patterns of inflammatory mediators in components 1 and 3. Interestingly, patient 32 of the mTLE + HS group did not cluster with the rest of the mTLE + HS group (Figure 7A). Neuropathological reassessment revealed only mild sclerosis (W2 score) for this patient (Table 1). Component 1 of the CX tissue contained sixteen inflammatory mediators, of which nine overlapped with the HC first component. Follow-up analyses of the components scores obtained from the PCA of the neocortical expression data (Figure 7B) also showed that the three patient groups could be discriminated, yet to a lesser degree, as only CX component 1 differed significantly between patient groups (Table 5B). Interestingly, two mTLE-HS patients clustered more with mTLE + HS patients (patients 20 and 28). We could not find any clinical parameters to explain this aberrant clustering (Table 1).

Subsequently, we investigated possible correlations between the top three principle components of the hippocampal PCA analysis and several clinical parameters.

Pearson's correlation analyses revealed a significant correlation between HC component 3 and seizure frequency (including and excluding clustered seizures, see Table 1) in mTLE-HS patients. No correlation was found with the occurrence of spikes on the iEcOG. Interestingly, the expression levels of the two inflammatory mediators with the strongest loadings in HC component 3; CCL3 and IL-10, showed a correlation with seizure frequency (correlation coefficient of >0.7 with a $P$ value below 0.05), however this correlation did not pass the strict Bonferroni correction for multiple testing.

In all, the data obtained from the PCA analyses showed that patient groups can be discriminated based on their expression profiles. The clustering in major components indicates that upregulation of inflammatory mediators in mTLE may involve multiple immunological pathways.

**Discussion**

Over recent years, it has become apparent that the immune system plays a role in the development of mTLE [9,15,16]. The focus of protein studies on the immune pathology in mTLE thus far has mostly been on single cyto- and chemokines. However, experimental data from microarray studies [10,11] suggest that probably a whole network of cyto -and chemokines is activated in mTLE. Therefore, this study used a multiplex immunoassay (MIA) approach to measure multiple proteins of the immune system in the same mTLE samples.

We find a broad upregulation of inflammatory mediators in both HC and CX tissue of mTLE patients compared to autopsy controls. Up-regulated mediators include inflammatory proteins previously identified in

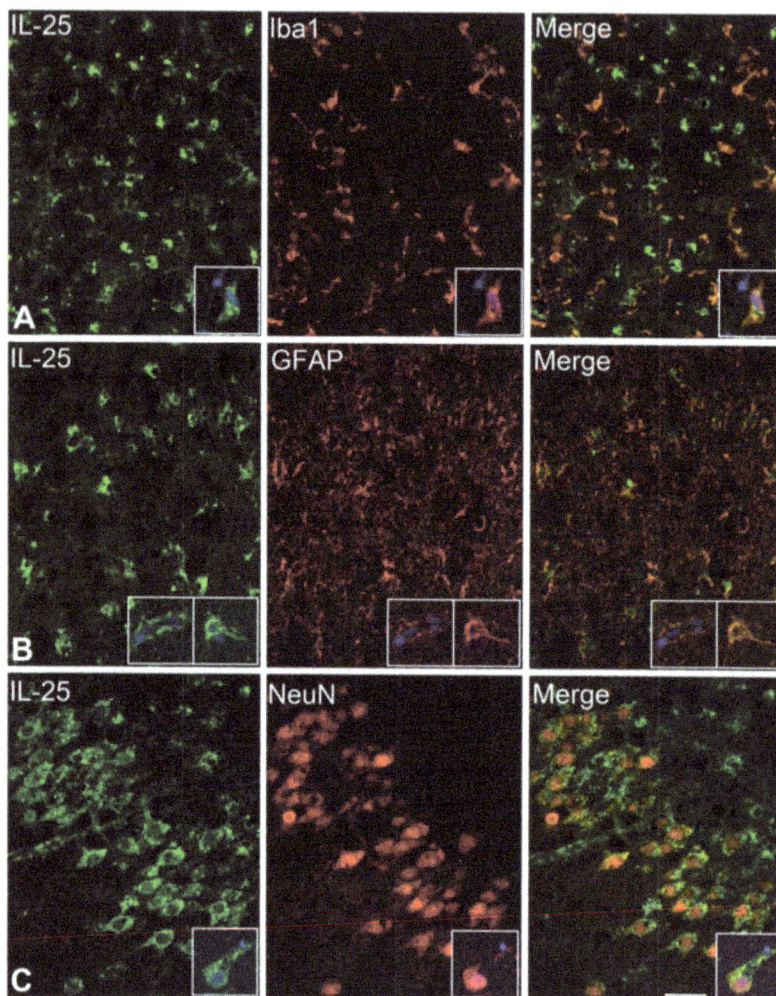

**Figure 4 IL-25 IR in neurons, astrocytes and microglia.** IFC reveals IL-25 IR (in green) co-localizing with three CNS cell type markers (red), (**A**) Iba1, a microglial marker, (**B**) GFAP, an astrocytic marker and (**C**) NeuN, a neuronal marker. **Panel A,B**: CA4; **Panel C**: dentate gyrus. Note that IL-25 IR is also present in the astrocytic endfeet surrounding the bloodvessels (**B**). The insets are higher power magnifications taken from a representative area, with the added nuclear marker DAPI (blue). Scale bar = 40 μm.

mTLE, but also proteins not previously associated with mTLE. Network analysis showed that within patient groups there are two main protein networks with a high degree of co-regulation. Three components, obtained with principle component analyses on data of protein expression in the hippocampus, revealed that the three studied groups could be distinguished based on their expression profile.

Our data indicate that in human mTLE there are complex networks of upregulated inflammatory mediators, which may exert both pro- and anti-epileptogenic influences on the brain.

### Distinct expression patterns of upregulated inflammatory mediators

We measured 40 inflammatory proteins in the hippocampus and neocortex of autopsy control and mTLE patients. In mTLE tissue, 35 of these proteins were expressed above the detection limit. Sixty percent of these detectable mediators were significantly upregulated in mTLE tissue compared to autopsy controls, the remaining 40% showed no significant difference between the three patient groups (Table 2). We could distinguish two main patterns of upregulation in mTLE patients. Inflammatory mediators showing the first pattern (for example, IL-10 and IL-25) were upregulated in mTLE + HS patients (Figure 1A, 1B and 1G) compared to mTLE-HS and autopsy controls. Mediators showing the second pattern (for example, CCL4 and IL-7) were upregulated in both mTLE patient groups (+ and −HS) compared to controls (Figure 1C, 1D and 1G). Significantly more proteins (71.4%) showed the second pattern (upregulation in hippocampus and cortex) than the first (23.8%). Only in 19% of the patients upregulation of inflammatory

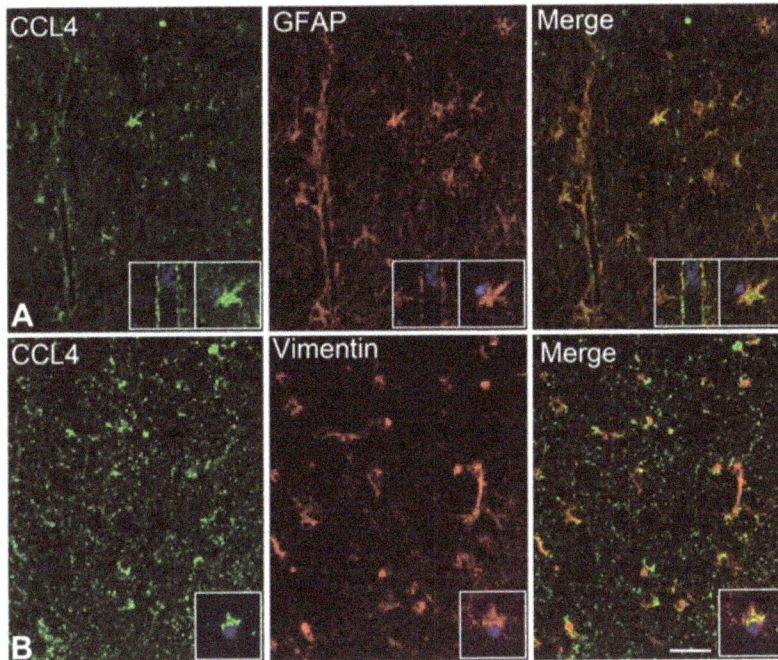

**Figure 5 CCL4 IR in astrocytes and reactive astrocytes.** IFC reveals CCL4 (in green) co-localizing with two types of glial cell markers (red), (**A**) astrocytic marker GFAP and (**B**) reactive astrocytic marker Vimentin. CCL4 IR is also present in the astrocytic endfeet of the GFAP positive astrocytes (**A**). Pictures are taken of representative areas in the CA4 region. The insets are higher power magnifications taken from the same anatomical area, with the added nuclear marker DAPI (blue). Scale bar = 40 μm.

mediators was confined to the hippocampus (Figure 1G, type A pattern). Thus, our results show that activation of inflammatory mediators is more widespread, and not restricted to the hippocampus, which often is the primary source of epileptic activity. Interestingly, IL1ra was upregulated only in the neocortex, but not in the

hippocampus. The significance of the upregulation of this endogenous anti-inflammatory protein [46] remains to be determined. Upregulation may be a response of the cortex to seizure activity. Alternatively, the lack of IL1ra upregulation in the hippocampus may contribute to the epileptic properties of the hippocampus.

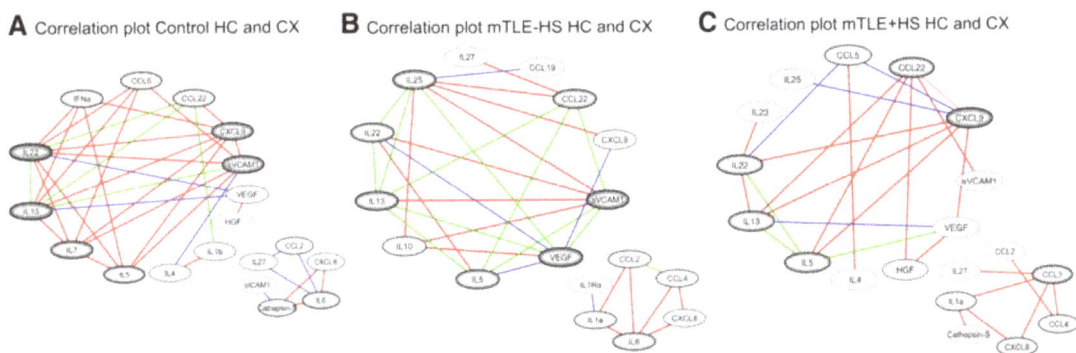

**Figure 6 Correlation network plots for all patient groups.** Network plots depicting significant correlations between levels of inflammatory mediators in Control patients (**A**), mTLE -HS patients (**B**) and mTLE + HS patients (**C**). Line (edge) color indicates in which tissue correlation was found: red = HC, blue = CX, green = HC & CX. Per patient group two main non-overlapping correlation networks were identified. Note that correlation networks are remarkably similar among the patient groups. Inflammatory mediators like IL-5, IL-13 and IL-22 all display >4 correlations with other inflammatory mediators. Only proteins that were in a network of more than 6 correlations (nodes) are depicted. In addition, 5 significant correlations were found in the total data set. In Control HC IL-10 & CCL3 correlated with IL-25 and in mTLE-HS CX Cathepsin-S correlated with ICAM1. All correlations had a correlation coefficient > 0.85 with a Bonferoni corrected p-value < 0.0017.

**Table 5 Summary principle component analysis**

**A**

**Component-HC**

| 1 37.7% | 2 13.4% | 3 11.1% | 4 7.5% | 5 6.7% | 6 5.3% | 7 3.7% | 8 3.2% |
|---|---|---|---|---|---|---|---|
| IL-13 | CCL4 | CCL3 | IL-6R | TIMP1 | CCL19 | TNFα | IL-23 |
| IL-5 | CCL2 | IL-10 | IL-18 | IL-6 | CCL5* | IL-1RA | CCL18 |
| IL-22 | IL-1α | ICAM1 | Adiponectin | Cathepsin-S | IL-1β * | IL-4 | |
| CCL19 | IL-8 | IL-27 | IL-1β | | MIF | | |
| VEGF | CCL3 | IL-25 | | | | | |
| CCL22 | CCL5 | IL-21 | | | | | |
| CXCL9 | | IFNα | | | | | |
| VCAM1 | | IL-6R | | | | | |
| IL-7 | | | | | | | |
| HGF | | | | | | | |
| IL-23 | | | | | | | |
| mTLE Δ control | mTLE Δ control | mTLE + HS Δ -HS & control | ND | ND | mTLE + HS Δ & control | ND | ND |

**B**

**Component-CX**

| 1 40.1% | 2 10% | 3 8.4% | 4 8% | 5 5.8% | 6 5% | 7 4% | 8 3.3% |
|---|---|---|---|---|---|---|---|
| IL-5 | IL-18 | CCL2 | Adiponectin | CXCL9 | TIMP1 | IL-1β | IL-25 |
| VEGF | IL-6R | CCL4 | ICAM1 | CCL5 | CXCL8.IL-8 | IL-6 | IL-21 |
| VCAM1 | MIF | Adiponectin | Cathepsin-S | HGF | IL-1α | IFNα | IL-4 |
| CCL3 | IL-1β | CXCL8.IL-8 | CCL18 | | TNFα | IL-23 | IL-10 |
| CCL19 | TNFα | | | | IL-4 | | |
| IL-1RA | | | | | | | |
| IL-27 | | | | | | | |
| IL-22 | | | | | | | |
| IL-13 | | | | | | | |
| IL-25 | | | | | | | |
| CCL22 | | | | | | | |
| IL-7 | | | | | | | |
| CXCL9 | | | | | | | |
| IL-1α | | | | | | | |
| IL-23 | | | | | | | |
| TNFα | | | | | | | |
| mTLE Δ control | ND | ND | ND | mTLE Δ control | mTLE + HS Δ & control | ND | mTLE + HS Δ -HS & control |

PCA identified 8 components in HC(A) and CX (B) that explain 88.5% (HC) and 84% (CX) of the variance in all the samples. The contribution of each component to the variance is given as percentage. Inflammatory mediators are listed in order of factor loading. Under each component list significant differences in this component between patient groups is indicated (delta). ND = no difference detected between component scores among the three patient groups.

The upregulation of a specific subset of inflammatory mediators in the hippocampus of mTLE + HS patients is most likely associated with hippocampal sclerosis. These data indicate that the increased expression in mTLE patients is not just caused by post mortem changes in the autopsy control tissue. This latter point is further substantiated by the fact that covariate analysis in the controls revealed no effects of post mortem delay on any

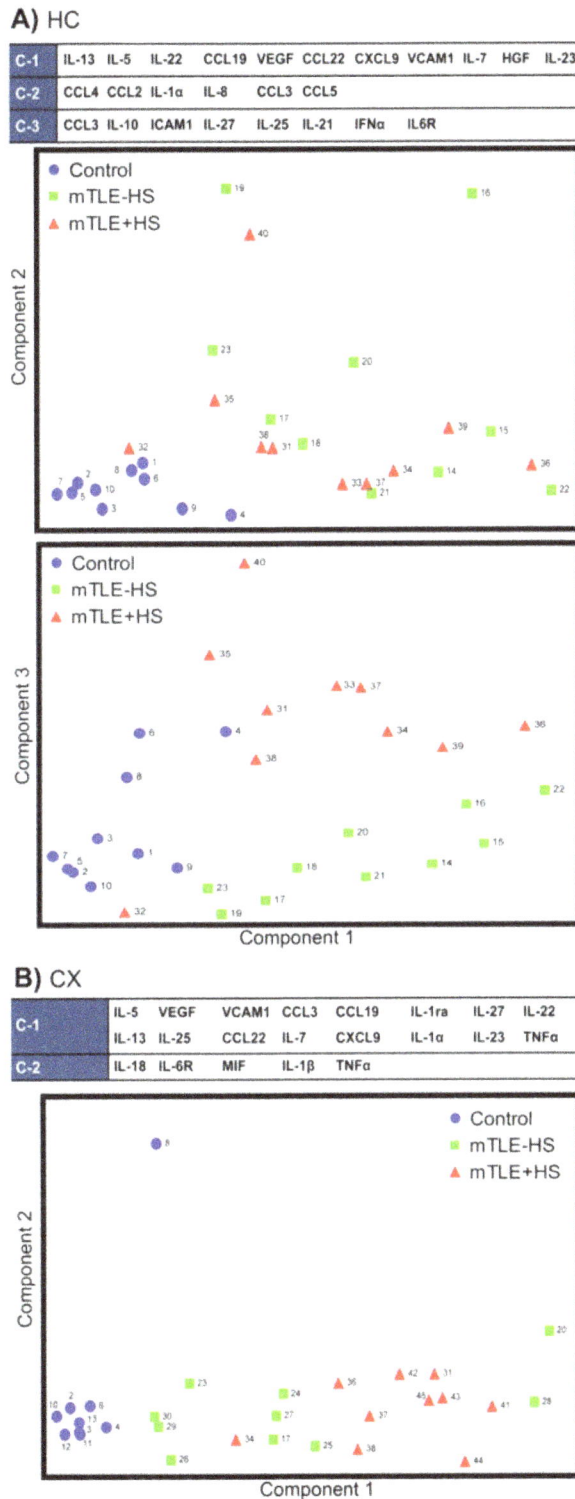

**Figure 7 Major components identified by principle component analyses reveal pathology-specific immunological networks in the HC and the CX.** PCA results for the main components identified by the analysis in the HC (**A**) and the CX (**B**). Proteins are depicted in sequence of factor loading, all depicted proteins of the components have a factor loading of >0.4 (is >16% of explained variance). Individual patient component scores were plotted against each other and revealed patient group-dependent clusters, component 1 versus 2 (**A**) segregated both mTLE patient groups from controls in HC (**A**) and CX (**B**), whereas the PCA plot for component 1 versus 3 in the HC segregated all three patient groups (**B**). C-1 to 3 = component 1 to 3.

of the parameters measured. The human tissue samples used in our study are from patients suffering from repetitive seizures over a prolonged period. Therefore, part of the effects observed may be seizure-induced rather than specific for the mTLE pathogenesis. Moreover, we cannot rule out effects of antiepileptic drugs when comparing autopsy control patients with mTLE patients, although no correlations with any AED were found in our study. Further studies, particularly in animal models for TLE will be required to analyze the role of individual or groups of inflammatory mediators in epileptogenesis. Animal studies will also be essential to establish whether upregulation of specific inflammatory mediators have epileptogenic, or rather anti-epileptogenic, properties.

Our data show upregulation of protein levels of several inflammatory mediators, which previously have been found upregulated in human mTLE tissue. These include IL1β, CCL2, CCL3, CCL4, VCAM1, ICAM1, and VEGF [10,11,18,20,47,48], which were found to have pro-epileptogenic properties in animal models for TLE (for references: see Table 6). Particularly, IL-1β has frequently been associated with pro-epileptogenic properties, a protein which affects neuronal $Ca^{2+}$ influx through NMDA-dependent signaling. As mentioned above, the endogenous antagonist of IL-1β, IL-1ra, has been attributed with seizure-inhibiting properties (Table 6).

Two proteins identified in this study have been described in human genetic studies before: single nucleotide polymorphisms (SNPs) present in IL-1α and IL-10 genes are associated with TLE and febrile seizures respectively (Table 6).

Our data showing upregulation of these pro-epileptogenic proteins in mTLE confirm that these genes are regulated, and that upregulation of transcripts translates into increased production of protein in mTLE tissue.

In this study, we identified a series of new inflammatory mediators that show increased protein levels in human mTLE tissue. These include CCL5, CCL19, CCL22, CXCL9, IL-5, IL-7, IL-13, IL-22, IL-25, IL-27, IFNα and HGF. As the majority of these new mTLE-associated inflammatory mediators have not been studied in animal models of TLE, information on pro- or anti-epileptogenic properties is limited. However, most of these proteins have previously been studied in relationship to other CNS pathologies. Processes such as neuroprotection, excitotoxicity through $Ca^{2+}$ influx, glutamate/GABA signaling and disruption of the BBB have been studied. These processes potentially can influence epileptogenesis [94-97]. Based on these studies, we categorized the newly identified inflammatory mediators in mTLE as potentially pro-epileptogenic or anti-epileptogenic (Table 6). Potentially pro-epileptogenic are all chemokines, the interleukins IL-5, 7 and 22, and the adhesion molecules VCAM1 and ICAM1. Potentially anti-epileptogenic are IL-1ra, IL-10,

13 and 25, IFNα and HGF. Studies on the potential role of IL-5, IL-7 and VEGF in processes related to epileptogenesis provide inconsistent information. [47,98].

IL-6 or TNFα protein levels did not differ between the three patient groups. Even though both cytokines have been implicated in epilepsy before [8,9,15,99], as we did not repeat the experiment with multiple antibodies, we cannot rule out technical issues. Our results however, are in line with data from mRNA profiling studies on human TLE tissue [10,11,14,15,100] as in these studies no significant differences in mRNA or protein were detected in brain tissue. Increased levels of IL-6, but not of TNFα, were found in plasma or cerebrospinal fluid (CSF) of TLE patients [101,102]. Therefore, increased IL-6 levels might not arise from brain tissue [103-105] but more likely from peripheral blood mononuclear cells (PMBCs). Indeed, upon stimulation, PMBCs from epileptic patients released increased amounts of IL-6 compared to controls [106].

Thus, our total set of upregulated inflammatory mediators comprises (potentially) pro- as well as anti-epileptogenic proteins in both mTLE patient groups.

Interestingly, we detected both CCL4 and IL-25 in glial cells surrounding blood vessels (Figures 4 and 5). Here, these proteins probably exert opposing influences on epileptogenesis, as CCL4 is thought to disrupt the blood–brain barrier (BBB) and attract immune cells across the BBB while IL-25 has been proposed to have a protective effect on the BBB (Table 6).

### Correlation and principle component analyses reveal complex immune networks in mTLE

To study co-regulation of inflammatory mediators, we first performed bivariate correlation network analysis on the datasets within each patient group. This analysis revealed co-regulation of inflammatory mediators in one large and one small network in each patient group (Figure 6). We observed that in most cases, patients with high levels of the smaller network components (for example, CCL2, CCL4, IL-8) had lower expression levels of larger network components (for example, IL-13, IL-5 CCL9) and vice versa. Subsequent PCAs on all investigated brain samples confirmed these networks and revealed eight components of clustered inflammatory proteins in both the HC and the CX separately (Figure 7, Table 5A and B). Each component typically contained both putative pro- and anti-epileptogenic proteins, suggesting that these proteins are co-regulated in all patient groups. We detected the majority of mTLE-specific differences in the HC of mTLE patients. Further analysis of the HC components shows that individual patients segregate into the three patient groups (Figure 7A), indicating that each patient group has a unique immune profile. The first two components, which explained the greatest variance of

**Table 6 Summary of potential pro-and anti-epileptogenic properties of inflammatory mediators**

| "Pro-epileptogenic" | | | "Anti-epileptogenic" | | |
|---|---|---|---|---|---|
| Protein | Function in CNS | reference | Protein | Function in CNS | reference |
| CCL2 | - contributes to immune-cell recruitment across the BBB | [49] | IL-1ra | - An anti-inflammatory protein with seizure inhibiting properties in experimental TLE | [50-53] |
| CCL3 | - Capable of inducing $Ca^{2+}$ transients in neuronal and microglial cultures.<br>- Inhibition of systemic receptor leads to decrease in seizure activity | [22,54] | IL-7 | Neurotrophic actions in embryonic brain cultures | [55,56] |
| CCL4 | - Capable of inducing $Ca^{2+}$ transients in neuronal and microglial cultures.<br><br>- Inhibition of systemic receptor leads to decrease in seizure activity | [22,54] | IL-10 | - Inhibits development of seizures in FS and a hypoxia model for epilepsy.<br>- SNPs that result in increased IL-10 are decreased in FS patients.<br><br>-Can give trophic support to neurons | [57-60] |
| CCL5 | - Capable of inducing $Ca^{2+}$ transients in neuronal and microglial cultures<br>- Glut release from CNS cells in hypothalamus<br>- contributes to immune-cell recruitment across the BBB<br>- Inhibition of systemic receptor leads to decrease in seizure activity | [22,49,54,61] | IL-13 | - Protects BBB integrity. | [62] |
| CCL19 | immune-cell recruitment across the BBB. | [63,64] | IL-25 | - Protects BBB integrity | [62,65] |
| CCL22 | -Immune-cell recruitment across the BBB. | [66,67] | IL-27 | Marked anti-inflammatory actions in EAE. | [68,69] |
| CXCL9 | -Immune-cell recruitment across the BBB. | [70-72] | IFNα | - Suppression of hippocampal CA1 neurons & LTP | [73,74] |
| IL-1α | Polymorphisms that lead to increased transcription are associated with TLE | [75-77] | HGF | - Enhances neuronal survival | [78,79] |
| IL-1β | - Increased NMDA R subunit NR2B phosphorylation leading to increased $Ca^{2+}$ influx<br><br>- Higher levels correlate with increased SRS after eFS | [80][25,52,81,82] | VEGF | - neuroprotective after experimental seizures<br>- reduces hippocampal excitability | [83-85] |
| IL-5 | - Implicated in BBB disruption in CNS tumor bloodvessels<br><br>- Induces microglial proliferation | [86-88] | IL-5 | - Anti-inflammatory actions in the periphery as a Th2 cytokine<br><br>- Induces microglial activation | [87-89] |
| IL-7 | Induces neuronal apoptosis in human NT2 cells | [90] | | | |
| IL-22 | - BBB disruption through down-regulation of occludin. | [91] | | | |
| VEGF | BBB disruption → reduction in tight junction proteins in kainate model for TLE | [92,93]. | | | |
| ICAM-1 | - implicated in BBB disruption | [20] | | | |
| VCAM-1 | - Immune-cell recruitment across the BBB | [20] | | | |

Abbreviations: *BBB* blood brain barrier, *CNS* central nervous system, *SRS* spontaneous recurrent seizure activity, *NMDA* N-methyl D-aspartate, *NR2B* N-methyl D-aspartate receptor subtype 2B, *eFS* experimental febrile seizures, *NT2* neuronal teratocarcinoma Tera 2, *FS* febrile seizures, *LTP* long term potentiation, *EAE* experimental autoimmune encephalitis, *SNP* single nucleotide polymorphism.

protein expression in the HC, contained only proteins of a type II pattern (that is, upregulated in both mTLE patient groups), whereas the majority of component 3 consists of proteins with a type I expression pattern, and this is clearly shown in the PCA plots (Figure 7A). As expected, the majority of HC component 1 consisted of proteins also detected in the large network detected in the bivariate correlation network analysis. HC component 2 comprises chemokines represented in the smaller correlation network (Figure 6).

The PCA analysis on the data set from the CX tissue also showed segregation of patients into patient groups (Figure 7B), although less pronounced, possibly due to the smaller number of regulated proteins. As expected, there was substantial overlap between the major clusters found in the HC and CX, as nine of the ten inflammatory mediators clustered in the HC component 1 were also present in the CX component 1 (Figure 7, Table 5).

The data obtained from the PCAs suggest that the activated immune system in mTLE is complex and may comprise different networks and pathways. The biological function and pathological outcome of activation of the immunological networks needs to be further investigated. Surprisingly, pro- and anti-epileptogenic inflammatory mediators cluster together, suggesting co-regulation of these two types of responses. Correlation analysis of upregulated whole networks with clinical parameters revealed a significant correlation between the HC component 3 and seizure frequency in the hippocampus of mTLE-HS patients. Indeed, the top two proteins in this component (CCL3 and IL-10) showed a weak correlation with seizure frequency in the hippocampi of mTLE-HS patients only. No correlations were found with iEcOG spikes. Larger patient populations will be required to further elucidate the relevance of upregulation of inflammatory networks or specific inflammatory mediators for patient pathology.

In summary, we observed a widespread upregulation of inflammatory mediators in the mTLE brain. Co-regulation of upregulated mediators indicates that they cluster in complex immunological networks. Within these networks we identified both pro- and anti-inflammatory mediators. Detailed analysis of these complex pathways in animal models will be required to assess their putative role in epileptogenesis. Our data suggests that the success of any future therapeutic strategies to treat mTLE will require a multifactorial approach aimed at blocking detrimental effects of proinflammatory pathways while promoting endogenous anti-inflammatory pathways. Promising targets for treatment would be, for instance, CCR5 receptors, which can be activated by a number of chemokines [54]. CCR5 inhibitors are currently being tested in clinical trials for HIV/AIDS treatment [107,108]. Treatment with CCR5

antagonists will inhibit the action of pro-epileptogenic chemokines CCL3, 4 and 5, the major chemokines in the second immunological network we identified in the HC. Inhibition of CCL3, 4 and 5 signaling, and in general proinflammatory pathways, may contribute to tipping the balance from a perturbed pro-epileptogenic to a more protective and anti-epileptogenic immune system in mTLE patients.

**Competing interests**
The authors certify that they have no competing financial interests.

**Authors' contributions**
The work presented here was carried out in collaboration between all authors. AK, ON and PG defined the research theme and designed the methods and experiments. AK and MW gathered and prepared the human tissues for the experiments. WJ carried out the multiplex ELISA and discussed and aided with the interpretation. AK performed the IHC and IFC. CH and MZ aided with the PCA analysis and the interpretation of the networks. PR and PG were the neurosurgeons responsible for the removal of brain tissue, CF carried out the intraoperative electrocorticography. AK drafted the manuscript and in conjunction with ON and PG presented this paper. All authors have read and approved the final version of the manuscript.

**Acknowledgements**
We wish to thank the patients who donated their tissue for our studies. We thank Frans S Leijten for helpful comments and grid EEG measurements and the Netherlands Brain Bank for providing tissue samples. We thank Kees van der Meulen for help with the tables in the manuscript. This work was supported by the National Epilepsy Fund of the Netherlands [NEF, grant number 06–09] and the Epilepsies of Childhood Foundation (EPOCH) (to PNE de Graan).

**Author details**
[1]Department of Neuroscience and Pharmacology, Rudolf Magnus Institute of Neuroscience, Universiteitsweg 100, 3584 CG, Utrecht, The Netherlands. [2]Department of Pediatric Immunology, University Medical Center Utrecht, Heidelberglaan 100, Utrecht, The Netherlands. [3]Department of Neurology and Neurosurgery, University Medical Center Utrecht, Heidelberglaan 100, Utrecht, The Netherlands. [4]Department of Child Neurology, University Medical Center Utrecht, Heidelberglaan 100, Utrecht, The Netherlands. [5]Laboratory of Neuroimmunology and Developmental Origins of Disease, University Medical Center Utrecht, Heidelberglaan 100, 3584 CX, Utrecht, The Netherlands.

**References**
1. Leonardi M, Ustun TB: The global burden of epilepsy. *Epilepsia* 2002, 43(Suppl 6):21–25.
2. Engel J Jr: A proposed diagnostic scheme for people with epileptic seizures and with epilepsy: report of the ILAE Task Force on Classification and Terminology. *Epilepsia* 2001, 42(6):796–803.
3. Kwan P, Brodie MJ: Clinical trials of antiepileptic medications in newly diagnosed patients with epilepsy. *Neurology* 2003, 60:S2–S12.
4. Cascino GD: When drugs and surgery don't work. *Epilepsia* 2008, 49(Suppl 9):79–84.
5. Proper EA, Oestreicher AB, Jansen GH, Veelen CW, van Rijen PC, Gispen WH, de Graan PN: Immunohistochemical characterization of mossy fibre sprouting in the hippocampus of patients with pharmaco-resistant temporal lobe epilepsy. *Brain* 2000, 123(Pt 1):19–30.
6. Houser CR: Neuronal loss and synaptic reorganization in temporal lobe epilepsy. *Adv Neurol* 1999, 79:743–761.
7. Rakhade SN, Jensen FE: Epileptogenesis in the immature brain: emerging mechanisms. *Nat Rev Neurol* 2009, 5:380–391.
8. Vezzani A, Granata T: Brain inflammation in epilepsy: experimental and clinical evidence. *Epilepsia* 2005, 46:1724–1743.
9. Vezzani A, French J, Bartfai T, Baram TZ: The role of inflammation in epilepsy. *Nat Rev Neurol* 2011, 7:31–40.

10. van Gassen KL, de Wit M, Koerkamp MJ, Rensen MG, van Rijen PC, Holstege FC, Lindhout D, de Graan PN: Possible role of the innate immunity in temporal lobe epilepsy. *Epilepsia* 2008, 49:1055–1065.

11. Lee TS, Mane S, Eid T, Zhao H, Lin A, Guan Z, Kim JH, Schweitzer J, King-Stevens D, Weber P, Spencer SS, Spencer DD, de Lanerolle NC: Gene expression in temporal lobe epilepsy is consistent with increased release of glutamate by astrocytes. *Mol Med* 2007, 13:1–13.

12. Ravizza T, Gagliardi B, Noe F, Boer K, Aronica E, Vezzani A: Innate and adaptive immunity during epileptogenesis and spontaneous seizures: Evidence from experimental models and human temporal lobe epilepsy. *Neurobiol Dis* 2008, 29:142–160.

13. Liimatainen S, Fallah M, Kharazmi E, Peltola M, Peltola J: Interleukin-6 levels are increased in temporal lobe epilepsy but not in extra-temporal lobe epilepsy. *J Neurol* 2009, 256:796–802.

14. Yamamoto A, Schindler CK, Murphy BM, Bellver-Estelles C, So NK, Taki W, Meller R, Simon RP, Henshall DC: Evidence of tumor necrosis factor receptor 1 signaling in human temporal lobe epilepsy. *Exp Neurol* 2006, 202:410–420.

15. Li G, Bauer S, Nowak M, Norwood B, Tackenberg B, Rosenow F, Knake S, Oertel WH, Hamer HM: Cytokines and epilepsy. *Seizure* 2011, 20:249–256.

16. Friedman A, Dingledine R: Molecular cascades that mediate the influence of inflammation on epilepsy. *Epilepsia* 2011, 52(Suppl 3):33–39.

17. Murdoch C, Finn A: Chemokine receptors and their role in inflammation and infectious diseases. *Blood* 2000, 95:3032–3043.

18. Fabene PF, Bramanti P, Constantin G: The emerging role for chemokines in epilepsy. *J Neuroimmunol* 2010, 224:22–27.

19. De Simoni MG, Perego C, Ravizza T, Moneta D, Conti M, Marchesi F, De Luigi A, Garattini S, Vezzani A: Inflammatory cytokines and related genes are induced in the rat hippocampus by limbic status epilepticus. *Eur J Neurosci* 2000, 12:2623–2633.

20. Fabene PF, Navarro MG, Martinello M, Rossi B, Merigo F, Ottoboni L, Bach S, Angiari S, Benati D, Chakir A, Zanetti L, Schio F, Osculati A, Marzola P, Nicolato E, Homeister JW, Xia L, Lowe JB, McEver RP, Osculati F, Sbarbati A, Butcher EC, Constantin G: A role for leukocyte-endothelial adhesion mechanisms in epilepsy. *Nat Med* 2008, 14:1377–1383.

21. Zeng LH, Rensing NR, Wong M: The mammalian target of rapamycin signaling pathway mediates epileptogenesis in a model of temporal lobe epilepsy. *J Neurosci* 2009, 29:6964–6972.

22. Louboutin JP, Chekmasova A, Marusich E, Agrawal L, Strayer DS: Role of CCR5 and its ligands in the control of vascular inflammation and leukocyte recruitment required for acute excitotoxic seizure induction and neural damage. *FASEB J* 2011, 25:737–753.

23. Marchi N, Fan Q, Ghosh C, Fazio V, Bertolini F, Betto G, Batra A, Carlton E, Najm I, Granata T, Janigro D: Antagonism of peripheral inflammation reduces the severity of status epilepticus. *Neurobiol Dis* 2009, 33:171–181.

24. Huang X, Zhang H, Yang J, Wu J, McMahon J, Lin Y, Cao Z, Gruenthal M, Huang Y: Pharmacological inhibition of the mammalian target of rapamycin pathway suppresses acquired epilepsy. *Neurobiol Dis* 2010, 40:193–199.

25. Maroso M, Balosso S, Ravizza T, Liu J, Aronica E, Iyer AM, Rossetti C, Molteni M, Casalgrandi M, Manfredi AA, Bianchi ME, Vezzani A: Toll-like receptor 4 and high-mobility group box-1 are involved in ictogenesis and can be targeted to reduce seizures. *Nat Med* 2010, 16:413–419.

26. Vezzani A: Inflammation and epilepsy. *Epilepsy Curr* 2005, 5:1–6.

27. Savarin-Vuaillat C, Ransohoff RM: Chemokines and chemokine receptors in neurological disease: raise, retain, or reduce? *Neurotherapeutics* 2007, 4:590–601.

28. Schwartz M: The emergence of a new science of the mind: immunology benefits the mind. *Mol Psychiatry* 2010, 15:337–338.

29. McClelland S, Flynn C, Dube C, Richichi C, Zha Q, Ghestem A, Esclapez M, Bernard C, Baram TZ: Neuron-restrictive silencer factor-mediated hyperpolarization-activated cyclic nucleotide gated channelopathy in experimental temporal lobe epilepsy. *Ann Neurol* 2011, 70:454–464.

30. Kan AA, van Erp S, Derijck AA, de Wit M, Hessel EV, O'Duibhir E, de Jager W, van Rijen PC, Gosselaar PH, de Graan PN, Pasterkamp RJ: Genome-wide microRNA profiling of human temporal lobe epilepsy identifies modulators of the immune response. *Cell Mol Life Sci* 2012, Epub ahead of print.

31. Debets RM, van Veelen CW, van Huffelen AV, van Emde BW: Presurgical evaluation of patients with intractable partial epilepsy: the Dutch epilepsy surgery program. *Acta Neurol Belg* 1991, 91:125–140.

32. Boer K, Spliet WG, van Rijen PC, Redeker S, Troost D, Aronica E: Evidence of activated microglia in focal cortical dysplasia. *J Neuroimmunol* 2006, 173:188–195.

33. Choi J, Nordli DR Jr, Alden TD, DiPatri A Jr, Laux L, Kelley K, Rosenow J, Schuele SU, Rajaram V, Koh S: Cellular injury and neuroinflammation in children with chronic intractable epilepsy. *J Neuroinflammation* 2009, 6:38.

34. Wyler AR, Dohan FC, Schweitzer JB, Berry AD: A grading system for mesial temporal pathology (hippocampal sclerosis) from anterior temporal lobectomy. *Journal of Epilepsy* 1992, 5:220–225.

35. Engel J, Van Ness PC, Rasmussen TB, Ojemann LM: *Outcome with respect to epileptic seizures.* New York: Raven; 1993:609–621.

36. Hulse RE, Kunkler PE, Fedynyshyn JP, Kraig RP: Optimization of multiplexed bead-based cytokine immunoassays for rat serum and brain tissue. *J Neurosci Methods* 2004, 136:87–98.

37. de Jager W, Te VH, Prakken BJ, Kuis W, Rijkers GT: Simultaneous detection of 15 human cytokines in a single sample of stimulated peripheral blood mononuclear cells. *Clin Diagn Lab Immunol* 2003, 10:133–139.

38. de Jager W, Prakken BJ, Bijlsma JW, Kuis W, Rijkers GT: Improved multiplex immunoassay performance in human plasma and synovial fluid following removal of interfering heterophilic antibodies. *J Immunol Methods* 2005, 300:124–135.

39. Romijn HJ, van Uum JF, Breedijk I, Emmering J, Radu I, Pool CW: Double immunolabeling of neuropeptides in the human hypothalamus as analyzed by confocal laser scanning fluorescence microscopy. *J Histochem Cytochem* 1999, 47:229–236.

40. Marengo E, Robotti E, Bobba M, Gosetti F: The principle of exhaustiveness versus the principle of parsimony: a new approach for the identification of biomarkers from proteomic spot volume datasets based on principal component analysis. *Anal Bioanal Chem* 2010, 397:25–41.

41. Loup F, Picard F, Yonekawa Y, Wieser HG, Fritschy JM: Selective changes in GABAA receptor subtypes in white matter neurons of patients with focal epilepsy. *Brain* 2009, 132:2449–2463.

42. Notenboom RG, Hampson DR, Jansen GH, van Rijen PC, van Veelen CW, van Nieuwenhuizen O, de Graan PN: Up-regulation of hippocampal metabotropic glutamate receptor 5 in temporal lobe epilepsy patients. *Brain* 2006, 129:96–107.

43. Proper EA, Hoogland G, Kappen SM, Jansen GH, Rensen MG, Schrama LH, van Veelen CW, van Rijen PC, van Nieuwenhuizen O, Gispen WH, de Graan PNE: Distribution of glutamate transporters in the hippocampus of patients with pharmaco-resistant temporal lobe epilepsy. *Brain* 2002, 125:32–43.

44. Aliashkevich AF, Yilmazer-Hanke D, Van Roost D, Mundhenk B, Schramm J, Blumcke I: Cellular pathology of amygdala neurons in human temporal lobe epilepsy. *Acta Neuropathol* 2003, 106:99–106.

45. Zattoni M, Mura ML, Deprez F, Schwendener RA, Engelhardt B, Frei K, Fritschy JM: Brain infiltration of leukocytes contributes to the pathophysiology of temporal lobe epilepsy. *J Neurosci* 2011, 31:4037–4050.

46. Dinarello CA: The interleukin-1 family: 10 years of discovery. *FASEB J* 1994, 8:1314–1325.

47. Rigau V, Morin M, Rousset MC, de Bock F, Lebrun A, Coubes P, Picot MC, Baldy-Moulinier M, Bockaert J, Crespel A, Lerner-Natoli M: Angiogenesis is associated with blood–brain barrier permeability in temporal lobe epilepsy. *Brain* 2007, 130:1942–1956.

48. Nakahara H, Konishi Y, Beach TG, Yamada N, Makino S, Tooyama I: Infiltration of T lymphocytes and expression of icam-1 in the hippocampus of patients with hippocampal sclerosis. *Acta Histochem Cytochem* 2010, 43:157–162.

49. dos Santos AC, Barsante MM, Arantes RM, Bernard CC, Teixeira MM, Carvalho-Tavares J: CCL2 and CCL5 mediate leukocyte adhesion in experimental autoimmune encephalomyelitis–an intravital microscopy study. *J Neuroimmunol* 2005, 162:122–129.

50. Vezzani A, Moneta D, Richichi C, Aliprandi M, Burrows SJ, Ravizza T, Perego C, De Simoni MG: Functional role of inflammatory cytokines and antiinflammatory molecules in seizures and epileptogenesis. *Epilepsia* 2002, 43(Suppl 5):30–35.

51. Auvin S, Shin D, Mazarati A, Sankar R: Inflammation induced by LPS enhances epileptogenesis in immature rat and may be partially reversed by IL1RA. *Epilepsia* 2010, 51(Suppl 3):34–38.

52. Heida JG, Pittman QJ: **Causal links between brain cytokines and experimental febrile convulsions in the rat.** *Epilepsia* 2005, **46:**1906–1913.

53. Vezzani A, Moneta D, Conti M, Richichi C, Ravizza T, De Luigi A, De Simoni MG, Sperk G, Andell-Jonsson S, Lundkvist J, De Simoni MG, Sperk G, Andell-Jonsson S, Lundkvist J, Iverfeldt K, Bartfai T: **Powerful anticonvulsant action of IL-1 receptor antagonist on intracerebral injection and astrocytic overexpression in mice.** *Proc Natl Acad Sci USA* 2000, **97:**11534–11539.

54. Biber K, de Jong EK, van Weering HR, Boddeke HW: **Chemokines and their receptors in central nervous system disease.** *Curr Drug Targets* 2006, **7:**29–46.

55. Michaelson MD, Mehler MF, Xu H, Gross RE, Kessler JA: **Interleukin-7 is trophic for embryonic neurons and is expressed in developing brain.** *Dev Biol* 1996, **179:**251–263.

56. Moors M, Vudattu NK, Abel J, Kramer U, Rane L, Ulfig N, Ceccatelli S, Seyfert-Margolies V, Fritsche E, Maeurer MJ: **Interleukin-7 (IL-7) and IL-7 splice variants affect differentiation of human neural progenitor cells.** *Genes Immun* 2010, **11:**11–20.

57. Ishizaki Y, Kira R, Fukuda M, Torisu H, Sakai Y, Sanefuji M, Yukaya N, Hara T: **Interleukin-10 is associated with resistance to febrile seizures: Genetic association and experimental animal studies.** *Epilepsia* 2009, **50:**761–767.

58. Levin SG, Godukhin OV: **Protective effects of interleukin-10 on the development of epileptiform activity evoked by transient episodes of hypoxia in rat hippocampal slices.** *Neurosci Behav Physiol* 2007, **37:**467–470.

59. Kurreeman FA, Schonkeren JJ, Heijmans BT, Toes RE, Huizinga TW: **Transcription of the IL10 gene reveals allele-specific regulation at the mRNA level.** *Hum Mol Genet* 2004, **13:**1755–1762.

60. Zhou Z, Peng X, Insolera R, Fink DJ, Mata M: **Interleukin-10 provides direct trophic support to neurons.** *J Neurochem* 2009, **110:**1617–1627.

61. Guyon A, Nahon JL: **Multiple actions of the chemokine stromal cell-derived factor-1alpha on neuronal activity.** *J Mol Endocrinol* 2007, **38:**365–376.

62. Kleinschek MA, Owyang AM, Joyce-Shaikh B, Langrish CL, Chen Y, Gorman DM, Blumenschein WM, McClanahan T, Brombacher F, Hurst SD, Kastelein RA: **IL-25 regulates Th17 function in autoimmune inflammation.** *J Exp Med* 2007, **204:**161–170.

63. Alt C, Laschinger M, Engelhardt B: **Functional expression of the lymphoid chemokines CCL19 (ELC) and CCL 21 (SLC) at the blood–brain barrier suggests their involvement in G-protein-dependent lymphocyte recruitment into the central nervous system during experimental autoimmune encephalomyelitis.** *Eur J Immunol* 2002, **32:**2133–2144.

64. Columba-Cabezas S, Serafini B, Ambrosini E, Aloisi F: **Lymphoid chemokines CCL19 and CCL21 are expressed in the central nervous system during experimental autoimmune encephalomyelitis: implications for the maintenance of chronic neuroinflammation.** *Brain Pathol* 2003, **13:**38–51.

65. Sonobe Y, Takeuchi H, Kataoka K, Li H, Jin S, Mimuro M, Hashizume Y, Sano Y, Kanda T, Mizuno T, Suzumura A: **Interleukin-25 expressed by brain capillary endothelial cells maintains blood–brain barrier function in a protein kinase Cepsilon-dependent manner.** *J Biol Chem* 2009, **284:**31834–31842.

66. Dogan RN, Long N, Forde E, Dennis K, Kohm AP, Miller SD, Karpus WJ: **CCL22 regulates experimental autoimmune encephalomyelitis by controlling inflammatory macrophage accumulation and effector function.** *J Leukoc Biol* 2011, **89:**93–104.

67. Galimberti D, Fenoglio C, Comi C, Scalabrini D, De Riz M, Leone M, Venturelli E, Cortini F, Piola M, Monaco F, Bresolin N, Scarpini E: **MDC/CCL22 intrathecal levels in patients with multiple sclerosis.** *Mult Scler* 2008, **14:**547–549.

68. Sweeney CM, Lonergan R, Basdeo SA, Kinsella K, Dungan LS, Higgins SC, Kelly PJ, Costelloe L, Tubridy N, Mills KH, Fletcher JM: **IL-27 mediates the response to IFN-beta therapy in multiple sclerosis patients by inhibiting Th17 cells.** *Brain Behav Immun* 2011, **25:**1170–1181.

69. Fitzgerald DC, Rostami A: **Therapeutic potential of IL-27 in multiple sclerosis?** *Expert Opin Biol Ther* 2009, **9:**149–160.

70. Muller M, Carter SL, Hofer MJ, Manders P, Getts DR, Getts MT, Dreykluft A, Lu B, Gerard C, King NJ, Campbell IL: **CXCR3 signaling reduces the severity of experimental autoimmune encephalomyelitis by controlling the parenchymal distribution of effector and regulatory T cells in the central nervous system.** *J Immunol* 2007, **179:**2774–2786.

71. Sorensen TL, Tani M, Jensen J, Pierce V, Lucchinetti C, Folcik VA, Qin S, Rottman J, Sellebjerg F, Strieter RM, Frederiksen JL, Ransohoff RM: **Expression of specific chemokines and chemokine receptors in the central nervous system of multiple sclerosis patients.** *J Clin Invest* 1999, **103:**807–815.

72. Kohler RE, Comerford I, Townley S, Haylock-Jacobs S, Clark-Lewis I, McColl SR: **Antagonism of the chemokine receptors CXCR3 and CXCR4 reduces the pathology of experimental autoimmune encephalomyelitis.** *Brain Pathol* 2008, **18:**504–516.

73. Camacho-Arroyo I, Lopez-Griego L, Morales-Montor J: **The role of cytokines in the regulation of neurotransmission.** *Neuroimmunomodulation* 2009, **16:**1–12.

74. Mendoza-Fernandez V, Andrew RD, Barajas-Lopez C: **Interferon-alpha inhibits long-term potentiation and unmasks a long-term depression in the rat hippocampus.** *Brain Res* 2000, **885:**14–24.

75. Salzmann A, Perroud N, Crespel A, Lambercy C, Malafosse A: **Candidate genes for temporal lobe epilepsy: a replication study.** *Neurol Sci* 2008, **29:**397–403.

76. Peltola J, Keranen T, Rainesalo S, Hurme M: **Polymorphism of the interleukin-1 gene complex in localization-related epilepsy.** *Ann Neurol* 2001, **50:**275–276.

77. Dominici R, Cattaneo M, Malferrari G, Archi D, Mariani C, Grimaldi LM, Biunno I: **Cloning and functional analysis of the allelic polymorphism in the transcription regulatory region of interleukin-1 alpha.** *Immunogenetics* 2002, **54:**82–86.

78. Akita H, Takagi N, Ishihara N, Takagi K, Murotomi K, Funakoshi H, Matsumoto K, Nakamura T, Takeo S: **Hepatocyte growth factor improves synaptic localization of the NMDA receptor and intracellular signaling after excitotoxic injury in cultured hippocampal neurons.** *Exp Neurol* 2008, **210:**83–94.

79. Tonges L, Ostendorf T, Lamballe F, Genestine M, Dono R, Koch JC, Bahr M, Maina F, Lingor P: **Hepatocyte growth factor protects retinal ganglion cells by increasing neuronal survival and axonal regeneration in vitro and in vivo.** *J Neurochem* 2011, **117:**892–903.

80. Dube CM, Ravizza T, Hamamura M, Zha Q, Keebaugh A, Fok K, Andres AL, Nalcioglu O, Obenaus A, Vezzani A, Baram TZ: **Epileptogenesis provoked by prolonged experimental febrile seizures: mechanisms and biomarkers.** *J Neurosci* 2010, **30:**7484–7494.

81. Viviani B, Bartesaghi S, Gardoni F, Vezzani A, Behrens MM, Bartfai T, Binaglia M, Corsini E, Di Luca M, Galli CL, Marinovich M: **Interleukin-1beta enhances NMDA receptor-mediated intracellular calcium increase through activation of the Src family of kinases.** *J Neurosci* 2003, **23:**8692–8700.

82. Balosso S, Maroso M, Sanchez-Alavez M, Ravizza T, Frasca A, Bartfai T, Vezzani A: **A novel non-transcriptional pathway mediates the proconvulsive effects of interleukin-1beta.** *Brain* 2008, **131:**3256–3265.

83. Cammalleri M, Martini D, Ristori C, Timperio AM, Bagnoli P: **Vascular endothelial growth factor up-regulation in the mouse hippocampus and its role in the control of epileptiform activity.** *Eur J Neurosci* 2011, **33:**482–498.

84. Nicoletti JN, Shah SK, McCloskey DP, Goodman JH, Elkady A, Atassi H, Hylton D, Rudge JS, Scharfman HE, Croll SD: **Vascular endothelial growth factor is up-regulated after status epilepticus and protects against seizure-induced neuronal loss in hippocampus.** *Neuroscience* 2008, **151:**232–241.

85. McCloskey DP, Croll SD, Scharfman HE: **Depression of synaptic transmission by vascular endothelial growth factor in adult rat hippocampus and evidence for increased efficacy after chronic seizures.** *J Neurosci* 2005, **25:**8889–8897.

86. Li Q, Oshige M, Zhen Y, Yamahara T, Oishi T, Seno T, Kawaguchi T, Numa Y, Kawamoto K: **Interleukin-5 and interleukin-10 are produced in central nervous system tumor cysts.** *J Clin Neurosci* 2009, **16:**437–440.

87. Liva SM, de Vellis J: **IL-5 induces proliferation and activation of microglia via an unknown receptor.** *Neurochem Res* 2001, **26:**629–637.

88. Ringheim GE: **Mitogenic effects of interleukin-5 on microglia.** *Neurosci Lett* 1995, **201:**131–134.

89. Mosmann TR, Cherwinski H, Bond MW, Giedlin MA, Coffman RL: **Two types of murine helper T cell clone. I. Definition according to profiles of lymphokine activities and secreted proteins.** *J Immunol* 1986, **136:**2348–2357.

90. Nunnari G, Xu Y, Acheampong EA, Fang J, Daniel R, Zhang C, Zhang H, Mukhtar M, Pomerantz RJ: **Exogenous IL-7 induces Fas-mediated human neuronal apoptosis: potential effects during human immunodeficiency virus type 1 infection.** *J Neurovirol* 2005, **11:**319–328.

91. Kebir H, Kreymborg K, Ifergan I, Dodelet-Devillers A, Cayrol R, Bernard M, Giuliani F, Arbour N, Becher B, Prat A: **Human TH17 lymphocytes promote**

blood–brain barrier disruption and central nervous system inflammation. *Nat Med* 2007, **13**:1173–1175.

92. Morin-Brureau M, Lebrun A, Rousset MC, Fagni L, Bockaert J, de Bock F, Lerner-Natoli M: **Epileptiform activity induces vascular remodeling and zonula occludens 1 downregulation in organotypic hippocampal cultures: role of VEGF signaling pathways.** *J Neurosci* 2011, **31**:10677–10688.

93. Suidan GL, Dickerson JW, Chen Y, McDole JR, Tripathi P, Pirko I, Seroogy KB, Johnson AJ: **CD8 T cell-initiated vascular endothelial growth factor expression promotes central nervous system vascular permeability under neuroinflammatory conditions.** *J Immunol* 2010, **184**:1031–1040.

94. Seiffert E, Dreier JP, Ivens S, Bechmann I, Tomkins O, Heinemann U, Friedman A: **Lasting blood–brain barrier disruption induces epileptic focus in the rat somatosensory cortex.** *J Neurosci* 2004, **24**:7829–7836.

95. Bittigau P, Ikonomidou C: **Glutamate in neurologic diseases.** *J Child Neurol* 1997, **12**:471–485.

96. Marchi N, Angelov L, Masaryk T, Fazio V, Granata T, Hernandez N, Hallene K, Diglaw T, Franic L, Najm I, Janigro D: **Seizure-promoting effect of blood–brain barrier disruption.** *Epilepsia* 2007, **48**:732–742.

97. van Vliet EA, da Costa AS, Redeker S, van Schaik R, Aronica E, Gorter JA: **Blood–brain barrier leakage may lead to progression of temporal lobe epilepsy.** *Brain* 2007, **130**:521–534.

98. Croll SD, Goodman JH, Scharfman HE: **Vascular endothelial growth factor (VEGF) in seizures: a double-edged sword.** *Adv Exp Med Biol* 2004, **548**:57–68.

99. Vezzani A, Aronica E, Mazarati A, Pittman QJ: **Epilepsy and brain inflammation.** *Exp Neurol* 2011, Epub ahead of print.

100. Lukasiuk K, Dabrowski M, Adach A, Pitkanen A: **Epileptogenesis-related genes revisited.** *Prog Brain Res* 2006, **158**:223–241.

101. Peltola J, Palmio J, Korhonen L, Suhonen J, Miettinen A, Hurme M, Lindholm D, Keranen T: **Interleukin-6 and interleukin-1 receptor antagonist in cerebrospinal fluid from patients with recent tonic-clonic seizures.** *Epilepsy Res* 2000, **41**:205–211.

102. Bauer S, Cepok S, Todorova-Rudolph A, Nowak M, Koller M, Lorenz R, Oertel WH, Rosenow F, Hemmer B, Hamer HM: **Etiology and site of temporal lobe epilepsy influence postictal cytokine release.** *Epilepsy Res* 2009, **86**:82–88.

103. Meisel C, Schwab JM, Prass K, Meisel A, Dirnagl U: **Central nervous system injury-induced immune deficiency syndrome.** *Nat Rev Neurosci* 2005, **6**:775–786.

104. Frost RA, Nystrom GJ, Lang CH: **Epinephrine stimulates IL-6 expression in skeletal muscle and C2C12 myoblasts: role of c-Jun NH2-terminal kinase and histone deacetylase activity.** *Am J Physiol Endocrinol Metab* 2004, **286**:E809–E817.

105. Febbraio MA, Pedersen BK: **Muscle-derived interleukin-6: mechanisms for activation and possible biological roles.** *FASEB J* 2002, **16**:1335–1347.

106. Pacifici R, Paris L, Di Carlo S, Bacosi A, Pichini S, Zuccaro P: **Cytokine production in blood mononuclear cells from epileptic patients.** *Epilepsia* 1995, **36**:384–387.

107. Lenz JC, Rockstroh JK: **Vicriviroc, a new CC-chemokine receptor 5 inhibitor for treatment of HIV: properties, promises and challenges.** *Expert Opin Drug Metab Toxicol* 2010, **6**:1139–1150.

108. Sayana S, Khanlou H: **Maraviroc: a new CCR5 antagonist.** *Expert Rev Anti Infect Ther* 2009, **7**:9–19.

# 15

# Analysis of plasma multiplex cytokines and increased level of IL-10 and IL-1Ra cytokines in febrile seizures

Kyungmin Kim[1], Byung Ok Kwak[1], Aram Kwon[1], Jongseok Ha[1], Soo-Jin Kim[2], Sun Whan Bae[2], Jae Sung Son[2], Soo-Nyung Kim[3] and Ran Lee[2,4]*

## Abstract

**Background:** Febrile seizures are the most common form of childhood seizures. Fever generation involves many cytokines, including both pro- and anti-inflammatory cytokines. Some of these cytokines also induce febrile seizures. We compared cytokine production in children with a fever alone (healthy control group) and febrile seizure children group. Also, we evaluated the cytokine level of children with a fever alone and febrile seizure history.

**Methods:** Fifty febrile seizure patients and 39 normal control patients who visited the emergency department of Konkuk University Hospital from December 2015 to December 2016 were included in this study. Blood was taken from the peripheral vessels of children in all groups within 1 h of the seizure, and serum was obtained immediately. Serum samples from patients with only a fever and a febrile seizure history ($N = 13$) and afebrile seizure controls ($N = 12$) were also analyzed.

**Results:** The serum IL-10 and IL-1Ra levels were significantly higher in the febrile seizure patients than in the fever-only control, fever only with a febrile seizure history, and afebrile seizure groups ($p < 0.05$). The serum IFN-γ and IL-6 levels were significantly higher in the febrile seizure patients than in the afebrile seizure group ($p < 0.05$). The serum IL-8 levels were higher in the febrile seizure patients than in the fever only controls ($p < 0.05$).

**Conclusions:** The serum levels of the IFN-γ, IL-6, and IL-8 pro-inflammatory cytokines and the serum levels of the IL-10 and IL-1Ra anti-inflammatory cytokines were significantly higher in the febrile seizure children. Furthermore, the serum level of IL-1Ra was more increased in the febrile seizure group than in the same patients with only a fever. Our data suggest that increased serum IL-10 and IL-1Ra may play potential roles as anti-inflammatory cytokines in a compensation mechanism that shortens the seizure duration or prevents a febrile seizure attack. Therefore, anti-inflammatory cytokines, including IL-10 and IL-1Ra, have potential as therapeutic targets for the prevention of seizures and nervous system development of children.

**Keywords:** Febrile seizures, Pro-inflammatory cytokines, Anti-inflammatory cytokines, IL-10, IL-1Ra

## Background

Febrile seizures (FSs) are the most common form of childhood seizures and occur in 2–5% of children before the age of 6 years [1]. FSs are seizures induced by fever (body temperature $\geq 38$ °C). These patients do not have any definitive causative diseases, such as a central nervous system infection, electrolyte imbalance, metabolic disorders, and history of afebrile seizures [2]. Although several cohort studies have suggested that the prognosis of FSs is good, epilepsy is observed in 5.4% of these patients [3]. The exact pathogenesis of FSs is not well understood. However, predisposing factors, genetic susceptibility, infection or immune-mediated factors, and a cytokine storm have been proposed [4]. A positive family history of FSs is the most meaningful risk factor, with more affected relatives resulting in a greater risk [5]. Cytokines act as mediators of the host response to

* Correspondence: 20050069@kuh.ac.kr
[2]Department of Pediatrics, Konkuk University Medical Center, Konkuk University School of Medicine, 120-1 Neungdong-ro (Hwayang-dong), Gwangjin-gu, Seoul 05030, Korea
[4]International Healthcare Research Institute, Konkuk University, Seoul, Korea
Full list of author information is available at the end of the article

infections and induce fever, leukocytosis, and acute-phase protein synthesis [6]. Recently, abnormalities in cytokine and immune cell expression have been observed in patients with seizures and in animal models of seizures. Many studies have shown that the production and release of cytokines are regulated by the immune system and that cytokines can aggravate brain damage when acting as mediators of seizures [7]. Cytokines can exert both pro-inflammatory and anti-inflammatory effects [4]. Fever is induced by pro-inflammatory cytokines, such as interleukin (IL)-1β, IL-6, and tumor necrosis factor (TNF)-α, during infections. The fever threshold temperature for FSs varies among individuals as well as by age and maturation [8].

Gallentien WB et al. has measured multiple cytokines and compared the results between children with FSs and controls [9]. Due to recent advances in technology, a small amount of serum can be applied to multiplex flow cytometry to obtain multiple cytokine levels. In this study, we hypothesized that the cytokine profiles might differ between patients with FSs and control groups, such as individuals with only fever without a FS history, only fever with a FS history, and afebrile seizures. This result would suggest that pro-inflammatory and anti-inflammatory cytokines play roles in the pathogenesis of FSs. Therefore, we assessed the correlation between cytokine levels and FSs.

## Methods
### Patient information
Fifty febrile seizure patients and 39 normal control patients who visited the emergency department of Konkuk University Hospital, Seoul, Korea from December 2015 to December 2016 were included in this study. All parents were provided information regarding the research method. The children included in the study underwent blood tests after their parent agreed and signed the informed consent form.

The inclusion criteria for the febrile seizure groups were (1) age between 6 months and 6 years, (2) body temperature $\geq 38$ °C, (3) C-reactive protein (CRP) < 3.0 mmol/dL, (4) presence of a simple febrile seizure (generalized seizure, usually tonic-clonic, lasting for < 15 min and not recurrent within a 24-h period), and (5) present no other identifiable cause of the seizure. Patients with a central nervous system infection, metabolic imbalance, and history of afebrile seizures were excluded. Laboratory findings, including complete blood counts (CBCs), blood chemistry, and CRP, were evaluated at the time of the seizure.

The control group included febrile children without seizures who visited our hospital for common febrile diseases, such as upper respiratory tract infections. Febrile diseases (viral or bacterial) were diagnosed according to the clinical manifestations. The control

groups were matched for age and temperature criteria and had no convulsions during the febrile illness and no known history of previous febrile seizures.

Blood was taken from the peripheral vessels of children in all groups, and serum was obtained by centrifugation at 3500 rpm for 5 min at 4 °C. The serum was immediately separated and stored in a deep freezer at − 70 °C. In the febrile seizure groups, blood samples were collected within 1 h after the occurrence of a seizure episode.

Additionally, blood serum sample was collected and frozen from children with an afebrile seizure attack ($N = 13$) and a febrile illness with a febrile seizure history ($N = 12$) to subtract the effects of the fever from the cytokine levels.

The study was approved by the Institutional Review Board at the Konkuk University Medical Center (30 October 2015–30 October 2017).

### Cytokine measurement
The concentrations of pro-inflammatory cytokines (IFN-γ, IL-1β, IL-2, IL-6, and IL-8) and anti-inflammatory cytokines (IL-10 and IL-1Ra) were measured using commercially available enzyme-linked immunosorbent assay (ELISA) kits (MILLIPLEX MAP KIT, human cytokine/chemokine magnetic bead panel—immunology multiplex assay, Cat #HCYTOMAG-60 K, EMD Millipore Corp. Billerica, MA, USA). All samples were measured in duplicate to improve the accuracy.

### Statistical analysis
The data were summarized using the mean ± standard deviation (SD) for clinical characteristics, whereas the cytokine levels were expressed as the median and range. The chi-square test was used to compare the clinical findings, and the Kruskal–Wallis test or Mann–Whitney $U$ test was performed to compare serum cytokine levels and laboratory findings among the FS, control, fever only with FS history, and afebrile seizure groups. Bonferroni correction was performed to account for multiple comparisons (corrected critical $p$ value $\leq 0.05$). Statistical calculations were performed using SPSS ver. 24. $p < 0.05$ was considered significant.

## Results
### Patient clinical profiles
Fifty patients with FSs and 39 healthy control children with febrile illness without seizures were included in this study. The demographic information and clinical characteristics of the children are summarized in Table 1. Although the mean age was younger in the FS group than in the control group ($27.3 \pm 13.2$ vs. $36.3 \pm 31.9$ months), the difference was not significant ($p = 0.327$). The proportion of boys and girls (26/34 vs. 20/19) and the body temperature at admission were similar in the FS and

**Table 1** Clinical findings of FS, control, fever only with FS history, and afebrile seizure groups

|  | Febrile seizure (N = 50) | Control (N = 39) | Fever only with FS history (N = 12) | Afebrile seizure (N = 13) | p value |
|---|---|---|---|---|---|
| Age (months) | 27.3 ± 13.2 | 36.3 ± 31.9 | 40.5 ± 32.6 | 95.9 ± 60.8 | 0.327 |
| Sex (male/female) | 26/24 | 20/19 | 8/4 | 7/6 |  |
| BT (°C) | 38.9 ± 0.5 | 38.6 ± 0.6 | 38.4 ± 0.5 | 36.8 ± 0.2 | 0.013 |
| WBC (/μL) | 10,861 ± 4,296 | 12,758 ± 6,023 | 10,642 ± 4,871 | 9750 ± 2,963 | 0.143 |
| CRP (mg/dL) | 0.55 ± 0.7 | 3.6 ± 2.6 | 4.8 ± 7.0 | 0.13 ± 0.1 | < 0.001 |

Data are presented as mean ± SD (standard deviation). The p value is about FS and control groups. A p value < 0.05 indicates a significant difference. Mann–Whitney U test

FS febrile seizure, BT body temperature, WBC whole blood cell, CRP C-reactive protein

control groups (38.9 ± 0.5 vs. 38.6 ± 0.6) ($p < 0.05$). The white blood cell (WBC) count was slightly increased in the control group compared to the FS group (10,861 ± 4296 vs. 12,758 ± 6023) ($p = 0.143$). The CRP was significantly higher in the control group than in the FS group (0.55 ± 0.7 vs. 3.6 ± 2.6) ($p < 0.001$). Furthermore, 13 children with fever only and with febrile seizure history and 12 children with afebrile seizures were included for comparison with the febrile seizure group. Boys were more prevalent than girls (8/4), and the CRP level was increased in the fever only with FS history group (4.8 ± 7.0). The mean age of the afebrile seizure patients was higher than the mean ages of the other groups (95.9 ± 60.8).

## Comparison of cytokines

A comparison of the plasma cytokines in the four groups (FS, febrile control, fever only with FS history and afebrile seizure) is shown in Table 2. IFN-γ, IL-10, IL-1Ra, IL-2, IL-6, and IL-8 were increased in the FS group ($p = 0.047$, <0.001, <0.001, 0.007, 0.001, and 0.030, respectively; Table 2). The remaining cytokines except IL-1β and IL-2 were significantly increased in the FS group when subjected to the Bonferroni multiple comparison correction test. The mean IFN-γ level was 48.3 pg/mL in the FS group and 13.7 pg/mL in the afebrile seizure group. Comparisons of the IFN-γ levels showed significantly higher levels in the FS group than in the only afebrile seizure group (corrected $p = 0.029$). The mean IL-10 level was 156.9 pg/mL in the FS group

and was significantly increased compared to the other three groups (febrile control, fever only with FS history and afebrile seizure) and had a significant corrected $p$ value within each group comparison. The IL-1Ra level was also higher in the FS group compared to the other three groups, with corrected $p$ values for each group comparison below 0.05. The mean IL-1β level was 3.8 pg/mL in the FS group and 4.5 pg/mL in the febrile control group. Comparisons of the IL-1β levels among the four groups showed no significant differences ($p = 0.300$, Table 3). The mean IL-2 level was 3.0 pg/mL in the FS group and 3.3 pg/mL in the febrile control group. The $p$ value was significantly lower when the IL-2 levels were compared among the four groups; however, this result was due to a difference between the afebrile seizure and febrile control group and did not affect the FS group. The mean IL-8 concentration was 109.1 pg/mL in the FS group and 33.8 pg/mL in the febrile control group. Comparisons of the IL-8 levels showed an increase in the FS group compared with the febrile control group (corrected $p = 0.042$). Interestingly, we also compared the serum cytokine levels between the same patients after a febrile seizure and when they had only a fever without a seizure (Table 3). The median IL-1Ra level was 638.9 pg/mL during febrile seizes and 177.6 pg/mL when the same patients only had a fever. The $P$ value was less than 0.05 and was significantly increased in the FS group. The median IL-2 level was 2.86 pg/mL in the febrile seizure group and 1.83 pg/mL in the same patients with only a fever. Comparison of the IL-2 levels between the FS and fever-only

**Table 2** Comparisons of cytokine levels in four groups including FS, control, fever only with FS history, and afebrile seizure children

| Cytokines | Febrile seizure (N = 50) | Control (N = 39) | Fever only with FS history (N = 12) | Afebrile seizure (N = 13) | p value |
|---|---|---|---|---|---|
| IFN-γ | 29.8(4–220) | 21.6(2.7–703) | 21(5.0–266) | 13.9(0.3–25.8) | 0.047 |
| IL-10 | 103.7(7.1–728) | 34.0(1.4–832.4) | 22.0(0.5–181) | 5.0(0.3–65.3) | < 0.001 |
| IL-1Ra | 652(144–5667) | 231(1.6–1461) | 202(34–422) | 200(0.3–3440) | < 0.001 |
| IL-1β | 2.8(2.8–16.2) | 2.9(0.4–47.4) | 2.2(0.4–25.4) | 1.1(0.2–61.6) | 0.300 |
| IL-2 | 2.8(2.8–5.3) | 2.8(0.3–17.1) | 1.7(0.2–27.2) | 0.9(0.1–42.2) | 0.007 |
| IL-6 | 16.9(1.3–798) | 7.9(0.2–104.2) | 6.5(0.2–71.4) | 0.8(0.2–31.5) | 0.001 |
| IL-8 | 43.3(2.3–1711) | 20.9(1.3–109.1) | 35.5(2.6–589) | 54.7(4.5–345.6) | 0.030 |

Data are presented as median (range), and the unit is pg/mL. Multiple comparison test (Bonferroni correction). A p value < 0.05 indicates a significant difference. Kruskal–Wallis test

**Table 3** Comparison of cytokine levels between febrile seizures and fever only in four patients

|  | Febrile seizure (N = 4) | Fever only with FSs history (N = 4) | p value |
|---|---|---|---|
| IFN-γ | 68.4(28.7–121.7) | 21.5(8.39–161.49) | 0.486 |
| IL-10 | 50.8(40.1–84.5) | 17.7(4.3–181.5) | 0.343 |
| IL-1Ra | 638.9(478–1244) | 177.6(40.9–281.7) | 0.029 |
| IL-1β | 3.4(2.8–4.7) | 1.88(1.2–3.9) | 0.114 |
| IL-2 | 2.86(2.8–3.6) | 1.83(0.4–2.2) | 0.029 |
| IL-6 | 17.27(6.4–96.5) | 4.43(0.4–7.6) | 0.057 |
| IL-8 | 27.2(11.4–59.4) | 39.6(14.9–144.1) | 0.486 |

Four patients of both groups are same children. Data are presented as median (range) and unit is pg/mL. A $p$ value < 0.05 indicates a significant difference. Mann–Whitney $U$ test

conditions showed a significant increase in the FS condition ($p = 0.029$, Table 3). The remaining cytokines excluding IL-1Ra and IL-2 showed no differences in their levels in the FS condition.

## Discussion

Although many studies have investigated the cause of febrile seizures, the actual cause of the disease is mostly unknown. Few studies have suggested the role of cytokines in febrile seizures [10]. Since FSs occur during the course of a high body temperature or a rapidly rising fever in susceptible individuals, various factors associated with fever generation could be involved in the possible causative mechanism of FSs. Fever generation involves many cytokines and endogenous mediators, including IL-1, IL-6, TNF-α, IL-1Ra, and IL-10, in response to exogenous pyrogens. Peripheral cytokines can impact brain functions as evidenced by CNS symptoms, such as fever, anorexia, lethargy, and a lower seizure threshold, during systemic inflammation, febrile illness, or sepsis. Although peripheral cytokine levels may not be an accurate reflection of CNS cytokine activity, there are mechanisms by which their presence may induce a reciprocal inflammatory response within the brain [11]. Several studies showed blood–brain barrier (BBB) failure after administration of IL-1, IL-6, TNF-α, and IFN-γ. This inflammation induces changes in the brain parenchyma, such as leakage of the BBB, which changes the functional properties of the BBB [12]. These changes in BBB permeability may favor the entry of peripheral cytokines as well as cells of the innate and adaptive immune response into the CNS, resulting in further activation of the inflammatory cascade within the brain [11]. The changes cause cell damage that contributes to neuronal hyperexcitability, which lowers the threshold for seizure induction and triggers epileptogenesis [12].

Another study reported that the plasma IL-1β and cerebrospinal fluid TNF-α levels were significantly higher in FS patients during the acute phase of the disease than in the controls [8, 13]. The chronic IL-1β expression during epileptogenesis highlights the possibility

that this cytokine may be involved in the mechanisms underlying the onset of spontaneous seizures [14]. Gallentine WB et al. compared the samples of children with febrile status epilepticus (FES) to children with fever. They found that as the balance shifts toward higher IL-1β and lower IL-1Ra, seizure threshold goes down and the likelihood of FSE increases. On the contrary, as the balance shifts toward lower IL-1β and higher IL-1Ra, seizure threshold is higher and the likelihood of FSE decreases [9].

In the present study, we analyzed a total of seven cytokines, including pro-inflammatory and anti-inflammatory cytokines, as described above. The multiplex cytokine analysis revealed no increase in serum IL-1β in our children with FSs compared to the controls. Therefore, in contrast to previous studies, these results conflict with the important role played by IL-1β in the mechanism of febrile seizures. This lack of an increase may be the result of excluding patients with presumptive bacterial infections, such as a low CRP level, because LPS is the main inducer of IL-1β synthesis [15]. Moreover, IL-1β is usually difficult to detect due to its binding to large proteins, such as α-2 microglobulin and complement. Furthermore, fever can occur independently of IL-1β activity during infections, possibly through the cytokine-like property of Toll-like receptor signal transduction [16]. The contradictory results reported by various studies may be due to the interference of confounding variables, such as time of sampling, severity of temperature, duration of fever, difficulty in measuring cytokines, type of infection, and sample size. Time of sampling is very important for measurement of the IL-1β levels. IL-1β increases within 1 h after a seizure, reaches its maximum level within 4–12 h after a seizure, and returns to its normal level after 24 h [17]. Thus, IL-1β is best measured within 12 h after the incidence of seizure. In the present study, samples were prepared within 1 h after the incidence of seizure. Therefore, in this study, low levels of IL-1β in patients with febrile seizures did not correlate with the time of sampling.

During the response to seizures, the IL-1β system induces IL-1Ra, which acts by limiting IL-1β-mediated pro-inflammatory actions. IL-1Ra has been shown to be a powerful anticonvulsant in various seizure models. IL-1Ra is induced by seizures several hours after IL-1β to rapidly terminate the effects of IL-1β. In another study, peak pro-inflammatory cytokine effects occurred 6 h after status epilepticus, whereas the peak effect of the anti-inflammatory cytokine IL-1Ra was delayed and occurred 24 h after IL-1β [18]. Therefore, IL-1Ra is induced by seizures several hours after IL-1β [19]. Changes in the IL-1Ra to IL-1 ratio act as a mechanism to control seizures after onset. During peripheral inflammatory reactions, IL-1Ra is generally produced at a 100-fold molar excess compared to IL-1 [14]. This change may be an effective pathophysiological mechanism to control seizures. In our study, IL-1Ra was significantly higher in the FS group than in the control, fever only with FS history, and afebrile seizure groups. This is contrary to Gallentine WB et al. that the IL-1Ra was not increased in FSE when comparing FSE to control patients. Because IL-1Ra has neuroprotective and anticonvulsant effects [20] and is closely correlated with the pro-convulsive cytokine IL-1β, we suggest that elevated IL-1Ra may be hyperreactive to IL-1β in response to the epileptogenic environment even though the IL-1β level does not change significantly. The IL-1β level is expected to react faster than the time presented in previous studies and will decrease in the usual range. Interestingly, the serum IL-1Ra level was also increased when we compared the cytokines between the same four patients in the presence of a febrile seizure and with a fever alone without a febrile seizure. Therefore, IL-1Ra is expected to increase the anti-inflammatory reaction and reduce the febrile convulsion duration and thus seems to be a more accurate indicator than IL-1β.

IL-6 is a cell signaling molecule that has been associated with many diseases, including inflammatory, neurological, vascular, and malignant processes [21]. The systemic concentration of IL-6 is mainly regulated at the level of expression, because IL-6 is rapidly cleared from the plasma and has a short plasma half-life of 20–60 min [22]. Many other studies have supported the potential immune modulatory effects of IL-6 and its importance as a major pro-inflammatory cytokine. The plasma IL-6 level was significantly higher in patients with FSs compared with the febrile control subjects, and the CSF IL-6 levels were detectable in all studied patients with FSs [23]. As expected, the current study showed that the serum IL-6 levels were markedly elevated in the patients with FSs compared to the afebrile seizure group. Our results together with other findings may support the proconvulsant action of IL-6 in FSs.

IL-10 is a multifunctional anti-inflammatory cytokine that is produced by monocytes, macrophages, lymphocytes, and microglia and inhibits the production of pro-inflammatory cytokines, including IL-1, IL-6, IL-8, and TNF-α [24]. Previous studies have shown lipopolysaccharide-induced increases in IL-10 production by peripheral blood mononuclear cells isolated from children with a history of FSs. Another group reported that the plasma IL-10 level did not differ between children with and without FSs. Therefore, little is known about the involvement of IL-10 in the pathogenesis of FSs [23]. However, the febrile seizure threshold temperatures were significantly higher in mice injected with recombinant human IL-10 to establish a hyperthermia-induced seizure model than in the control group [25]. As expected, in the present study, the IL-10 levels were higher in the FS group than in control, fever only with FS history, and afebrile seizure groups. These findings may reflect compensatory activation of the anti-inflammatory role or an anti-convulsive mechanistic effect of IL-10 in FSs.

Interestingly, IL-8 was also elevated in our study. IL-8 exhibits trophic-like activity and is implicated in the maintenance of normal neuronal populations as well as the promotion of neuronal survival and regeneration. IL-8 is also a known neutrophil activation peptide and is produced by monocyte-derived macrophages, microglia, and astrocytes [26]. IL-8 strongly promotes leukocyte migration to inflammatory foci in the CNS by inducing neutrophil–endothelial adhesions and contributes to BBB breakdown during acute brain injury. Therefore, the present study suggests that IL-8 may contribute to the proconvulsant environment and possibly promote epileptogenesis.

IL-2 plays an important role in regulating the immune response by driving T cell growth, augmenting NK cytolytic activity, inducing the differentiation of regulatory T cells, and mediating activation-induced cell death [27]. Intraventricular administration of IL-2 in DBA/2 mice promotes seizure generation in various models of experimental epilepsy [28]. However, the IL-2 levels in the plasma and CSF remained unchanged in patients with prolonged FSs with or without encephalopathy during the acute stage [29]. As shown in our results, the IL-2 dose level did not significantly differ between the children with FSs and the control group. However, the serum IL-2 level was increased when we compared serum cytokines between the same four patients after a febrile seizure and when there was fever only without a febrile seizure. Although the number of patients in the case is small, we suggest that IL-2 is also correlated with febrile seizures as a pro-inflammatory cytokine.

## Conclusions

In conclusion, pro-inflammatory cytokines, including IFN-γ, IL-6, and IL-8 and anti-inflammatory cytokines, including IL-1Ra and IL-10, were increased in children with FSs. Furthermore, the serum level of IL-1Ra was more increased in the febrile seizure group than in the same patients with only a fever. If pro-inflammatory cytokines are produced by the IL-1 systemic cascade in the febrile condition, peripheral cytokines enter the CNS and lower the seizure threshold. Pro-inflammatory cytokine production may promote seizures, further exacerbate epilepsy, and cause subsequent intractable epilepsy. Anti-inflammatory cytokines were also elevated in children with FSs as a compensatory mechanism to prevent FS attacks. The symptom of seizures improved within 5 min in almost all of the children with FSs due to the effects of anti-inflammatory cytokines. Therefore, anti-inflammatory cytokines, including IL-10 and IL-1Ra, may play critical roles and represent therapeutic targets for the prevention of seizures and for nervous system development in children.

There are two reasons why our research results, which are different from other studies, are more meaningful. First, we selected both a group of healthy children accompanied only by fever and a group of children with a fever only and a FS history to compare the cytokine levels. Second, by comparing the levels of cytokines during an FS episode and during fever alone in the same patient, various factors that occurred when comparing different patients could be eliminated. Although the number of samples compared in the same patient was small, the results supported the results compared with the fever-only healthy children control group. Subsequently, by further increasing the number of samples, other cytokines related to FSs could be clearly identified, especially IL-10 and IL-1Ra.

## Abbreviations
BBB: Blood–brain barrier; CBC: Complete blood count; COX: Cyclooxygenase; CRP: C-reactive protein; FS: Febrile seizure; IL: Interleukin; LPS: Lipopolysaccharide; PGE: Prostaglandin E; TNF: Tumor necrosis factor; WBC: Whole blood cell

## Authors' contributions
KK carried out the molecular genetic studies, participated in the sequence alignment and drafted the manuscript. BK carried out the immunoassays. AK and JH participated in the sequence alignment. KK and SYK participated in the design of the study and performed the statistical analysis. SJK, SB, and JS participated in the design of the study. RL conceived of the study and participated in its design and coordination. All authors read and approved the final manuscript.

## Funding
Not applicable

## Consent for publication
Not applicable

## Competing interests
The authors declare that they have no competing interest.

## Author details
[1]Department of Pediatrics, Konkuk University Medical Center, Seoul, Korea. [2]Department of Pediatrics, Konkuk University Medical Center, Konkuk University School of Medicine, 120-1 Neungdong-ro (Hwayang-dong), Gwangjin-gu, Seoul 05030, Korea. [3]Department of Obstetrics and Gynecology, Konkuk University Medical Center, Konkuk University School of Medicine, Seoul, Korea. [4]International Healthcare Research Institute, Konkuk University, Seoul, Korea.

## References
1. Baumann RJ, Duffner PK. Treatment of children with simple febrile seizures: the AAP practice parameter. Pediatr Neurol. 2000;23:11–7.
2. Sugai K. Current management of febrile seizures in Japan: an overview. Brain Dev. 2010;32:64–70.
3. Graves RC, Oehler K, Tingle LE. Febrile seizures: risks, evaluation, and prognosis. Am Fam Physician. 2012;85
4. M-H H, Huang G-S, C-T W, Lin J-J, Hsia S-H, Wang H-S, Lin K-L. Analysis of plasma multiplex cytokines for children with febrile seizures and severe acute encephalitis. J Child Neurol. 2014;29:182–6.
5. Nur BG, Kahramaner Z, Duman O, Dundar NO, Sallakcı N, Yavuzer U, Haspolat S. Interleukin-6 gene polymorphism in febrile seizures. Pediatr Neurol. 2012;46:36–8.
6. Soltani S, Zare-Shahabadi A, Shahrokhi A, Rezaei A, Zoghi S, Zamani GR, Mohammadi M, Ashrafi MR, Rezaei N. Association of interleukin-1 gene cluster and interleukin-1 receptor polymorphisms with febrile seizures. J Child Neurol. 2016;31:673–7.
7. Li G, Bauer S, Nowak M, Norwood B, Tackenberg B, Rosenow F, Knake S, Oertel WH, Hamer HM. Cytokines and epilepsy. Seizure. 2011;20:249–56.
8. Choi J, Min HJ, Shin JS. Increased levels of HMGB1 and pro-inflammatory cytokines in children with febrile seizures. J Neuroinflammation. 2011;8:135.
9. Gallentine WB, Shinnar S, Hesdorffer DC, Epstein L, Nordli DR, Lewis DV, Frank LM, Seinfeld S, Shinnar RC, Cornett K: Plasma cytokines associated with febrile status epilepticus in children: a potential biomarker for acute hippocampal injury. Epilepsia 2017.
10. Mahyar A, Ayazi P, Orangpour R, Daneshi-Kohan MM, Sarokhani MR, Javadi A, Habibi M, Talebi-Bakhshayesh M. Serum interleukin-1beta and tumor necrosis factor-alpha in febrile seizures: is there a link? Korean J Pediatr. 2014;57:440–4.
11. Gallentine WB, Shinnar S, Hesdorffer DC, Epstein L, Nordli DR, Jr., Lewis DV, Frank LM, Seinfeld S, Shinnar RC, Cornett K, et al: Plasma cytokines associated with febrile status epilepticus in children: a potential biomarker for acute hippocampal injury. Epilepsia 2017, 58:1102-1111.
12. Youn Y, Sung IK, Lee IG. The role of cytokines in seizures: interleukin (IL)-1β, IL-1Ra, IL-8, and IL-10. Korean J Pediatr. 2013;56:271–4.
13. Tütüncüoğlu S, Kütükçüler N, Kepe L, Çoker C, Berdeli A, Tekgül H. Proinflammatory cytokines, prostaglandins and zinc in febrile convulsions. Pediatr Int. 2001;43:235–9.
14. Vezzani A, Balosso S, Ravizza T. The role of cytokines in the pathophysiology of epilepsy. Brain Behav Immun. 2008;22:797–803.
15. Heida JG, Moshé SL, Pittman QJ. The role of interleukin-1β in febrile seizures. Brain and Development. 2009;31:388–93.
16. Dinarello CA. Review: infection, fever, and exogenous and endogenous pyrogens: some concepts have changed. J Endotoxin Res. 2004;10:201–22.
17. Haspolat S, Mihçi E, Coşkun M, Gümüslü S, Özbenm T, Yegin O. Interleukin-1β, tumor necrosis factor-α, and nitrite levels in febrile seizures. J Child Neurol. 2002;17:749–51.
18. Vezzani A, Moneta D, Richichi C, Aliprandi M, Burrows SJ, Ravizza T, Perego C, De Simoni MG. Functional role of inflammatory cytokines and antiinflammatory molecules in seizures and epileptogenesis. Epilepsia. 2002; 43(Suppl 5):30–5.
19. De Simoni MG, Perego C, Ravizza T, Moneta D, Conti M, Marchesi F, De Luigi A, Garattini S, Vezzani A. Inflammatory cytokines and related genes are induced in the rat hippocampus by limbic status epilepticus. Eur J Neurosci. 2000;12:2623–33.
20. Sinha S, Patil S, Jayalekshmy V, Satishchandra P. Do cytokines have any role in epilepsy? Epilepsy Res. 2008;82:171–6.
21. Azab SF, Abdalhady MA, Ali A, Amin EK, Sarhan DT, Elhindawy EM, Almalky MA, Elhewala AA, Salam MM, Hashem MI, et al. Interleukin-6 gene polymorphisms in Egyptian children with febrile seizures: a case-control study. Ital J Pediatr. 2016;42:31.

22. Fischer CP. Interleukin-6 in acute exercise and training: what is the biological relevance. Exerc Immunol Rev. 2006;12:41.

23. Virta M, Hurme M, Helminen M. Increased plasma levels of pro- and anti-inflammatory cytokines in patients with febrile seizures. Epilepsia. 2002;43:920–3.

24. Williams K, Dooley N, Ulvestad E, Becher B, Antel JP. IL-10 production by adult human derived microglial cells. Neurochem Int. 1996;29:55–64.

25. Ishizaki Y, Kira R, Fukuda M, Torisu H, Sakai Y, Sanefuji M, Yukaya N, Hara T. Interleukin-10 is associated with resistance to febrile seizures: genetic association and experimental animal studies. Epilepsia. 2009;50:761–7.

26. Asano T, Ichiki K, Koizumi S, Kaizu K, Hatori T, Fujino O, Mashiko K, Sakamoto Y, Miyasho T, Fukunaga Y. IL-8 in cerebrospinal fluid from children with acute encephalopathy is higher than in that from children with febrile seizure. Scand J Immunol. 2010;71:447–51.

27. Liao W, Lin J-X, Leonard WJ. IL-2 family cytokines: new insights into the complex roles of IL-2 as a broad regulator of T helper cell differentiation. Curr Opin Immunol. 2011;23:598–604.

28. De Sarro G, Rotiroti D, Audino MG, Gratteri S, Nisticó G. Effects of interleukin-2 on various models of experimental epilepsy in DBA/2 mice. Neuroimmunomodulation. 1994;1:361–9.

29. Ichiyama T, Suenaga N, Kajimoto M, Tohyama J, Isumi H, Kubota M, Mori M, Furukawa S. Serum and CSF levels of cytokines in acute encephalopathy following prolonged febrile seizures. Brain and Development. 2008;30:47–52.

# 16

# Activation of brain indoleamine 2,3-dioxygenase contributes to epilepsy-associated depressive-like behavior in rats with chronic temporal lobe epilepsy

Wei Xie[1,2,3*†], Lun Cai[2,3,4†], Yunhong Yu[5], Liang Gao[3], Limin Xiao[3], Qianchao He[4], Zhijun Ren[2] and Yuanzheng Liu[2]

## Abstract

**Background:** Depression has most often been diagnosed in patients with temporal lobe epilepsy (TLE), but the mechanism underlying this association remains unclear. In this study, we report that indoleamine 2,3-dioxygenase 1 (IDO1), a rate-limiting enzyme in tryptophan metabolism, plays a key role in epilepsy-associated depressive-like behavior.

**Methods:** Rats which develop chronic epilepsy following pilocarpine status epilepticus exhibited a set of interictal disorders consistent with depressive-like behavior. Changes of depressive behavior were examined by taste preference test and forced swim test; brain IL-1β, IL-6 and IDO1 expression were quantified using real-time reverse transcriptase PCR; brain kynurenine/tryptophan and serotonin/tryptophan ratios were analyzed by liquid chromatography-mass spectrometry. Oral gavage of minocycline or subcutaneous injection of 1-methyltryptophan (1-MT) were used to inhibit IDO1 expression.

**Results:** We observed the induction of IL-1β and IL-6 expression in rats with chronic TLE, which further induced the upregulation of IDO1 expression in the hippocampus. The upregulation of IDO1 subsequently increased the kynurenine/tryptophan ratio and decreased the serotonin/tryptophan ratio in the hippocampus, which contributed to epilepsy-associated depressive-like behavior. The blockade of IDO1 activation prevented the development of depressive-like behavior but failed to influence spontaneous seizures. This effect was achieved either indirectly, through the anti-inflammatory tetracycline derivative minocycline, or directly, through the IDO antagonist 1-MT, which normalizes kynurenine/tryptophan and serotonin/tryptophan ratios.

**Conclusion:** Brain IDO1 activity plays a key role in epileptic rats with epilepsy-associated depressive-like behavior.

**Keywords:** 1-methyltryptophan, Minocycline, Kynurenine, Tryptophan, Serotonin, Interleukin-1β, Interleukin-6, Taste preference test, Forced swim test, Epilepsy, Depression

## Introduction

Depression represents one of the most common comorbidities of temporal lobe epilepsy (TLE) and has a profoundly negative impact on the quality of life of TLE patients [1]. However, the causes and mechanisms of depression in TLE remain poorly understood. It has been reported that

IL-6 mRNA is elevated in the brain of epileptic rats [2,3] and IL-1β expression is also elevated in the brains [4-6] of chronic epileptic animals and children with mesial TLE [6]. Proinflammatory cytokines, such as IL-1β, IL-6 and INF-γ, stimulate indoleamine 2,3-dioxygenase 1 (IDO1) in the brain [7-9]. IDO1 is a rate-limiting enzyme in tryptophan (TRY) metabolism. IDO1 activity has been associated with decreased serotonin (5-HT) content and increased kynurenine (KYN) content and neuroplastic changes through the effect of KYN derivatives, such as quinolinic acid (QUIN), on glutamate receptors, which are all associated with depression [10,11]. IDO1 activation plays a key

* Correspondence: xieweizn@fimmu.com
†Equal contributors
[1]Department of Traditional Chinese Medicine, Nanfang Hospital, Southern Medical University, Guangzhou, People's Republic of China
[2]School of Traditional Chinese Medicine, Southern Medical University, Guangzhou, People's Republic of China
Full list of author information is available at the end of the article

role in the development of depressive-like behavior. It has been suggested that chronic epilepsy induces the expression of proinflammatory cytokines which, in turn, induce IDO1 expression in the brain. The activation of IDO1 could alter brain TRY metabolism, which contributes to epilepsy-associated depressive-like behavior in rats with chronic TLE.

It has been reported that rats that develop chronic epilepsy following pilocarpine status epilepticus (SE) exhibited a set of interictal disorders consistent with depression [1,12,13]. This model has been further validated as a model of comorbidity between chronic TLE and depression [13]. We examined this hypothesis using a pilocarpine-induced model of chronic TLE in rats.

## Materials and methods
### Animals and treatments
#### Animals
The experiments were performed using 45- to 50-day-old male Wistar rats (Southern Medical University, Guangzhou, People's Republic of China). The animals were housed and handled in strict accordance with the guidelines of the institutional and national Committees of Animal Use and Protection. Rats were housed in a temperature- (23 to 25°C) and humidity- (45 to 55%) controlled environment with a 12/12-hour modified dark–light cycle (light on 7.00 am to 7.00 pm). The protocol was approved through the Committee on the Ethics of Animal Experiments of the Southern Medical University (Permit Number: SCXK 2013–021).

Study design is outlined in Figure 1.

#### Status epilepticus
SE was induced as previously described [1,12,13]. Briefly, the rats received an intraperitoneal injection of LiCl (130 mg/kg, #310468, Sigma, Buchs, Switzerland). The next day, the animals received a subcutaneous injection of pilocarpine hydrochloride (40 mg/kg, #P0472, Sigma). SE was characterized by continuous limbic seizures which started 10 to 15 minutes after pilocarpine injection. The severity of seizures was evaluated using the Racine [14] scale: (i) motor arrest and twitching vibrissae; (ii) chewing, head bobbing; (iii) forelimb clonus; (iv) forelimb clonus and rearing; and (v) rearing and falling. Rats exhibiting continuous generalized clonic-tonic seizures (which corresponded to stages 4 to 5 on the Racine scale), lasting at least 2 hours, were used for further studies (of 73 pilocarpine-treated rats, 66 met the requirements). After 3 and 8 hours of seizure onset, the rats were injected intraperitoneally with diazepam (5 mg/kg) and phenytoin (50 mg/kg) to alleviate further seizures and increase survival. Control animals received injections of LiCl, diazepam, phenytoin, and saline in lieu of pilocarpine.

### Monitoring spontaneous seizures
To select the proper time points for the forced swim test (FST) and evaluate the effects of treatment on seizure frequency in chronic TLE-induced depression, the behavior of the rats was continuously recorded at 3 and 6 weeks after SE using a digital camera with night vision that could record seizures in the dark (Figure 1A). For experiments using 1-MT (Figure 1B) or minocycline (Figure 1C) to inhibit IDO expression from 6 weeks after SE until the end of the experiment, the behavior of the rats was continuously recorded. Focal seizures (motor arrest, facial twitches and mastication), and generalized clonic or clonic-tonic seizures (all body clonus, rearing or rearing and falling) [1] were analyzed offline. The spontaneous seizure counts were recorded for two consecutive 2-week periods: the first recording was obtained immediately preceding 1-MT/saline or minocycline/distilled water treatment, and the second recording was obtained during the 1-MT/saline or minocycline/distilled water treatment. To analyze the data obtained from post-SE rats treated with 1-MT/saline or minocycline/distilled water, we compared the seizure counts before treatment with those obtained during treatment.

### Behavioral testing
We evaluated depressive behavior using two consecutive tests: taste preference test (TPT) to examine a behavioral correlate of anhedonia (that is, inability to experience pleasure) [1,12,13,15], and FST to study the ability to adapt active strategy in an inescapable stressful situation [1,12,13,16,17]. To examine chronic TLE-induced depressive behavior, we performed FST and TPT at 0, 3 and 6 weeks after SE. For experiments using 1-MT or minocycline to inhibit IDO expression, TPT and FST were performed at 4 days before and after treatment. To avoid the potential immediate effects of seizures, FST was only performed when no seizures had developed for at least 6 hours prior to the test (determined by reviewing video recordings).

TPT was performed using the saccharin solution consumption test as previously described [1,12,13]. Briefly, the animals had free access to a standard rodent diet. On the first day of the experiment (habituation), each cage was supplied with two water bottles containing 250 ml of water. The next day (test), one of the bottles was replaced with 0.1% saccharin (#109185, Sigma) diluted in tap water. The test was initiated at 6.00 pm and ran for 24 hours. TPT was expressed as a percentage of the volume of saccharin solution intake relative to the total water intake (saccharin plus regular water) over 24 hours. The loss of preference for saccharin is indicative of anhedonia [1,12,13,15].

Subsequently, we employed a modified version of the FST in a single 5-minute trial. This modification of the

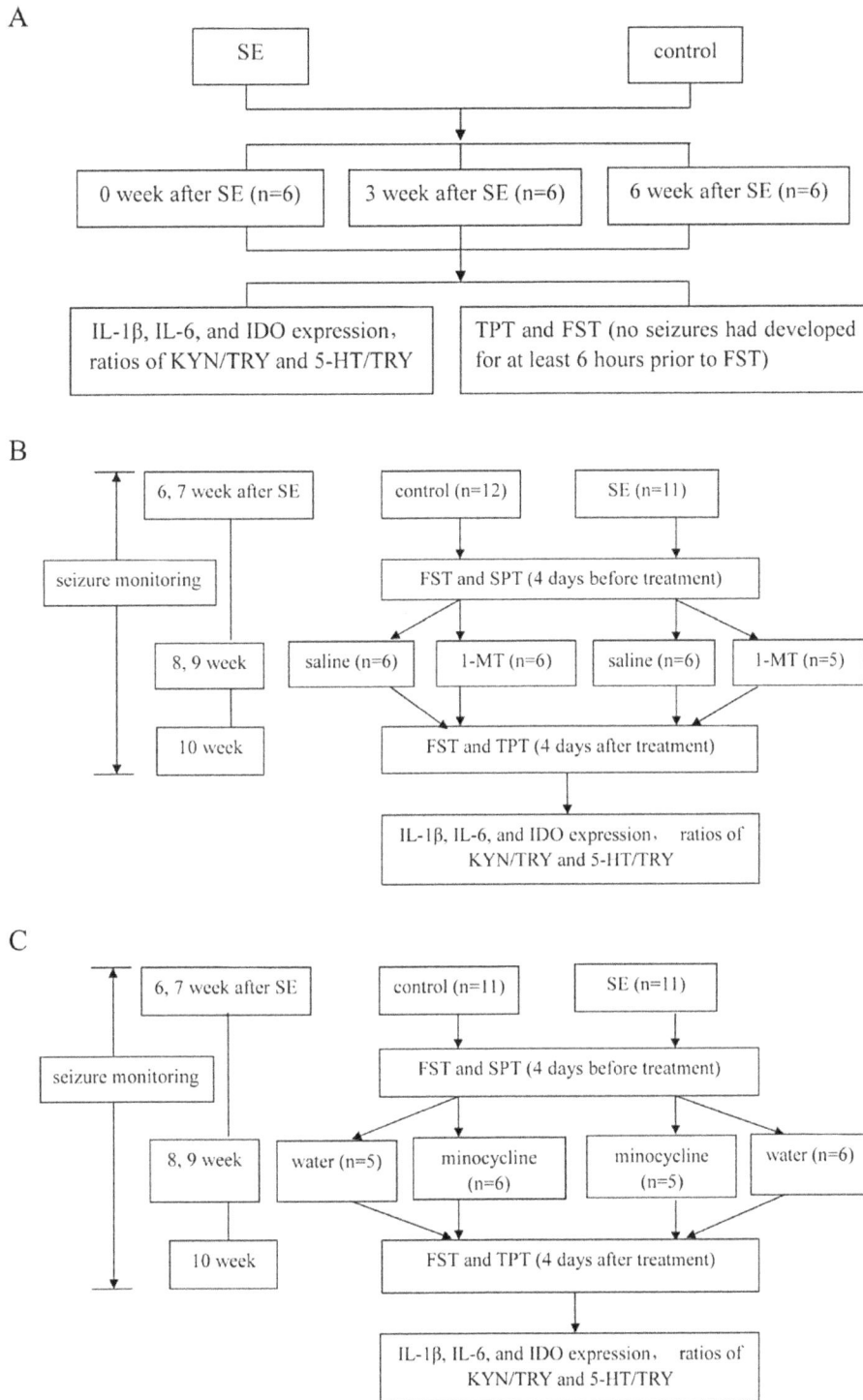

**Figure 1 Study designs. (A)** Study design 1: chronic temporal lobe epilepsy induces depressive behavior. **(B)** Study design 2: 1-methyltryptophan inhibits indoleamine 2,3-dioxygenase 1 directly. **(C)** Study design 3: minocycline inhibits indoleamine 2,3-dioxygenase 1 indirectly.1-MT, 1-methyltryptophan; 5-HT, serotonin; FST, forced swim test; IDO, indoleamine 2,3-dioxygenase; KYN, kynurenine; SE, status epilepticus; TPT, taste preference test; TRY, tryptophan.

classic test was shown to be relevant for examining a depressive-like state, with the increased immobility time indicating the state of despair [1,12,13,16,17]. Between 4.00 pm and 6.00 pm, the rat was placed for 5 minutes in a glass container (60 cm in height and 30 cm in width) filled with tap water to a height of 45 cm and maintained at 22 to 25°C. The swimming behavior was videotaped and analyzed offline by an investigator blinded to treatment, and the total immobility time was calculated.

### Minocycline and 1-methyltryptophan treatments

Minocycline (#M9511, Sigma) was administered at 120 mg/kg in distilled water through gavage in a dose volume of 10 ml/kg, twice daily, at 12-hour intervals. Previous studies have demonstrated minocycline effectively attenuated IL-1β expression in the brain [8,18].

1-MT (#860646, Sigma) was administered through subcutaneous injection at 50 mg/kg in a dose volume of 5 ml/kg. The injections were administered twice daily at 12-hour intervals, in accordance with the methods of Professor Keith W Kelley, who had administered 50 mg/kg of 1-MT to mice twice a day, and the effect was equal to that observed in studies using 5 mg/day pellets [8]. We prepared 1-MT using 0.1 M NaOH and adjusted the pH to 9.0 using 1 M HCl.

### Real-time reverse transcriptase PCR

Total RNA was extracted from the brain samples using TRIzol reagent (TaKaRa Bio, Dalian, China). The reverse transcriptase reactions were performed on a Stratagene Robocycler Gradient 96 Thermal Cycler (Stratagene, California, USA) using a reverse transcriptase kit (TaKaRa Bio, Dalian, China) according to the manufacturer's instructions. The single-stranded cDNA was amplified through comparative quantitative real-time reverse transcriptase PCR using a SYBR green Master Mix kit (Thermo Scientific, California, USA; Cat. No. #K0251) on an Mx3005 (Stratagene). The following primers were used: β-actin, (forward) 5′-GCA GGA GTA CGA TGA GTC CG-3′ and (reverse) 5′-ACG CAG CTC AGT AAC AGT CC-3′; IDO1, (forward) 5′-AGC ACT GGA GAA GGC ACT GT-3′ and (reverse) 5′-ACG TGG AAA AAG GTG TCT GG-3′; IL-1β, (forward) 5′-AAA TGC CTC GTG CTG TCT GAC C-3′ and (reverse) 5′-GGT GGG TGT GCC GTC TTT CAT C-3′; and IL-6, (forward) 5′-AGC CCA CCA GGA ACG AAA G-3′ and (reverse) 5′-GGA AGG CAG TGG CTG TCA A-3′. The mRNA expression levels of the target genes were normalized to those of β-actin.

### Liquid chromatography-mass spectrometry

#### Chemicals

Serotonin hydrochloride (#H9523), L-tryptophan (#PHR 1176), L-kynurenine (#K8625), and high-performance liquid chromatography-grade methanol were purchased from Sigma. Ultrapure water was generated using a Milli-Q Gradient water purification system (Millipore, Molsheim, France).

#### Apparatus

Liquid chromatography-mass spectrometry (LC-MS) comprised a Prominence 20A series UFLC System (Shimadzu, Kyoto, Japan) and an API 4000 Qtrap MS System (ABSciex, Massachusetts, USA). The analysis was performed using a $100 \times 2.1$-mm Restek C18 Aqueous column (Restek, Pennsylvania, USA). The LC-MS detection parameters and mobile phases were prepared as previously described [19].

#### Sample preparation

The brain samples were prepared as previously described [20]. Briefly, the frozen brain was dissected on ice into the different regions (prefrontal cortex, midbrain, hippocampus, and thalamus). The samples were subsequently homogenized in a 10-fold volume of a 0.1 M formic acid solution. The homogenates were centrifuged at $18,000 \times$ g for 20 minute at 4°C. The supernatants were collected and stored at −80°C until chromatographic analysis.

### Statistical analysis

All results were expressed as means ± SEM. The statistical analysis was performed using Statistical Product and Service Solutions (SPSS 19.0, Chicago, USA) software (independent samples $t$-test, paired $t$-test, one-way analysis of variance, Wilcoxon test, Mann–Whitney test or Kruskal-Wallis test).

### Results

#### Time-dependent induction of depressive-like behavior in chronic epileptic rats

Chronic TLE induces depressive-like behavior in rats at 6 weeks after SE, but not at 3 weeks after SE, in the FST (Figure 2A, $P < 0.01$) and the TPT (Figure 2B, $P < 0.01$).

#### IL-1β and IL-6 expression are induced through spontaneous seizure in the hippocampus of rats with chronic temporal lobe epilepsy

The IL-1β (Figure 2C, $P < 0.05$) mRNA levels were increased at 3 weeks after SE in the seizure group but not in the control group. At 6 weeks after SE, the difference between IL-1β (Figure 2C, $P < 0.01$) and IL-6 (Figure 2D, $P < 0.01$) expression was significant in the hippocampus of rats with coexisting chronic TLE and depressive behavior.

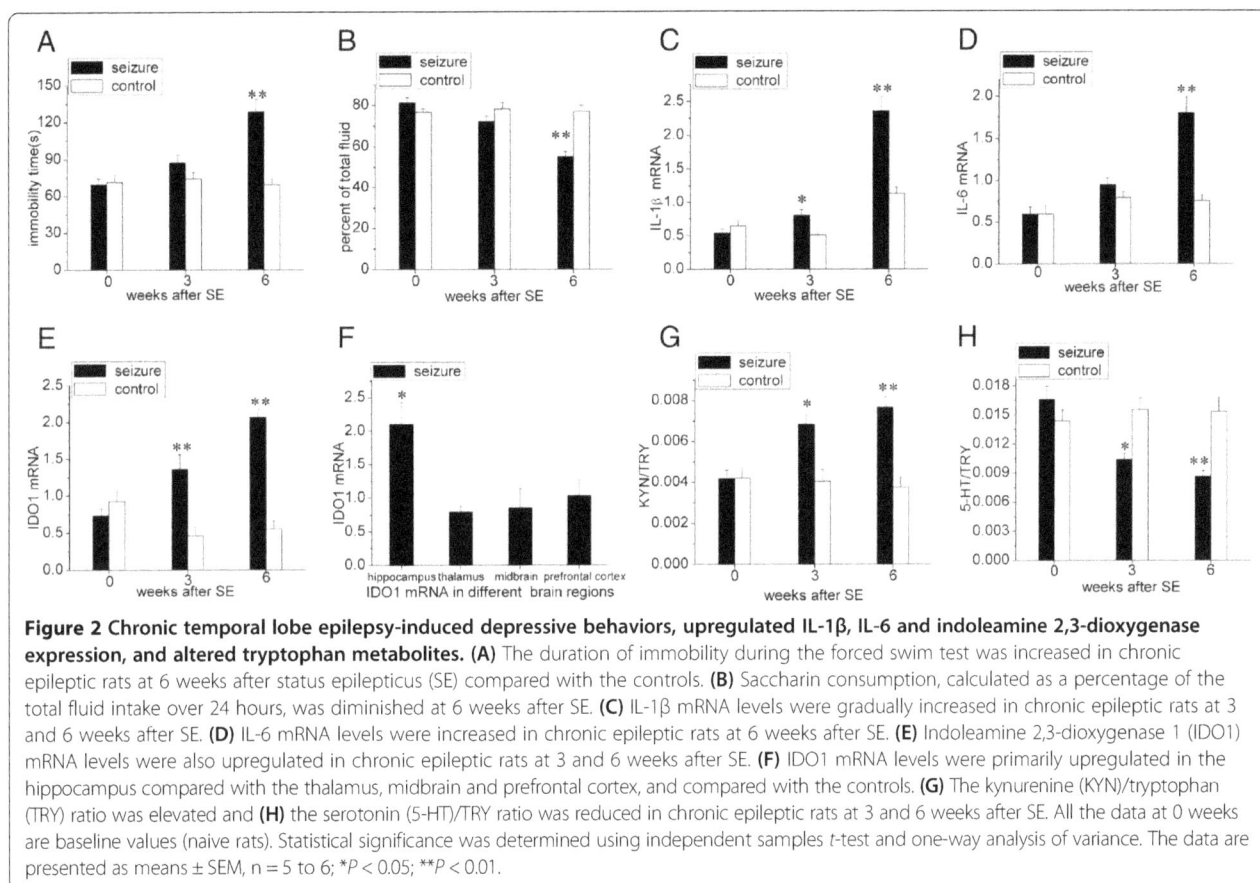

**Figure 2** Chronic temporal lobe epilepsy-induced depressive behaviors, upregulated IL-1β, IL-6 and indoleamine 2,3-dioxygenase expression, and altered tryptophan metabolites. **(A)** The duration of immobility during the forced swim test was increased in chronic epileptic rats at 6 weeks after status epilepticus (SE) compared with the controls. **(B)** Saccharin consumption, calculated as a percentage of the total fluid intake over 24 hours, was diminished at 6 weeks after SE. **(C)** IL-1β mRNA levels were gradually increased in chronic epileptic rats at 3 and 6 weeks after SE. **(D)** IL-6 mRNA levels were increased in chronic epileptic rats at 6 weeks after SE. **(E)** Indoleamine 2,3-dioxygenase 1 (IDO1) mRNA levels were also upregulated in chronic epileptic rats at 3 and 6 weeks after SE. **(F)** IDO1 mRNA levels were primarily upregulated in the hippocampus compared with the thalamus, midbrain and prefrontal cortex, and compared with the controls. **(G)** The kynurenine (KYN)/tryptophan (TRY) ratio was elevated and **(H)** the serotonin (5-HT)/TRY ratio was reduced in chronic epileptic rats at 3 and 6 weeks after SE. All the data at 0 weeks are baseline values (naive rats). Statistical significance was determined using independent samples $t$-test and one-way analysis of variance. The data are presented as means ± SEM, n = 5 to 6; $*P < 0.05$; $**P < 0.01$.

## IDO1 expression is activated through the upregulation of IL-1β and IL-6 expression in the hippocampus of rats with coexisting chronic temporal lobe epilepsy and depressive behavior

IDO1 expression was significantly upregulated at both 3 and 6 weeks after SE (Figure 2E, $P < 0.01$ compared with controls). An examination of the IDO1 expression in different regions showed a significant increase in the hippocampus, compared with the thalamus, midbrain and prefrontal cortex (Figure 2F, $P < 0.05$). These results verified that the hippocampus was a vital region for the upregulation of IDO1 expression. We also observed that, compared with saline treatment, 1-MT specifically inhibited IDO1 expression (Figure 3E, $P < 0.01$) without affecting IL-1β (Figure 3C, $P > 0.05$) and IL-6 (Figure 3D, $P > 0.05$) expression in the post-SE group; compared with distilled water treatment, minocycline inhibited the expression of IDO1 (Figure 4E, $P < 0.01$), IL-1β (Figure 4C, $P < 0.01$) and IL-6 (Figure 4D, $P < 0.01$) in the post-SE group. These results showed that IL-1β and IL-6 induced IDO1 expression.

## Ratios of hippocampal tryptophan metabolites are altered through increased IDO1 enzyme activity

To examine the role of IDO1 enzyme activity in TRY metabolism in both the post-SE and control groups, we first measured TRY, 5-HT, and KYN concentrations in the hippocampus using LC-MS and subsequently determined the ratio of 5-HT or KYN to TRY. There were no baseline differences in the KYN/TRY or 5-HT/TRY ratios between the two groups (Figure 2G and H). However, at 3 and 6 weeks after SE, the KYN/TRP ratio was increased (Figure 2G, $P < 0.05$ at 3 weeks after SE and $P < 0.01$ at 6 weeks after SE) and the 5-HT/TRP ratio was decreased (Figure 2H, $P < 0.05$ at 3 weeks after SE and $P < 0.01$ at 6 weeks after SE) in the post-SE group compared with the control group.

## Both minocycline and 1-methyltryptophan inhibit upregulated IDO1 expression to normalize ratios of hippocampal tryptophan metabolites and block chronic temporal lobe epilepsy-induced depressive-like behavior

To examine whether the inhibition of IDO1 activity influences hippocampal TRY metabolites and depressive behaviors in epileptic rats, we administered the IDO1 inhibitor l-MT (50 mg/kg) or physiological saline twice daily (at 12-hour intervals) for a period of 2 weeks, and the treatments were administered at 8 weeks after SE. The spontaneous seizure counts before or during 1-MT treatment were within the same statistical range in the two chronic TLE groups (Table 1). Treatment with 1-MT,

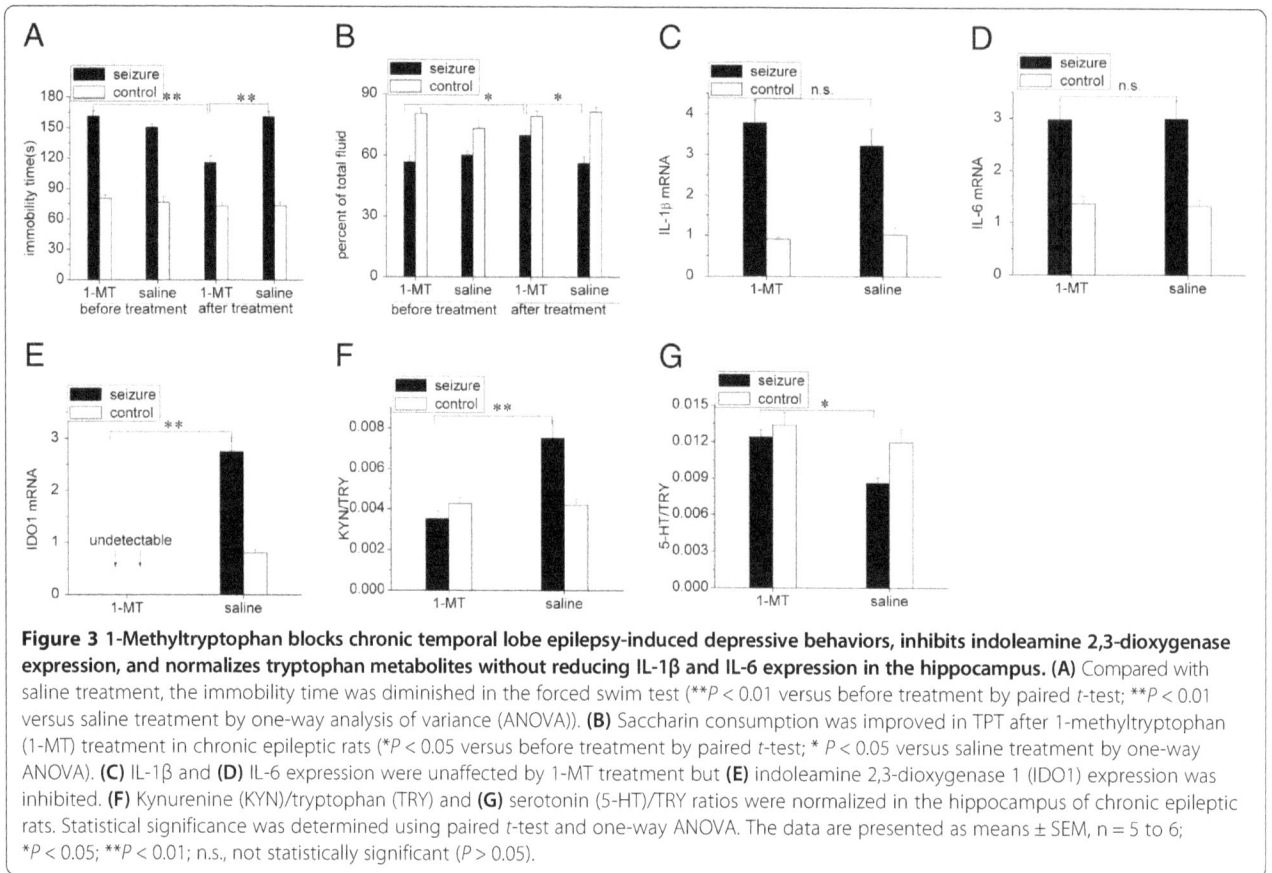

**Figure 3** 1-Methyltryptophan blocks chronic temporal lobe epilepsy-induced depressive behaviors, inhibits indoleamine 2,3-dioxygenase expression, and normalizes tryptophan metabolites without reducing IL-1β and IL-6 expression in the hippocampus. **(A)** Compared with saline treatment, the immobility time was diminished in the forced swim test (**$P < 0.01$ versus before treatment by paired $t$-test; **$P < 0.01$ versus saline treatment by one-way analysis of variance (ANOVA)). **(B)** Saccharin consumption was improved in TPT after 1-methyltryptophan (1-MT) treatment in chronic epileptic rats (*$P < 0.05$ versus before treatment by paired $t$-test; * $P < 0.05$ versus saline treatment by one-way ANOVA). **(C)** IL-1β and **(D)** IL-6 expression were unaffected by 1-MT treatment but **(E)** indoleamine 2,3-dioxygenase 1 (IDO1) expression was inhibited. **(F)** Kynurenine (KYN)/tryptophan (TRY) and **(G)** serotonin (5-HT)/TRY ratios were normalized in the hippocampus of chronic epileptic rats. Statistical significance was determined using paired $t$-test and one-way ANOVA. The data are presented as means ± SEM, n = 5 to 6; *$P < 0.05$; **$P < 0.01$; n.s., not statistically significant ($P > 0.05$).

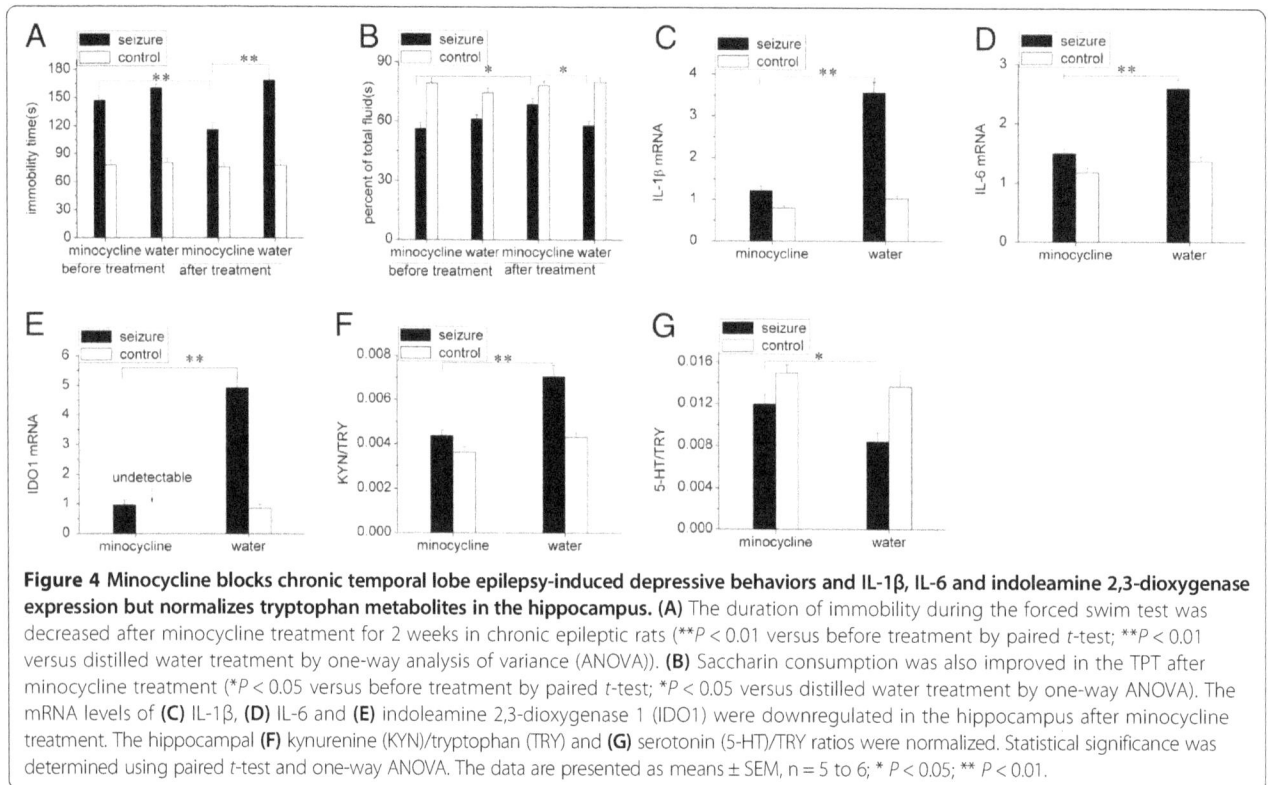

**Figure 4** Minocycline blocks chronic temporal lobe epilepsy-induced depressive behaviors and IL-1β, IL-6 and indoleamine 2,3-dioxygenase expression but normalizes tryptophan metabolites in the hippocampus. **(A)** The duration of immobility during the forced swim test was decreased after minocycline treatment for 2 weeks in chronic epileptic rats (**$P < 0.01$ versus before treatment by paired $t$-test; **$P < 0.01$ versus distilled water treatment by one-way analysis of variance (ANOVA)). **(B)** Saccharin consumption was also improved in the TPT after minocycline treatment (*$P < 0.05$ versus before treatment by paired $t$-test; *$P < 0.05$ versus distilled water treatment by one-way ANOVA). The mRNA levels of **(C)** IL-1β, **(D)** IL-6 and **(E)** indoleamine 2,3-dioxygenase 1 (IDO1) were downregulated in the hippocampus after minocycline treatment. The hippocampal **(F)** kynurenine (KYN)/tryptophan (TRY) and **(G)** serotonin (5-HT)/TRY ratios were normalized. Statistical significance was determined using paired $t$-test and one-way ANOVA. The data are presented as means ± SEM, n = 5 to 6; * $P < 0.05$; ** $P < 0.01$.

## Table 1 Behavioral spontaneous seizure count in post-status epilepticus rats

| Treatment group | Before treatment | During treatment |
| --- | --- | --- |
| 1-MT | 2 | 1 |
| | 1 | 2 |
| | 7 | 4 |
| | 30 | 18 |
| | 5 | 3 |
| Saline | 14 | 17 |
| | 7 | 8 |
| | 4 | 2 |
| | 0 | 0 |
| | 13 | 9 |
| | 5 | 3 |
| Minocycline | 5 | 2 |
| | 0 | 1 |
| | 4 | 0 |
| | 27 | 15 |
| | 9 | 5 |
| Distilled water | 9 | 7 |
| | 14 | 17 |
| | 2 | 0 |
| | 17 | 18 |
| | 7 | 10 |
| | 3 | 2 |

Before and during minocycline and distilled water treatments, the cumulative spontaneous seizure count in post-status epilepticus rats over two consecutive 2-week periods indicated that no differences were observed between the two periods for each of the groups ($P > 0.05$, both Wilcoxon and Mann–Whitney tests for paired and unpaired comparisons), and across the groups ($P > 0.05$, Kruskal-Wallis test). Similar results were also observed between or across the groups (both $P > 0.05$) with 1-methyltryptophan (1-MT) and saline treatments.

but not saline, lowered the KYN/TRY ratio (Figure 3F, $P < 0.01$), elevated the 5-HT/TRY ratio (Figure 3G, $P < 0.05$) in the hippocampus, reduced the duration of immobility in FST (Figure 3A, $P < 0.01$), and increased saccharin consumption in TPT (Figure 3B, $P < 0.05$).

Similar results were obtained after treatment with the cytokine inhibitor minocycline (100 mg/kg) or distilled water twice daily (at 12-hour intervals) for 2 weeks (administered at 8 weeks after SE). No significant difference in the spontaneous seizure count between the two chronic TLE groups (Table 1) was observed, and treatment with minocycline, but not distilled water, also lowered the KYN/TRY ratio (Figure 4F, $P < 0.01$), elevated the 5-HT/TRY ratio (Figure 4G, $P < 0.01$) in the hippocampus, reduced the duration of immobility in FST (Figure 4A, $P < 0.01$, and increased saccharin consumption in TPT (Figure 4B, $P < 0.05$).

Consistent with the fluctuation of IDO1 expression and depressive behavior in the post-SE group, these results suggest that altered ratios of TRY metabolites in the hippocampus indicate increased IDO1 enzyme activity in the hippocampus, which plays a key role in chronic TLE-induced depressive behavior.

### Effect of minocycline and 1-methyltryptophan inhibition on seizures

Before and during minocycline and distilled water treatments, the cumulative spontaneous seizure count in post-SE rats over two consecutive 2-week periods indicated that no differences were observed between the two periods for each of the groups (Table 1, $P > 0.05$) and across the groups (Table 1, $P > 0.05$).

Similar results were also observed between or across the groups (Table 1, both $P > 0.05$) with 1-MT and saline treatments.

### Discussion

Here, we demonstrated that IL-1β, IL-6 and IDO1 expression were selectively upregulated in the hippocampus of rats with chronic TLE and depressive behavior. The blockade of IDO1 activation, either indirectly, with the anti-inflammatory tetracycline derivative minocycline, or directly, with the IDO antagonist 1-MT, prevents the development of depressive-like behavior but failed to affect the occurrence of spontaneous seizures. Both minocycline and 1-MT normalize the KYN/TRY and 5-HT/TRY ratios in the hippocampus of chronic epileptic rats exhibiting depressive behaviors. These results indicated that brain IDO activity plays a critical role in epileptic rats with epilepsy-associated depressive-like behavior.

Epilepsy-associated depression has long been recognized [1,21]. Most studies have focused on the hypothalamo-pituitary-adrenocortical axis, monoaminergic system and various other neurotransmitters/neuromodulators, including GABA and brain-derived neurotrophic factor [22,23]. Despite some progress, the pathogenic mechanisms of epilepsy-associated depression are not completely understood. Although neuroinflammatory pathogenic mechanisms have been identified in rats with coexisting chronic TLE and depression [1], alteration of inflammation in the brain has not been concluded in detail nor completely. To our knowledge, the present study provides the first evidence that experimental chronic TLE is accompanied by interictal IDO upregulation and also verifies alterations in hippocampal inflammation in rats with epilepsy-associated depressive-like behavior.

The data obtained in the present study suggest a novel mechanistic link between epilepsy and depression via IDO1 expression in the hippocampus. The regulation of hippocampal IDO1 expression is likely mediated through upregulated pro-inflammatory cytokines, as the inhibition of IDO1 activity through 1-MT treatment did not prevent the elevation of pro-inflammatory cytokine expression, but the expression of pro-inflammatory cytokines was inhibited with minocycline treatment, which also blocks IDO expression. The data also indicate that pro-inflammatory cytokines are likely induced through chronic TLE. These findings are consistent with previous reports that pro-inflammatory cytokines are elevated in the hippocampus of animal models [1,24-26] and patients [26,27]. In the present study, we also observed that IDO1 was notably upregulated in the hippocampus. These findings are consistent with previous reports that certain brain regions, including the hippocampus, play a critical role in the integration of mood changes and chronic TLE [1,28,29].

KYN and 5-HT are two major TRY metabolites produced through the regulation of metabolic enzymes, including IDO. The results of the present study verified that KYN/TRY and 5-HT/TRY ratios in the hippocampus were regulated through IDO1 activity. Increased IDO1 activity lowers endogenous 5-HT levels; however, this activity also increases KYN derivatives, such as QUIN, a depressogenic glutamate receptor agonist which activates oxidative pathways, causing mitochondrial dysfunctions, and exhibits neuroexcitatory and neurotoxic effects that might lead to neurodegeneration [30]. Moreover, inadequate endogenous 5-HT levels and detrimental increases in the concentration of KYN derivatives lead to depressive symptoms [7,30,31]. Thus, IDO plays a key role in the TRY metabolic pathway, and IDO activation modulates the level of endogenous KYN and 5-HT, leading to epilepsy-associated depressive-like behavior. The proposed mechanism is supported by studies showing that blocks of IDO1 activation either indirectly or directly normalize the increased KYN/TRY ratio and decreased 5-HT/TRY ratio caused by IDO upregulation in the hippocampus. Future studies should address the relationship between IDO expression and other derivatives of TRY metabolism to determine the role of this enzyme in epilepsy-associated depressive-like behavior.

It has been previously reported that pro-inflammatory cytokines might play an important role in epileptogenesis [32-34]. Considering that pro-inflammatory cytokines also play a key role in the pathophysiology of depression [30,35], verified in the present study, these molecules might contribute to the comorbidity between epilepsy and depression. Previous studies have indicated that minocycline might block the epileptogenic process [32,36] or depressive-like behaviors [37,38] through an anti-inflammatory effect. However, in the present study, minocycline administration did not affect spontaneous seizures, as baseline seizure frequencies were relatively low, which likely prohibit the modifying effects of therapeutic interventions. These findings are consistent with those of previous reports [12]. The results of the present study also suggested that the attenuation of depressive symptoms through minocycline administration was not

an epiphenomenon of the anticonvulsant effects of this drug.

Although the observed effects of minocycline treatment were different from the 1-MT-meadiated attenuation of depressive symptoms, the anti-epileptic effect of this drug was not verified in the present study. Indeed, IDO1 activation increases KYN derivatives, such as QUIN, a glutamate receptor agonist with neuroexcitatory and neurotoxic effects that induce epilepsy [39,40]. However, this effect has been previously observed in the pathophysiology of depression. Thus, IDO1 activation increases KYN derivatives and likely contributes to the comorbidity between epilepsy and depression. In the present study, 1-MT administration attenuates depressive symptoms through the inhibition of IDO1 activation, which normalizes KYN/TRY and 5-HT/TRY ratios in the hippocampus. However, 1-MT did not affect spontaneous seizures, reflecting either the relatively low baseline seizure frequencies observed in the present study [12] or other mechanisms involved in the described phenomenon. Notably, the experimental protocol used in the present study might not be suitable for the reliable examination of anti-epileptic therapies [1]. Thus, future studies will focus on effects of the TRY pathway and 1-MT treatment on epilepsy.

In conclusion, the results of the present study implicate hippocampal IDO1 activation in epilepsy-associated depressive-like behavior, suggesting that depression in TLE patients could be treated through the regulation of brain inflammation and IDO1 activity. Although the mechanism underlying the relationship between epilepsy and depression is most likely complex and involves other neurotransmitters and neuromodulators [16,18], the results of the present suggest a new strategy for the prevention and reversal of depression in TLE patients through a mechanism involving altered endogenous TRY metabolite ratios via upregulated pro-inflammatory cytokines and IDO expression in certain brain regions.

## Abbreviations

1-MT: 1-methyltryptophan; 5-HT: serotonin; FST: forced swim test; IDO1: indoleamine 2,3-dioxygenase 1; IL: interleukin; INF: interferon; KYN: kynurenine; LC-MS: liquid chromatography-mass spectrometry; PCR: polymerase chain reaction; QUIN: quinolinic acid; SE: status epilepticus; TLE: temporal lobe epilepsy; TPT: taste preference test; TRY: tryptophan.

## Competing interests
The authors declare that they have no competing interests.

## Authors' contributions
WX contributed to the study design. LC contributed to the study design and participated in the acquisition and analysis of data, the statistical analysis and the manuscript drafting and revision. LG, YY, LX and QH participated in the data analysis and manuscript revision. ZR and YL participated in data acquisition and manuscript drafting and revision. All authors have read and approved the final version of the manuscript.

## Authors' information
Wei Xie and Lun Cai are co-first authors.

## Acknowledgments
The authors would like to thank Professor Jan L Du Preez and Professor Francois. The authors would also like to thank Viljoen for assistance with tryptophan metabolite detection and Professor KW Kelley for assistance with 1-MT preparation. We thank Elsevier for the professional English language editing. This work was supported through research grants from the China Natural Science Foundation (81173458).

## Author details
[1]Department of Traditional Chinese Medicine, Nanfang Hospital, Southern Medical University, Guangzhou, People's Republic of China. [2]School of Traditional Chinese Medicine, Southern Medical University, Guangzhou, People's Republic of China. [3]Southern Medical University, Guangzhou, People's Republic of China. [4]Department of Encephalopathy, The first affiliated hosipital of Guangxi University of Chinese Medicine, Guangxi University of Chinese Medicine, Nanning, People's Republic of China. [5]Department of Traditional Chinese Medicine, Guangdong General Hospital, Guangdong Academy of Medical Sciences, Guangdong Geriatric Institute, Guang Zhou 510080, China.

## References
1. Mazarati AM, Pineda E, Shin D, Tio D, Taylor AN, Sankar R: Comorbidity between epilepsy and depression: role of hippocampal interleukin-1β. *Neurobiol Dis* 2010, 37:461–478.
2. Minami M, Kuraishi Y, Satoh M: Effects of kainic acid on messenger RNA levels of IL-1 beta, IL-6, TNF alpha and LIF in the rat brain. *Biochem Biophys Res Commun* 1991, 176:593–598.
3. Lehtimäki KA, Peltola J, Koskikallio E, Keränen T, Honkaniemi J: Expression of cytokines and cytokine receptors in the rat brain after kainic acid-induced seizures. *Mol Brain Res* 2003, 110:253–260.
4. De Simoni MG, Perego C, Ravizza T, Moneta D, Conti M, Marchesi F, De Luigi A, Garattini S, Vezzani A: Inflammatory cytokines and related genes are induced in the rat hippocampus by limbic status epilepticus. *Eur J Neurosci* 2000, 12:2623–2633.
5. Minami M, Kuraishi Y, Yamaguchi T, Nakai S, Hirai Y, Satoh M: Convulsants induce interleukin-1 beta messenger RNA in rat brain. *Biochem Biophys Res Commun* 1990, 171:832–837.
6. Omran A, Peng J, Zhang C, Xiang QL, Xue J, Gan N, Kong H, Yin F: Interleukin-1β and microRNA-146a in an immature rat model. *Epilepsia* 2012, 53:1215–1224.
7. Schwarcz R, Bruno JP, Muchowski PJ, Wu HQ: Kynurenines in the mammalian brain: when physiology meets pathology. *Nat rev Neurosci* 2012, 13:465–477.
8. O'Connor JC, Lawson MA, André C, Moreau M, Lestage J, Castanon N, Kelley KW, Dantzer R: Lipopolysaccharide-induced depressive-like behavior is mediated by indoleamine 2,3-dioxygenase activation in mice. *Mol Psychiatry* 2009, 14:511–522.
9. Kim H, Chen L, Lim G, Sung B, Wang S, McCabe MF, Rusanescu G, Yang L, Tian Y, Mao J: Brain indoleamine 2,3-dioxygenase contributes to the comorbidity of pain and depression. *J Clin Invest* 2012, 122:2940–2954.
10. Sublette ME, Postolache TT: Neuroinflammation and depression: the role of indoleamine 2,3-dioxygenase (IDO) as a molecular pathway. *Psychosom Med* 2012, 74:668–672.
11. Myint AM: Kynurenines: from the perspective of major psychiatric disorders. *FEBS J* 2012, 279:1375–1385.
12. Mazarati AM, Siddarth P, Baldwin RA, Shin D, Caplan R, Sankar R: Depression after status epilepticus: behavioural and biochemical deficits and effects of fluoxetine. *Brain* 2008, 131:2071–2083.
13. Mazarati AM, Shin D, Kwon YS, Bragin A, Pineda E, Tio D, Taylor AN, Sankar R: Elevated plasma corticosterone level and depressive behavior in experimental temporal lobe epilepsy. *Neurobiol Dis* 2009, 34:457–461.
14. Racine RJ: Modification of seizure activity by electrical stimulation: II. Motor seizures. *Electroencephalogr Clin Neurophysiol* 1972, 32:281–294.
15. Pucilowski O, Overstreet DH: Effect of chronic antidepressant treatment on responses to apomorphine in selectively bred rat strains. *Brain Res Bull* 1993, 32:471–475.
16. Pucilowski O, Overstreet DH, Rezvani AH, Janowsky DS: Chronic mild stress-induced anhedonia: greater effect in a genetic rat model of depression. *Physiol Behav* 1993, 54:1215–1220.
17. Overstreet DH, Pucilowski O, Rezvani AH, Janowsky DS: Administration of antidepressants, diazepam and psychomotor stimulants further confirms the utility of Flinders Sensitive Line rats as an animal model of depression. *Psychopharmacology (Berl)* 1995, 121:27–37.
18. Zhao F, Cai TJ, Liu MC, Zheng G, Luo W, Chen J: Manganese induces dopaminergic neurodegeneration via microglial activation in a rat model of manganism. *Toxicol Sci* 2009, 107:156–164.
19. Möller M, Du Preez JL, Harvey BH: Development and validation of a single analytical method for the determination of tryptophan, and its kynurenine metabolites in rat plasma. *J Chromatogr B Analyt Technol Biomed Life Sci* 2012, 898:121–129.
20. Gonzalez RR, Fernandez RF, Vidal JL, Frenich AG, Perez ML: Development and validation of an ultra-high performance liquid chromatography-tandem mass-spectrometry (UHPLC-MS/MS) method for the simultaneous determination of neurotransmitters in rat brain samples. *J Neurosci Methods* 2011, 198:187–194.
21. Fiest KM, Dykeman J, Patten SB, Wiebe S, Kaplan GG, Maxwell CG, Bulloch AG, Jette N: Depression in epilepsy: a systematic review and meta-analysis. *Neurology* 2013, 80:590–599.
22. Pineda E, Shin D, Sankar R, Mazarati AM: Comorbidity between epilepsy and depression: experimental evidence for the involvement of serotonergic, glucocorticoid, and neuroinflammatory mechanisms. *Epilepsia* 2010, 51(Suppl 3):110–114.
23. Kanner AM, Schachter SC, Barry JJ, Hersdorffer DC, Mula M, Trimble M, Hermann B, Ettinger AE, Dunn D, Caplan R, Ryvlin P, Gilliam F: Depression and epilepsy: epidemiologic and neurobiologic perspectives that may explain their high comorbid occurrence. *Epilepsy Behav* 2012, 24:156–168.
24. Järvelä JT, Lopez-Picon FR, Plysjuk A, Ruohonen S, Holopainen IE: Temporal profiles of age-dependent changes in cytokine mRNA expression and glial cell activation after status epilepticus in postnatal rat hippocampus. *J Neuroinflammation* 2011, 8:29.
25. Pernot F, Heinrich C, Barbier L, Peinnequin A, Carpentier P, Dhote F, Baille V, Beaup C, Depaulis A, Dorandeu F: Inflammatory changes during epileptogenesis and spontaneous seizures in a mouse model of mesiotemporal lobe epilepsy. *Epilepsia* 2011, 52:2315–2325.
26. Ashhab MU, Omran A, Kong H, Gan N, He F, Peng J, Yin F: Expressions of tumor necrosis factor alpha and microRNA-155 in immature rat model of status epilepticus and children with mesial temporal lobe epilepsy. *J Mol Neurosci* 2013, 51:950–958.
27. Teocchi MA, Ferreira AÉ, da Luz de Oliveira EP, Tedeschi H, D'Souza-Li L: Hippocampal gene expression dysregulation of Klotho, nuclear factor kappa B and tumor necrosis factor in temporal lobe epilepsy patients. *J Neuroinflammation* 2013, 10:53.
28. Valente KD, Busatto FG: Depression and temporal lobe epilepsy represent an epiphenomenon sharing similar neural networks: clinical and brain structural evidences. *Arq Neuropsiquiatr* 2013, 71:183–190.
29. Martinez A, Finegersh A, Cannon DM, Dustin I, Nugent A, Herscovitch P, Theodore WH: The 5-HT 1A receptor and 5-HT transporter in temporal lobe epilepsy. *Neurology* 2013, 80:1465–1471.
30. Maes M, Leonard BE, Myint AM, Kubera M, Verkerk R: The new '5-HT' hypothesis of depression: cell-mediated immune activation induces indoleamine 2,3-dioxygenase, which leads to lower plasma tryptophan and an increased synthesis of detrimental tryptophan catabolites (TRYCATs), both of which contribute to the onset of depression. *Prog Neuro-Psychopharmacol Biol Psychiatry* 2011, 35:702–721.
31. Christmas DM, Potokar JP, Davies SJ: A biological pathway linking inflammation and depression: activation of indoleamine 2,3-dioxygenase. *Neuropsychiatr Dis Treat* 2011, 7:431–439.
32. Riazi K, Galic MA, Kuzmiski BJ, Ho W, Sharkey KA, Pittman QJ: Microglial activation and TNF-α production mediate altered CNS excitability following peripheral inflammation. *Proc Natl Acad Sci U S A* 2008, 105:17151–17156.
33. Andrzejczak D: Epilepsy and pro-inflammatory cytokines. Immunomodu-lating properties of antiepileptic drugs. *Neurol Neurochir Pol* 2011, 45:275–285.
34. Vezzani A: The role of inflammation in epilepsy. *Nat Rev Neurol* 2011, 7:31–40.
35. Leonard B, Maes M: Mechanistic explanations how cell-mediated immune activation, inflammation and oxidative and nitrosative stress pathways and their sequels and concomitants play a role in the pathophysiology of unipolar depression. *Neurosci Biobehav Rev* 2012, 36:764–785.

36. Abraham J, Fox PD, Condello C, Bartolini A, Koh S: **Minocycline attenuates microglia activation and blocks the long-term epileptogenic effects of early-life seizures.** *Neurobiol Dis* 2012, **46:**425–430.

37. Pae CU, Marks DM, Han C, Patkar AA: **Does minocycline have antidepressant effect?** *Biomed Pharmacother* 2008, **62:**308–311.

38. Soczynska JK, Mansur RB, Brietzke E, Swardfager W, Kennedy SH, Woldeyohannes HO, Powell AM: **Novel therapeutic targets in depression: minocycline as a candidate treatment.** *Behav Brain Res* 2012, **235:**302–317.

39. Russi MA, Vandresen-Filho S, Rieger DK, Costa AP, Lopes MW, Cunha RM, Teixeira EH, Nascimento KS, Cavada BS, Tasca CI, Leal RB: **ConBr, a lectin from Canavalia brasiliensis seeds, protects against quinolinic acid-induced seizures in mice.** *Neurochem Res* 2012, **37:**288–297.

40. Ganzella M, Faraco RB, Almeida RF, Fernandes VF, Souza DO: **Intracerebroventricular administration of inosine is anticonvulsant against quinolinic acid-induced seizures in mice: an effect independent of benzodiazepine and adenosine receptors.** *Pharmacol Biochem Behav* 2011, **100:**271–274.

# Effects of rapamycin and curcumin on inflammation and oxidative stress in vitro and in vivo — in search of potential anti-epileptogenic strategies for temporal lobe epilepsy

C. M. Drion[1], J. van Scheppingen[2], A. Arena[3], K. W. Geijtenbeek[2], L. Kooijman[1], E. A. van Vliet[1,2], E. Aronica[2,4] and J. A. Gorter[1*]

## Abstract

**Background:** Previous studies in various rodent epilepsy models have suggested that mammalian target of rapamycin (mTOR) inhibition with rapamycin has anti-epileptogenic potential. Since treatment with rapamycin produces unwanted side effects, there is growing interest to study alternatives to rapamycin as anti-epileptogenic drugs. Therefore, we investigated curcumin, the main component of the natural spice turmeric. Curcumin is known to have anti-inflammatory and anti-oxidant effects and has been reported to inhibit the mTOR pathway. These properties make it a potential anti-epileptogenic compound and an alternative for rapamycin.

**Methods:** To study the anti-epileptogenic potential of curcumin compared to rapamycin, we first studied the effects of both compounds on mTOR activation, inflammation, and oxidative stress in vitro, using cell cultures of human fetal astrocytes and the neuronal cell line SH-SY5Y. Next, we investigated the effects of rapamycin and intracerebrally applied curcumin on status epilepticus (SE)—induced inflammation and oxidative stress in hippocampal tissue, during early stages of epileptogenesis in the post-electrical SE rat model for temporal lobe epilepsy (TLE).

**Results:** Rapamycin, but not curcumin, suppressed mTOR activation in cultured astrocytes. Instead, curcumin suppressed the mitogen-activated protein kinase (MAPK) pathway. Quantitative real-time PCR analysis revealed that curcumin, but not rapamycin, reduced the levels of inflammatory markers IL-6 and COX-2 in cultured astrocytes that were challenged with IL-1β. In SH-SY5Y cells, curcumin reduced reactive oxygen species (ROS) levels, suggesting anti-oxidant effects. In the post-SE rat model, however, treatment with rapamycin or curcumin did not suppress the expression of inflammatory and oxidative stress markers 1 week after SE.

**Conclusions:** These results indicate anti-inflammatory and anti-oxidant properties of curcumin, but not rapamycin, in vitro. Intracerebrally applied curcumin modified the MAPK pathway in vivo at 1 week after SE but failed to produce anti-inflammatory or anti-oxidant effects. Future studies should be directed to increasing the bioavailability of curcumin (or related compounds) in the brain to assess its anti-epileptogenic potential in vivo.

**Keywords:** Rapamycin, Curcumin, Inflammation, Oxidative stress, Temporal lobe epilepsy, mTOR, MAPK

* Correspondence: j.a.gorter@uva.nl
[1]Center for Neuroscience, Swammerdam Institute for Life Sciences, University of Amsterdam, Amsterdam, The Netherlands
Full list of author information is available at the end of the article

## Background

Temporal lobe epilepsy (TLE) is the most common form of acquired epilepsy in adults [1]. TLE is characterized by progressive development of spontaneous seizures after an initial insult, often associated with hippocampal sclerosis, mossy fiber sprouting, and blood-brain barrier dysfunction [2]. About 30% of TLE patients do not respond to treatment with anti-epileptic drugs (AEDs) that are used to suppress seizures [3, 4]. Therefore, there is a need to develop treatments that interfere with epileptogenic mechanisms (anti-epileptogenic strategies).

In recent years, the mammalian target of rapamycin (mTOR) pathway has been studied as a possible target for anti-epileptogenic strategies [5–7]. The mTOR pathway regulates a large number of cellular processes [8, 9], and mTOR hyperactivation occurs in TLE patients and in several experimental models for epilepsy [10]. Several studies have shown potential anti-epileptogenic properties of mTOR pathway inhibitor rapamycin in different experimental models of TLE [11–14].

Still, the mechanisms mediating possible anti-epileptogenic effects of rapamycin remain to be elucidated. In the electrical post-status epilepticus (SE) rat model for TLE, where the SE is the equivalent of the initial insult, it was shown that chronic treatment with the mTOR inhibitor rapamycin suppressed spontaneous seizures and reduced cell death, mossy fiber sprouting, and blood-brain barrier leakage after SE [14]. Since rapamycin was able to reduce SE-induced microgliosis in rats after pilocarpine-induced SE [15] and kainic acid-induced SE [16] and has been shown to be neuroprotective after traumatic brain injury [17, 18] and stroke [19], it was proposed that rapamycin might have anti-epileptogenic effects through anti-inflammatory actions, possibly mediated by inhibition of the mTOR pathway.

However, rapamycin is effective in suppressing epileptogenesis only when treatment is continued, and rapamycin blood levels remain sufficiently high [20]. Moreover, prolonged treatment with rapamycin produces unwanted side effects, primarily on growth [14, 20, 21]. Therefore, there is a growing interest for alternative anti-epileptogenic treatments through mTOR inhibition. In this context, curcumin is considered. Curcumin is the main component of turmeric from the *Curcuma longa* plant. It is known for anti-inflammatory and neuroprotective properties [22–24], but it has also been reported to inhibit the mTOR pathway [25] and the mitogen-activated kinase (MAPK) pathways (extracellular signal-regulated kinase (ERK)1/2 and p38 pathway) [26]. In addition, curcumin has anti-oxidant effects [23, 27, 28]. No adverse effects of curcumin have been reported in phase 1 clinical studies [29, 30]. Because of its rapid degradation, curcumin has a low bioavailability in vivo [31] which could pose a challenge for its use as an anti-epileptogenic drug. Still, its anti-inflammatory, anti-oxidant, and mTOR-inhibiting properties make curcumin potentially anti-epileptogenic and possibly an interesting alternative to rapamycin.

Here, we aim to elucidate anti-inflammatory and anti-oxidant effects of curcumin compared to rapamycin in the context of epileptogenesis. We first studied the effects of both compounds on inflammation in vitro. Next, we studied anti-inflammatory and anti-oxidant effects of rapamycin and curcumin in vivo, in the early phase of epileptogenesis after SE in rats. With this combined approach, we aim to shed light on the anti-epileptogenic potential of curcumin compared to rapamycin and study the possible anti-inflammatory and anti-oxidant actions as potential underlying mechanisms.

## Methods

### Effects of rapamycin and curcumin on inflammation and oxidative stress in vitro

To assess the effects of rapamycin and curcumin on inflammation in vitro, we used primary human fetal astrocyte cell cultures and studied the levels of pro-inflammatory cytokines after challenging the cultures with interleukin 1-β (IL-1β). To study the effects of curcumin on oxidative stress in vitro, we studied the reactive oxygen species (ROS) levels in human primary neuronal cultures.

### Astrocyte cell cultures

Primary astrocyte-enriched cell cultures were made from human fetal brain tissue (cortex, 14–19 gestational weeks) obtained from medically induced abortions. A written informed consent for the use of the tissue for research purposes was given by all donors to the Bloemenhove Clinic. The tissue was obtained in accordance with the Declaration of Helsinki and the Academic Medical Center (AMC) Research Code provided by the Medical Ethics Committee of the AMC. Cell isolation was performed as described in Additional file 1 and elsewhere [32]. Cultures were incubated with Dulbecco's modified Eagle's medium (DMEM)/HAM F10 (1:1) medium (Gibco, Life Technologies, Grand Island, NY, USA), supplemented with 1% penicillin/streptomycin and 10% fetal calf serum (FCS; Gibco, Life Technologies, Grand Island, NY, USA). Cultures were refreshed twice a week and reached confluence after 2–3 weeks. Secondary astrocyte cultures for experimental manipulation were established by trypsinizing confluent cultures and re-plating onto poly-L-lysine (PLL; 15 µg/ml, Sigma-Aldrich; St. Louis, MO, USA)-precoated 12 and 24-well plates (Costar, Cambridge, MA, USA; $10 \times 10^4$ cells/well in a 12-well plate for RNA isolation and quantitative real-time PCR; $5 \times 10^4$ cells/well in a 24-well plate for immunocytochemistry). Astrocytes were used for analyses at passages 2–4. Cell cultures were stimulated with human recombinant (r)IL-1β (Peprotech, Rocky Hill, NJ, USA; 10 ng/ml) for 24 h. Treatment of astrocytes with rapamycin (100 nM) or curcumin

(10 μM) in 0.05% dimethyl sulfoxide (DMSO) was either started 24 h before, and continued during IL-1β stimulation (pre-treatment), or given simultaneously with IL-1β stimulation (simultaneous treatment). Concentrations of rapamycin (100 nm) and curcumin (10 μM) were selected based on previous work [33–36], and we selected the concentrations used in the experiments (100 nm rapamycin and 10 μM curcumin) after testing multiple concentrations with cell viability assays—see Additional file 1 and Additional file 2: Figure S1). Cells were harvested 24 h after stimulation with IL-1β.

## Human neuronal culture

To study the effects of curcumin on oxidative stress, we used the human neuroblastoma SH-SY5Y cell line, which is widely used for studying oxidative stress in vitro [37]. SH-SY5Y cells were cultured in Dulbecco's modified Eagle's medium (DMEM)/HAM F12 (1:1) (Gibco, Life Technologies, Grand Island, NY, USA) supplemented with 1% penicillin/streptomycin and 10% FCS (Gibco, Life Technologies, Grand Island, NY, USA). The cells were seeded into 96-well cell culture plates at a density of $10 \times 10^3$ cells per well and allowed to adhere for 24 h in a 5% $CO_2$ incubator at 37 °C. The culture medium was then replaced with either fresh medium containing 0.05% DMSO alone (vehicle) or with different concentrations of curcumin (1, 5, 10, and 20 μM) in 0.05% DMSO, and cell cultures were incubated in a 5% $CO_2$ incubator for 30 min. For cell viability analysis, see Additional file 1 and Additional file 3: Figure S2).

## Oxidative stress assay

Intracellular ROS levels were measured in SH-SY5Y cells after treatment with the different concentrations (1, 5, 10, and 20 μM) of curcumin using the 2′7′-dichloro-fluorescein (DCF, Sigma-Aldrich, St Louis, MO, USA) method, which is described in Additional file 1. The formation of DCF due to the ROS-driven oxidation of H2DCFH was measured using a microplate reader with excitation and emission wavelengths of 485 nm (bandwidth 5 nm) and 535 nm (bandwidth 5 nm), respectively. In this assay, the levels of DCF fluorescence are directly proportional to intracellular ROS levels and reported as a fold change compared to the control samples. All assays were performed in triplicate for each condition.

## Effects of rapamycin and curcumin on inflammation in the post-SE rat model for TLE

To study whether rapamycin and curcumin could be anti-inflammatory in early stages of epileptogenesis, we tested the effects of 1-week treatment with rapamycin or curcumin following electrically induced SE in rats.

## Animals

Adult male Sprague Dawley rats (Harlan Netherlands, Horst, The Netherlands) weighing 250–350 g at the start of the experiment were used. Rats were housed individually in a controlled environment (21 ± 1 °C, 60% humidity, 12-h light/dark cycle with lights on 08:00 AM–8:00 PM), with water and food (standard laboratory chew) available ad libitum. All animal procedures were approved by the Animal Ethics Committee of the University of Amsterdam, according to Dutch law, and performed in accordance with the guidelines of the European Community Council Directives 2010/63/EU.

## Status epilepticus induction

Rats were implanted with intracranial electrodes for stimulation and EEG recording using surgical procedures that are described in Additional file 1 and elsewhere [38]. After several weeks of recovery, the rats underwent tetanic stimulation of the angular bundle in the form of a succession of trains of 50-Hz pulses every 13 s. Each train lasted 10 s and consisted of biphasic pulses of 0.5 ms with a minimal intensity of 300 μA and a maximal intensity of 700 μA. Stimulation was stopped when the rats displayed sustained forelimb clonus and salivation for several minutes, which usually occurred within 1 h. If not, stimulation was continued but never lasted longer than 110 min. SE was defined electrographically by the occurrence of periodic epileptiform discharges (PEDs) of 1–2 Hz in the hippocampal EEG immediately after termination of stimulation. Behavior was observed during electrical stimulation and several hours thereafter.

## Rapamycin and curcumin treatment

Stock solutions of 150 mg/ml rapamycin (LC Laboratories, Woburn, MA, USA) were prepared in 100% ethanol and stored at − 20 °C until use. Prior to use, rapamycin stock was diluted in a vehicle solution (5% Tween 80 + 5% polyethylene glycol 400) resulting in a 4% ethanol containing solution. Rats ($n = 5$) were injected intraperitoneally with 6 mg/kg rapamycin solution, starting 4 h after SE and once daily for 7 days thereafter. A vehicle post-SE group ($n = 5$) was injected with vehicle solution following the same paradigm. To allow for intracerebral ventricle (icv) injections for curcumin treatment, a stainless steel cannula was placed on the cortex of the rats during electrode implantation at 1.0 mm AP and 2.5 mm ML from Bregma and secured to the skull with dental cement. Curcumin (70%, Sigma-Aldrich, Zwijndrecht, The Netherlands) was stored at − 20 °C and freshly prepared (diluted in DMSO) on each treatment day. Rats ($n = 7$) were injected via the icv cannula with 2 μl of 2 mM curcumin solution, and a vehicle post-SE group ($n = 4$) was injected with a vehicle solution (DMSO, Sigma) using the same paradigm. Similar to the rapamycin treatment, curcumin injections started 4 h after SE and continued with daily injections for 7 days after SE. Based on the estimates of the cerebrospinal fluid (CSF) volume in the rat [39, 40], the end concentration of curcumin was estimated at a range of ~ 20–40 µM, which is comparable with in vitro levels reported previously [33] and in our vitro data in the supplementary results (Additional file 3: Figure S2). The end concentration of DMSO in the cerebrospinal fluid was ~ 1–2%. Control rats were included that were not stimulated or treated.

One week after SE, the rats were killed by decapitation under isoflurane anesthesia, and the hippocampal sections were dissected and stored in – 80 °C until use. This time point was chosen because it coincides with the activation of microglia and astrocytes and the upregulation of various pro-inflammatory markers, according to previous findings [41, 42].

### RNA isolation and quantitative real-time quantitative PCR

For RNA isolation, cell culture material was homogenized in Qiazol Lysis Reagent (Qiagen Benelux, Venlo, The Netherlands). Total RNA was isolated using the miRNeasy Mini kit (Qiagen Benelux, Venlo, The Netherlands) according to the manufacturer's instructions. For rat hippocampal tissue sections, total RNA was isolated using the TRIzol® LS Reagent, following the manufacturer's instructions (Invitrogen—Life Technologies, Breda, The Netherlands). Concentration and purity of RNA were determined at 260/280 nm using a NanoDrop 2000 spectrophotometer (Thermo Fisher Scientific, Wilmington, DE, USA). To evaluate mRNA expression, 200–500 ng (for cell culture-derived total RNA) or 2500 ng (for rat hippocampal total RNA) was reverse-transcribed into cDNA using oligo dT primers. Quantitative RT-PCRs were run on a Roche Lightcycler 480 thermocycler (Roche Applied Science, Basel, Switzerland) using the following primers: for human cell cultures: IL-6 (forward: ctcagccctgagaaaggaga; reverse: tttcagccatctttggaagg), COX-2 (forward: gaatggggtgatgagcagtt; reverse: gccactcaagtgttgcacat), EF1a (forward: atccacctttgggtcgcttt; reverse: ccgcaactgtctgtctcatatcac), and C1orf43 (forward: gatttccctgggtttccagt; reverse: attcgactctccagggttca). For rat hippocampal samples: IL-1β (forward: aaaaatgcctcgtgctgtct; reverse: tcgttgcttgtctctccttg), IL-6 (forward: gccagagtcattcagagcaa; reverse: cattggaagttggggtagga), TGF-β (forward: cctggaaagggctcaacac; reverse: cagttcttctctgtggagctga), Hmox-1 (forward: caaccccaccaagttcaaaca; reverse: aggcggtcttagcctcctctg), HMGB-1 (forward: gtaattttccgcgcgcttttgt; reverse: tcatccaggactcatgttcagt), cyclophilin A (CycA) (forward: cccaccgtgttcttcgacat; reverse: aaacagctcgaagcagacgc), and GAPDH (forward: atgactctacccacggcaag; reverse: tactcagcaccagcatcacc).

Quantification of data was performed using the computer program LinRegPCR in which linear regression on the Log (fluorescence) per cycle number data is applied to determine the amplification efficiency per sample [43]. The starting concentration of each specific product was divided by the geometric mean of the starting concentration of the reference genes (EF1a and C1orf43 for cell cultures and CycA or GAPDH for hippocampal sections), and this ratio was compared between groups. For the in vivo experiments, ratios were normalized to not-stimulated control group values. If treatment groups were not different from their corresponding vehicle group, the vehicle and treatment groups were pooled to make one post-SE group to compare to the corresponding not-stimulated control group.

### Western blot

Cells in culture or rat hippocampal tissue sections were homogenized in lysis buffer containing 10 mM Tris (pH 8.0), 150 mM NaCl, 10% glycerol, 1% NP-40, 0.4 mg/ml Na-orthovanadate, 5 mM EDTA (pH 8.0), 5 mM NaF, and protease inhibitors (cocktail tablets, Roche Diagnostics, Mannheim, Germany). Protein content was determined using the bicinchoninic acid method. For electrophoresis, an equal amount of proteins (10 or 15 µg/lane for cell cultures and rat hippocampal sections, respectively) were separated by sodium dodecyl sulfate-polyacrylamide gel electrophoresis (SDS-PAGE, 12% acrylamide). Separated proteins were transferred to nitrocellulose paper by electroblotting for 1 h and 30 min (BioRad, Transblot SD, Hercules, CA, USA). After blocking for 1 h in TBST (20 mM Tris, 150 mM NaCl, 0.1% Tween, pH 7.5)/5% non-fat dry milk, blots were incubated overnight at 4 °C with the primary antibodies (phosphorylated S6 (pS6) #5364, rabbit monoclonal, Cell Signaling Technology, Danvers, MA, USA, 1:1000; MAPK #9102, rabbit monoclonal, Cell Signaling Technology, 1:1500; phosphorylated MAPK (pMAPK) #4370, rabbit monoclonal, Cell Signaling Technology, 1:1500; β-tubulin, mouse monoclonal, Sigma, St. Louis, MO, USA; 1: 50,000). After several washes in TBST, the membranes were incubated in TBST/5% non-fat dry milk, containing the goat anti-rabbit or rabbit anti-mouse antibodies coupled to horseradish peroxidase (1:2500; Dako, Glostrup, Denmark) for 1 h. After washes in TBST, immunoreactivity was visualized using ECL Western blotting detection reagent (Thermo Fisher Scientific, Wilmington, DE, USA). For the culture experiments, for each condition, two wells were analyzed from a total of two donors.

### Data analysis

Data were analyzed using non-parametric testing (Kruskal--Wallis followed by Dunn's tests for multiple comparisons, or Mann-Whitney $U$ tests), using GraphPad™ Prism v.5

(GraphPad Software, Inc. La Jolla, CA, USA). $p < 0.05$ was assumed to indicate a significant difference.

## Results

### Effects of curcumin and rapamycin on inflammation and oxidative stress in vitro

Anti-inflammatory effects of rapamycin and curcumin were tested in vitro by measuring COX-2 and IL-6 mRNA expression in astrocyte cultures that were challenged with IL-1β stimulation (Fig. 1). IL-1β stimulation increased the expression of COX-2 and IL-6 in cultured astrocytes ($p < 0.005$ for both markers). The increase in IL-6 could be reduced by 10 μM curcumin, both with pre-treatment and simultaneous treatment ($p < 0.01$), whereas rapamycin did not affect the IL-1β-induced increase in IL-6 expression. The IL-1β-induced increase in COX-2 expression was reduced by simultaneous curcumin (10 μM) treatment ($p < 0.005$), but not by pre-treatment. Rapamycin (both pre- and simultaneous treatment with 100 nM) further increased the expression of COX-2, compared to IL-1β stimulation ($p < 0.005$).

To investigate the involvement of the mTOR pathway, the effect of rapamycin (100 nM) and curcumin (10 μM) on the downstream target of mTOR, phosphorylated S6 (pS6), was evaluated by Western blot (Fig. 2). Rapamycin, but not curcumin, suppressed pS6 levels in cultured astrocytes, in the presence of IL-1β, and without IL-1β stimulation. We next investigated whether curcumin could suppress the MAPK (ERK1/2) pathway, using Western blot for phospho-(p)MAPK (ERK1/2) and found that curcumin (10 μM) suppressed the levels of pMAPK in cultured astrocytes (Fig. 3).

Next, we assessed the anti-oxidant effects of curcumin in vitro, by studying reactive oxygen species (ROS) in human SH-SY5Y cell cultures using a DCF assay. Curcumin (10 and 20 μM) reduced ROS levels after 30 min acute treatment compared to control (10 μM, $p < 0.05$; 20 μM, $p < 0.001$, Fig. 4).

### Effects of curcumin and rapamycin on inflammation and oxidative stress in post-SE rats

We then set out to test the effects of rapamycin and curcumin in vivo, in the post-SE rat model for TLE. Rapamycin (6 mg/kg) and curcumin (~ 40 μM, see the "Methods" section) treatment was given for 1 week, starting 4 h after SE. Gene expression of inflammatory markers IL-1β, IL-6, TGF-β, Hmox-1, and HMGB-1 in the hippocampus was analyzed using quantitative RT-PCR 1 week after SE (Fig. 5). The expression of IL-1β, IL-6, and TGF-β was increased 1 week after SE compared to non-stimulated control rats. Expression of IL-1β, IL-6, and TGF-β was not different between treatment (rapamycin or curcumin) and their corresponding vehicle groups. Expression of HMGB-1 was not different

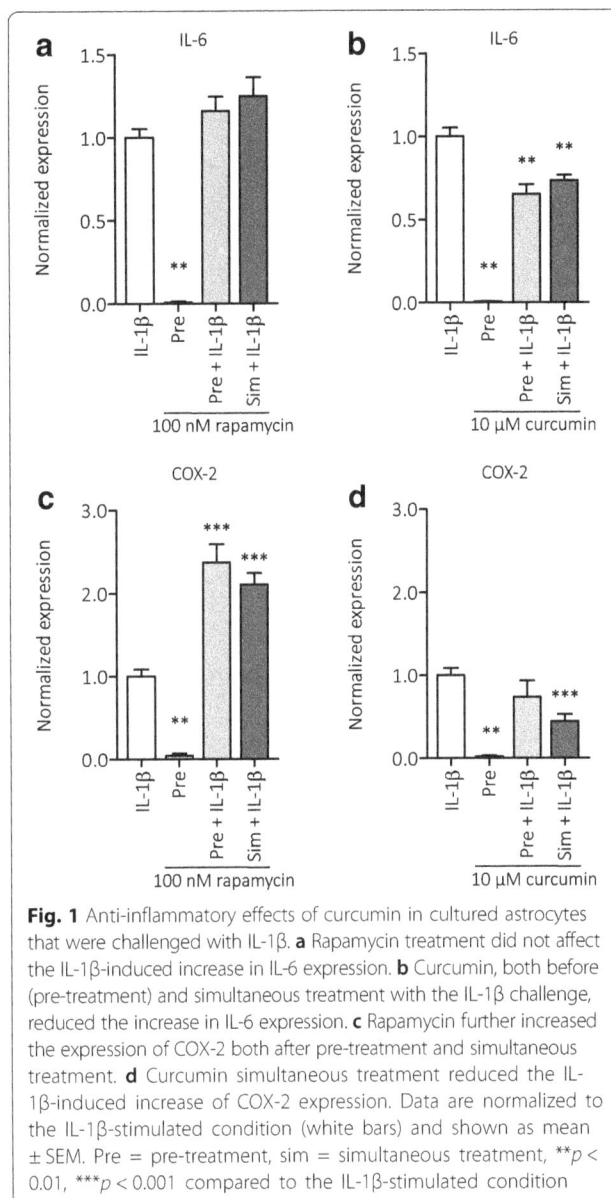

**Fig. 1** Anti-inflammatory effects of curcumin in cultured astrocytes that were challenged with IL-1β. **a** Rapamycin treatment did not affect the IL-1β-induced increase in IL-6 expression. **b** Curcumin, both before (pre-treatment) and simultaneous treatment with the IL-1β challenge, reduced the increase in IL-6 expression. **c** Rapamycin further increased the expression of COX-2 both after pre-treatment and simultaneous treatment. **d** Curcumin simultaneous treatment reduced the IL-1β-induced increase of COX-2 expression. Data are normalized to the IL-1β-stimulated condition (white bars) and shown as mean ± SEM. Pre = pre-treatment, sim = simultaneous treatment, $**p < 0.01$, $***p < 0.001$ compared to the IL-1β-stimulated condition

between not-stimulated control rats and post-SE rats. Expression of Hmox-1 was increased 1 week after SE compared to non-stimulated control rats. Levels of Hmox-1 expression were not different between treatment (rapamycin or curcumin) groups and their corresponding vehicle groups.

### Effect of curcumin on pMAPK levels in post-SE rats

To verify that icv-applied curcumin was able to inhibit the MAPK pathway in vivo, as was seen in vitro, hippocampal sections of post-SE rats were used for Western blot analysis. The 42-kDa band of pMAPK (p42) was suppressed in curcumin-treated versus vehicle-treated rats, whereas the 44-kDa band (p44 MAPK) was enhanced in the curcumin group (Fig. 6)

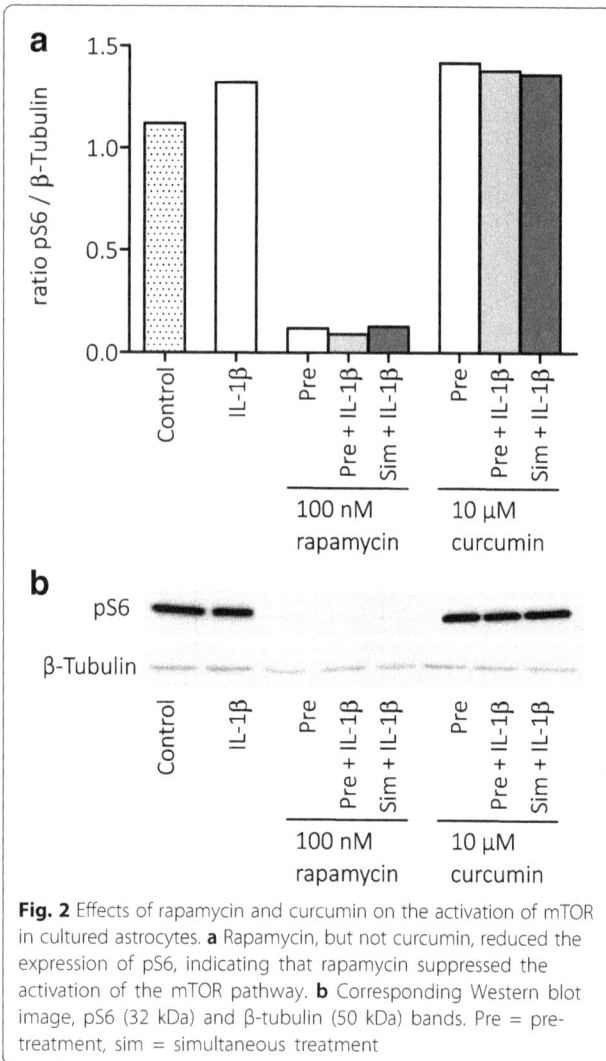

**Fig. 2** Effects of rapamycin and curcumin on the activation of mTOR in cultured astrocytes. **a** Rapamycin, but not curcumin, reduced the expression of pS6, indicating that rapamycin suppressed the activation of the mTOR pathway. **b** Corresponding Western blot image, pS6 (32 kDa) and β-tubulin (50 kDa) bands. Pre = pre-treatment, sim = simultaneous treatment

indicating that curcumin reached the hippocampus in sufficient concentrations to influence the MAPK pathway.

## Discussion

We compared anti-inflammatory and anti-oxidant effects of curcumin and rapamycin to investigate whether curcumin has anti-epileptogenic potential that could make it an alternative for mTOR inhibitor rapamycin. We found anti-inflammatory and anti-oxidant effects of curcumin in vitro but not in vivo in the post-SE rat model.

When we assessed mTOR inhibition in vitro in the astrocyte cultures, we found that only rapamycin was able to reduce phosphorylated S6 levels, indicating that rapamycin, but not curcumin, inhibited the mTOR pathway. Instead, curcumin suppressed pMAPK (ERK1/2) in the astrocyte cultures. The activity of the MAPK pathway has been associated with different experimental

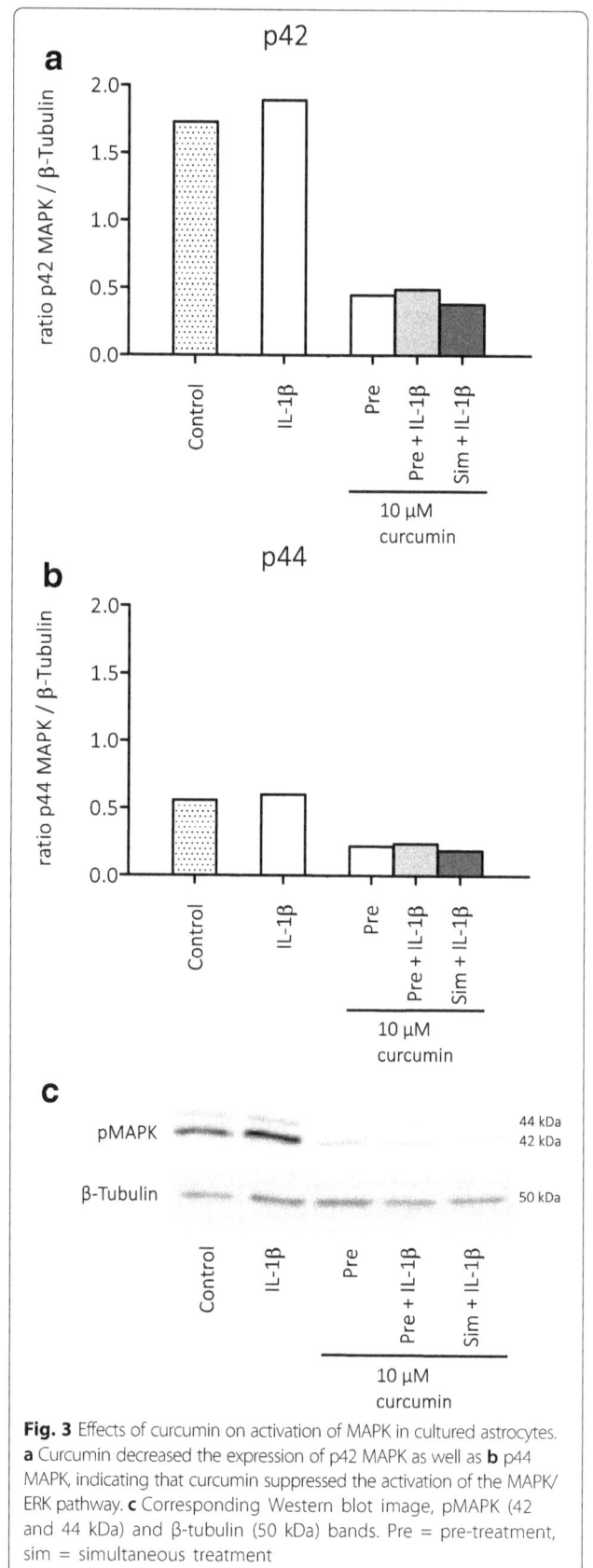

**Fig. 3** Effects of curcumin on activation of MAPK in cultured astrocytes. **a** Curcumin decreased the expression of p42 MAPK as well as **b** p44 MAPK, indicating that curcumin suppressed the activation of the MAPK/ERK pathway. **c** Corresponding Western blot image, pMAPK (42 and 44 kDa) and β-tubulin (50 kDa) bands. Pre = pre-treatment, sim = simultaneous treatment

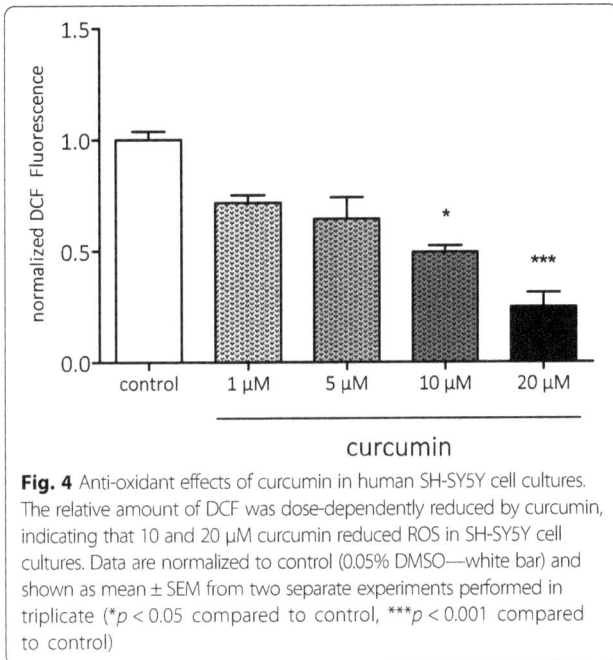

**Fig. 4** Anti-oxidant effects of curcumin in human SH-SY5Y cell cultures. The relative amount of DCF was dose-dependently reduced by curcumin, indicating that 10 and 20 μM curcumin reduced ROS in SH-SY5Y cell cultures. Data are normalized to control (0.05% DMSO—white bar) and shown as mean ± SEM from two separate experiments performed in triplicate (*$p < 0.05$ compared to control, ***$p < 0.001$ compared to control)

models of epilepsy and seizures [44–50]. Increased MAPK activity could contribute to cell death [51, 52] and inflammation [53], and previous studies suggested that the neuroprotective effects of curcumin could be mediated by the MAPK pathway [26, 54, 55].

Anti-inflammatory effects differed between rapamycin and curcumin in the astrocyte cultures. Rapamycin did not suppress inflammatory cytokine IL-6 expression and even further increased COX-2 expression after the IL-1β challenge. This is in line with a previous study in rat astrocyte cultures that also showed increased COX-2 immunoreactivity [56] in microglia and increased IL-6 production after rapamycin treatment [57]. Since we used IL-1β as a trigger to mimic inflammation, we did not test rapamycin effects on the Il-1β mRNA level itself, but an effect by rapamycin on IL-1β and other inflammatory associated proteins (than IL6 and COX-2) cannot be excluded. Curcumin on the other hand suppressed IL-6 and COX-2, which is in line with the previously reported anti-inflammatory effects [23, 54, 55, 58, 59]. Curcumin only suppressed COX-2 when treatment was applied simultaneously with the IL-1β challenge. The findings that curcumin inhibits MAPK pathway and inflammatory cytokines in these experiments support the

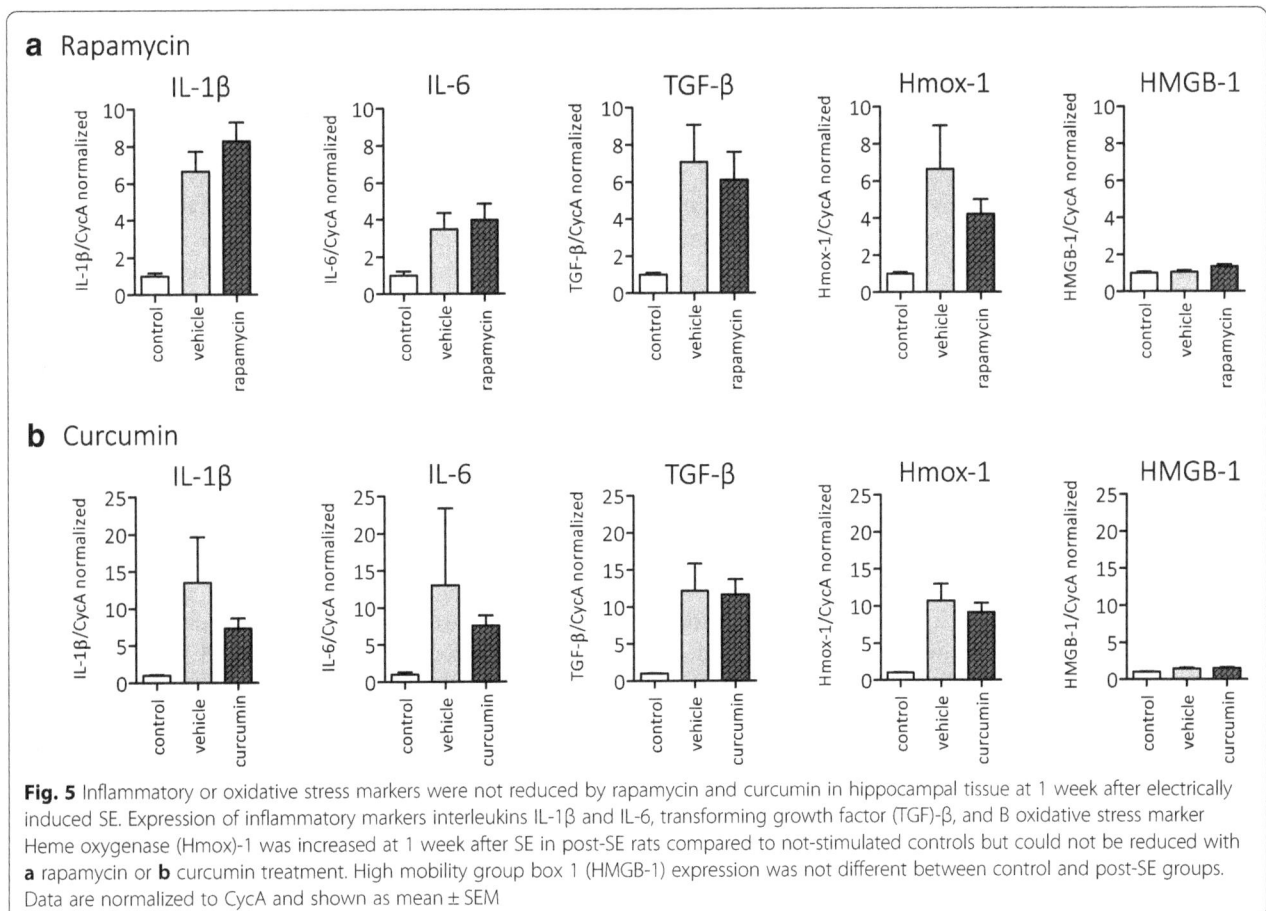

**Fig. 5** Inflammatory or oxidative stress markers were not reduced by rapamycin and curcumin in hippocampal tissue at 1 week after electrically induced SE. Expression of inflammatory markers interleukins IL-1β and IL-6, transforming growth factor (TGF)-β, and B oxidative stress marker Heme oxygenase (Hmox)-1 was increased at 1 week after SE in post-SE rats compared to not-stimulated controls but could not be reduced with **a** rapamycin or **b** curcumin treatment. High mobility group box 1 (HMGB-1) expression was not different between control and post-SE groups. Data are normalized to CycA and shown as mean ± SEM

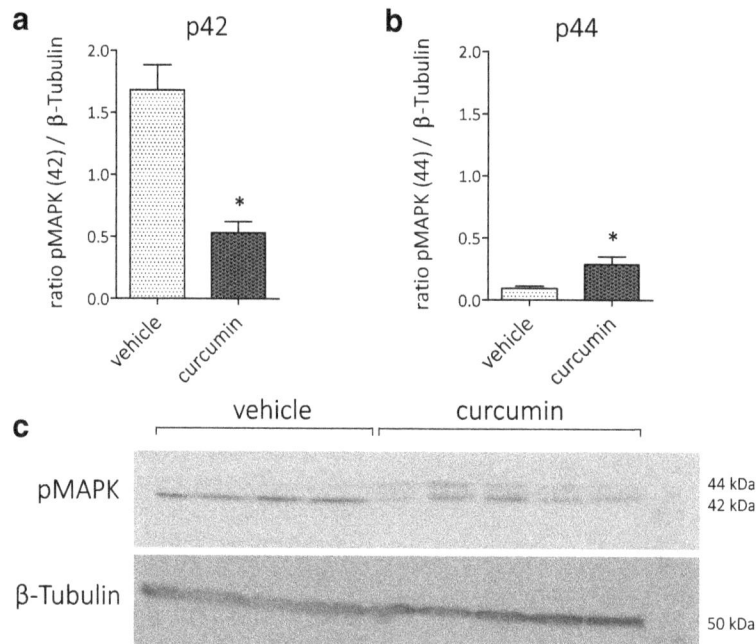

**Fig. 6** Effects of icv-applied curcumin on activation of the MAPK pathway in rat hippocampus 1 week after SE. **a**, **b** Curcumin reduced the expression of p42 MAPK and increased the expression of p44 MAPK, indicating that curcumin modified the activation of the MAPK/ERK pathway. **c** Corresponding Western blot image, pMAPK (42 and 44 kDa) and β-tubulin (50 kDa) bands (*p < 0.05 compared to vehicle)

idea that curcumin could have anti-inflammatory effects mediated by the MAPK pathway in astrocytes, as suggested by previous studies [54, 55].

In SH-SY5Y cell cultures, we found anti-oxidant effects of curcumin, as shown by reduced ROS levels. Anti-oxidant effects of curcumin are likely mediated via induction of Heme oxygenase (Hmox-1), which can protect against damage by free radicals and programmed cell death [60]. Curcumin is a known inducer of Hmox-1 [27, 28, 61], which could contribute to its neuroprotective effects.

We then tested whether curcumin and rapamycin could interfere with inflammation during early epileptogenesis by measuring the expression of several inflammatory markers (after treatment during the first week after SE). Reduced inflammation would explain the seizure modifying effects of rapamycin observed later during epileptogenesis and would be in line with the anti-inflammatory actions of curcumin. At 1 week after electrically induced SE, there is an increase of activation of microglia and astrocytes, which is accompanied by the upregulation of various pro-inflammatory markers [41, 42]. Accordingly, we found that mRNA levels of inflammatory cytokines IL-1β, IL-6, and TGF-β were increased at this time point in post-SE rats compared to control rats. Upregulation of Hmox-1, indicative of oxidative stress, was also increased at 1 week after SE. We did not detect any effect of rapamycin or curcumin on inflammatory and oxidative stress markers at 1 week

after SE. For rapamycin, this is in line with our findings in vitro. However, the lack of anti-inflammatory effects in vivo could also be explained by the recent findings that rapamycin can contribute to blood-brain barrier leakage at this early time point (but not in the chronic phase) after SE [16]. Blood-brain barrier leakage could initially contribute to the enhanced levels of inflammatory markers since it is known that peripheral immune cells and serum proteins that enter the central nervous system enhance inflammatory responses [62–64]. Alternatively, starting treatment 4 h after SE could have been too late for both curcumin and rapamycin to exert anti-inflammatory effects.

In another study using pentylenetetrazole (PTZ)-induced model for chronic epilepsy, curcumin did have anti-inflammatory and had anti-oxidant effects after oral administration [65, 66]. In the electrical post-SE rat model, however, we have not been able to detect effects of curcumin on the exhibition of spontaneous seizures when we administered curcumin orally [20]. Curcumin is known to have a low bioavailability due to rapid systemic degradation [31]. To circumvent these problems in the current study, we administered curcumin intracerebrally and found that curcumin did influence pMAPK at 1 week after SE but was not able to suppress brain inflammation. Possibly, SE induces too severe damage to be restored by curcumin treatment, or the dosing, location, and timing of the curcumin treatment were not sufficient to reverse the SE-induced inflammation and oxidative stress.

## Conclusions

Taken together, we found that 1-week post-SE treatment with rapamycin or curcumin did not alter SE-induced upregulation of markers of inflammation and oxidative stress, while in vitro, curcumin displayed anti-inflammatory and anti-oxidant effects. Since these in vitro results are promising, the anti-epileptogenic potential of curcumin deserves further investigation, possibly employing different TLE models and administration strategies to optimize bioavailability.

## Abbreviations

COX-2: Cyclooxygenase 2; DMSO: Dimethylsulfoxide; EEG: Electroencephalogram; ERK: Extracellular signal-regulated kinase; H2DCF-DA: 2′,7′-Dichlorofluorescein diacetate; HMGB-1: High mobility box group 1; Hmox-1: Heme oxygenase 1; icv: Intracerebroventricular; IL-6/IL-1β: Interleukin 6/IL-β; MAPK: Mitogen-activated protein kinase; mTOR: Mammalian target of rapamycin; ROS: Reactive oxygen species; SE: Status epilepticus; TGF-β: Transforming growth factor β; TLE: Temporal lobe epilepsy

## Acknowledgements

We acknowledge the HIS Mouse Facility of the Academic Medical Center, Amsterdam, and the Bloemenhove Clinic (Heemstede, The Netherlands) for providing the fetal tissues. We also acknowledge Grazia Forte and Anand Iyer for their contributions at the beginning of the experiment.

## Funding

The research leading to these results has received funding from the Dutch Epilepsy Foundation, project number EF 14-08 (CD, JAG) and the European Union's Seventh Framework Programme (FP7/2007-2013) under grant agreement no. 602391 (EPISTOP; JvS, EA) and no. 602102 (EPITARGET; EA, JAG, EAvV).

## Authors' contributions

Experiments with astrocyte cultures were performed by JvS and KG. Experiments with SY-SY5Y cells were performed by AA. The post-SE experiments were carried out by CD, LK, and EAvV. qPCR of the post-SE material was performed by CD and LK, and the Western blot was performed by CD. The data was analyzed by KG, JvS, AA, and CD. CD drafted and prepared the manuscript. JG and EA supervised the study and participated in the experiment design, coordination, and manuscript writing. EAvV, JG, and EA revised and contributed to the manuscript. All authors read and approved the final manuscript.

## Consent for publication

Not applicable

## Competing interests

The authors declare that they have no competing interests.

## Author details

[1]Center for Neuroscience, Swammerdam Institute for Life Sciences, University of Amsterdam, Amsterdam, The Netherlands. [2]Department of (Neuro) Pathology, Amsterdam UMC, University of Amsterdam, Amsterdam, The Netherlands. [3]Department of Biochemical Sciences, Sapienza University of Rome, Rome, Italy. [4]Stichting Epilepsie Instellingen Nederland (SEIN), Heemstede, The Netherlands.

## References

1. Banerjee PN, Filippi D, Allen Hauser W. The descriptive epidemiology of epilepsy—a review. Epilepsy Res. 2009;85:31–45.
2. Pitkänen A, Lukasiuk K. Mechanisms of epileptogenesis and potential treatment targets. Lancet Neurol. 2011;10:173–86.
3. Schuele SU, Lüders HO. Intractable epilepsy: management and therapeutic alternatives. Lancet Neurol. 2008;7:514–24.
4. Kwan P, Arzimanoglou A, Berg AT, Brodie MJ, Hauser WA, Mathern G, et al. Definition of drug resistant epilepsy: consensus proposal by the ad hoc Task Force of the ILAE Commission on Therapeutic Strategies. Epilepsia. 2010;51: 1069–77.
5. McDaniel SS, Wong M. Therapeutic role of mammalian target of rapamycin (mTOR) inhibition in preventing epileptogenesis. Neurosci Lett. 2011;497: 231–9.
6. Sadowski K, Kotulska-Jóźwiak K, Jóźwiak S. Role of mTOR inhibitors in epilepsy treatment. Pharmacol Reports. 2015;67:636–46.
7. Galanopoulou AS, Gorter JA, Cepeda C. Finding a better drug for epilepsy: the mTOR pathway as an antiepileptogenic target. Epilepsia. 2012;53:1119–30.
8. Switon K, Kotulska K, Janusz-Kaminska A, Zmorzynska J, Jaworski J. Molecular neurobiology of mTOR. Neuroscience. 2017;341:112–53.
9. Swiech L, Perycz M, Malik A, Jaworski J. Role of mTOR in physiology and pathology of the nervous system. Biochim Biophys Acta - Proteins Proteomics. 2008;1784:116–32.
10. Sha L-Z, Xing X-L, Zhang D, Yao Y, Dou W-C, Jin L-R, et al. Mapping the spatio-temporal pattern of the mammalian target of rapamycin (mTOR) activation in temporal lobe epilepsy. PLoS One. 2012;7:e39152.
11. Buckmaster PS, Ingram EA, Wen X. Inhibition of the mammalian target of rapamycin signaling pathway suppresses dentate granule cell axon sprouting in a rodent model of temporal lobe epilepsy. J Neurosci. 2009;29: 8259–69.
12. Huang X, Zhang H, Yang J, Wu J, McMahon J, Lin Y, et al. Pharmacological inhibition of the mammalian target of rapamycin pathway suppresses acquired epilepsy. Neurobiol Dis. 2010;40:193–9.
13. Zeng L-H, Rensing NR, Wong M. The mammalian target of rapamycin signaling pathway mediates epileptogenesis in a model of temporal lobe epilepsy. J Neurosci. 2009;29:6964–72.
14. van Vliet EA, Forte G, Holtman L, den Burger JCG, Sinjewel A, de Vries HE, et al. Inhibition of mammalian target of rapamycin reduces epileptogenesis and blood-brain barrier leakage but not microglia activation. Epilepsia. 2012; 53:1254–63.
15. Brewster AL, Lugo JN, Patil VV, Lee WL, Qian Y, Vanegas F, et al. Rapamycin reverses status epilepticus-induced memory deficits and dendritic damage. PLoS One. 2013;8:e57808.
16. van Vliet EA, Otte WM, Wadman WJ, Aronica E, Kooij G, de Vries HE, et al. Blood-brain barrier leakage after status epilepticus in rapamycin-treated rats II: potential mechanisms. Epilepsia. 2016;57:70–8.
17. Erlich S, Alexandrovich A, Shohami E, Pinkas-Kramarski R. Rapamycin is a neuroprotective treatment for traumatic brain injury. Neurobiol Dis. 2007;26: 86–93.
18. Park J, Zhang J, Qiu J, Zhu X, Degterev A, Lo EH, et al. Combination therapy targeting Akt and mammalian target of rapamycin improves functional outcome after controlled cortical impact in mice. J Cereb Blood Flow Metab. 2012;32:330–40.
19. Chauhan A, Sharma U, Jagannathan NR, Reeta KH, Gupta YK. Rapamycin protects against middle cerebral artery occlusion induced focal cerebral ischemia in rats. Behav Brain Res. 2011;225:603–9.
20. Drion CM, Borm LE, Kooijman L, Aronica E, Wadman WJ, Hartog AF, et al. Effects of rapamycin and curcumin treatment on the development of epilepsy after electrically induced status epilepticus in rats. Epilepsia. 2016; 57:688–97.
21. Sliwa A, Plucinska G, Bednarczyk J, Lukasiuk K. Post-treatment with rapamycin does not prevent epileptogenesis in the amygdala stimulation model of temporal lobe epilepsy. Neurosci Lett. 2012;509:105–9.
22. Beevers CS, Chen L, Liu L, Luo Y, Webster NJG, Huang S. Curcumin disrupts the mammalian target of rapamycin-raptor complex. Cancer Res. 2009;69: 1000–8.
23. Maheshwari RK, Singh AK, Gaddipati J, Srimal RC. Multiple biological activities of curcumin: a short review. Life Sci. 2006;78:2081–7.
24. Zhou HS, Beevers C, Huang S. Targets of curcumin. Curr Drug Targets. 2011; 12:332–47.
25. Beevers CS, Li F, Liu L, Huang S. Curcumin inhibits the mammalian target of

rapamycin-mediated signaling pathways in cancer cells. Int J Cancer. 2006; 119:757–64.

26. Shi X, Zheng Z, Li J, Xiao Z, Qi W, Zhang A, et al. Curcumin inhibits Aβ-induced microglial inflammatory responses in vitro: involvement of ERK1/2 and p38 signaling pathways. Neurosci Lett. 2015;594:105–10.

27. Parada E, Buendia I, Navarro E, Avendao C, Egea J, Lpez MG. Microglial HO-1 induction by curcumin provides antioxidant, antineuroinflammatory, and glioprotective effects. Mol Nutr Food Res. 2015;59:1690–700.

28. Motterlini R, Foresti R, Bassi R, Green CJ. Curcumin, an antioxidant and anti-inflammatory agent, induces heme oxygenase-1 and protects endothelial cells against oxidative stress. Free Radic Biol Med. 2000;28:1303–12.

29. Cheng A, Hsu C, Lin J, Hsu M, Ho Y, Shen T, et al. Phase I clinical trial of curcumin, a chemopreventive agent, in patients with high-risk or pre-malignant lesions. Anticancer Res. 2001;21:2895–900.

30. Hsu CH, Cheng AL. Clinical studies with curcumin. Adv Exp Med Biol. 2007; 595:471–80.

31. Chen Y, Wu Q, Zhang Z, Yuan L, Liu X, Zhou L. Preparation of curcumin-loaded liposomes and evaluation of their skin permeation and pharmacodynamics. Molecules. 2012;17:5972–87.

32. van Scheppingen J, Iyer AM, Prabowo AS, Mühlebner A, Anink JJ, Scholl T, et al. Expression of microRNAs miR21, miR146a, and miR155 in tuberous sclerosis complex cortical tubers and their regulation in human astrocytes and SEGA-derived cell cultures. Glia. 2016;64:1066–82.

33. Xie L, Li X-K, Funeshima-Fuji N, Kimura H, Matsumoto Y, Isaka Y, et al. Amelioration of experimental autoimmune encephalomyelitis by curcumin treatment through inhibition of IL-17 production. Int Immunopharmacol. 2009;9:575–81.

34. Codeluppi S, Svensson CI, Hefferan MP, Valencia F, Silldorff MD, Oshiro M, et al. The Rheb-mTOR pathway is upregulated in reactive astrocytes of the injured spinal cord. J Neurosci. 2009;29:1093–104.

35. Ji Y-F, Zhou L, Xie Y-J, Xu S-M, Zhu J, Teng P, et al. Upregulation of glutamate transporter GLT-1 by mTOR-Akt-NF-small ka, CyrillicB cascade in astrocytic oxygen-glucose deprivation. Glia. 2013;61:1959–75.

36. Pla A, Pascual M, Guerri C. Autophagy constitutes a protective mechanism against ethanol toxicity in mouse astrocytes and neurons. PLoS One. 2016; 11:e0153097.

37. Faria J, Barbosa J, Queirós O, Moreira R, Carvalho F, Dinis-Oliveira RJ. Comparative study of the neurotoxicological effects of tramadol and tapentadol in SH-SY5Y cells. Toxicology. 2016;359–360:1–10.

38. Gorter JA, van Vliet EA, Aronica E, Lopes da Silva FH. Long-lasting increased excitability differs in dentate gyrus vs. CA1 in freely moving chronic epileptic rats after electrically induced status epilepticus. Hippocampus. 2002;12:311–24.

39. Pardridge WM. Drug transport in brain via the cerebrospinal fluid. Fluids Barriers CNS. 2011;8:7.

40. Murtha LA, Yang Q, Parsons MW, Levi CR, Beard DJ, Spratt NJ, et al. Cerebrospinal fluid is drained primarily via the spinal canal and olfactory route in young and aged spontaneously hypertensive rats. Fluids Barriers CNS. 2014;11:12.

41. Gorter JA, van Vliet EA, Aronica E, Breit T, Rauwerda H, Lopes da Silva FH, et al. Potential new antiepileptogenic targets indicated by microarray analysis in a rat model for temporal lobe epilepsy. J Neurosci. 2006;26: 11083–110.

42. Gorter JA, Mesquita ARM, van Vliet EA, da Silva FHL, Aronica E. Increased expression of ferritin, an iron-storage protein, in specific regions of the parahippocampal cortex of epileptic rats. Epilepsia. 2005;46:1371–9.

43. Ruijter JM, Ramakers C, Hoogaars WMH, Karlen Y, Bakker O, van den Hoff MJB, et al. Amplification efficiency: linking baseline and bias in the analysis of quantitative PCR data. Nucleic Acids Res. 2009;37:e45.

44. Gass P, Kiessling M, Bading H. Regionally selective stimulation of mitogen activated protein (MAP) kinase tyrosine phosphorylation after generalized seizures in the rat brain. NeurosciLett. 1993;162:39–42.

45. Gorter JA, Iyer A, White I, Colzi A, van Vliet EA, Sisodiya S, et al. Hippocampal subregion-specific microRNA expression during epileptogenesis in experimental temporal lobe epilepsy. Neurobiol Dis. 2013;62:508–20.

46. Korotkov A, Mills JD, Gorter JA, Van Vliet EA, Aronica E. Systematic review and meta- analysis of differentially expressed miRNAs in experimental and human temporal lobe epilepsy. Sci Rep. 2017;7(1):11592.

47. Lopes MW, Soares FMS, De Mello N, Nunes JC, De Cordova FM, Walz R, et al. Time-dependent modulation of mitogen activated protein kinases and

AKT in rat hippocampus and cortex in the pilocarpine model of epilepsy. Neurochem Res. 2012;37:1868–78.

48. McNamara JO, Huang YZ, Leonard AS. Molecular signaling mechanisms underlying epileptogenesis. Sci STKE. 2006;2006:re12.

49. Pernice HF, Schieweck R, Kiebler MA, Popper B. mTOR and MAPK: from localized translation control to epilepsy. BMC Neurosci. 2016;17:73.

50. Yamagata Y, Kaneko K, Kase D, Ishihara H, Nairn AC, Obata K, et al. Regulation of ERK1/2 mitogen-activated protein kinase by NMDA-receptor-induced seizure activity in cortical slices. Brain Res. 2013;1507:1–10.

51. Choi Y-S, Horning P, Aten S, Karelina K, Alzate-Correa D, Arthur JSC, et al. Mitogen- and stress-activated protein kinase 1 regulates status epilepticus-evoked cell death in the hippocampus. ASN Neuro. 2017;9:175909141772660.

52. Liou AKF, Clark RS, Henshall DC, Yin XM, Chen J. To die or not to die for neurons in ischemia, traumatic brain injury and epilepsy: a review on the stress-activated signaling pathways and apoptotic pathways. Prog Neurobiol. 2003;69:103–42.

53. Kaminska B. MAPK signalling pathways as molecular targets for anti-inflammatory therapy—from molecular mechanisms to therapeutic benefits. Biochim Biophys Acta, Proteins Proteomics. 2005:253–62.

54. Kim G-Y, Kim K-H, Lee S-H, Yoon M-S, Lee H-J, Moon D-O, et al. Curcumin inhibits immunostimulatory function of dendritic cells: MAPKs and translocation of NF-B as potential targets. J Immunol. 2005;174:8116–24.

55. Cho J-W, Lee K-S, Kim C-W. Curcumin attenuates the expression of IL-1beta, IL-6, and TNF-alpha as well as cyclin E in TNF-alpha-treated HaCaT cells; NF-kappaB and MAPKs as potential upstream targets. Int J Mol Med. 2007;19: 469–74.

56. de Oliveira AC, Candelario-Jalil E, Langbein J, Wendeburg L, Bhatia HS, Schlachetzki JC, et al. Pharmacological inhibition of Akt and downstream pathways modulates the expression of COX-2 and mPGES-1 in activated microglia. J Neuroinflammation. 2012;9:2.

57. Codeluppi S, Fernandez-Zafra T, Sandor K, Kjell J, Liu Q, Abrams M, et al. Interleukin-6 secretion by astrocytes is dynamically regulated by PI3K-mTOR-calcium signaling. PLoS One. 2014;9:e92649.

58. Plummer SM, Holloway KA, Manson MM, Munks RJ, Kaptein A, Farrow S, et al. Inhibition of cyclo-oxygenase 2 expression in colon cells by the chemopreventive agent curcumin involves inhibition of NF-kappaB activation via the NIK/IKK signalling complex. Oncogene. 1999;18:6013–20.

59. Jobin C, Bradham CA, Russo MP, Juma B, Narula AS, Brenner DA, et al. Curcumin blocks cytokine-mediated NF-kB activation and proinflammatory gene expression by inhibiting inhibitory factor I-kB kinase activity. J Immunol. 1999;163:3474–83.

60. Gozzelino R, Jeney V, Soares MP. Mechanisms of cell protection by Heme oxygenase-1. Annu Rev Pharmacol Toxicol. 2010;50:323–54.

61. Scapagnini G. Caffeic acid phenethyl ester and curcumin: a novel class of Heme oxygenase-1 inducers. Mol Pharmacol. 2002;61:554–61.

62. Gorter JA, Van Vliet EA, Aronica E. Status epilepticus, blood-brain barrier disruption, inflammation, and epileptogenesis. Epilepsy Behav. 2015;49:13–6.

63. Iori V, Frigerio F, Vezzani A. Modulation of neuronal excitability by immune mediators in epilepsy. Curr Opin Pharmacol. 2016;26:118–23.

64. Riazi K, Galic MA, Pittman QJ. Contributions of peripheral inflammation to seizure susceptibility: cytokines and brain excitability. Epilepsy Res. 2010;89:34–42.

65. Kaur H, Patro I, Tikoo K, Sandhir R. Curcumin attenuates inflammatory response and cognitive deficits in experimental model of chronic epilepsy. Neurochem Int. 2015;89:40–50.

66. Kaur H, Bal A, Sandhir R. Curcumin supplementation improves mitochondrial and behavioral deficits in experimental model of chronic epilepsy. Pharmacol Biochem Behav. 2014;125:55–64.

# Permissions

All chapters in this book were first published in JN, by BioMed Central; hereby published with permission under the Creative Commons Attribution License or equivalent. Every chapter published in this book has been scrutinized by our experts. Their significance has been extensively debated. The topics covered herein carry significant findings which will fuel the growth of the discipline. They may even be implemented as practical applications or may be referred to as a beginning point for another development.

The contributors of this book come from diverse backgrounds, making this book a truly international effort. This book will bring forth new frontiers with its revolutionizing research information and detailed analysis of the nascent developments around the world.

We would like to thank all the contributing authors for lending their expertise to make the book truly unique. They have played a crucial role in the development of this book. Without their invaluable contributions this book wouldn't have been possible. They have made vital efforts to compile up to date information on the varied aspects of this subject to make this book a valuable addition to the collection of many professionals and students.

This book was conceptualized with the vision of imparting up-to-date information and advanced data in this field. To ensure the same, a matchless editorial board was set up. Every individual on the board went through rigorous rounds of assessment to prove their worth. After which they invested a large part of their time researching and compiling the most relevant data for our readers.

The editorial board has been involved in producing this book since its inception. They have spent rigorous hours researching and exploring the diverse topics which have resulted in the successful publishing of this book. They have passed on their knowledge of decades through this book. To expedite this challenging task, the publisher supported the team at every step. A small team of assistant editors was also appointed to further simplify the editing procedure and attain best results for the readers.

Apart from the editorial board, the designing team has also invested a significant amount of their time in understanding the subject and creating the most relevant covers. They scrutinized every image to scout for the most suitable representation of the subject and create an appropriate cover for the book.

The publishing team has been an ardent support to the editorial, designing and production team. Their endless efforts to recruit the best for this project, has resulted in the accomplishment of this book. They are a veteran in the field of academics and their pool of knowledge is as vast as their experience in printing. Their expertise and guidance has proved useful at every step. Their uncompromising quality standards have made this book an exceptional effort. Their encouragement from time to time has been an inspiration for everyone.

The publisher and the editorial board hope that this book will prove to be a valuable piece of knowledge for researchers, students, practitioners and scholars across the globe.

# List of Contributors

**Peiyuan F Hsieh, Mei-Lin Shen, Ching-Huei Lin, Ya-Yun Chao and Ming-Hong Chang**
Division of Neurology, Taichung Veterans General Hospital, Taichung, Taiwan

**Peiyuan F Hsieh**
Graduate Institute of Biomedicine and Biomedical Technology, National Chi Nan University, Nantou, Taiwan

**Chien-Wei Hou, Pei-Wun Yao, Szu-Pei Wu and Yu-Fen Peng**
Department of Biotechnology Yuanpei University, Hsinchu, Taiwan

**Kee-Ching Jeng**
Department of Physical Education Office, Yuanpei University, Hsinchu, Taiwan
Department of Medical Research, Taichung Veterans General Hospital, Taichung, Taiwan

**Allen D. DeSena**
Division of Neurology, Department of Pediatrics, Cincinnati Children's Hospital Medical Center, University of Cincinnati College of Medicine, 3333 Burnet Ave, MLC 2015, Cincinnati, OH 45229, USA

**Thuy Do and Grant S. Schulert**
Division of Rheumatology, Department of Pediatrics, Children's Hospital Medical Center, University of Cincinnati College of Medicine, 3333 Burnet Ave, MLC 4010, Cincinnati, OH 45229, USA

**Ludmyla Kandratavicius, Jose Eduardo Peixoto-Santos, Mariana Raquel Monteiro, Renata Caldo Scandiuzzi, Jaime Eduardo Hallak and Joao Pereira Leite**
Department of Neurosciences and Behavior, Ribeirao Preto Medical School, University of Sao Paulo (USP), Av Bandeirantes 3900, CEP 14049-900 Ribeirao Preto, SP, Brazil

**Ludmyla Kandratavicius**
Center for Interdisciplinary Research on Applied Neurosciences (NAPNA), USP, Ribeirao Preto, Brazil

**Carlos Gilberto Carlotti Jr and Joao Alberto Assirati Jr**
Department of Surgery, Ribeirao Preto Medical School, USP, Ribeirao Preto, Brazil

**Jaime Eduardo Hallak**
National Institute of Science and Technology in Translational Medicine (INCT-TM - CNPq), Ribeirao Preto, Brazil

**Matilda Ahl, Una Avdic, Idrish Ali, Deepti Chugh and Christine T Ekdahl**
Inflammation and Stem Cell Therapy Group, Division of Clinical Neurophysiology, Lund University, BMC A11, Sölvegatan 17, SE-221 84 Lund, Sweden

**Matilda Ahl, Una Avdic, Idrish Ali, Deepti Chugh and Christine T Ekdahl**
Lund Epilepsy Center, Lund University, SE-221 85 Lund, Sweden

**Ulrica Englund Johansson and Cecilia Skoug**
Division of Ophthalmology, Department of Clinical Sciences, Lund University, SE-221 85 Lund, Sweden

**Ming-Tao Yang**
Department of Pediatrics, Far Eastern Memorial Hospital, New Taipei City, Taiwan
Department of Chemical Engineering and Materials Science, Yuan Ze University, Taoyuan, Taiwan

**Yi-Chin Lin, Whae-Hong Ho and Wang-Tso Lee**
Department of Pediatric Neurology, National Taiwan University Children's Hospital, No. 7 Chung-Shan South Road, Taipei 100, Taiwan

**Yi-Chin Lin and Wang-Tso Lee**
Graduate Institute of Brain and Mind Science, National Taiwan University, Taipei, Taiwan

**Chao-Lin Liu**
Department of Chemical Engineering, Ming Chi University of Technology, New Taipei City, Taiwan
College of Engineering, Chang Gung University, Taoyuan, Taiwan

**Yao-Chung Chuang, Tsu-Kung Lin, Wen-Neng Chang, Chia-Wei Liou, Shang-Der Chen, Alice YW Chang and Samuel HH Chan**
Department of Neurology, Kaohsiung Chang Gung Memorial Hospital and Chang Gung University College of Medicine, Kaohsiung 83301, Taiwan

**Yao-Chung Chuang, Shang-Der Chen, Alice YW Chang and Samuel HH Chan**
Center for Translational Research in Biomedical Sciences, Kaohsiung Chang Gung Memorial Hospital and Chang Gung University College of Medicine, Kaohsiung 83301, Taiwan

**Hsuan-Ying Huang**
Department of Pathology, Kaohsiung Chang Gung Memorial Hospital and Chang Gung University College of Medicine, Kaohsiung 83301, Taiwan

**Adriana Fernanda K. Vizuete, Fernanda Hansen, Elisa Negri, Marina Concli Leite, Diogo Losch de Oliveira and Carlos-Alberto Gonçalves**
Department of Biochemistry, Instituto de Ciências Básicas da Saúde, Universidade Federal do Rio Grande do Sul, Ramiro Barcelos, 2600-Anexo, Porto Alegre, RS 90035-003, Brazil

**Olesya Okuneva, Zhilin Li, Inken Körber, Saara Tegelberg, Tarja Joensuu and Anna-Elina Lehesjoki**
Folkhälsan Institute of Genetics, Haartmaninkatu 8, 00014 Helsinki, Finland

**Olesya Okuneva, Inken Körber, Saara Tegelberg, Tarja Joensuu and Anna-Elina Lehesjoki**
Research Program's Unit, Molecular Neurology, University of Helsinki, Haartmaninkatu 8, 00014 Helsinki, Finland

**Olesya Okuneva, Zhilin Li, Inken Körber, Saara Tegelberg, Tarja Joensuu, Li Tian and Anna-Elina Lehesjoki**
Neuroscience Center, University of Helsinki, Viikinkaari 4, 00014 Helsinki, Finland

**Li Tian**
Beijing Huilongguan Hospital, Peking University teaching hospital, Beijing, China

**Bo Gao, Yu Wu, Wei-Zu Li, Kun Dong, Yan-Yan Yin and Wen-Ning Wu**
Department of Pharmacology, School of Basic Medical Sciences, Key Laboratory of Anti-inflammatory and Immunopharmacology, Anhui Medical University, Hefei 230032, People's Republic of China

**Yuan-Jian Yang**
Department of Psychiatry and Medical Experimental Center, Jiangxi Mental Hospital/Affiliated Mental Hospital of Nanchang University, Nanchang 330029, People's Republic of China

**Jun Zhou**
Department of Pharmacy, Xi'an Chest Hospital, Shaanxi University of Chinese Medicine, Xi'an 710061, People's Republic of China

**Da-Ke Huang**
Synthetic Laboratory, School of Basic Medical Sciences, Anhui Medical University, Hefei 230032, People's Republic of China

**Beatriz O. Amorim, Luciene Covolan, Elenn Ferreira, José Geraldo Brito, Diego P. Nunes and David G. de Morais**
Disciplina de Neurofisiologia, Universidade Federal de São Paulo, Rua Botucatu, 862 5 andar, 04023-062 São Paulo, Brazil

**José N. Nobrega and Clement Hamani**
Behavioural Neurobiology Laboratory, Centre for Addiction and Mental Health, Toronto, Canada

**Antonio M. Rodrigues and Antonio Carlos G. deAlmeida**
Departamento de Engenharia de Biossistemas, Universidade Federal de São João del-Rei, São João del-Rei, MG 36301-160, Brazil

**Clement Hamani**
Division of Neurosurgery, Toronto Western Hospital, University of Toronto, Toronto, Canada

**Ji-Eun Kim, Hea Jin Ryu and Tae-Cheon Kang**
Department of Anatomy and Neurobiology, Institute of Epilepsy Research, College of Medicine, Hallym University, Chunchon, Kangwon-Do 200-702, South Korea

**Ji-Eun Kim**
Ji-Eun Kim, Department of Neurology, UCSF, and Veterans Affairs Medical Center, San Francisco, California 94121, USA

**Wen-di Luo, Jia-wei Min, Xin Wang, Yuan-yuan Peng and Bi-Wen Peng**
Department of Physiology, Hubei Provincial Key Laboratory of Developmentally Originated Disorder, School of Basic Medical Sciences, Wuhan University, Hubei Donghu Rd 185#, Wuhan 430071, Hubei, China

**Wen-Xian Huang**
Department of Pathology, Renmin Hospital, Wuhan University, Wuhan, China

**Song Han, Jun Yin and Xiao-Hua He**
Department of Pathophysiology, School of Basic Medical Sciences, Wuhan University, Wuhan, China

**Wan-Hong Liu**
Department of Immunology, School of Basic Medical Sciences, Wuhan University, Wuhan, China

**Elena Avignone, Marilyn Lepleux, Julie Angibaud and U. Valentin Nägerl**
Interdisciplinary Institute for Neurosciences, CNRS UMR 5297, 33077 Bordeaux, France
Université de Bordeaux, CNRS UMR 5297, 33077 Bordeaux, France

**Anne A Kan, Marina de Wit, Ellen Hessel and Pierre N E de Graan**
Department of Neuroscience and Pharmacology, Rudolf Magnus Institute of Neuroscience, Universiteitsweg 100, 3584 CG, Utrecht, The Netherlands

**Wilco de Jager**
Department of Pediatric Immunology, University Medical Center Utrecht, Heidelberglaan 100, Utrecht, The Netherlands

**Cyrill Ferrier, Peter Gosselaar and Peter van Rijen**
Department of Neurology and Neurosurgery, University Medical Center Utrecht, Heidelberglaan 100, Utrecht, The Netherlands

**Onno van Nieuwenhuizen**
Department of Child Neurology, University Medical Center Utrecht, Heidelberglaan 100, Utrecht, The Netherlands

**Cobi Heijnen and Mirjam van Zuiden**
Laboratory of Neuroimmunology and Developmental Origins of Disease, University Medical Center Utrecht, Heidelberglaan 100, 3584 CX, Utrecht, The Netherlands

**Kyungmin Kim, Byung Ok Kwak, Aram Kwon and Jongseok Ha**
Department of Pediatrics, Konkuk University Medical Center, Seoul, Korea

**Soo-Jin Kim, Sun Whan Bae, Jae Sung Son and Ran Lee**
Department of Pediatrics, Konkuk University Medical Center, Konkuk University School of Medicine, 120-1 Neungdong-ro (Hwayang-dong), Gwangjin-gu, Seoul 05030, Korea

**Soo-Nyung Kim**
Department of Obstetrics and Gynecology, Konkuk University Medical Center, Konkuk University School of Medicine, Seoul, Korea

**Ran Lee**
International Healthcare Research Institute, Konkuk University, Seoul, Korea

**Wei Xie**
Department of Traditional Chinese Medicine, Nanfang Hospital, Southern Medical University, Guangzhou, People's Republic of China

**Wei Xie, Lun Cai, Zhijun Ren and Yuanzheng Liu**
School of Traditional Chinese Medicine, Southern Medical University, Guangzhou, People's Republic of China

**Wei Xie, Lun Cai, Liang Gao and Limin Xiao**
Southern Medical University, Guangzhou, People's Republic of China

**Lun Cai and Qianchao He**
Department of Encephalopathy, The first affiliated hosipital of Guangxi University of Chinese Medicine, Guangxi University of Chinese Medicine, Nanning, People's Republic of China

**Yunhong Yu**
Department of Traditional Chinese Medicine, Guangdong General Hospital, Guangdong Academy of Medical Sciences, Guangdong Geriatric Institute, Guang Zhou 510080, China

**C. M. Drion, L. Kooijman, E. A. van Vliet and J. A. Gorter**
Center for Neuroscience, Swammerdam Institute for Life Sciences, University of Amsterdam, Amsterdam, The Netherlands

**J. van Scheppingen, K. W. Geijtenbeek and E. Aronica**
Department of (Neuro) Pathology, Amsterdam UMC, University of Amsterdam, Amsterdam, The Netherlands

**A. Arena**
Department of Biochemical Sciences, Sapienza University of Rome, Rome, Italy

**E. Aronica**
Stichting Epilepsie Instellingen Nederland (SEIN), Heemstede, The Netherlands

# Index